MasterCases
Orthopaedic Trauma

MasterCases
Orthopaedic Trauma

Clayton R. Perry, M.D.
Associate Clinical Professor of Orthopaedic Surgery
U.S. Center for Sports Medicine
St. Louis University Hospital
St. Louis, Missouri

Charles M. Court-Brown, M.D., F.R.C.S., Ed. (ORTH)
Consultant Orthopaedic Surgeon
The Royal Infirmary of Edinburgh
Edinburgh, Scotland

1999
Thieme
New York • Stuttgart

Thieme New York
333 Seventh Avenue
New York, NY 10001

Executive Editor: Jane Pennington, Ph.D.
Editorial Director: Avé McCracken
Developmental Editor: Kathleen P. Lyons
Assistant Editor: Jinnie Kim
Production Editor: Eric Gladstone
Director of Production and Manufacturing: Maxine Langweil
President: Brian D. Scanlan
Marketing Director: Phyllis D. Gold
Sales Manager: David Bertelsen
Chief Financial Officer: Seth S. Fishman

MasterCases: Orthopaedic Trauma
Clayton R. Perry, M.D.
Charles M. Court-Brown, M.D.

Library of Congress Cataloging-in-Publication Data
Perry, Clayton.
Mastercases : orthopaedic trauma / Clayton R. Perry, Charles M. Court-Brown.
p. cm.
Includes bibliographical references and index.
ISBN 0-86577-782-9 (TNY).—ISBN 3-13-115121-8 (GTV)
1. Musculoskeletal system—Wounds and injuries—Case studies.
2. Orthopedic surgery—Case studies. I. Court-Brown, Charles M.
II. Title. III. Title: Orthopaedic trauma.
[DNLM: 1. Fractures case studies. 2. Dislocations case studies.
WE 175 P462m 1999]
RD680.P47 1999
617.4'7044—dc21
DNLM/DLC
for Library of Congress 98-31524
CIP

Important note: Medical knowledge is ever-changing. As new research and clinical experience broaden our knowledge, changes in treatment and drug therapy may be required. The authors and the editors of the material herein have consulted sources believed to be reliable in their efforts to provide information that is complete and in accord with the standards accepted at the time of publication. However, in view of the possibility of human error by the authors, editors, or publisher of the work herein, or changes in medical knowledge, neither the authors, editors, publisher, nor any other party who has been involved in the preparation of this work, warrants that the information contained herein is in every respect accurate or complete, and they are not responsible for any errors or omissions or for the results obtained from use of such information. Readers are encouraged to confirm the information contained herein with other sources. For example, readers are advised to check the product information sheet included in the package of each drug they plan to administer to be certain that the information contained in this publication is accurate and that changes have not been made in the recommended dose or in the contraindications for administration. This recommendation is of particular importance in connection with new or infrequently used drugs.

Printed in the United States of America
Composition by Compset Inc.; Printed by Maple-Vail Press

5 4 3 2 1

TNY ISBN 0–86577–782–9
GTV ISBN 3–13–115121–8

CONTENTS

Foreword by Robert A. Winquist vii
Preface ix

SECTION I: UPPER EXTREMITY

CASE 1. Intraarticular Fracture of the Glenoid 3
CASE 2. Fracture of the Body of the Scapula 8
CASE 3. Fracture of the Proximal Clavicular Physis 12
CASE 4. Fractures of the Clavicle and Glenoid Neck 16
CASE 5. Mid-diaphyseal Clavicular Fracture 21
CASE 6. Distal Clavicular Fracture 27
CASE 7. Posterior Fracture Dislocation 32
CASE 8. Two Part Surgical Neck Fracture 40
CASE 9. Four Part Proximal Humeral Fracture 47
CASE 10. Fracture of the Humerus with Radial Nerve Palsy 54
CASE 11. Fracture of the Humerus with Bone Loss 59
CASE 12. Distal Humeral Intercondylar Fracture 66
CASE 13. Transcondylar Distal Humeral Fracture 74
CASE 14. Open Distal Humeral Fracture with Bone Loss 79
CASE 15. Elbow Fracture Dislocation 87
CASE 16. Open Elbow Dislocation with Humeral and Forearm Fractures 92
CASE 17. Elbow Dislocation with Radial Head Fracture 98
CASE 18. Isolated Radial Head Fracture 105
CASE 19. Fracture of the Proximal Radius with Radioulnar Dissociation, Essex-Lopresti Lesion 110
CASE 20. Comminuted Proximal Ulnar Fracture with Proximal Radial Damage 117
CASE 21. Monteggia Fracture Dislocation 126
CASE 22. Segmental Fracture of Both Bones of the Forearm 135
CASE 23. Closed Distal Radial and Ulnar Fractures in an Adolescent 142
CASE 24. Extraarticular Distal Radial Fracture 148
CASE 25. Intraarticular Distal Radial Fracture 157

SECTION II: LOWER EXTREMITY

CASE 1. Open Pelvic Fracture 167
CASE 2. Displaced Subcapital Fracture in an Elderly Patient 174
CASE 3. Reverse Obliquity Peritrochanteric Fracture 182
CASE 4. Unstable Intertrochanteric Fracture 189
CASE 5. Open Proximal Femoral Fracture 196
CASE 6. Comminuted Subtrochanteric Fracture 203

CASE 7. Subtrochanteric Fracture of Osteomyelitic Bone **208**
CASE 8. Ipsilateral Femoral Diaphyseal and Neck Fractures **216**
CASE 9. Open Femoral Diaphyseal Fracture **222**
CASE 10. Femoral Diaphyseal Fractures in a Patient with Metabolic Bone Disease **230**
CASE 11. Bilateral Femoral Fractures in a Multiple Injured Patient **238**
CASE 12. Fracture of the Femur Distal to a Well Fixed Femoral Prosthesis **246**
CASE 13. Fracture of the Femur Distal to a Loose Hip Arthroplasty **253**
CASE 14. Supracondylar Femoral Fracture in an Elderly Patient **258**
CASE 15. Intercondylar Femoral Fracture **267**
CASE 16. Intercondylar Femoral Fracture in a Patient with Factor VIII Resistant Hemophilia **272**
CASE 17. Open Intercondylar Fracture with Bone Loss **278**
CASE 18. Distal Femoral Physeal Fracture **287**
CASE 19. Femoral Fracture Proximal to a Knee Arthroplasty **293**
CASE 20. Comminuted Fracture of the Patella **300**
CASE 21. Osteoporotic Proximal Tibial Fracture **305**
CASE 22. High Energy Fracture of the Proximal Tibia **313**
CASE 23. Proximal Diaphyseal Fracture of the Tibia **321**
CASE 24. Fracture of the Tibia Below a Knee Prosthesis **329**
CASE 25. Closed Tibial Fracture with Compartment Syndrome **335**
CASE 26. Gustilo IIIb Open Tibial Fracture **344**
CASE 27. Gustilo IIIc Open Tibial Fracture **355**
CASE 28. Pathological Tibial Fracture after Irradiation **361**
CASE 29. Tibial Plafond Fracture with Diaphyseal Extension **367**
CASE 30. Ankle Fracture with Talar Shift **374**
CASE 31. Distal Tibial Fracture with Overlying Burn **381**
CASE 32. Comminuted Talar Neck Fracture **386**
CASE 33. Talar Body Fracture **391**
CASE 34. Open Subtalar Fracture Dislocation **397**
CASE 35. Calcaneal Fracture Dislocation **403**
CASE 36. Intraarticular Calcaneal Fracture **408**
CASE 37. Unreconstructable Calcaneal Fracture **415**
CASE 38. Midtarsal (Chopart's) Dislocation of the Foot **423**
CASE 39. Open Lisfranc Dislocation **429**

INDEX **435**

FOREWORD

Caring for the individual patient is the essence of medicine. *MASTERCASES: Orthopaedic Trauma* creates a novel approach to orthopaedic learning and essentially makes one think about one patient at a time. Instead of a lecture or a treatise, this book is an interactive collection of case presentations, requiring thought by the author and reader every step of the way.

The reader is presented with the mechanism and magnitude of injury as well as the patient's medical and social conditions. Classification of the fracture is defined, at which point the reader should pause. After synthesizing the information and agreeing or disagreeing with the authors, the reader should select his or her own treatment of choice. As the reader continues through the case, the text provides an excellent brief synopsis of the subject with current treatment options, including their advantages and disadvantages. The audience may agree or disagree at each step. This is learning at its best.

This outstanding book includes the upper and lower extremities, with both common, simple injuries as well as uncommon, complex injuries. Some patients do well and some have complications, which take the reader through further thought-provoking steps. Because Drs. Perry and Court-Brown live on both sides of the Atlantic, this work expands the accepted forms of treatment and provides an up-to-date global approach to these injuries.

Anyone managing patients with orthopaedic injuries should be interested in these *MASTERCASES*. Students in medicine and nursing will quickly comprehend the overall subject surrounding each case. General orthopaedists may use this as an updated guide to rapidly review treatment options for their patients. Even a trauma specialist will enjoy mentally sparring with the authors over each phase of treatment in these *MASTERCASES*. I strongly recommend *MASTERCASES: Orthopaedic Trauma* to all orthopaedic care givers.

Robert A. Winquist, M.D.
Clinical Professor of Orthopedic Surgery
University of Washington School of Medicine
Seattle, Washington

PREFACE

Problem fractures and dislocations are always of interest to orthopaedic surgeons. They not only allow us to use unusual techniques, but more importantly they encourage us to have an understanding of the pathogenesis of the fractures and all of the treatment methods that might be appropriate for their management. More important still is the fact that there is usually no one answer to problem cases, and accordingly orthopaedic surgeons can spend a great deal of time debating the issues.

In MASTERCASES, we have collected a number of interesting and problematic fractures and dislocations. We do not pretend to have treated them all correctly. Indeed in a few cases we would have liked to try again! However, we hope that readers will find the cases instructive and be able to adapt some of our surgical strategies in their daily practice.

In addition to presenting a number of obviously unusual fractures and dislocations, we have also included some conditions that surgeons may feel are relatively straightforward. Their inclusion is deliberate as, not infrequently, the results of their management are not as good as we would wish. New techniques have improved the management of many straightforward cases, and hopefully the inclusion of these cases will engender debate.

For each fracture problem we present a complete work-up of the patient. This takes the reader from *History and Physical Examination* to *Radiologic Findings* and then *Diagnosis.* From there *Surgical Management* is discussed in detail, outlining specific surgical techniques. To present a balanced overview, we have a tabulated section for each case outlining the *Alternative Methods of Management* with their corresponding advantages and disadvantages. The interspersed *Pearls* and *Pitfalls* that are highlighted in the margins will hopefully prove to be useful practical guidelines for daily surgical practice.

The content of the book should provide some insight and perhaps a different perspective to surgeons who are faced with challenging trauma. We also believe that for those in training, MASTERCASES will present the sequential steps involved for total patient care (patient evaluation, diagnostic tests, surgical management, and postoperative care) and supportive information about why specific surgical procedures are implemented.

The book assumes a degree of orthopaedic knowledge, and accordingly we have abbreviated many of the clinical findings. It would have been repetitive to have done otherwise, and we hope that readers will accept this.

Clayton R. Perry, M.D.
Charles M. Court-Brown, M.D., F.R.C.S., Ed. (ORTH)

Section 1

Upper Extremity

Case 1

History and Physical Examination

A 48-year-old male was brought to the emergency department approximately 15 minutes after being shot in the shoulder. The patient was awake but disoriented and in acute distress. The patient's shirt was cut away, revealing an entrance wound anteriorly over the deltoid. An exit wound was not identified. Breath sounds were equal bilaterally. The neurovascular examination of the right upper extremity was within the limits of normal. Toxicology was positive for ethanol (ETOH) and cocaine. No other injuries were identified.

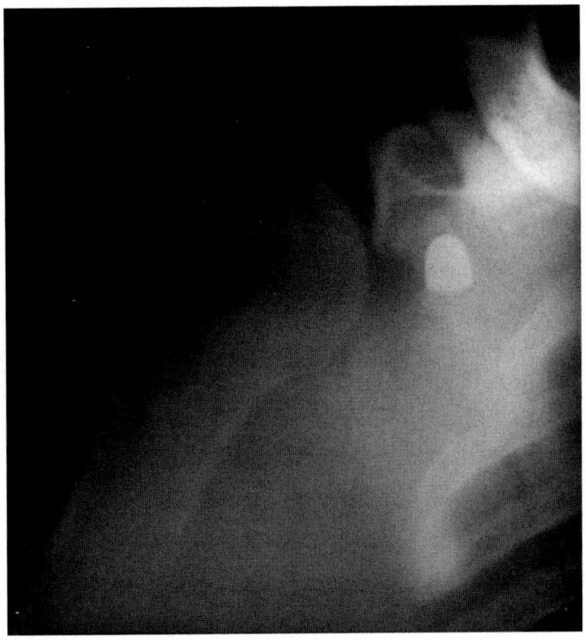

Figure 1–1. An anteroposterior radiograph of the shoulder indicating a fracture of the glenoid due to a gunshot. The bullet is seen overlying the glenoid. The inferior half of the glenoid is displaced distally, beneath the humeral head.

Radiologic Findings

Radiograph of the shoulder revealed a comminuted fracture of the lower half of the glenoid (Fig. 1–1). The articular surface was displaced, and the bullet was seen overlying the scapula. The humeral head was located in the remaining glenoid. Radiologic evidence of a pneumothorax was not present. Spurring of the acromioclavicular joint and extraarticular calcification indicated the presence of osteoarthritis and long-standing rotator cuff irritation.

Diagnosis

Isolated fracture of the inferior half of the glenoid secondary to a gunshot. OTA classification: 09–B2.2.

Surgical Management

The wound was cultured, and a second generation cephalosporin was administered. The arm was supported in a sling.

PEARL

- The vascular examination of the upper extremity is extremely important. A missed hemopneumothorax or injury of the axillary artery is potentially life threatening. The presence of decreased breath sounds, an expanding hematoma in the axilla, and decreased peripheral pulses indicate possible hemopneumothorax and arterial injury.

The day after injury, the patient was awake and oriented. He was taken to the operating room where a general anesthetic was administered. The patient was placed in the "beach chair position" with the head supported in a Mayfield headrest. The fracture was exposed via the deltopectoral interval. The subscapularis was detached from the lesser tuberosity of the humerus and reflected medially, exposing the remnants of the joint capsule. The capsule was debrided and elevated, exposing the glenoid. The bullet tract was irrigated and free fragments of bone were removed. The inferior portion of the glenoid was palpated distally, grasped with a Kocher clamp, and reduced to the intact superior portion. The origin of the long head of the triceps remained attached to the posterior aspect of the glenoid fragment; reduction was facilitated by extending the elbow. The major fragment was held in place with small fragment screws (Fig. 1–2). Following reduction, a defect was present in the glenoid anteriorly secondary to the impact of the bullet. It was not possible to repair the joint capsule of the shoulder. The subscapularis was reattached to the lesser tuberosity of the humerus, and the wound was closed.

Postoperative Management

Antibiotics were continued for 2 days. The arm was supported and maintained in internal rotation in a sling. At 3 weeks, circumduction exercises in the sling were initiated. At 6 weeks, gentle active and passive range of motion was started, and at 8 weeks all restrictions were discontinued. One year following injury, minimal glenohumeral motion was present. Radiographs indicated degenerative arthritis, with resorbtion of the fractured fragment of the glenoid (Fig. 1–3). However, the shoulder was painless and the humerus remained located.

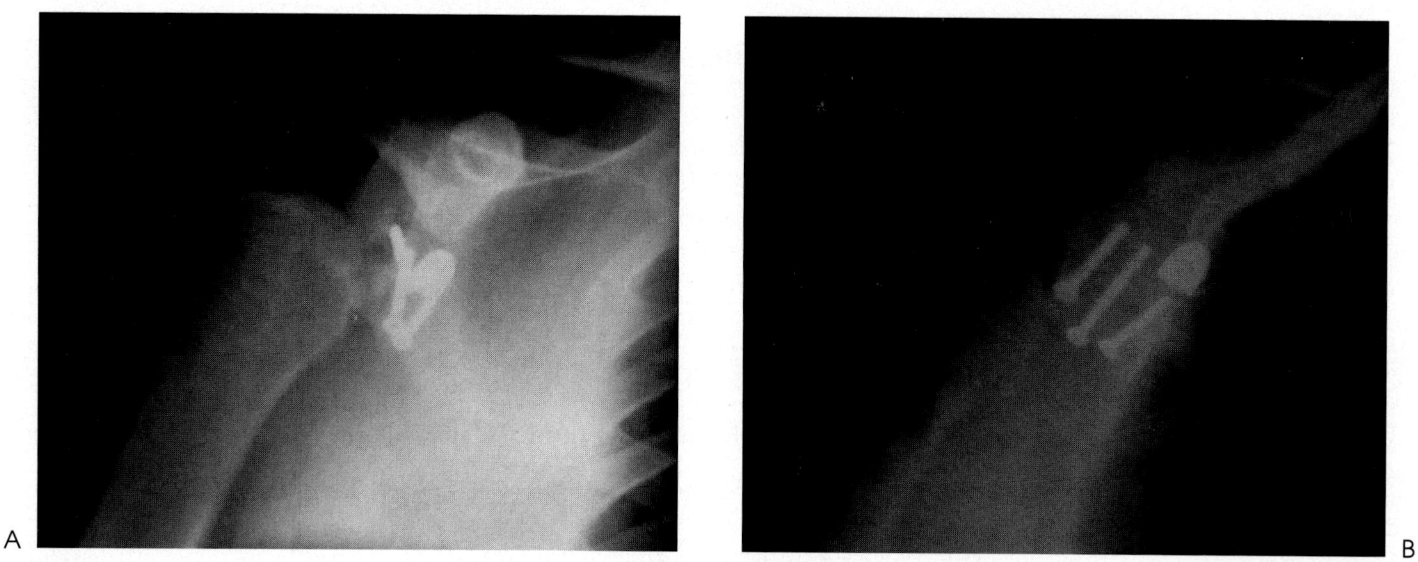

Figure 1–2. Anteroposterior (A) and oblique (B) radiographs of the shoulder following reduction and internal fixation of the glenoid with three screws. Although overall alignment is anatomic, a defect in the articular surface is clearly evident.

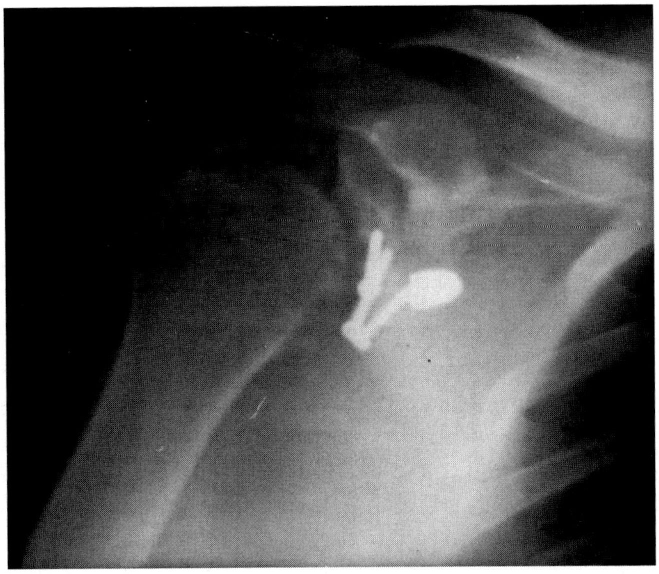
A

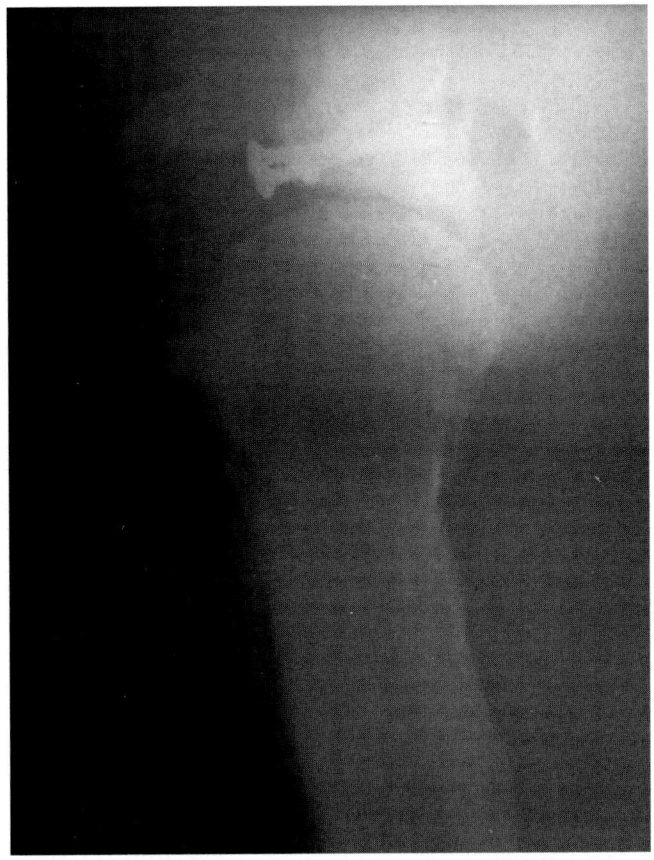
B

Figure 1–3. Anteroposterior (A) and axillary (B) radiographs obtained 1 year after the injury. Degenerative changes of the glenohumeral joint are present, and the fracture fragment appears to have undergone avascular necrosis and collapse.

Discussion

Management could be criticized because the wound was not debrided emergently, even though this was an open fracture. On the other hand, the presence of ETOH and cocaine may have made a general anesthetic more of a risk for the patient than delaying debridement of this low velocity gunshot wound. Indications for immediate debridement would have been a high energy gunshot wound (i.e., shotgun or high velocity), concomitant injury of the lung, and injury of the brachial or subclavian artery or vein.

Alternative Methods of Management

The alternatives to debridement followed by open reduction and fixation are closed management, debridement and stabilization of the glenohumeral articulation with a transarticular pin or external fixator, and debridement with reconstruction of the glenoid with a bone block.

Debridement followed by open reduction and stable fixation of the glenoid minimizes the risk of instability and late osteoarthritis. The disadvantages of open reduction and fixation are an increased risk of infection due to the extensive surgical exposure and the presence of the screws, inability to reconstruct the articular surface of the glenoid anatomically (as we found in this case), and the potential of avascular necrosis of the fracture fragment.

Closed management spares the patient a surgical procedure, but does not address the open, potentially contaminated wound and the potential instability of the glenohumeral articulation resulting from displacement of the lower half of the glenoid.

Debridement and stabilization of the glenohumeral articulation with a transarticular pin or external fixator would be performed if the glenoid could not be reduced or stabilized and if there were demonstrable glenohumeral instability. These methods are useful in severe injuries involving the shoulder, but were not required in this case because instability did not become a deciding factor.

Debridement followed by reconstruction of the inferior portion of the glenoid with a bone block would have been performed with a tricortical fragment of autogenous iliac crest or an allograft if it had not been possible to reduce the fracture and if glenohumeral instability had occurred. In this case, it was possible to reduce and stabilize the fracture, thus restoring glenohumeral stability. Use of a large avascular segment of bone in this case would increase the risk of infection.

Type of Management	Advantages	Disadvantages	Comments
Debridement and open reduction and internal fixation (ORIF)	Minimizes the risk of instability and posttraumatic arthritis	Technically difficult procedure, risk of infection due to extensive exposure	Best balance of risk vs. benefit
Closed management	No surgical procedure	Does not address infection, instability, or posttraumatic arthritis	Not an acceptable alternative unless extenuating circumstances are present
Debridement and stabilization with external fixator or transarticular pin	Guarantees a located glenohumeral joint, best method to avoid recurrent dislocation	Will result in significant loss of motion	Not necessary in this case because stability was restored
Debridement and reconstruction with bone block	Best method to restore stability if glenoid is severely comminuted, could be used with external fixator or transarticular pin	Increased risk of infection due to large segment of avascular bone	Not necessary in this case because the glenoid was reconstructable

Complications

The potential complications of open reduction and fixation of this glenoid fracture are posttraumatic arthritis, infection, and inferior instability. Posttraumatic arthritis occurs because of damage sustained by the articular cartilage and underlying bone during injury and because anatomic reduction of the articular surface was not achieved. Once posttraumatic arthritis has occurred, management is conservative with nonsteroidal antiinflammatories and local steroid injections. In cases in which conservative therapy is not successful, the glenohumeral joint can be debrided arthroscopically, an arthroplasty can be performed, or the glenohumeral joint can be arthrodesed. Arthroscopic debridement will yield only temporary relief. In this case, arthroplasty is not indicated because of the patient's age and social history. Arthrodesis is a major undertaking and should be considered only if the shoulder is very painful.

Management of infection consists of drainage of abscesses, continuation of implants that are providing stability, and suppression of the symptoms of infection with intravenous and then oral antibiotics. When the fracture is healed, the implants are removed and the area debrided. Systemic antibiotics are administered for 4 to 6 weeks.

Inferior instability of the glenohumeral articulation results from loss of the inferior half of the glenoid. Management involves reconstruction of the inferior half of the glenoid with an appropriately contoured allograft or autograft iliac crest.

Suggested Readings

Aston JW Jr, Gregory CF: Dislocation of the shoulder with significant fracture of the glenoid. J Bone Joint Surg 1973; 55A:1531–1533.

Aulicino PL, Reinert C, Kornberg M, Williamson S: Displaced intra-articular glenoid fractures treated by open reduction and internal fixation. J Trauma 1986; 26:1137–1141.

Goss TP: Fractures of the glenoid cavity. Current concepts Review. J Bone Joint Surg 1992; 74A:299–305.

Hardegger FH, Simpson LA, Weber BG: The operative treatment of scapular fractures. J Bone Joint Surg 1984; 66B, 5:725–731.

Case 2

History and Physical Examination

A 54-year-old man was an unrestrained driver in an automobile accident. The automobile left the road at a high rate of speed and rolled several times. He was extracted from the wreckage and arrived in the emergency department 1 hour and 15 minutes after the accident. The patient had been unconscious at the scene of the accident. His right lower extremity was shortened and externally rotated. Echymosis were present over the right side of the chest and back. Breath sounds were equal bilaterally, and there were no signs of a pneumothorax. Other injuries of the abdomen, spine, or extremities were not present.

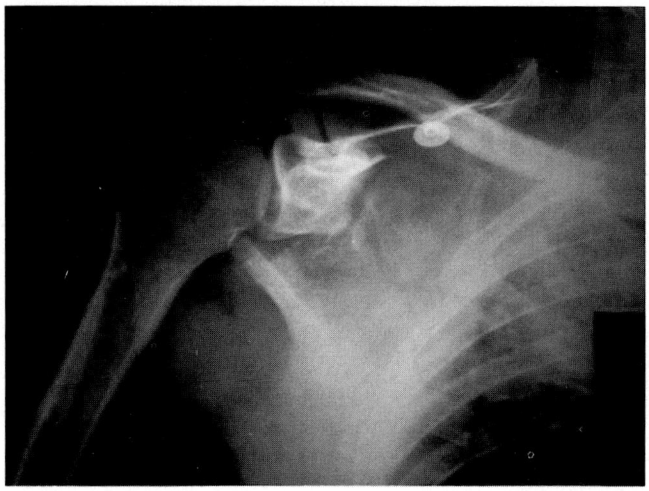

Figure 2–1. An anteroposterior radiograph of the shoulder indicating a comminuted extraarticular fracture of the scapula involving the body, the neck of the glenoid, and the acromion. The glenoid is displaced approximately 2 cm medially. A spike of bone consisting of the lateral border of the scapula appears to be impinging on the humeral head.

Radiologic Findings

Radiographs of the right femur, chest, and right scapula indicated a transverse fracture of the femoral diaphysis, a fracture of the body of the scapula, and fractured ribs. The scapular fracture was comminuted and involved the neck of the glenoid and the acromion. The glenoid was displaced medially approximately 2 cm (Fig. 2–1). There were no signs of a pneumothorax.

Diagnosis

Closed head injury, transverse fracture of the femoral diaphysis, and displaced extraarticular fracture of the scapula. OTA classification: 09–A3.3.

Surgical Management

The head injury was managed by neurosurgeons. The right lower extremity was placed in skeletal traction and the right arm placed in a sling. Twelve hours after injury, the patient was stable enough to undergo fixation of his femur with an intramedullary rod.

PEARLS

- A displaced scapular fracture is a high energy injury that is frequently accompanied by other life-threatening visceral injuries. Pneumothorax is the most commonly associated visceral injury, but other injuries such as cardiac contusion and aortic tear must also be ruled out.
- The two nerves at risk with this approach are the suprascapular nerve and the axillary nerve. The suprascapular nerve enervates the infraspinatous muscle. It enters the infraspinous fossae just lateral to the spine of the scapula. Exposure of the proximal scapula lateral to its spine is limited by risk of injury to this nerve. To protect the suprascapular nerve, the infraspinatous must be elevated subperiosteally. The axillary nerve enters the back of the shoulder via the quadrilateral space and supplies the deltoid muscle. The axillary nerve runs beneath the deltoid muscle. Overzealous retraction of the deltoid muscle laterally or distally may injure the axillary nerve.

Seven days after the injury the patient had recovered completely from his head injury. Repeat radiographs indicated persistent displacement of the scapular fracture fragments. The patient was taken to the operating room where a general anesthetic was administered. He was rolled to the prone position. The arm and shoulder were prepped free. An L-shaped incision was made, extending from the acromion along the spine of the scapula and angling distally over the medial border of the scapula. The posterior third of the deltoid was elevated from its origin on the spine of the scapula and gently retracted laterally. The infraspinatus was elevated subperiosteally from the fracture fragments starting medially and proceeding laterally. The fracture was reduced and stabilized with a large fragment reconstruction plate. The infraspinatus and deltoid muscles were reattached to the medial border of the scapula and scapular spine, respectively, and the wound was closed over a drain.

Postoperative Management

Postoperatively, the arm was supported in a sling for 3 weeks. At 3 weeks following surgery, gentle passive motion was initiated. At 4 weeks active range of motion in the sling was begun. At 6 weeks the sling was discontinued. One year postinjury the scapula was healed with a shortened glenoid neck. The range of motion of the glenohumeral articulation was: internal rotation 45 degrees; external rotation 45 degrees; forward flexion 90 degrees; extension 80 degrees; and abduction 90 degrees (Fig. 2–2).

Discussion

This type of displaced fracture of the scapula has been termed the *explosion fracture.* In most cases, explosion fractures are caused by direct impact. The energy imparted by the impact accounts for the frequency of associated visceral injuries. Explosion fractures of the scapula have a much better prognosis than a fracture due to scapulothoracic dissociation. This is because the neurological and vascular injuries that are invariably associated with a scapulothoracic dissociation are seldom associated with an explosion fracture. The vast majority of extraarticular scapular fractures are adequately treated by closed methods. The amount of displacement seen in this case is rare and may have resulted in impingement of the glenohumeral articulation by the lateral border of the scapula, or even nonunion.

One of the major problems encountered when attempting to internally fix fractures of the scapula is stability. Excluding its lateral border, the glenoid and its spine, the scapula is quite thin in the anteroposterior plane. This limits screw purchase. An additional problem is that the muscles of the shoulder all tend to shorten the neck of the glenoid, making anatomical reduction difficult. In most cases the goals of surgery are limited to removal of spikes of bone that may impinge on the glenohumeral articulation and alignment of the fragments in such a way that they will heal.

Alternative Methods of Management

The only alternative to open reduction and internal fixation is closed management in the form of a sling or shoulder immobilizer. Open reduction and fixation require

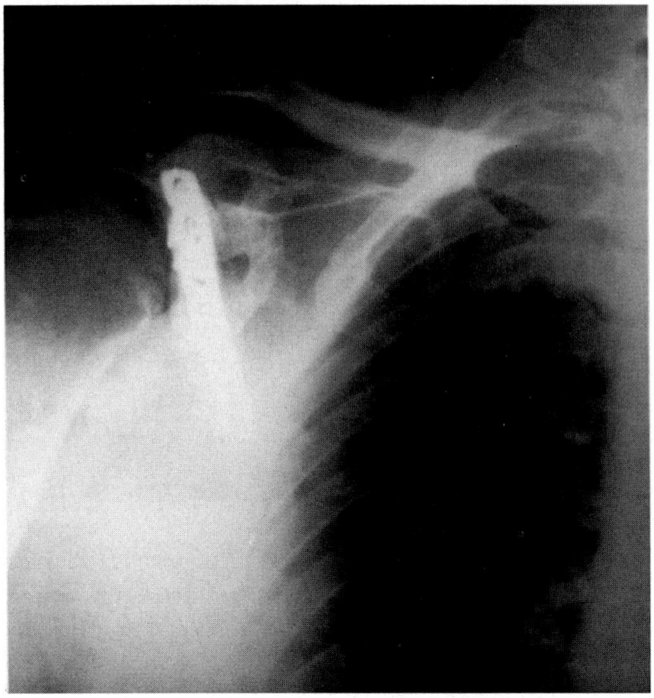
A

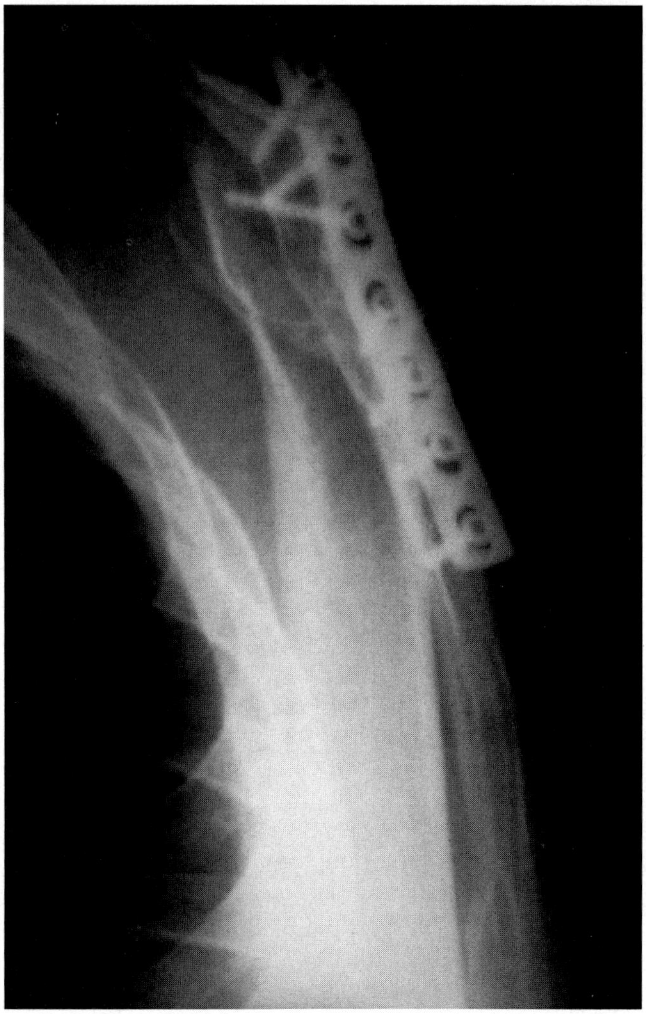
B

Figure 2–2. Anteroposterior (A) and lateral (B) radiographs of the scapula obtained 1 year after injury. The fracture is healed with 1 cm of residual medial displacement of the glenoid. The lateral border of the scapula has healed in good position.

an operative procedure, but have the best chance of restoring function. Closed management does not subject the patient to surgery, but one would expect a major limitation of shoulder function if the fragments healed in their displaced position or failed to unite.

Type of Management	Advantages	Disadvantages	Comments
Open reduction and fixation	Restores the anatomy of the scapula	Exposes the patient to the risk of surgery	Marked displacement is an unusual indication for open reduction and fixation of an extraarticular scapular fracture
Closed management	Surgery not required	Fracture will heal malaligned or go on to nonunion	An acceptable method of management

Complications

Complications of internal fixation of a scapular fracture are nonunion, infection, and loss of motion of the shoulder. Nonunion is very rare; it would be managed conservatively unless symptomatic. A symptomatic nonunion with displacement of the fragments would be managed by open reduction, stabilization with plates, and possible autogenous bone grafting.

Infection is managed like any other bone and joint infection with local control of symptoms until the fracture has healed, followed by debridement and organism-specific systemic antibiotic administration.

Loss of motion of the shoulder is expected after an injury of this severity and in all probability is due to adhesive capsulitis. Computerized axial tomography or examination under fluoroscopy might help rule out other causes. Unless there is a definable block to motion, such as a spike of bone impinging on the capsule of the shoulder or heterotopic ossification, management of loss of motion is in the form of physical therapy.

Suggested Readings

Armstrong CP, Van der Spuy: The fractured scapula: importance and management based on a series of 62 patients. Injury 1984; 15(5):324–329.

Guttentag IJ, Rechtine GR: Fractures of the scapula. A review of the literature. Orthop Rev 1988; 17:1147–1158.

Harris RD, Harris JH Jr: The prevalence and significance of missed scapular fractures in blunt trauma. Am J Rheum 1988; 151:747–750.

Ideberg R, Grevsten S, Larsson S: Epidemiology of scapular fractures. Incidence and classification of 338 fractures. Acta Orthop Scand 1995; 66(5):395–397.

Case 3

History and Physical Examination

A 19-year-old male presented at the emergency department after being injured while playing field hockey. He had fallen on his outstretched left arm and felt immediate pain in his upper sternum. Examination showed a prominence over the left sternoclavicular joint that was very tender on palpation. Movement of the left shoulder caused pain over the sternoclavicular area.

Examination of vascular supply of the left arm showed no abnormality, with a normal radial pulse being palpated. There was no neurological deficit in the arm.

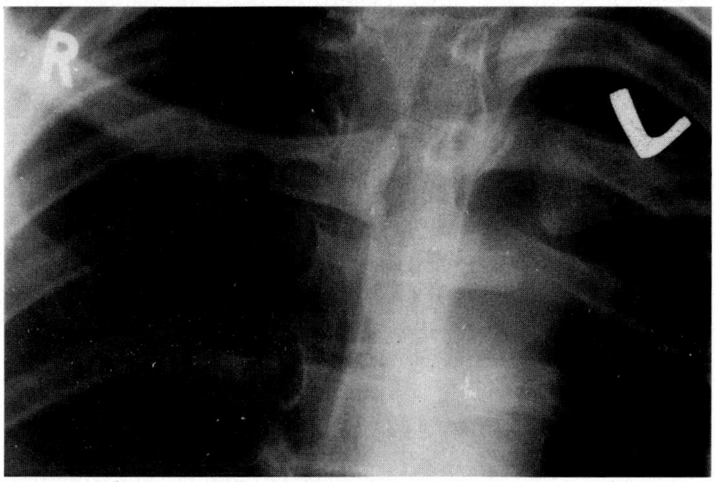

Figure 3–1. A radiograph of the sternoclavicular joints merely demonstrating incongruity.

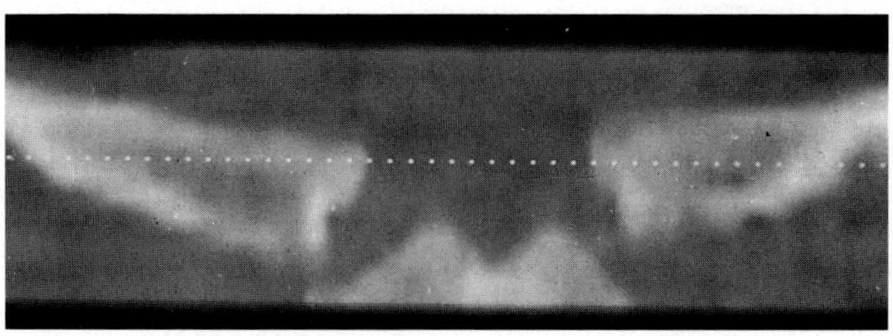

Figure 3–2. A CAT scan showed an apparent subluxation of the left sternoclavicular joint.

Radiologic Findings

An anteroposterior view of the sternum showed incongruity of the two sternoclavicular joints (Fig. 3–1). The proximal clavicular physes were not calcified. A subsequent computerized axial tomography (CAT) scan appeared to demonstrate anterior subluxation of the left sternoclavicular joint (Fig. 3–2) but the precise diagnosis could not be made by imaging.

PEARL

- A physeal fracture separation is much easier to treat than an anterior dislocation of the sternoclavicular joint. Thus, operative management should be considered in any patient under 25 years of age if the patient is concerned about cosmesis.

PITFALL

- Closed Kirschner wiring should never be used to treat sternoclavicular fractures and dislocations. The presence of vessels makes this technique dangerous.

Diagnosis

This patient either had a fracture of the proximal clavicular physis with anterior displacement of the proximal end of the clavicle or an anterior dislocation of the sternoclavicular joint. The former diagnosis was more likely in view of the patient's age.

Surgical Management

The patient was taken to the operating room and placed in a beach chair position. The upper chest was prepped and draped for surgery and an incision was made over the proximal clavicle, extending obliquely downward over the upper end of the sternum. Cautery was used to expose the end of the clavicle and the presence of a Salter-Harris II proximal epiphyseal fracture confirmed. The physis was maintained in its correct alignment with the proximal sternum but the proximal clavicular metaphysis had displaced anteriorly. It was a relatively simple matter to reduce the fracture by depressing the clavicle. The fracture was adequately held by passing two transosseous number 1 absorbable sutures through the physis and the proximal clavicular metaphysis and tightening them. This resulted in good fracture fixation. The wound was closed and dressings were applied.

Postoperative Management

In view of the nature of the fixation that had been employed, the patient's left arm was placed in an immobilizer for 3 weeks. A physiotherapy regime was then instituted and he quickly regained his shoulder motion. There was no recurrence of the deformity and 6 months after fracture he was asymptomatic and discharged from follow-up.

Discussion

The proximal clavicular physis is the last physis in the body to close and it may remain open until the patient is 23 to 25 years of age. The physis may not calcify and therefore appear on radiographs until the patient is about 18 years of age, rendering the condition difficult to visualize on either radiographs or CAT scans. The condition is much more common than many surgeons imagine and if a patient less than 25 years of age presents with what looks like an anterior or posterior sternoclavicular dislocation the presence of a Salter-Harris I or II physeal fracture should be suspected.

The mechanism of the injury and the succeeding repair process is illustrated in Figure 3–3. As the physis fractures and the clavicle dislocates anteriorly, the periosteum on the undersurface of the clavicle is stripped away from the bone. New bone will form between the periosteum and the clavicle, stabilizing the joint again. However, the sternoclavicular swelling will usually remain, although there may be some remodeling in younger patients. The suturing technique used in this case resulted in fracture reduction and therefore minimized the cosmetic deformity.

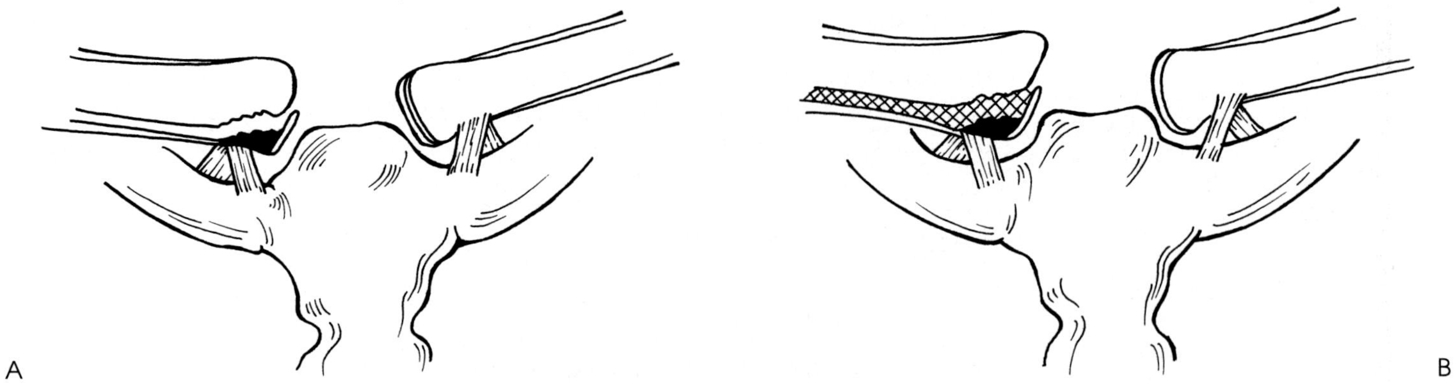

Figure 3–3. (A) The etiology of a Salter-Harris II proximal physeal fracture. (B) The normal repair process of the fracture.

Alternative Methods of Management

The obvious alternative method to the suture technique used in this case is nonoperative management. This will result in joint stabilization but probably not in removal of the cosmetic deformity. Because this is perhaps the main difference between treatments, the role of operative treatment must be discussed with the patient. Many patients will not be too concerned about the cosmetic abnormality associated with the sternoclavicular swelling and it must always be remembered that surgical intervention will leave the patient with a scar. If surgery is to be undertaken, it should never be performed blind or with Kirschner wires because of the risk of damage to the major vessels lying under the sternoclavicular joint. Nonoperative management or open suturing is recommended.

Type of Management	Advantages	Disadvantages	Comments
Nonoperative	Good results	Cosmesis	Probably the method of choice in most patients
Bone suture	Good results; removal of sternoclavicular swelling	Presence of a scar	Currently there is no indication as to which method of management is the best

Complications

Few complications are associated with either the use of nonoperative management or bone suturing techniques. Complications may arise if the surgeon elects to use Kirschner wires for fixation in view of the presence of the great vessels behind the sternoclavicular joint. Kirschner wires also tend to migrate and have been detected at considerable distances from their point of insertion!

Suggested Readings

Levinsohn EM, Bunnell WP, Hansen AY: Computed tomography in the diagnosis of dislocations of the sternoclavicular joint. Clin Orthop 1979; 140:12–14.

Neer CS: Injuries to the sternoclavicular joint. In: Rockwood CA, Green DP (eds): Fractures in Adults, pp 910–950. JP Lippincott, Philadelphia, 1984.

Case 4

History and Physical Examination

A 32-year-old male fell from a height, injuring his right shoulder and chest. He arrived at the emergency department 30 minutes after the injury. On physical examination no obvious deformity or open wounds were noted. The patient complained of pain with motion of the right upper extremity and with palpation along the clavicle and back. The patient also complained of pleuritic pain with breathing. Examination of the chest revealed that breath sounds were equal bilaterally. The neurovascular examination of the upper extremity was within the limits of normal. The examination of the abdomen was within the limits of normal.

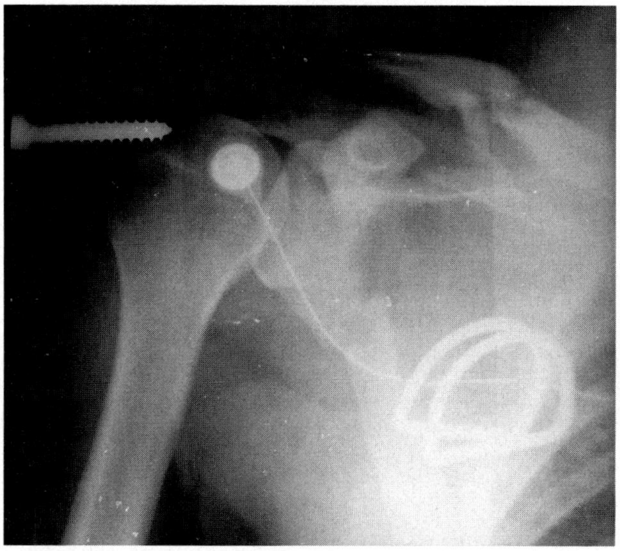

Figure 4–1. Anteroposterior radiograph of the shoulder obtained 1 hour after injury. There are minimally displaced and angulated fractures of the midclavicle and neck of the glenoid.

Radiologic Findings

Radiographs of the shoulder indicated a fracture of the right midshaft clavicle and right glenoid neck. Both fractures were minimally displaced and extraarticular (Fig. 4–1). Radiographs of the chest indicated minimally displaced fractures of the first through third ribs. There were no radiographic signs of pneumothorax or mediastinal widening.

Diagnosis

Minimally displaced fracture of the right clavicle and glenoid neck. In addition, and acutely more important, the patient sustained a lung contusion and fractured ribs.

Surgical Management

Initial management was focused on the lung contusion. The patient was admitted for observation. He developed pneumonitis, which was treated successfully with an-

PEARL

- Fracture of the scapula is a high energy injury frequently associated with life-threatening visceral injuries. It is imperative to rule out pneumothorax, aortic injury, and intraabdominal bleed.

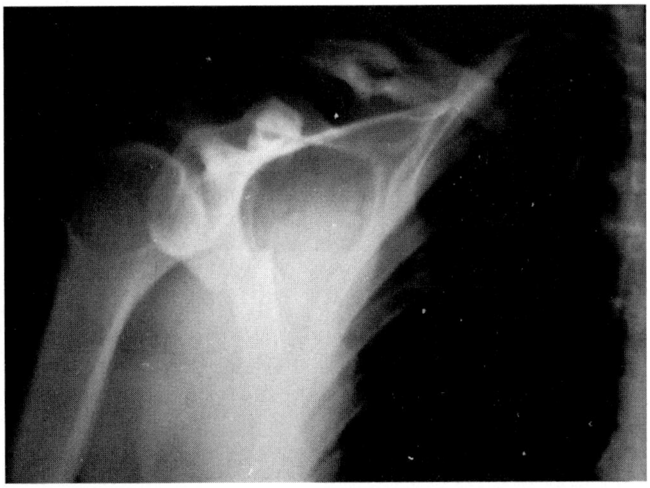

Figure 4–2. Anteroposterior radiograph of the shoulder obtained 1 week after injury. Displacement and angulation of the clavicular and scapular fractures are now present.

tibiotics and nasal oxygen. The right arm was placed in a sling. Radiographs obtained at 1 week postinjury indicated increased angulation of the clavicle fracture and increased displacement of the glenoid neck fracture (Fig. 4–2).

The patient was taken to the operating room and a general anesthetic administered. He was turned with his right side up. The arm, shoulder, back, and chest were

A

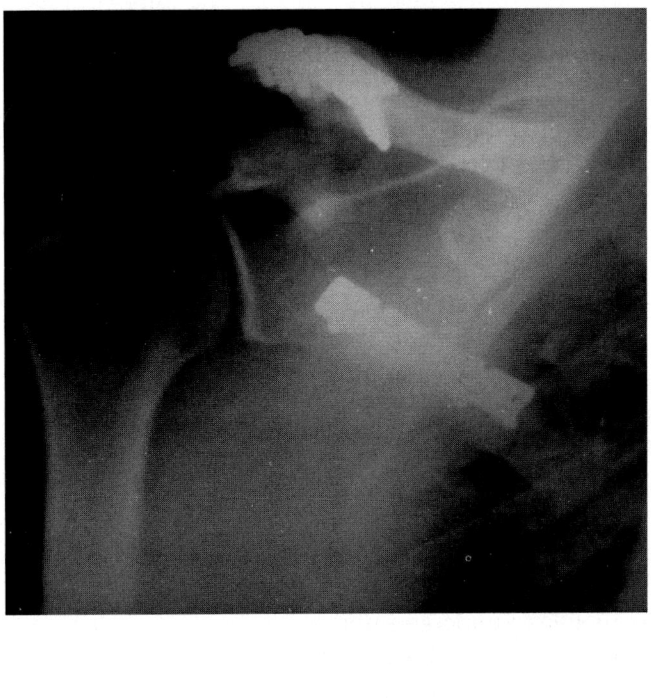

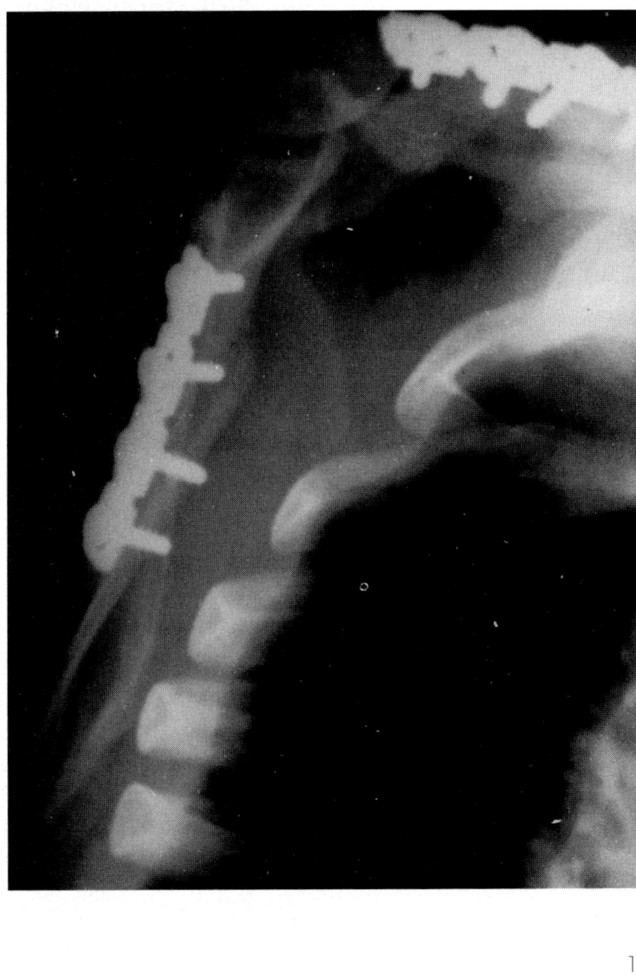

B

Figure 4–3. Anteroposterior (A) and lateral (B) radiographs of the shoulder indicated reduction and internal fixation of both the clavicle and glenoid neck.

prepped and draped. First, the clavicle was addressed. The shoulders were turned in a semisupine position. An incision was made along the clavicle. The fracture was reduced and stabilized with a small fragment reconstruction plate. The shoulders were then rotated to the semiprone position. An L-shaped incision was made along the medial border of the scapula extending laterally along the spine of the scapula. The infraspinatus was detached medially, leaving a cuff of tissue to which it could be reattached, and elevated off the scapula from medial to lateral. The fracture of the neck of the glenoid was identified, reduced, and stabilized with a small fragment reconstruction plate applied to the relatively thick bone of the lateral border of the scapula (Fig. 4–3). Both wounds were closed and the arm placed in a sling.

Postoperative Management

At 3 days following surgery, circumduction exercises of the shoulder and active exercises of the elbow and wrist were initiated. At 6 weeks, the sling was discontinued and active strengthening and range of motion exercises of the shoulder were initiated. One year after injury the plate was removed from the clavicle (Fig. 4–4).

Discussion

Acute management of this high energy injury is focused on the identification and management of life-threatening visceral trauma, in this case the lung contusion. Sling immobilization of the upper extremity constitutes adequate initial management of the shoulder injury. The combination of an ipsilateral clavicle and scapula fracture has been called the "floating shoulder" by Herscovici et al. (1992). They described seven cases of this injury and noted that the fractures are extremely unstable. Fractures treated nonoperatively were likely to displace further, resulting in a drooping shoulder. Herscovici et al. recommended stabilization of the fractures as the optimum definitive treatment.

Alternative Methods of Management

The management options were continued closed management with a sling or shoulder immobilizer, open reduction and stabilization of the clavicle alone, and open reduction and stabilization of the clavicle and glenoid neck. The advantage of closed management is that there is no surgical trauma; the disadvantage is that there is likely to be further displacement with eventual loss of shoulder function and potential nonunion of the clavicle. Closed management may be the only option in polytraumatized patients who are unable to undergo surgery.

Open reduction and stabilization of the clavicle alone will prevent further displacement of the glenoid and minimize the surgical trauma. The disadvantages of stabilization of the clavicle alone are that the glenoid is not stabilized and therefore rehabilitation is prolonged due to pain; the glenoid is not reduced anatomically, although the degree of displacement usually does not affect shoulder function; and increased stresses placed on the clavicular fixation may lead to its failure (Fig. 4–5).

Open reduction of the clavicle and glenoid neck has the advantages of aiding rehabilitation because both fractures are immobilized and preventing further dis-

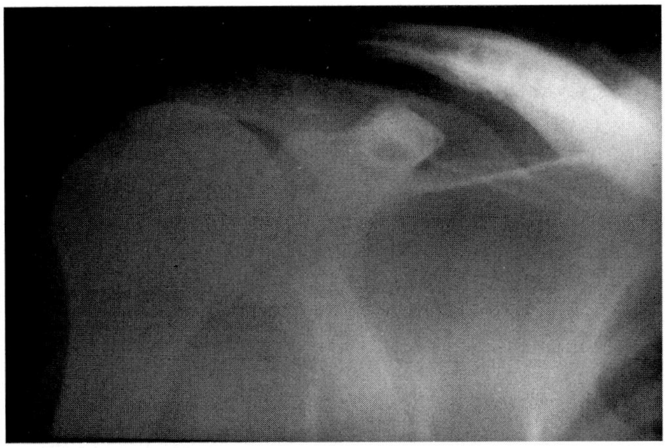

Figure 4–4. Anteroposterior radiograph obtained 1 year after injury following plate removal from the clavicle.

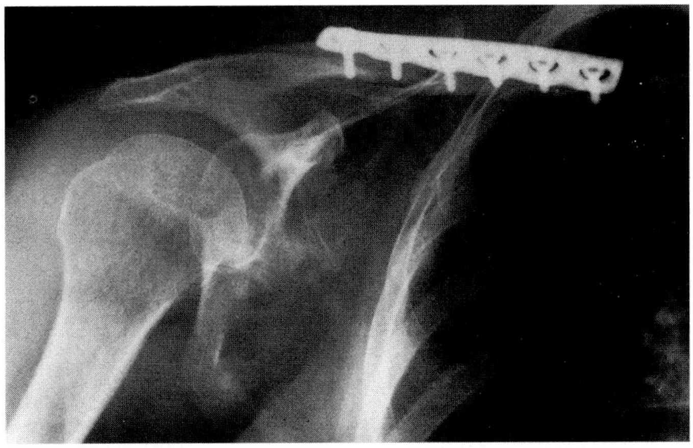

Figure 4–5. Plating the clavicle alone is an alternative method of treatment. There is a malunion of the scapula with at least 2 cm of shortening of the glenoid neck.

placement of the glenoid and resultant loss of shoulder function. The disadvantages of fixation of both fractures are the extensive surgical exposure, the unfamiliarity most surgeons have with the exposure of the posterior scapula, and the difficulty achieving stable fixation of the scapula.

Type of Management	Advantages	Disadvantages	Comments
Closed management	No surgical trauma	Continued displacement may occur	Often only option with multiply traumatized patients
Fixation of clavicle	Minimizes surgical trauma	Fixation may fail; rehabilitation slowed by motion through glenoid neck	Often a good "middle of the road" management
Fixation of clavicle and glenoid neck	Most stable method of fixation, allows early rehabilitation	Extensive surgical procedure	Optimum method of management if patient can withstand surgical trauma

Complications

Complications of fixation of the clavicle and glenoid neck include loss of fixation, nonunion of the clavicle, and infection. Loss of fixation of the clavicle and glenoid neck occurs simultaneously. In cases in which the fracture fragments remain in acceptable alignment, management is immobilization of the upper extremity in a shoulder immobilizer until the glenoid fracture heals. If the clavicle has not healed, its fixation is revised and the fracture is grafted with autogenous cancellous bone. In cases in which fixation has failed and the fracture fragments are no longer in acceptable alignment, fixation is revised and the arm is immobilized postoperatively.

Nonunion of the clavicle with healing of the glenoid neck is managed with revision plating and grafting of the clavicle with autogenous cancellous bone. Infection of the clavicle and glenoid is managed like other infected fractures (i.e., the infection is controlled with oral antibiotics or simply dressing changes until the fractures have healed). When healing has occurred, the implants are removed, infected and necrotic tissue is debrided, and systemic antibiotics are administered for 4 to 6 weeks. In cases in which infection and loss of fixation have occurred, the fixation is revised, and systemic antibiotics are administered for 4 to 6 weeks postoperatively. When the fractures have healed, the implants are removed.

Suggested Readings

Hardegger FH, Simpson, LA, Weber BG: The operative treatment of scapular fractures. J Bone Joint Surg 1984; 66B, 5:725–731.

Harris RD, Harris JH Jr: The prevalence and significance of missed scapular fractures in blunt trauma. Am J Rheum 1988; 151:747–750.

Herscovici D Jr, Fiennes AG, Allgower M, Ruedi TP: The floating shoulder: ipsilateral clavicle and scapular neck fractures. J Bone Joint Surg 1992; 74B:362–364.

Ruedi TP, Chapman MW: Fractures of the scapula and clavicle. In: Operative Orthopaedics, pp 197–202. JB Lippincott, Philadelphia, 1988.

Case 5

History and Physical Examination

A 21-year-old male admitted to the emergency department had fallen off a mountain bike while descending a mountain at high speed. His only significant injury was to his right shoulder and on admission it was noted that he had marked swelling over his right clavicle and all movement of his right shoulder was extremely painful. Examination of the right arm showed no neurological abnormality and in particular no evidence of a brachial plexus lesion. The vascular supply to the arm was normal.

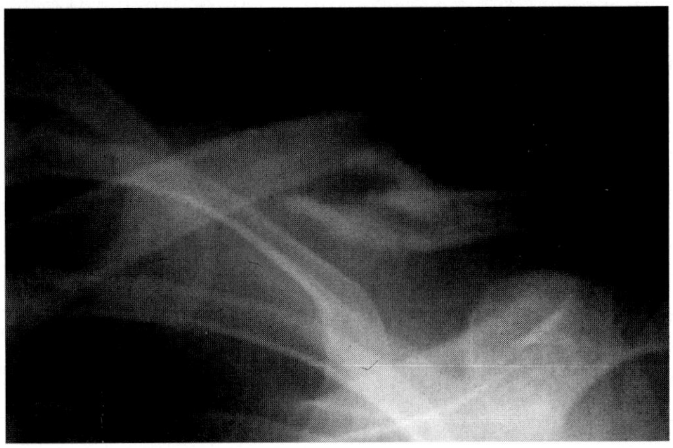

Figure 5–1. A midshaft fracture of the clavicle. There are two intermediate fragments that may well have reduced vascularity.

Radiologic Findings

An anteroposterior radiograph of the right clavicle showed a comminuted fracture of the middle third of the bone (Fig. 5–1). The proximal clavicle was overriding the distal segment and there were two intermediate fragments.

Diagnosis

A comminuted fracture of the right clavicle. Using the OTA modification of the AO classification, this is a 06B3 fracture.

Surgical Management

The patient was supplied with a sling with which to rest the right shoulder and arm. The sling was maintained for 2 weeks and then gradual shoulder mobilization was introduced. A further anteroposterior radiograph was taken 6 weeks after the injury (Fig. 5–2) by which time the patient had less pain but commented that the fracture still felt mobile. The radiograph showed no evidence of union. A further anteroposterior radiograph was obtained at 12 weeks after the injury (Fig. 5–3). This suggested that there was evidence of union radiologically, but clinical examination demonstrated that the fracture site remained mobile.

A diagnosis of clavicular nonunion was made and the patient was admitted for plating with or without bone grafting. Surgery was undertaken with the patient in

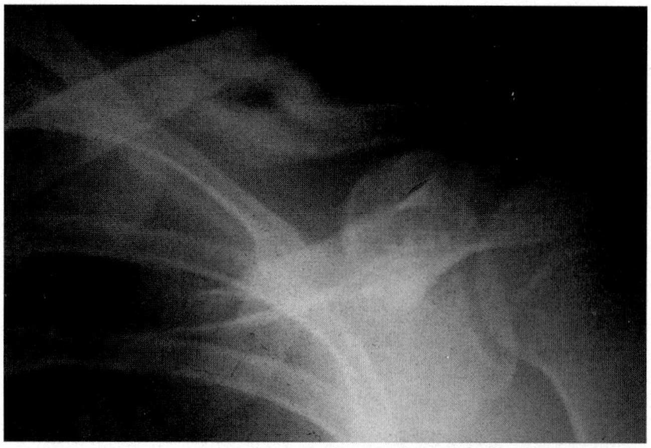

Figure 5–2. After 6 weeks there is no sign of bone union.

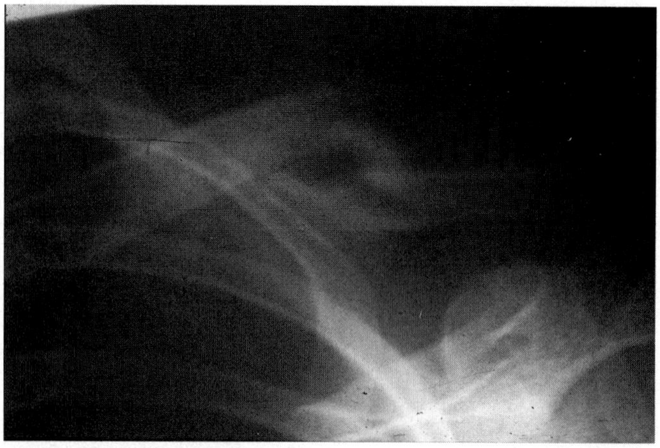

Figure 5–3. By 12 weeks there is evidence of healing, but clinically the fracture remained mobile.

the beach chair position. An incision was made over the middle two thirds of the clavicle and cutting cautery used to expose the bone ends. It was noted that the two intermediate fragments had united with the distal clavicle but that there was no sign of union to the proximal clavicle. After exposure of the two ends of the clavicle using cutting cautery, bone nibblers were used to trim the bone spike produced by the union of the distal intermediate fragment to the distal clavicle. It was impossible to regain length and a saw was therefore used to osteotomize the clavicle to allow reduction and produce two flat bone surfaces. The bone was then reduced and a six-hole reconstruction plate applied (Fig. 5–4).

PEARL

- It is conventional merely to take an anteroposterior radiograph of a clavicular fracture. This may give a good indication of the degree of overlap if, as in this case, the proximal clavicle overlies the distal clavicle. However, surgeons must remember that the ends of the clavicle may both be in the horizontal plane and it may require an oblique radiograph, angled downward, to illustrate the degree of overlap.

Postoperative Management

The right arm was placed in a shoulder immobilizer for 2 weeks following which a program of shoulder mobilization was commenced under physiotherapy supervision. The patient regained full shoulder mobility 4 weeks after surgery. Eight

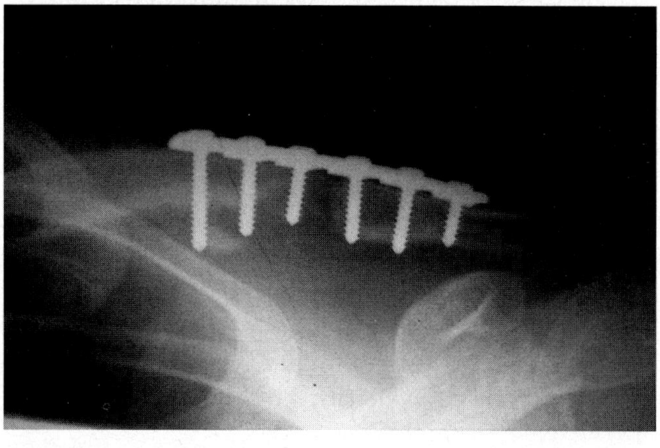

Figure 5–4. An osteotomy was undertaken and held with a six-hole reconstruction plate.

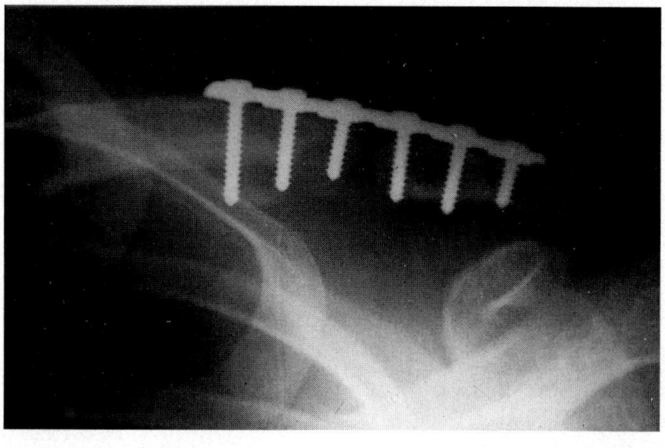

Figure 5–5. Twelve weeks after surgery a bridge of bone was noted on the inferior surface of the clavicle.

PEARL

- Many overlapped clavicular nonunions will follow oblique or spiral fractures (OTA classification 06-A1 or 06-A2). Surgeons may be tempted to try to gain union by merely compressing the oblique ends of the nonunion together and inserting intrafragmentary screws. This technique will not work. The shear forces across the fracture will interfere with union. The bone ends should be cut transversely and opposed before the plate is applied.

PITFALL

- Care must be taken inserting bone screws into the clavicle. The proximity of the subclavian vessels means that the drill must not be allowed to travel into the soft tissues on the undersurface of the clavicle. Thus, a sharp drill bit must be used, and the surgeon must not apply excessive pressure to the drill to expedite its passage through the bone. Care must also be taken when using the tap and depth gauge.

weeks after surgery it was noted that he was painfree, and 4 weeks later a radiograph (Fig. 5–5) showed a good bridge of bone across the osteotomy. The plate was not removed.

Discussion

Clavicle fractures have received scant attention in the orthopedic literature in recent years. The perceived wisdom is that adult clavicle fractures will heal with minimal treatment in the vast majority of cases. Nonunion rates have been stated to be between 0.1 and 5%, but it is likely that this is a gross underestimate of the true situation.

It is logical to assume that clavicle fractures will behave like any other long-bone injury and that the more severe the fracture and the coexisting soft tissue damage the higher the incidence of nonunion. This has been reported by White et al. (1989) who found a 23% incidence of union problems in high energy clavicle fractures. In a recent retrospective study Hill et al. (1997) found that 15% of adult displaced fractures of the middle third of the clavicle developed nonunions and that 31% of patients reported unsatisfactory results. They examined a number of parameters to see if they could predict nonunion and reported that initial shortening of more than 18 mm was associated with nonunion in all cases. They consequently advocated primary open reduction and internal fixation of these fractures. The literature therefore leaves surgeons in a quandry. The early articles suggested a benign prognosis. However, the landmark articles of Neer (1960) and Rowe (1968) did not separate adult fractures from pediatric fractures and later articles certainly point toward a higher incidence of nonunion in displaced clavicular fractures in adults. It seems likely that there are two main types of displaced clavicle fracture in adults that may give rise to nonunion. The displaced fracture described by Hill et al. (1997) is undoubtedly associated with a significant incidence of nonunion and the high energy comminuted fracture illustrated in this case also has a potential for nonunion. However, the true incidence of nonunion has yet to be properly defined in a large prospective study and indeed it may prove difficult to define the exact incidence because anteroposterior radiographs are often difficult to interpret and angled radiographs, which show the nonunion site, are infrequently obtained. In addition, a number of patients with fibrous nonunion are asymptomatic and do not report back to outpatient clinics.

The treatment of nonunion is reasonably well established. Intramedullary pin fixation can be used, but most surgeons prefer plating. The technique, however, is de-

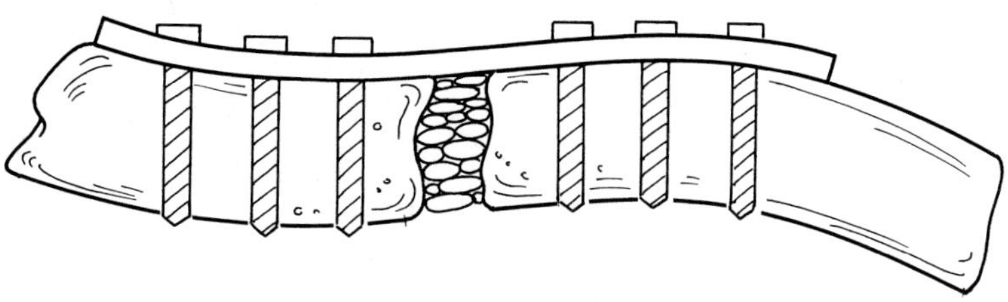

Figure 5–6. Bone graft can be used to fill a complete bone deficit. As shown, the plate may have to be bent to achieve an appropriate contour. To facilitate this reconstruction, plates are preferred to dynamic compression plates.

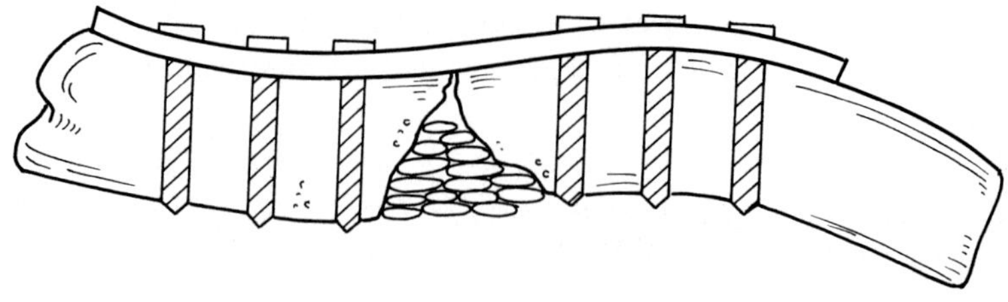

Figure 5–7. More commonly, a wedge defect will be present. This can be grafted with good results.

manding. Even though the clavicle is subcutaneous, the presence of the underlying subclavian vein means that great care must be taken with mobilization of the bone ends and screw insertion. It is suggested that cutting cautery be used to mobilize the bone ends because the area is extremely vascular. Not infrequently the proximal clavicle will overlay the distal clavicle and must be mobilized before the distal clavicle can even be adequately visualized. Often there is considerable overlap and reduction of the clavicle is impossible. Under these circumstances, the ends of the clavicle must be cut so that end to end apposition is possible. A plate can then be applied.

In the fragmented wedge fracture illustrated in this case it is not unusual to find that intermediate bone fragments are avascular. These fragments should be excised and the resulting defect treated by the insertion of autograft from the iliac crest.

Bone graft is used in two circumstances. There may be an avascular segment of clavicle that may need to be removed, resulting in a complete bone defect as shown in (Fig. 5–6). A similar bone defect may also be seen in an atrophic nonunion that has been left for a considerable period of time. These defects will require grafting. The clavicle can be shortened easily, but it seems unwise to excessively shorten the bone; the results of grafting nonunions with bone defects are good.

The second situation where bone graft can be used is with a wedge or fragmented wedge fracture. If the wedge is avascular and consists almost entirely of cortical bone, it should be removed and bone graft used to fill the defect. Again, the results of this procedure are good. This is illustrated in Figure 5–7.

Alternative Methods of Management

There is widespread agreement that displaced midshaft clavicle fractures should be treated primarily by nonoperative means. Hill et al. (1997) may be correct in stating that grossly overlapped clavicular fractures should be fixed primarily, but further clinical research is required before this view is widely accepted. There are certain indications for primary fixation: open clavicle fractures, fractures where the overlying skin is compromised by an underlying bone spike, and those where there is associated vascular or severe neurological injury. Most brachial plexus lesions associated with clavicle fractures will recover spontaneously, but if there is a closed shoulder dissociation with a brachial plexus lesion and a clavicular fracture, some stability will be regained by plating the clavicle.

Once a nonunion is established, the principal treatment methods are either plating or intramedullary pinning.

Intramedullary pinning has been reported to be successful in the management of clavicular nonunion. It is usually performed as an open technique by passing a Steinmann pin antegrade through the fracture site out of the anterior clavicular wall

PEARL
- If the bone defect is over 1 cm in length, using an eight-hole plate is suggested to gain adequate stability.

at the junction of the middle and distal thirds of the clavicle. The fragments are then reduced and the pin advanced over the fracture site. This technique is well described by Capicotto et al. (1994), who reported on the management of 14 clavicular nonunions in an 8-year period. They did not report infection or pin migration, but did have two refractures through osteopenic bone.

If intramedullary pinning is used in the clavicle, it is suggested that a large pin, such as a Steinmann pin, be used. If Kirschner wires are used, there is a high incidence of pin migration and Lyons and Rockwood (1990) have documented pins migrating from the shoulder into the heart, subclavian artery, ascending aorta, pulmonary artery, lung, and mediastinum.

Little has been documented in recent years about the use of external skeletal fixation in clavicular fractures. It can be used, but care must be exercised in placing pins because of the underlying vascular structures. There is also an incidence of clavicular fracture through the pin tracks if the pins are placed eccentrally.

Type of Management	Advantages	Disadvantages	Comments
Nonoperative management	Easy; low infection rate	High incidence of nonunion in high energy fractures	There is as yet insufficient evidence that operative management is indicated for most displaced clavicle fractures
Plating	Good reduction	Infection; vascular damage	There is some evidence that primary plating may be indicated for grossly overlapped fractures
External fixation	Closed technique	Clavicle fracture; vascular damage; pin tract infection	More work is required before the usefulness of external fixation in displaced clavicle fractures can be determined
Intramedullary pinning	No indication for the primary management of clavicular fractures	Difficult technique; pin migration; secondary fracture	Of use in the management of nonunion, but not indicated for primary fixation

Complications

As already detailed, the most common complication of displaced clavicular fractures in adults is nonunion. This may be asymptomatic, although it is likely that many "asymptomatic" nonunions can be shown to be symptomatic if the appropriate questions are asked. Other complications include skin penetration by an underlying bone fragment, brachial plexus damage, and local vascular injury.

There is debate about the effect on shoulder function of a short clavicle. Eskola et al. (1986) demonstrated abductor weakness in patients who had shortening of the clavicle averaging 17 mm. However, many surgeons believe that shortening of the clavicle is associated with minimal functional deficit.

The complications of surgery for clavicular nonunion should be few. The area is well vascularized and, if the bone ends are well reduced, the results should be good.

Infection must be treated rigorously using techniques described elsewhere in this book. If infection is diagnosed and treated late, the subcutaneous location of the bone means that the overlying atrophic skin may have to be resected and a skin flap used to cover the defect.

If there is a gap between the bone ends after plating, it is important that bone grafts be used to fill this bone defect, otherwise nonunion will persist.

Suggested Readings

Capicotto PN, Heiple KG, Wilbur JH: Mid-shaft clavicle non-unions treated with intramedullary Steinmann pin fixation and onlay bone grafts. J Orthop Trauma 1994; 8:88–93.

Eskola A, Vainiopaa S, Myllynen P, Patiala H, Rokkanen P: Surgery for un-united clavicular fracture. Acta Orthop Scand 1986; 57:366–367.

Hill JM, McGuire MH, Crosby LA: Closed treatment of displaced middle third fractures of the clavicle gives poor results. J Bone Joint Surg [Br]1997; 79B: 537–539.

Lyons FA, Rockwood CA: Migration of pins used in operations on the shoulder. J Bone Joint Surg [Am]1990; 72A:1262–1267.

Neer CS: Nonunion of the clavicle. JAMA 1960; 172:1006–1011.

Rowe CR: An atlas of anatomy and treatment of mid-clavicular fractures. Clin Orthop 1968; 68:29–42.

White RR, Anson PS, Kristiansen T, Healy W: Adult clavicle fractures: relationship between mechanism of injury and healing. Orthop Trans 1989; 13:514–515.

Case 6

History and Physical Examination

A 35-year-old male injured his right shoulder wrestling with a friend. The injury occurred when he was pushed onto his shoulder while his arm was adducted. There was immediate onset of pain and swelling of the anterior and superior aspect of the shoulder. The patient arrived in the emergency department approximately 6 hours after injury. Physical examination revealed swelling of the anterior aspect of the shoulder, but no obvious deformity. There was pain and crepitation with palpation of the distal clavicle and anterior shoulder. Any active or passive motion of the shoulder was painful. The neurovascular examination of the upper extremity was within the limits of normal. The patient's history was significant in that he had sustained a fracture of the neck of the glenoid 3 years prior to this injury. The fracture of the glenoid neck had been managed conservatively with a sling. Clinically, his shoulder had been asymptomatic for the last 2 years.

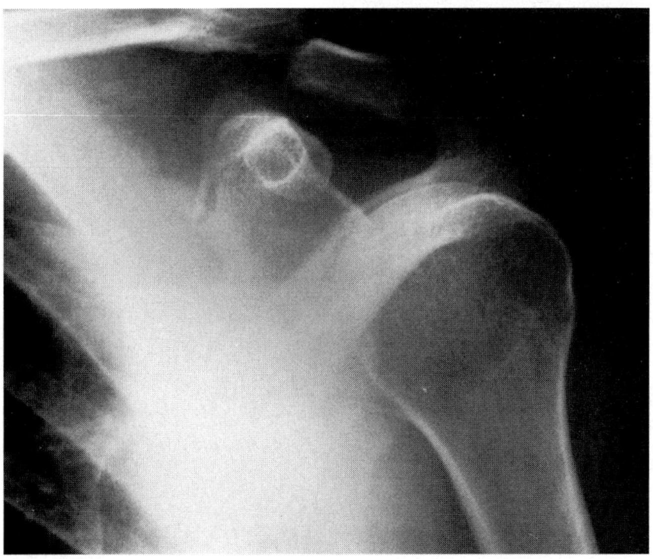

Figure 6–1. An anteroposterior radiograph of the shoulder indicating a transverse fracture of the distal clavicle. A fracture of the coracoid is evident, but not well visualized. The acromioclavicular joint appears intact.

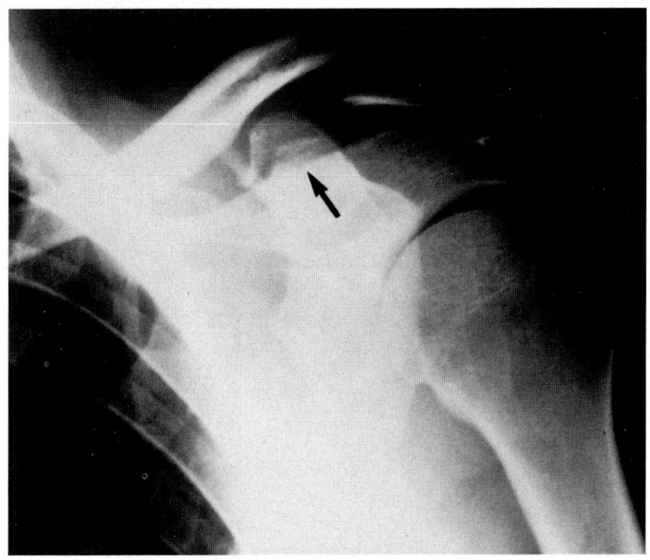

Figure 6–2. Cephalic tilt radiograph of the shoulder shows the fracture of the coracoid (arrow) and cephalad displacement of the proximal fragment of the clavicle.

Radiologic Findings

In addition to a routine anteroposterior radiograph, a radiograph with the beam directed 20 degrees cephalad was obtained. This "cephalic tilt" projection profiles the clavicle and eliminates overlying bony anatomy of the scapula and ribs from the radiograph. A fracture of the distal clavicle was present with cephalad displacement of the proximal portion. The coracoid was fractured through its base and displaced cephalad. The acromioclavicular joint and proximal humerus appeared intact. The neck of the glenoid had been fractured previously and was healed with approximately 5 mm of shortening (Figs. 6–1 and 6–2).

Diagnosis

Interligamentous fracture of the distal clavicle with avulsion of the corocoid process.

Surgical Management

The patient was taken to the operating room the day after injury. A general anesthetic was administered and he was placed in the "beach chair" position with his head supported in a Mayfield headrest. The fracture was exposed via a deltopectoral incision that was extended medially along the clavicle. The clavicle was exposed subperiosteally, taking care to preserve the coracoclavicular ligaments. The coracoid process and conjoined tendon were exposed via the deltopectoral interval. The clavicle fracture was reduced and stabilized with a small fragment reconstruction plate and screws. The coracoid was reduced, overdrilled, and stabilized with a large fragment cortical screw (Fig. 6–3).

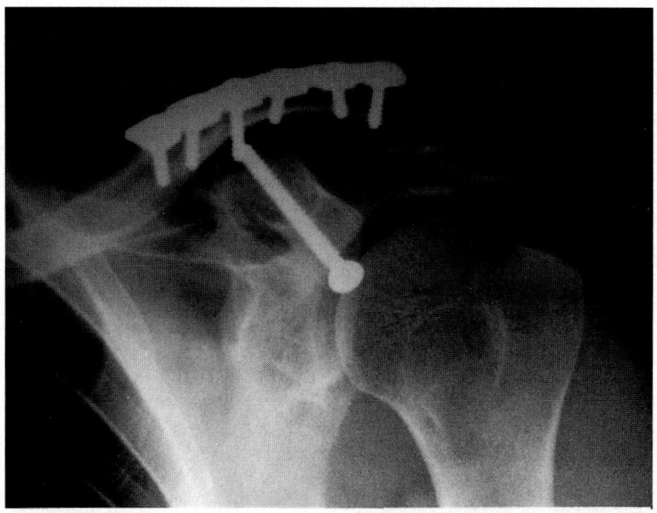

Figure 6–3. An anteroposterior radiograph of the shoulder following plating of the clavicle and fixation of the coracoid with a lag screw.

Postoperative Management

Postoperatively the arm was supported in a sling for 6 weeks. At 1 week gentle circumduction exercises of the shoulder in the sling were initiated. At 4 weeks gentle passive range of motion of the shoulder was initiated. At 6 weeks active and passive ranges of motion of the shoulder were initiated.

Discussion

The clavicle is the only bony connection between the shoulder girdle and the body. The clavicle functions as a fulcrum against which the muscles of the shoulder girdle work. Without it, contraction of the muscles, which take origin from the chest and insert on the scapula and humerus (e.g., the serratus and pectoralis major), would simply approximate the shoulder to the chest. For the clavicle to function as a fulcrum, its articulation with the acromion must be intact. Fractures of the distal third or dislocations of the clavicle potentially compromise this function.

Fractures of the distal third of the clavicle have been classified into three types by Neer (1984). Type I fractures occur lateral to the coracoclavicular ligament. They are minimally displaced, and the coracoclavicular ligament and acromioclavicular joint capsule are intact. Type II fractures are displaced oblique fractures with the coracoclavicular ligament and acromioclavicular joint capsule intact and remaining attached to the distal fragment. Type III fractures are intraarticular fractures of the distal clavicle with the ligaments and joint capsule intact.

There are two types of distal clavicle fractures in addition to those described by Neer. The first is a fracture lateral to the coracoclavicular ligaments with an associated tear of the coracoclavicular ligaments. The second is a fracture lateral to the coracoclavicular ligaments with a bony avulsion of the coracoid process or of the clavicular origin of the ligament. These two types of fractures along with the Neer type II fractures share one of the major characteristics of acromioclavicular joint separations—namely, the forces displacing the fracture fragments and acromioclavicular joint separations are identical (i.e., the trapezius and sternocleidomastoid displace the medial clavicle proximally, while the weight of the arm displaces the lateral fragment distally). However, unlike acromioclavicular separations, displacement of fracture fragments must be addressed or there is a significant risk of nonunion. On the other hand, if the fracture is reduced and heals, the intact acromioclavicular joint capsule will hold the clavicle reduced and restore its function as a fulcrum.

In this case the clavicle fracture was reduced and stabilized with a plate. The fixation was augmented by fixation of the coracoid process, thus reestablishing the coracoclavicular ligaments.

Alternative Methods of Management

Alternative methods of management are operative with an intramedullary pin or intraosseous wires and conservative with a Kenny Howard sling.

Type of Management	Advantages	Disadvantages	Comments
Operative with plating	Technically simple	When fixation fails reconstruction is difficult	Probably the most commonly used method of management.
Operative with intramedullary pin or interosseous wires	Interosseous wiring is technically simple	Technically difficult to place intramedullary pin between tables of acromion; failure of pin because bending stresses; interosseous wires fail	The risk of failure of fixation and migration of the fixation device to the lung or heart limits the application of these methods.
Conservative with a Kenny Howard sling	Closed procedure	Patient compliance is limited; reduction is usually lost	Indicated for patients who cannot be managed operatively

Complications

The complications of distal clavicle fractures are nonunion and arthritis of the acromioclavicular joint. The complication unique to internal fixation of a distal clavicle fracture is loss of fixation.

PEARL

- Stability of fixation is completely dependent on the pullout strength of the screws lateral to the fracture or nonunion. Pullout strength of these screws is decreased by a small distal clavicle fragment into which only one screw can be inserted.

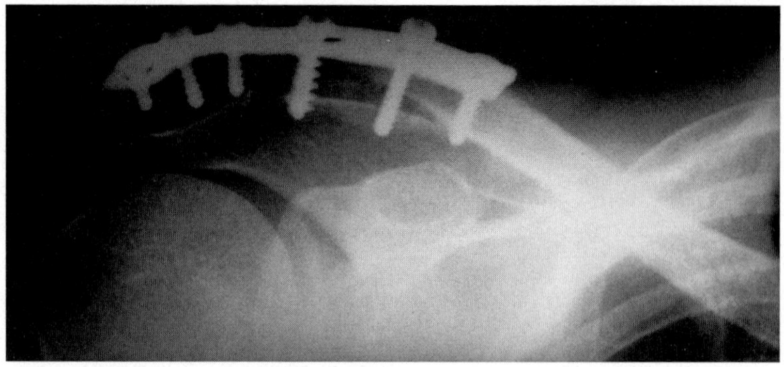

Figure 6–4. Alternative fixation of the clavicle with a "T" plate that spans the acromioclavicular joint. Fixation is limited by the pullout strength of the screws distal to the fracture. The acromion is surprisingly thin and provides minimal additional purchase.

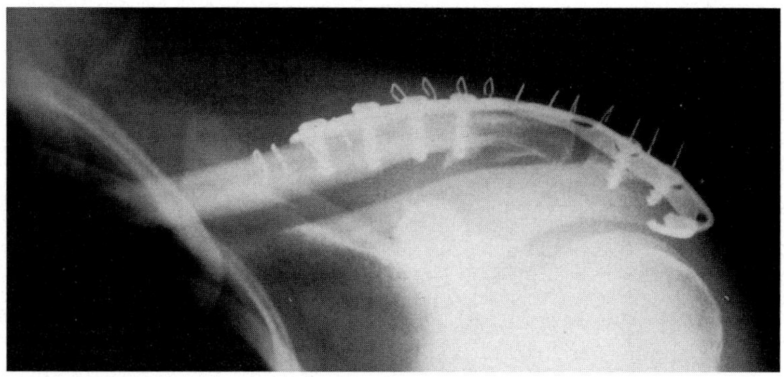

Figure 6–5. Alternative fixation of the clavicle with a "hook" plate. The plate is bent around the lateral border of the acromion and must be removed after the clavicle is healed to prevent impingement on the rotator cuff.

Nonunion of a distal clavicle fracture results from persistent displacement. Invariably, the proximal fragment is displaced proximally and the distal fragment is displaced distally. Management of a displaced nonunion is open reduction, removal of intervening fibrous tissue, autogenous bone grafting, and plating. In cases in which the distal fragment of clavicle is very small, a Mumford procedure is performed (see below).

Arthritis of the acromioclavicular joint follows type III fractures more frequently than the other types of distal clavicle fractures. When arthritis occurs, a trial of conservative management with nonsteroidal antiinflammatories and local steroid injections is warranted. When conservative management fails, a Mumford procedure is performed. The distal clavicle is resected and the coracoacromial ligament detached from the acromion and reattached to the end of the clavicle. The coracoacromial ligament substitutes for the disrupted coracoclavicular ligaments and prevents the clavicle from displacing proximally.

Loss of fixation following plating is due to pullout of the screws.

To decrease the incidence of failure of fixation, a T-shaped plate can be used to increase the number screws laterally; the acromioclavicular joint can be bridged (Fig.

6–4); the plate can be bent around the tip of the acromion (the plate should be removed following healing to prevent impingement) (Fig. 6–5); and postoperatively the arm should be supported in a sling that supports the arm until some healing has occurred (at least 3 weeks). Support of the arm counteracts the major deforming force across the fracture. When failure of fixation has occurred, management is either acceptance of the deformity and nonunion or revision of fixation and autogenous bone grafting.

Suggested Readings

Allman FL: Fractures and ligamentous injuries of the clavicle and its articulations. J Bone Joint Surg 1967; 49A:774–784.

Hak DJ, Johnson EE: Avulsion fracture of the coracoid associated with acromioclavicular dislocation. J Orthop Trauma 1993; 7(4):381–383.

Neer CS: Injuries to the acromioclavicular joint. In: Rockwood CA, Green DP (eds): Fractures in Adults, p 895. JB Lippincott, Philadelphia, 1984.

Post M: Current concepts in the treatment of fractures of the clavicle. CORR August 1989; 245:89–101.

Sim E, Schwarz N, Hocker K, Berzlanovich A: Repair of complete acromioclavicular separations using the acromioclavicular-hook plate. CORR 1995; 314:134–142.

Wurtz LD, Lyons FA, Rockwood CA: Fracture of the middle third of the clavicle and dislocation of the acromioclavicular joint. J Bone Joint Surg 1992; 74A, 1: 133–137

Zenni EJ, Krieg JK, Rosen MJ: Open reduction and internal fixation of clavicular fractures. J Bone Joint Surg 1981; 63A:147–151.

Case 7

History and Physical Examination

A 58-year-old patient presented to the emergency department following a fall. She had fallen on her outstretched right arm and after the incident she was unable to move her right shoulder. There was no other injury. Examination of the shoulder showed no obvious deformity, but it was noted that the patient was unable to move the joint in any direction. There was no evidence of a distal neurovascular deficit in the arm.

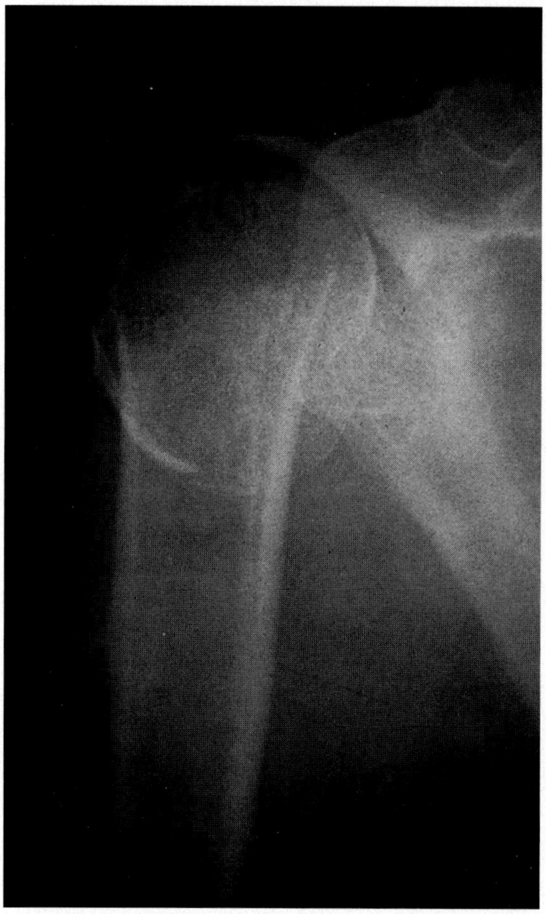

Figure 7–1. An anteroposterior radiograph of a proximal humerus. This is an inadequate X ray that shows the presence of a fracture and raises the possibility of a dislocation.

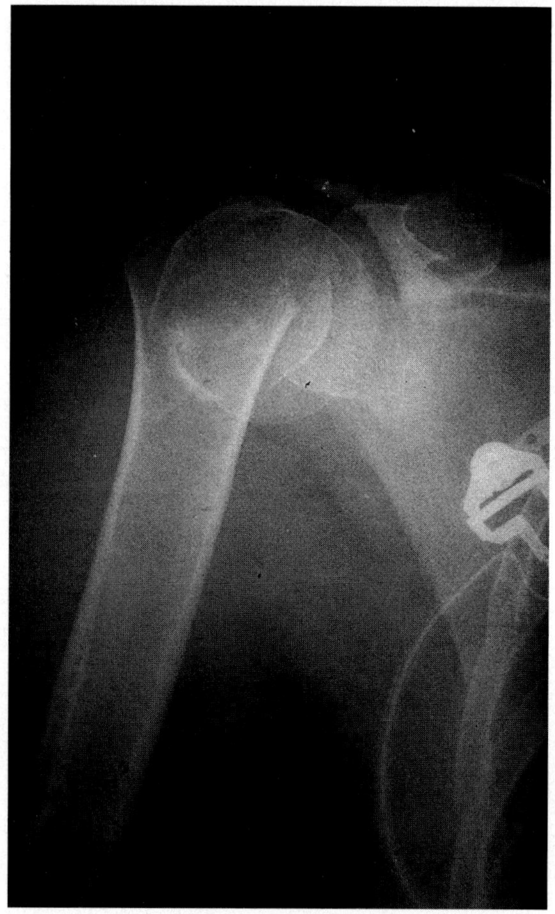

Figure 7–2. A second anteroposterior radiograph that delineates the proximal humeral fractures and strongly suggests the presence of a posterior dislocation.

Radiologic Findings

An anteroposterior radiograph was obtained and interpreted as showing evidence of a proximal humeral fracture (Fig. 7–1). The examining physician thought that the

PITFALL

- The Neer classification of proximal humeral fractures is often misused. Although surgeons usually remember the four parts of the proximal humerus—the two tuberosities, the head, and the shaft—they forget about the importance of displacement. It is not uncommon for minimally displaced fractures to be diagnosed as two, three, or four part fractures.

head of the humerus had rotated but was not absolutely sure about the precise diagnosis. Another view of the proximal humerus was obtained (Fig. 7–2). This view was thought to show a three part fracture of the proximal humerus; fractures of the surgical neck and lesser tuberosity were noted. One further attempt was made to take a lateral view of the proximal humerus, but this was thought merely to corroborate the diagnosis of proximal humeral fracture.

Diagnosis

Three part fracture of the proximal humerus involving the surgical neck and lesser tuberosity (tentative). This is a B3.3 fracture in the AO classification.

Surgical Management

The patient was given a broad arm sling in the emergency department. The diagnosis of a proximal humeral fracture was explained to her and she was discharged with an appointment for an orthopedic follow-up review clinic 3 weeks later. At the follow-up clinic further anteroposterior and axial radiographs were taken (Fig. 7–3). The anteroposterior view indicated some apparent overlap of the head of the humerus over the glenoid and the axial view clearly showed the presence of a posterior dislocation of the glenohumeral joint. Analysis of these two X rays confirms the presence of fractures of the surgical neck and the lesser tuberosity; if Neer's criteria are used, this is a two part fracture dislocation with significant displacement of the lesser tuberosity only. The surgical neck is fractured, but it is neither displaced by more than 1 cm or angulated by more than 45 degrees. The axial view is not diagnostic of an impaction fracture of the humeral head but certainly suggests that one is present.

The patient was admitted to the orthopedic unit the next day for an open reduction and internal fixation of this posterior fracture dislocation. However, a preoperative medical assessment suggested that the patient had a localized hypertrophic obstructive cardiomyopathy and a cardiologist thought that more tests were required before surgery could be permitted. Unfortunately, the tests were protracted and it was a further 2 weeks before a reduction could be undertaken.

Five weeks after the posterior fracture dislocation had occurred the patient was taken to the operating room. An anterior deltopectoral incision was made and 2 in of the cephalic vein was mobilized, ligated, and removed. The space between the deltoid and pectoralis major muscles was then opened and the underlying musculature exposed. Dissection was continued proximally to expose the coracoid process which was predrilled to take a small fragment cancellous screw. The coracoid process was then cut using a power saw and turned downward and medially. This allowed exposure of the underlying subscapularis muscle that was opened between two sets of absorbable stay sutures. This exposure permitted a good view of the glenoid and the proximal humerus that had internally rotated to lie behind the gle-

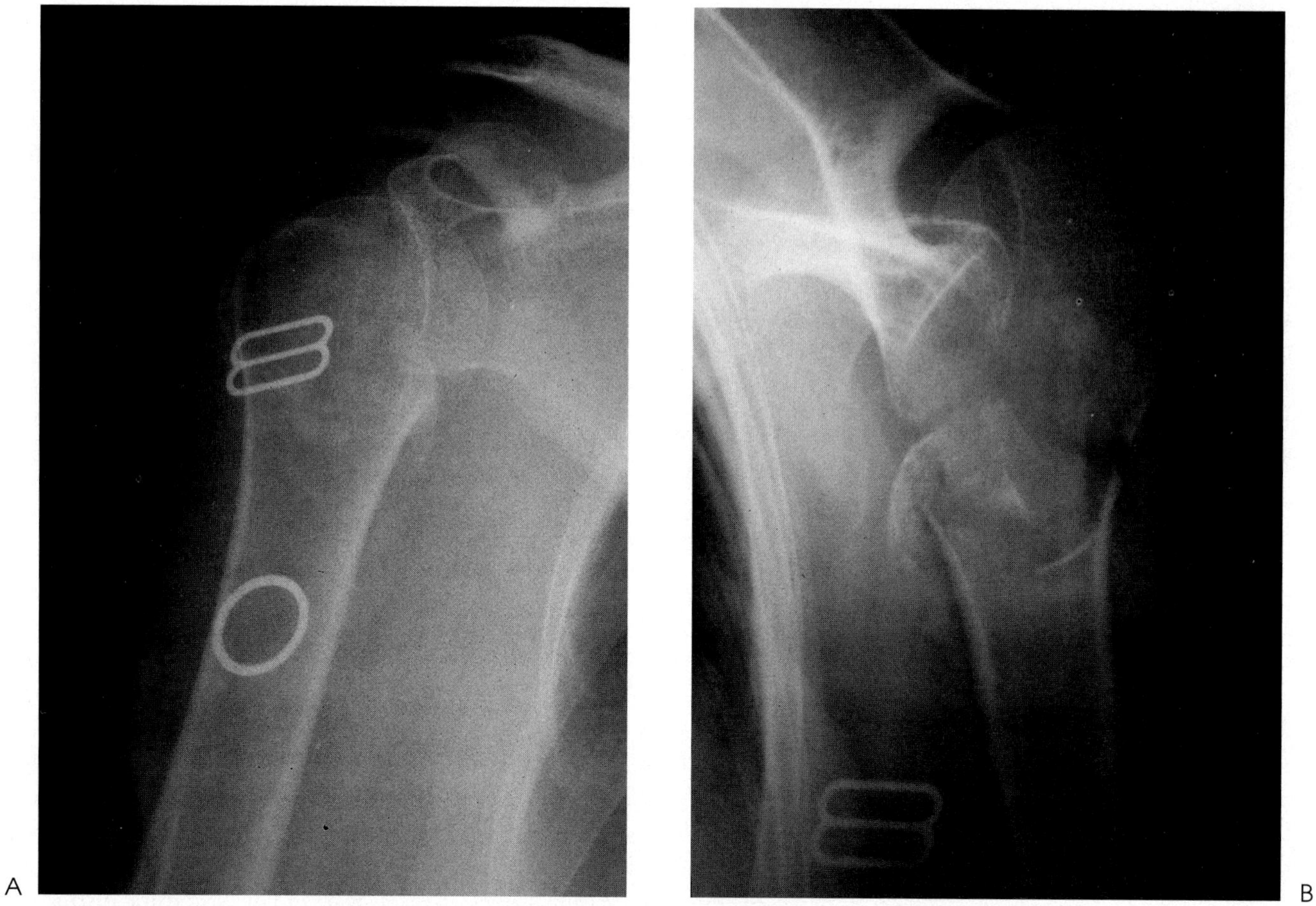

Figure 7–3. Anteroposterior (A) and axial (B) radiographs that confirm the dislocation. The axial view confirms the displacement of the lesser tuberosity and that the surgical neck fracture is beginning to unite.

noid. The initial plan was to internally fix the surgical neck fracture, but after 5 weeks it had united sufficiently to make fixation unnecessary. It proved impossible to reduce the humeral head without applying a lever between it and the glenoid; even after it was reduced, a combination of the shortening of the posterior soft tissues, the impaction fracture, and the posterior soft tissue defect resulted in the humeral head resuming its dislocated position unless the arm was placed in extreme external rotation.

It was considered that the difficulty of holding the humeral head in position combined with the damage to the articular surface mitigated against achieving a good result from an open reduction and stabilization and a hemiarthroplasty was therefore inserted. The insertion of the hemiarthroplasty was a relatively straightforward procedure, although care had to be taken when deciding on the correct angle and retroversion of the humeral head. Placing the humeral head in the usual 30 degree retroversion resulted in dislocation. Consequently, the humeral head was placed in about a 10 degree retroversion. To facilitate the correct placement of the humeral head, a prosthesis with a narrow stem was used to prevent binding of the prosthetic stem on the endosteal surface of the humerus. The soft tissues were then repaired and the skin closed.

The initial radiographs taken after surgery showed an apparent inferior subluxation of the humeral head in the glenoid (Fig. 7–4) but an anteroposterior film taken two months later (Fig. 7–5) indicated that the subluxation had reduced, although the joint was not completely congruous.

A physiotherapy regime was instituted after surgery, but progress was slow. Six months after surgery the patient reported no pain in her shoulder but she only had 40 degrees of abduction, 60 degrees of flexion, and 10 degrees of external rotation. She could only internally rotate her right arm so that her hand could reach the area of the fifth lumbar vertebrae. Because she was righthanded she was left with a significant functional deficit and experienced difficulty in dressing, toileting, and carrying out her normal household activities.

Discussion

It is quite clear that the posterior dislocation was missed by the examining physician in the emergency room. Posterior fracture dislocations and pure posterior disloca-

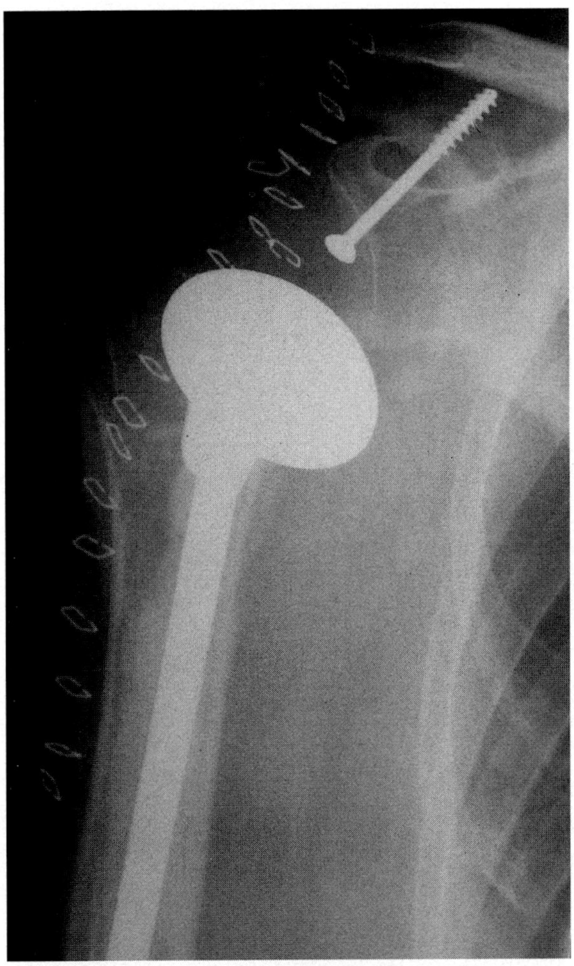

Figure 7–4. A postoperative radiograph after the insertion of a Neer's hemiarthroplasty. Note the subluxation caused by a transient deltoid paralysis.

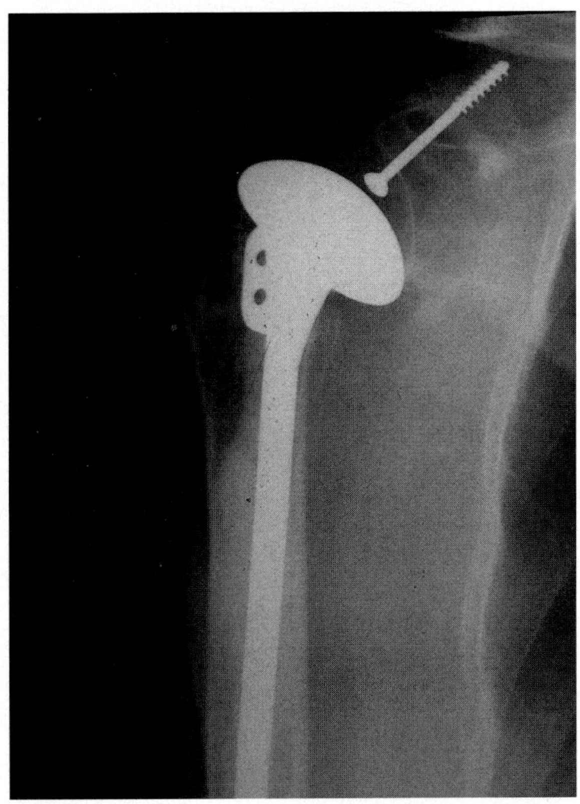

Figure 7–5. The subluxation is improving, although the joint is not as yet congruous.

PITFALL

- The objective of treatment should be to restore function. All too often the surgeon is satisfied with gaining fracture union or implanting a prosthesis. Patients should be followed up to assess that treatment has been successful in regaining function.

tions of the shoulder are very rare, with posterior dislocation comprising only about 2% of all dislocations of the glenohumeral joint. It is likely that between 60 and 80% of all posterior dislocations are missed at the initial examination because the emergency doctor is looking for the typical radiological signs of an anterior dislocation. However, it is important to take the correct radiographs and many hospital emergency departments do not include an adequate axial view of the shoulder as a routine. Two views of the shoulder, anteroposterior and axial views, will suffice to allow a correct diagnosis of all proximal humeral fractures and dislocations.

The key to the radiological diagnosis of a posterior dislocation on an anteroposterior radiograph is the incongruity of the glenohumeral joint. Figure 7–6A shows that there is marked overlap of the proximal humerus over the glenoid, suggesting a dislocation. Overlap depends on the degree of internal rotation of the proximal humerus and the angle of the X rays. An overlap may not be obvious. If there is marked internal rotation, the anteroposterior radiograph may take a lateral view of the tuberosities and show the classical "light bulb" sign. Increased distance between the anterior lip of the glenoid and the medial aspect of the humeral head may also be seen. The importance of a small alteration in the angle of the X-ray beam is seen in Figure 7–6B. This view was taken after the X ray shown in Figure 7–6A and clearly indicates a posterior dislocation. The key is joint incongruity; if there is any

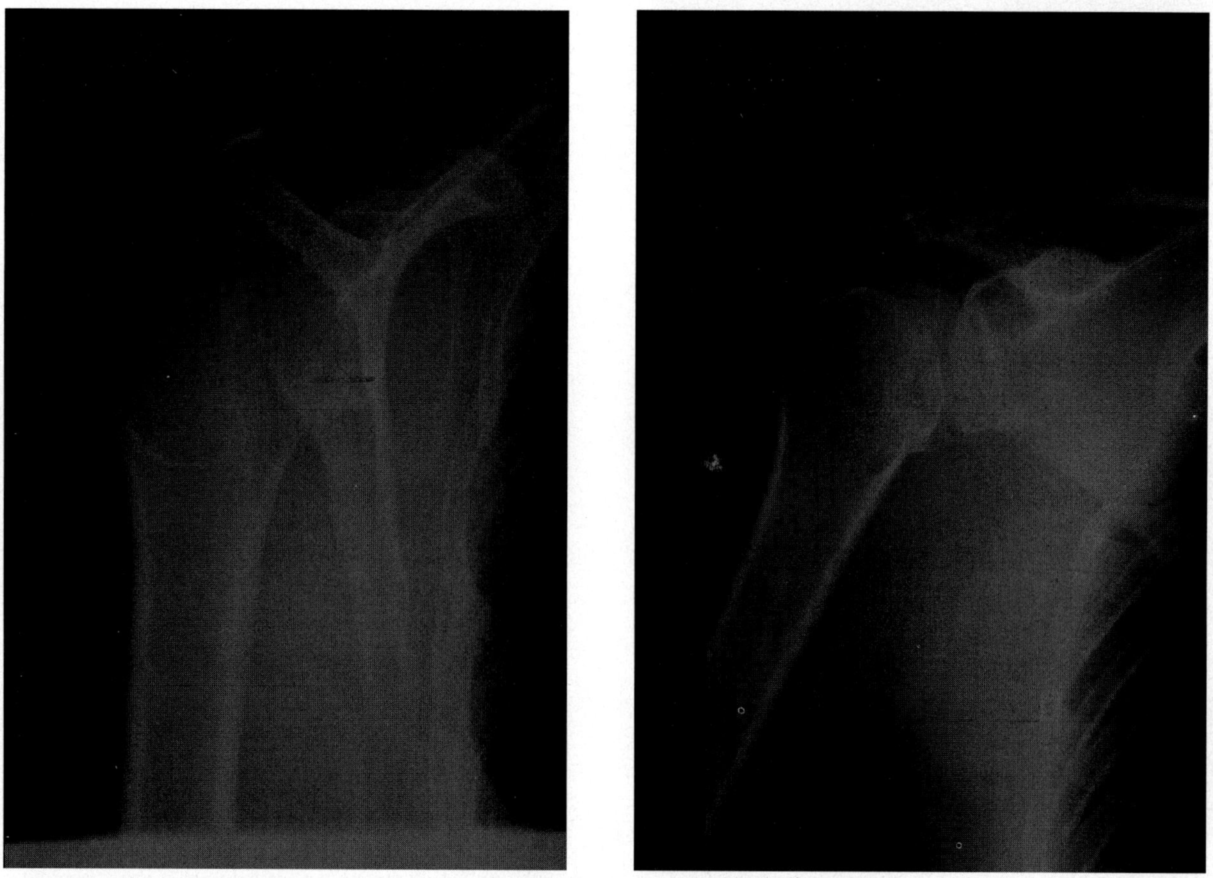

A B

Figure 7–6 (A, B) Two anteroposterior radiographs of a patient with a posterior dislocation. They illustrate the importance of altering the angle of the X-ray beam.

suspicion of this, further views or a computerized axial tomography scan should be obtained because the hazards of missing a posterior dislocation are considerable.

It is also obvious that the patient was not adequately examined in the emergency room. Physical signs may be difficult to elicit in overweight patients, but in general the clinical signs of a posterior dislocation are characteristic. The examining doctor will see flattening of the anterior aspect of the shoulder with a posterior prominence. The coracoid is usually much more apparent on the dislocated side and there is a complete block to external rotation with the patient holding the arm in internal rotation. This is usually accentuated by asking the patient to flex the elbow to 90 degrees when the fixed internal rotation of the affected arm will become apparent.

The importance of recognizing and treating a posterior dislocation early is obvious in that the prognosis for missed dislocations treated late is very much worse. When detected early, the treatment is closed reduction and immobilization with the prospect of achieving an excellent result. If, as in this case, the diagnosis is missed, open surgery is required and the prognosis is frequently poor.

Alternative Methods of Management

If the surgeon has to open the joint to reduce the dislocation, there are a number of possible methods of maintaining joint reduction. A shoulder spica can be applied with the arm in external rotation and a degree of abduction. This is a reasonable alternative, but patients find the spica uncomfortable and difficult to wear. The joint can also be held in a reduced position by external fixation (Fig. 7–7). External fixation of the shoulder is difficult because pin fixation can be problematic. Pins will need to be placed in the clavicle, acromion, and scapula if sufficiently rigid fixation is to be obtained. Immobilization is usually maintained for 3 to 4 weeks and, as with plaster spicas, patients find the external fixator tedious to wear. After this period the shoulder will stay in joint unless there is a large associated impaction fracture. However, the joint will almost certain remain stiff. Other alternatives are a lesser tuberosity transfer or a McLaughlin subscapularis transfer. There is no universally accepted policy of treating missed posterior dislocations, but Hawkins and Neer (1984) and Rockwood suggest a protocol based on the size of the impaction

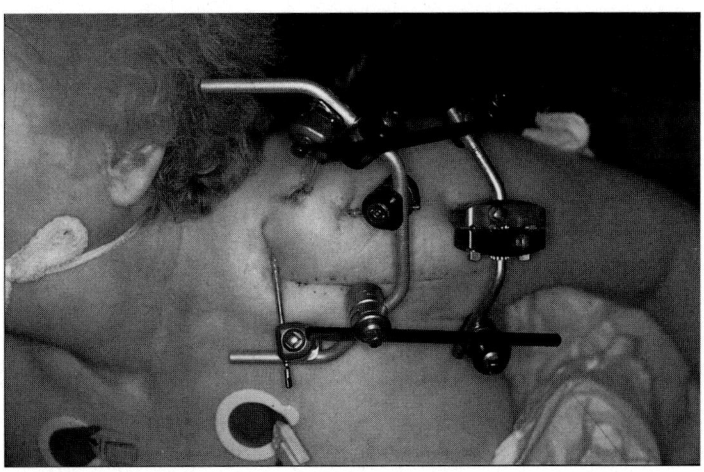

Figure 7–7. The application of an external fixator to the shoulder in a patient with a missed posterior dislocation.

defect of the humeral head and the duration of the dislocation. If the patient is elderly, debilitated, and dependent, it is probably advisable not to treat a missed posterior dislocation provided the patient is not in pain.

Type of Management	Advantages	Disadvantages	Comments
Closed reduction and immobilization	Straightforward technique; good results if condition diagnosed early	Usually impossible after 2 weeks	Closed reduction should be attempted, but unfortunately it is often impossible after 2 weeks
Open reduction and external fixation using spica or external fixator	No requirement for hemiarthroplasty or muscle transfer	Both shoulder spica and external fixator unpleasant to wear; arm held in external rotation; pin tract sepsis; joint stiffness	Both techniques are difficult for the patient and are associated with poor results
Hemiarthroplasty	Definitive management usually painfree	Joint stiffness	Particularly useful if there is a large impaction fracture of the humeral head
Tuberosity transfer/ subscapularis transfer	Maintains the humeral head	Joint stiffness; occasional recurrent dislocation	Useful technique, but questionable whether it is better than hemiarthroplasty

Complications

We have described a number of the complications of treating late posterior dislocations and fracture dislocations of the shoulder. Patients' principle complaints are pain and stiffness. Unfortunately, these are all too common after missed posterior dislocations. Pain is best treated by the use of analgesics, nonsteroidal antiinflammatory medication, and occasional use of steroid injections into the anterior rotator cuff if there is an impingement syndrome. Pain and stiffness frequently co-exist and physiotherapy may help both. Rarely shoulder arthrodesis will be required for patients who have intractable pain in a stiff shoulder.

Suggested Readings

Flatow, EL, Ulrich C (eds): Humerus. Butterworth Heinemann, Oxford, 1996.

Hawkins, RJ, Neer CS: Missed posterior dislocations of the shoulder. In: Bateman JE, Welsh RP (eds): Surgery of the Shoulder, pp 117–120. BC Decker, Philadelphia, 1984.

Kelly I (ed): The Practice of Shoulder Surgery. Butterworth Heinemann, Oxford, 1993.

McLaughlin HL: Posterior dislocation of the shoulder. J Bone Joint Surg (Am) 1952; 34A:584–590.

Neer CS, Rockwood CA: Fractures about the shoulder. In: Rockwood CA, Greene DP (eds): Fractures in Adults, pp 675–985. JB Lippincott, Philadelphia, 1984.

Norris TR: Fractures of the proximal humerus and dislocations of the shoulder. In: Browner BD, Jupiter JB, Levine AM, Trafton PG (eds): Skeletal Trauma, pp 1201–1290. WB Saunders, Philadelphia, 1992.

Case 8

History and Physical Examination

A 76-year-old woman fell in the street and was unable to move her right shoulder after the incident. She was taken to the emergency department where her right shoulder was seen to be swollen and painful and it was noted that no movement was possible. There was no evidence of neurovascular dysfunction in the arm and she had no other injury.

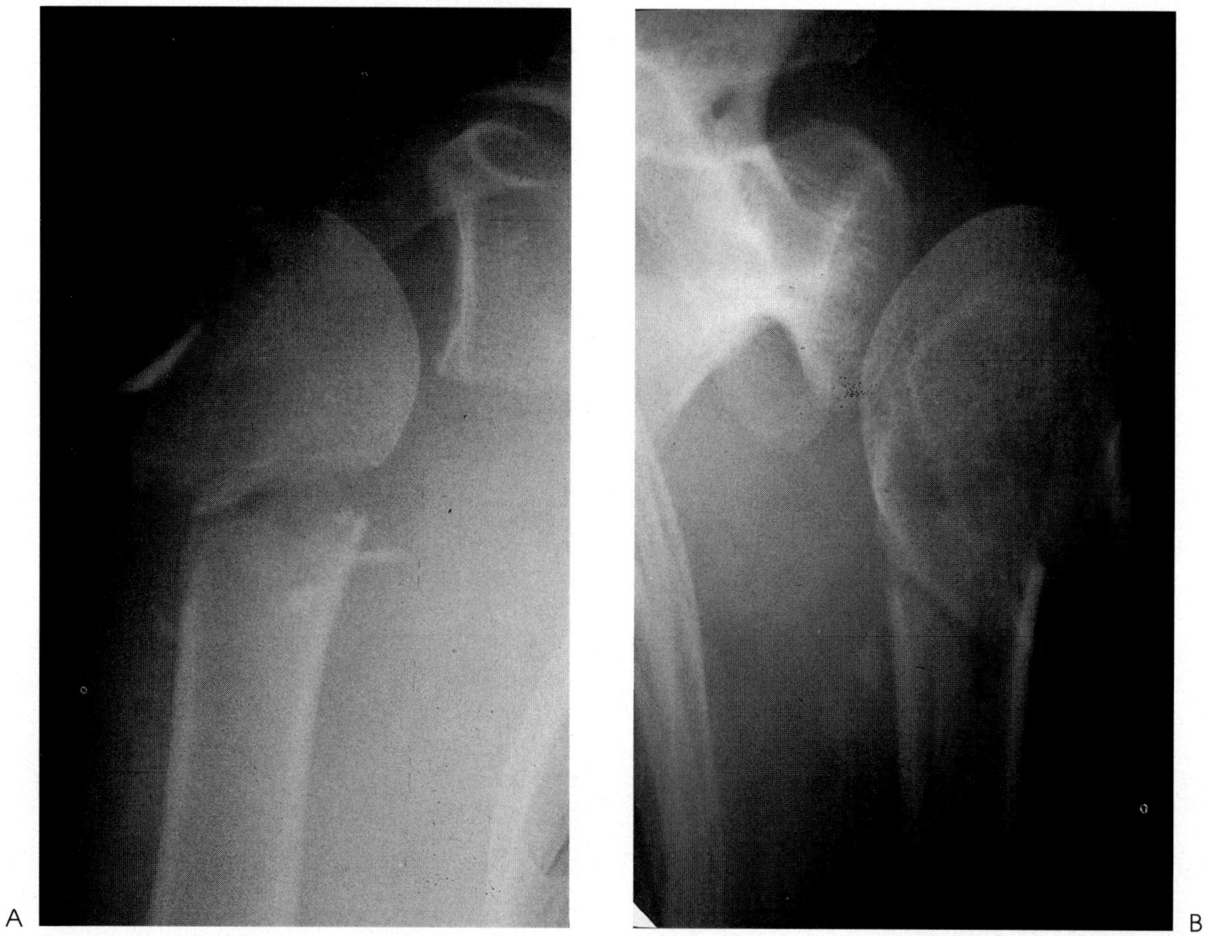

Figure 8–1. Anteroposterior (A) and axilary (B) views of a translated two part proximal humeral fracture. Note the complete displacement and varus angulation.

Radiologic Findings

Anteroposterior and modified axilary radiographs showed a displaced two part fracture of the proximal humerus (Fig. 8–1). The anteroposterior radiograph showed complete displacement of the surgical neck of the humerus with some varus angulation of the head of the humerus.

PITFALL

- It is important that the surgeon be aware of the timing of patients' recovery from fractures. In the elderly it may take over 9 months to recover good shoulder movement and there is no evidence that surgery accelerates rehabilitation.

Diagnosis

A translated two part fracture of the proximal humerus. AO classification: 11–A3.2 fracture.

Treatment

No surgical treatment was thought necessary. The patient was treated with immobilization of the arm in a collar and cuff for 2 weeks. At this time a physiotherapy regime was instituted that was continued for 3 months. The patient was formally assessed using Neer's shoulder outcome criteria at 6 weeks, 13 weeks, 26 weeks, and 1 year after the injury. At 6 weeks the Neer score was 48 and at 13 weeks it was 62. By 26 weeks the patient had a Neer score of 78 and at 1 year the score was 92. At 1 year physical examination, the patient had only some restriction of internal rotation. She could only get her hand to her fifth lumbar vertebra. No other physical abnormality was noted. The radiographs at 1 year showed good union with a lateral bone buttress (Fig. 8–2).

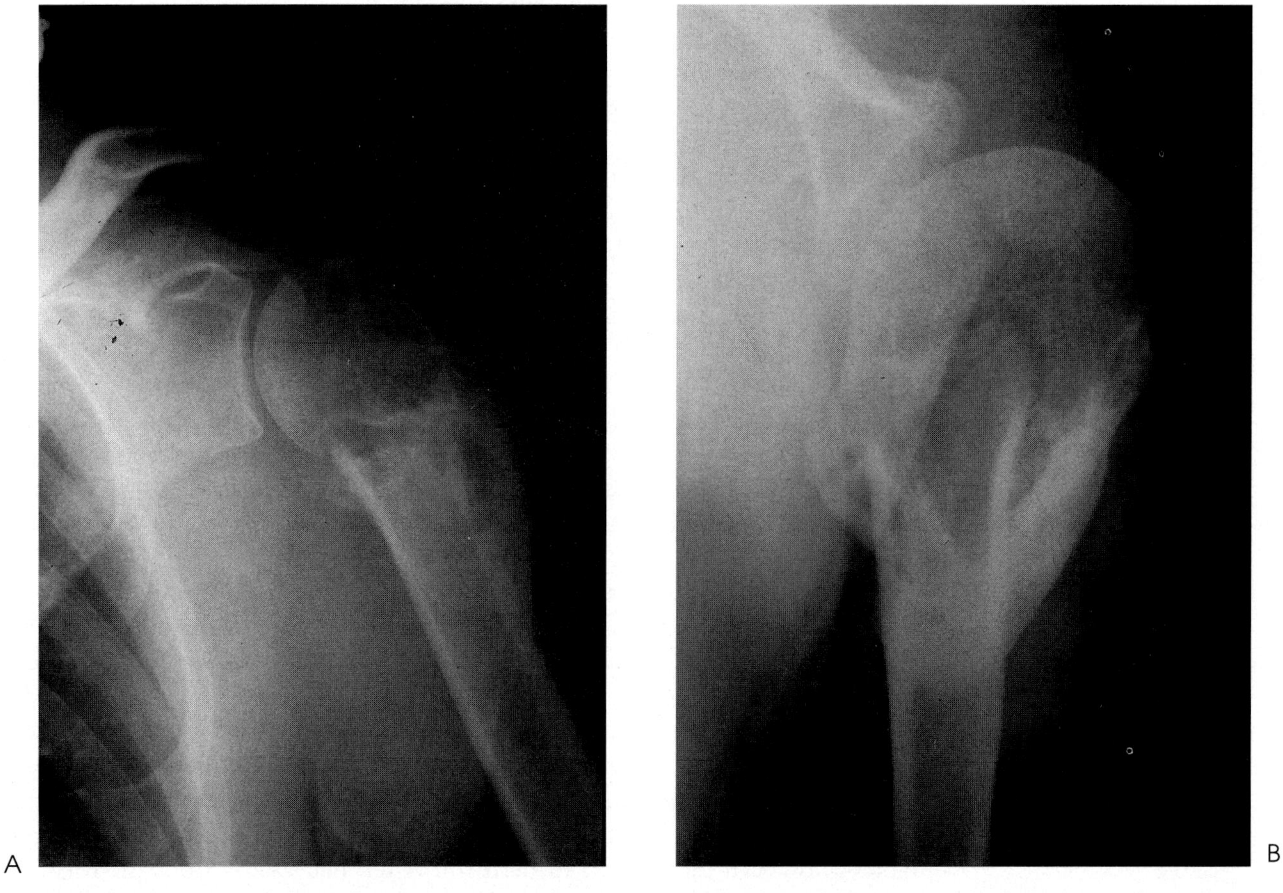

Figure 8–2. Anteroposterior (A) and axilary (B) radiographs at 1 year show good union. The patient had an excellent result.

PEARL

- If this technique is used, the positioning of the patient is important. To visualize the shoulder, the patient may have to be positioned so that the shoulder is over the side of the table. A radiolucent board under the patient's torso will facilitate this.

Discussion

There is considerable confusion in the literature about the treatment of proximal humeral fractures. About 55% of all proximal humeral fractures are minimally displaced according to Neer's criteria and require no operative intervention. At the other end of the spectrum most surgeons would accept that four part fractures, head splitting fractures, and complex fracture dislocations are probably best treated using a hemiarthroplasty prosthesis. It is the intermediate fractures that cause debate about the role of fixation. The most common proximal humeral fractures, after the minimally displaced fractures, are displaced at two part surgical neck fractures that comprise about 27% of all proximal humeral fractures. Many surgeons believe that these fractures should be internally fixed because the degree of displacement mitigates against a successful result if they are treated nonoperatively. When considering this philosophy, it is important to define the patient population with which one is dealing. Proximal humeral fractures are an osteoporotic fracture and are only infrequently encountered in young patients. A recent prospective study of 1000 consecutive proximal humeral fractures in the orthopedic trauma unit in Edinburgh has shown that only 6% of proximal humeral fractures occur in patients aged less than 30 years. The average age of the proximal humeral fracture population is 65 years, with the average age in women being 69 years.

The age of the fracture population is important because the techniques that are employed for fractures in young patients may not be applicable to older patients and the results in the young and the elderly may well be very different. In this case the results at 1 year were excellent, with virtually no residual functional deficit. These results have been good because the patient had a low velocity injury occurring adjacent to a joint with considerable potential for movement. Almost all two part fractures in the elderly will have a good outcome with nonoperative management. In the older patient surgery should be reserved for those patients who present with displacement between the humeral head and the diaphysis such that there is no bony contact whatsoever.

This philosophy does not apply to younger patients. Most proximal humeral fractures in younger patients follow high energy trauma and are associated with more soft tissue damage. In this group of patients displaced two part fractures should be internally fixed to allow early movement. There are a variety of surgical techniques available to the orthopedic surgeon for the treatment of displaced two part fractures in younger patients.

In adolescents Salter-Harris II fractures of the proximal humeral epiphysis are occasionally encountered. These may be treated by closed manipulation and the application of a shoulder spica with the arm placed in abduction. However, it is not possible to adequately reduce the fracture or maintain it in the reduced position with a shoulder spica and fixation is often required. If the surgeon elects to internally fix this fracture, he or she can choose from a number of techniques. One option is to use percutaneous Kirschner wires, introduced under fluoroscopic control (Fig. 8–3). Superficially, this is an attractive operation because open surgery is avoided, but can be difficult to perform. After anaesthesia the patient should be placed in the beach chair position with the C-arm positioned to give an anteroposterior view of the shoulder. A thin Steinmann pin can be placed into the humeral epiphysis that can then be maneuvered into a reduced position. Once the reduction has been achieved, three or four percutaneous Kirschner wires can be inserted

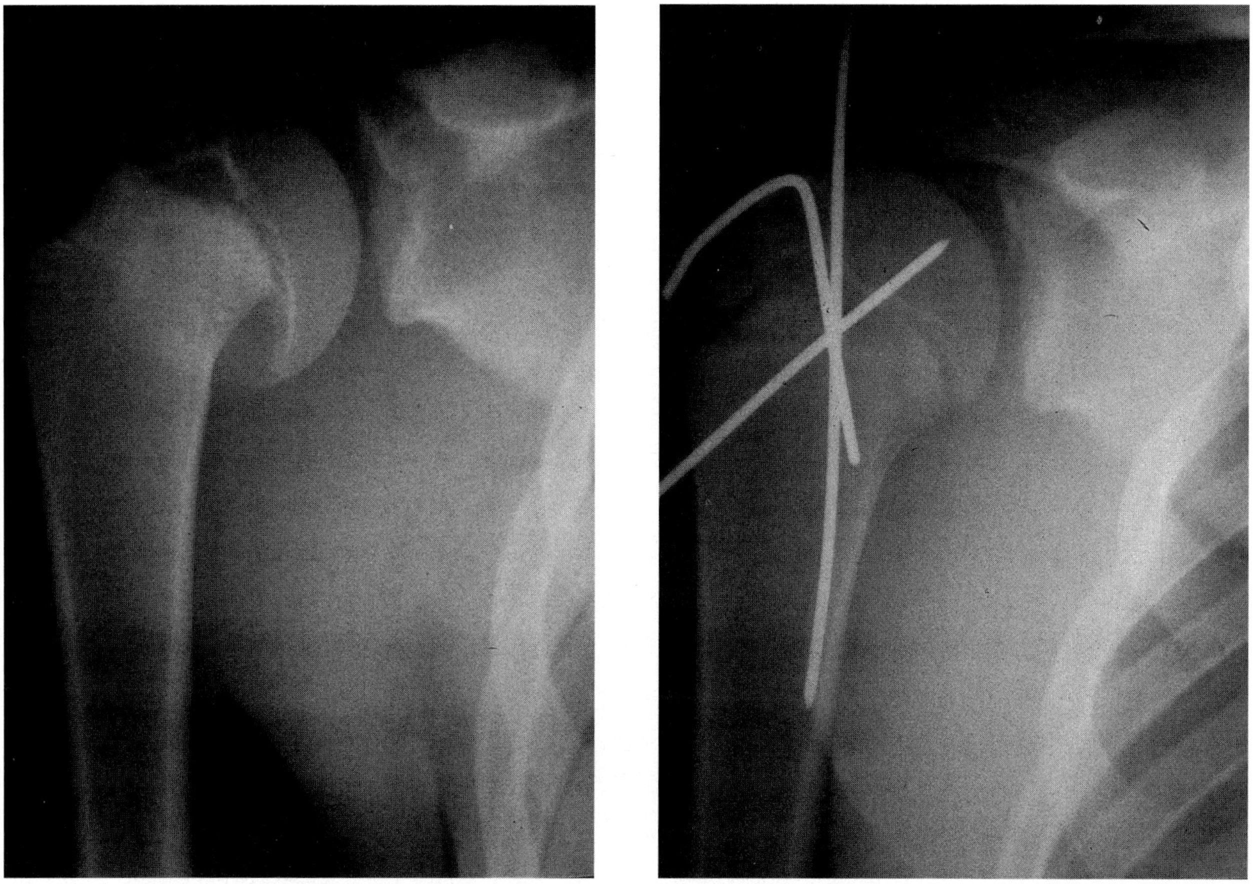

Figure 8–3. A Salter-Harris II physeal fracture (A) fixed with percutaneous Kirschner wires (B).

under fluoroscopic control to maintain the reduction. It is remarkably easy to insert the wires into the soft tissues around the humerus and care must be taken to pass the wires across the fracture site. Care must also be taken that the wires do not migrate because they can be very difficult to locate when they disappear under the skin.

Two other methods used to internally fix two part proximal humeral fractures in young patients are either fixation with a plate, commonly a T-plate (Fig. 8–4), or wiring with a figure of eight wire loop (Fig. 8–5). The T-plate is inserted through a deltopectoral incision. This is a relatively straightforward technique, although the surgeon must be careful not to damage the deltoid by mobilizing it from the clavicle. Care must also be taken to avoid damage to the axillary nerve and the long head of biceps and not place the proximal screws into the glenohumeral joint.

An alternative technique involves the use of an anterolateral figure of eight wire. This technique depends on the presence of an intact soft tissue bridge on the posteromedial aspect of the proximal humerus. This is present in all epiphyseal fractures in adolescents. The surgeon merely exposes the proximal humerus through a deltopectoral incision, reduces the fracture, and places a figure of eight wire loop over the physis. Excellent fixation is obtained and early motion is per-

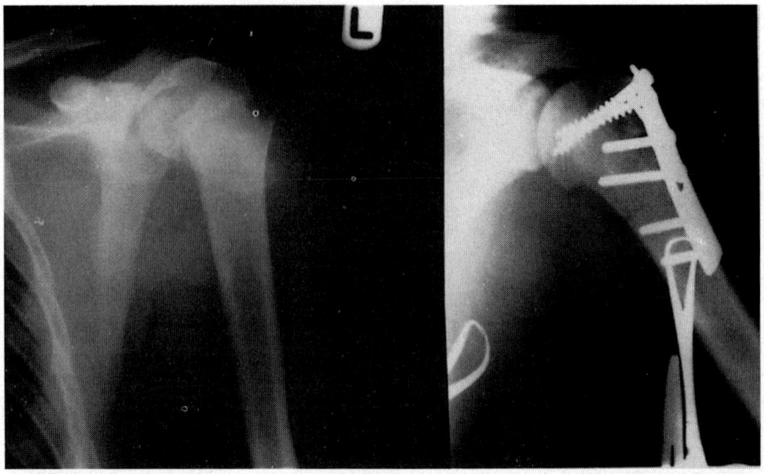

A B

Figure 8–4. A Salter-Harris II physeal fracture (A) in a young patient treated with a T-plate (B).

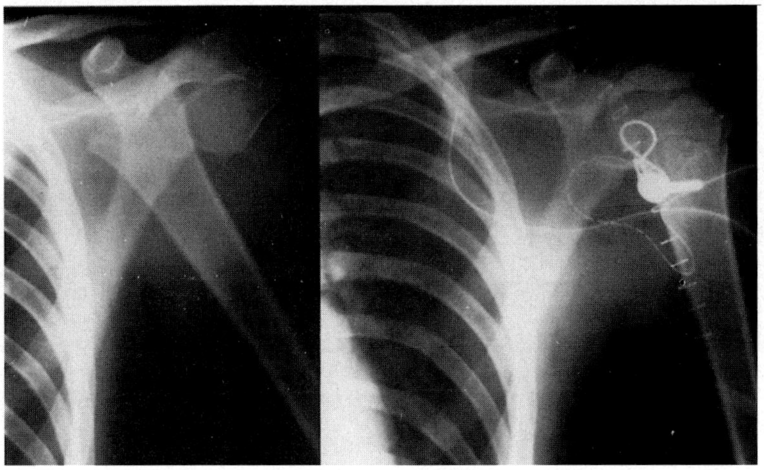

A B

Figure 8–5. A translated two part proximal humeral fracture (A) treated with a wire loop to provide good fixation (B). This technique is only applicable in young patients with an intact posteromedial soft tissue bridge.

mitted. The advantage of this technique is that the wire loop need not be removed whereas the proximal humeral T-plate usually has to be removed at a second operation.

Alternative Methods of Management

If internal fixation of the displaced two part fracture is to be performed in elderly patients, the surgeon will usually need to use different techniques. Bone screws frequently fail to hold in osteoporotic bone and an intramedullary technique is often employed. One technique is to use two Rush pins or modified Enders nails and secure them to the humeral shaft using a figure of eight wire (Fig. 8–6). Alternatively, a humeral nail and a specially designed flexible washer can be used to envelop the humeral head. Both techniques have the same problem—damage to the rotator cuff musculature. These techniques may be the only ones available in osteoporotic bone, but it is suggested that their use be confined to those fractures with wide separation of the head and shaft. Even fractures such as the one illustrated here can be treated nonoperatively with good results.

Type of Management	Advantages	Disadvantages	Comments
Nonoperative management	Easy; good results in elderly patients	Not applicable to displaced fractures following high energy trauma	Should be used for low energy fractures in elderly patients
Rigid fixation	Early motion; good results in young patients	Poor fixation in the elderly; intramedullary techniques better	Useful in young patients but less so in elderly patients. Intramedullary techniques damage the rotator cuff
External fixation	None	Difficult; unnecessary	No advantage over internal fixation or nonoperative techniques
Hemiarthroplasty	None	Unnecessary surgery	Not required in the primary management of two part fracture

Complications

The two complications that surgeons encounter most frequently in the management of displaced two part proximal humeral fractures are failure of the implant to hold an osteoporotic fracture in an elderly patient and nonunion of the surgical neck. If fixation failure is encountered, the surgeon will have to treat each case on its merits, taking into account the age and psychological status of the patient and the degree of bony damage caused by the failure of the implant. Refixation is probably the method of choice, although the surgeon may decide that this is technically impossible. An alternative is to use a hemiarthroplasty prosthesis, but this may prove to be a difficult operation if the surgical neck fracture remains ununited. If a hemiarthroplasty is to be used, care must be taken to osteotomize both tuberosities and rebuild the proximal humerus around the prosthetic head. It is also important to

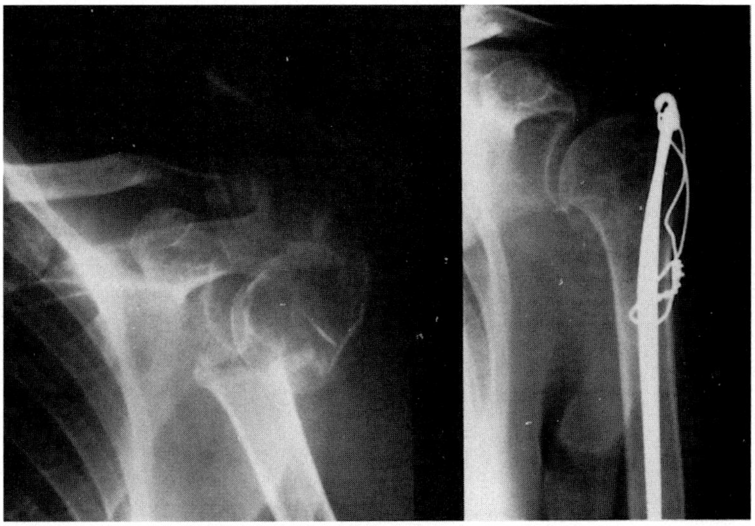

A B

Figure 8–6. A displaced two part fracture in an elderly patient (A) treated with rush pins and wire (B).

seat the prosthetic head correctly because it is likely that the surgeon will be faced with a shortened humerus.

Nonunion of the surgical neck of the proximal humerus is uncommon, but may be difficult to treat. Usually several months have elapsed before the diagnosis of proximal humeral nonunion is confidently made. By this time the soft tissues around the glenohumeral joint have become stiff and the proximal humeral fragment will not move in the glenoid with all of the apparent shoulder movement occurring at the site of the nonunion. Many of these patients will be elderly and several will have significant medical and social problems. Treatment should be aimed at controlling pain because it is highly unlikely that any form of surgery will result in improved glenohumeral movement. Thus many patients do not require treatment at all and it should be explained to them that although surgery might heal the nonunion it might also stiffen their shoulder. If the nonunion is causing pain, either bone grafting and internal fixation or the use of a hemiarthroplasty can be undertaken.

The surgeon may encounter other complications. The use of a T-plate may cause an impingement syndrome and actually obstruct abduction and flexion of the joint. Under these circumstances the implant must be removed. It is also likely that the various forms of intramedullary fixation will need to be removed. Not only will they damage the rotator cuff but they will restrict glenohumeral motion (Fig. 8–6) and removal is usually indicated although it does not always ensure increased shoulder mobility.

Infection can occur after any surgical operation. If it occurs after proximal humeral fracture fixation before the fracture has united, it is important not to remove the implant and thereby destabilize the fracture. Treatment is by high dose antibiotics, joint lavage, and debridement.

Suggested Readings

Court-Brown CM, Copeland SA: Fractures of the shoulder girdle. In: Kelly I (ed): The Practice of Shoulder Surgery, pp 99–138. Butterworth Heinemann, Oxford, 1993.

Flatow EL, Ulrich C (eds): Humerus. Butterworth Heinemann, Oxford, 1996.

Kristiansen B, Christensen SW: Plate fixation of proximal humeral fractures. Acta Orthop Scand 1986; 57:320–323.

Neer CS: Displaced proximal humeral fractures. Parts I and II. J Bone Joint Surg (Am) 1970; 52A:1077–1103.

Norris TR: Fractures of the proximal humerus and dislocations of the shoulder. In: Browner BD, Jupiter JB, Levine AM, Trafton PG (eds): Skeletal Trauma, pp 1201–1290. WB Saunders, Philadelphia, 1992.

Schatzker J, Tile M (eds): Rationale of operative fracture care. Springer Verlag, Berlin, 1988.

Case 9

History and Physical Examination

A 78-year-old woman was admitted to the emergency department following a fall. She had slipped on a wet floor and fallen on her right side. After the fall she complained of severe pain in her right shoulder and could not move the joint. Examination showed no evidence of neurovascular damage in the right arm. No other injury was noted.

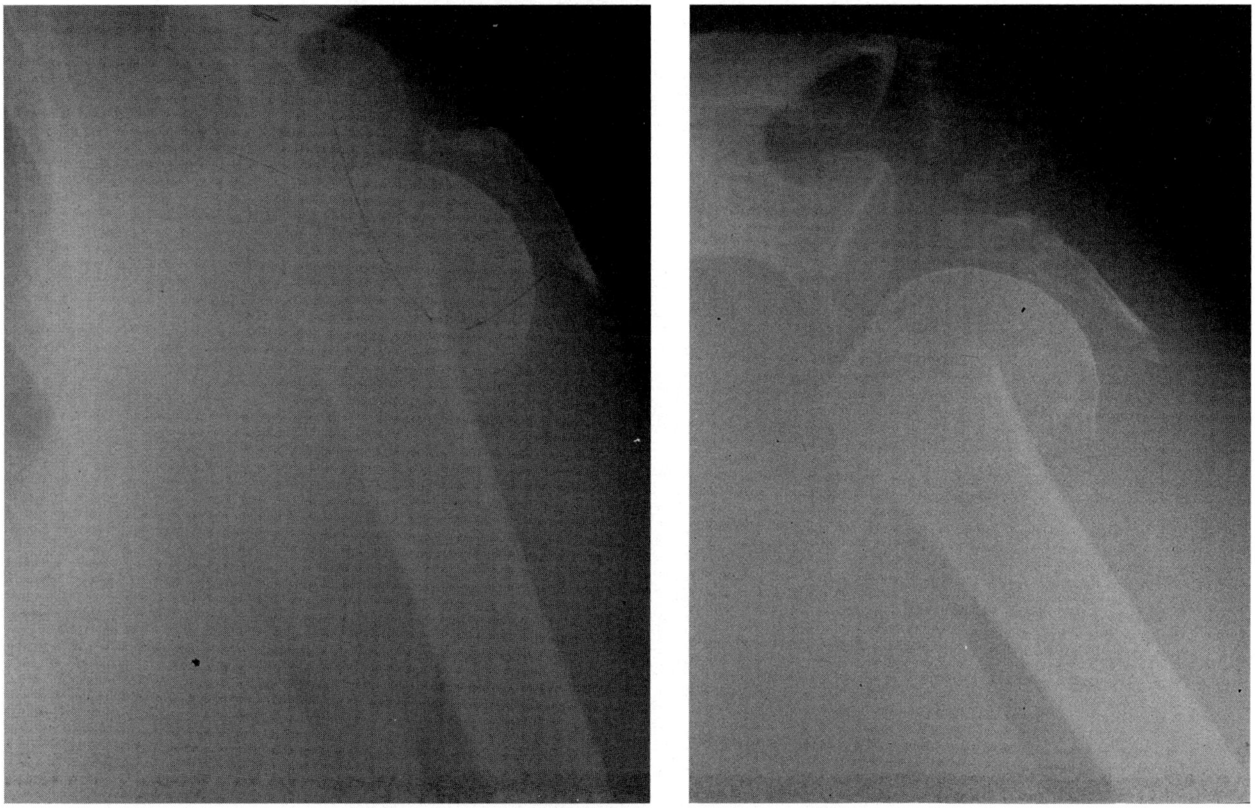

A B

Figure 9–1. Anteroposterior (A) and oblique (B) radiographs showing a four part proximal humeral fracture.

Radiologic Findings

Anteroposterior and oblique radiographs (Fig. 9–1) showed that the patient had a four part proximal humeral fracture. There is obvious rotation of the humeral head and the greater and lesser tuberosities are displaced by more than 1 cm.

Diagnosis

A four part fracture of the proximal humerus. AO classification: 11–C2.1.

Surgical Management

The patient was admitted to the orthopedic unit and prepared for surgery. She was taken to the operating room where she was anesthetized and placed in the beach chair position. Her arm was prepped and draped so that it was freely mobile and the shoulder joint was approached through a deltopectoral incision. A Neer's hemiarthroplasty was inserted and the wound closed (Fig. 9–2). Dressings and an arm immobilizer were applied.

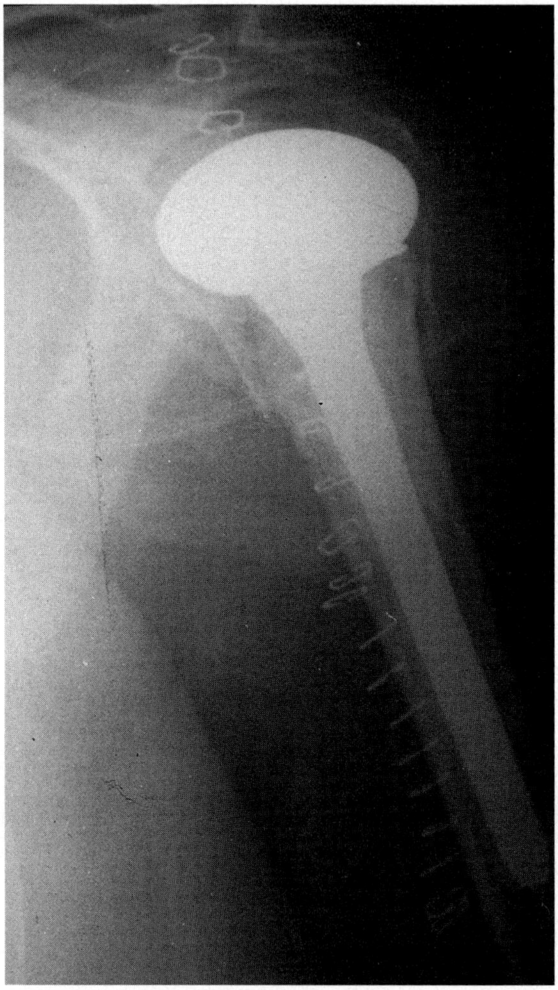

Figure 9–2. A Neer's hemiarthroplasty has been inserted.

Postoperative Management

Postoperatively, a standard mobilization regime was instituted. Initially passive and active assisted exercises were instituted. These were followed by active exercises and the patient slowly regained her shoulder function. Six months after surgery she had 80 degrees of abduction, 90 degrees of flexion, and 30 degrees of extension. She had 20 degrees of external rotation and could internally rotate her right arm such that her hand could get to her fifth lumbar vertebrae. By 1 year her movements had improved somewhat, but she was left with some functional impairment. She tended to

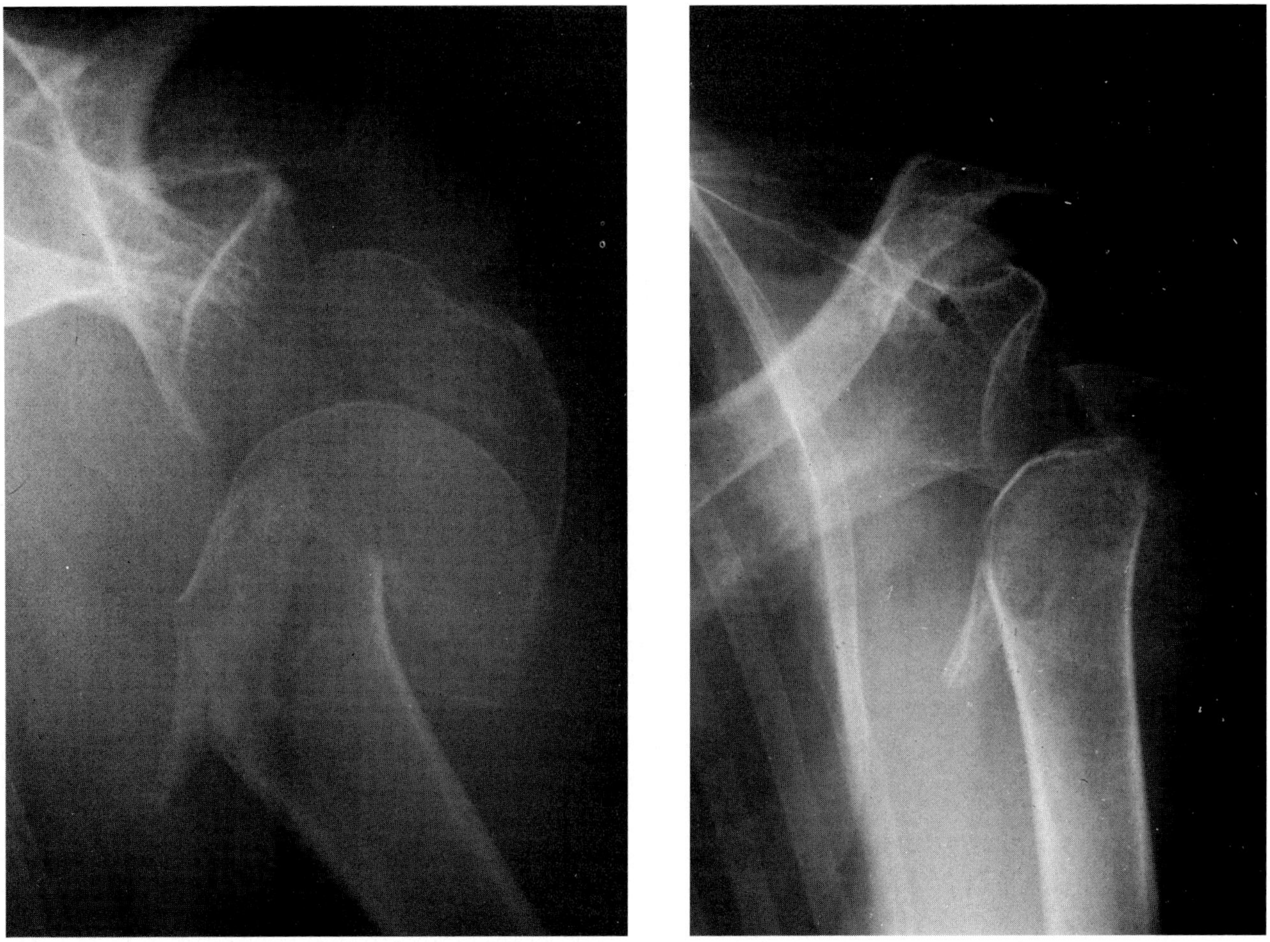

A B

Figure 9–3. Anteroposterior (A) and oblique (B) radiographs showing a fracture similar to that seen in Figure 9–1. However, the greater tuberosity fragment is much larger and this could be defined as a head splitting fracture. Much of the greater tuberosity fragment must be removed before it can be fixed to the prosthesis.

use her left arm for activities that required her to work above her shoulder level and had some problems with dressing and undertaking all her household chores. She did not complain of any pain. The patient's Neer scores were documented throughout her convalescence. At 6 weeks the Neer score was 35, with 49 recorded at 3 months. By 6 months the score had risen to 62 and the final score at 1 year was 74.

Discussion

It is accepted by most surgeons that the insertion of a hemiarthroplasty prosthesis is the best method of managing a four part fracture in the elderly patient. The reason for this relates to the vascularity of the humeral head. The humeral head derives virtually all its blood supply through the two tuberosities and the humeral shaft; when they are separated from the head by more than about 1 cm the blood supply to the head is virtually abolished. Neer (1970) showed in his classic article that the results of internal fixation of four part fractures were poor and strongly advocated the use of a hemiarthroplasty.

PEARL

- Exposure of the proximal humerus is facilitated by a partial release of the deltoid insertion, abduction of the arm, and gentle digital dissection to free the deltoid from the underlying tissues.

PITFALL

- It is important to remember that the humeral head, unlike the femoral head, is in retroversion. If the prosthetic head is inserted in neutral version or anteversion, dislocation is likely.

The operative technique is well documented. It is easiest to insert a hemiarthroplasty prosthesis with the patient semisitting in the beach chair position. A deltopectoral incision is made and the cephalic vein is identified and either retracted medially or ligated and about 3 in of its length removed. The surgeon then opens the space between pectoralis major and deltoid muscles. The two muscles should be separated as far proximally as the clavicle, but under no circumstances should the deltoid be mobilized from the clavicle to facilitate exposure. Instead, the distal insertion of pectoralis major can be mobilized and the arm abducted to allow the surgeon access to the humeral head.

Care must be taken not to damage the rotator cuff. Occasionally the surgeon will encounter a patient who has a chronic rotator cuff tear that greatly facilitates exposure but usually the surgeon will have to gently mobilize the greater and lesser tuberosities with their attached rotator cuff muscles away from the humeral head. The head can then be removed. Sometimes the greater tuberosity has a portion of the articular surface attached to it; this should also be removed to facilitate the later reattachment of the greater tuberosity to the hemiarthroplasty prosthesis (Fig. 9–3). Wire loops are passed through the greater and less tuberosity fragments and the appropriate size of humeral prosthesis selected. This is cemented into position, bearing in mind that the head of the humerus is usually retroverted by about 30 degrees. The tuberosities are then attached to the prosthesis by the previously inserted wires. The surgeon should be careful to try to gauge the correct humeral length when inserting the prosthesis and the tuberosities must be brought round so that the neck of the prosthesis is enclosed within the rebuilt proximal humeral metaphysis.

A number of articles dealing with the results of hemiarthroplasty report a high proportion of good and excellent results. However, surgeons must be careful to examine in which age group the good results are being achieved. Experience suggests that good results can be achieved following hemiarthroplasty, but these tend to be in the younger fitter patients who are able and willing to cooperate with what is an arduous rehabilitation regime. In the elderly population the operation is successful in that a painless stable shoulder is often achieved but usually there is diminished glenohumeral motion. However, in this group of patients the functional goals are less than in younger patients and many elderly patients are satisfied with the results of surgery. A prospective analysis in Edinburgh, Scotland, of 20 elderly patients who had their four part proximal humeral fractures treated by hemiarthroplasty showed that the average Neer score at 6 weeks was 32 and at 3 months was 47. By 6 months the average score had risen to 58, but at one year it was only 65. However, almost all the patients reported that they had only minimal discomfort and most had given up their physiotherapy regimes at a relatively early stage.

The only real option to hemiarthroplasty in the elderly patient with a four part fracture is nonoperative management. Unfortunately this often results in a very stiff painful shoulder with an incongruent glenohumeral joint (Fig. 9–4). The functional disability is often very great. Stableforth (1984) undertook a prospective comparison of nonoperative management with hemiarthroplasty and concluded that the latter technique was much better and resulted in less pain and better function than if nonoperative management was employed. It is suggested that nonoperative management be reserved for the very debilitated elderly patient who has a poor prognosis.

Four part fractures in young patients are extremely rare and few surgeons will have to treat more than one or two during their career. There is little information in

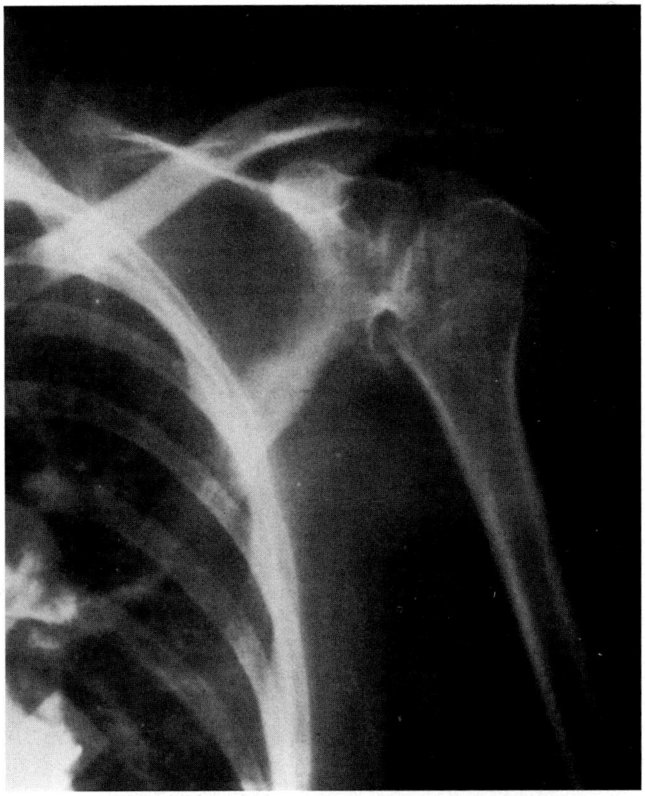

Figure 9–4. A vascular necrosis after nonoperative management of a four part fracture. The patient had a painful stiff shoulder.

the literature about the results of either internal fixation or hemiarthroplasty in the management of four part fractures in young patients and as a result the information that is available tends to be anecdotal and is often based on one or two good results. Some surgeons recommend that four part fractures in the young patient should be internally fixed; this belief is often based on hearsay and there is little theoretical evidence to suggest that it is a correct treatment method. It is unfortunately not uncommon for surgeons to incorrectly apply the Neer classification and inappropriately refer to four part fractures when there is little or no displacement of the fractures. Surgeons should always remember that a genuine four part fracture will almost always result in avascular necrosis and there is no logical reason why internal fixation should be more useful in the young patient than in the elderly patient. If the surgeon chooses to internally fix a four part fracture, he or she will be left having to undertake a secondary hemiarthroplasty in a stiff shoulder and the results are almost certain to be poor.

There is, however, one variant of the four part fracture where internal fixation can be considered. This is the impacted valgus four part fracture originally described by Jakob (1991). An example is shown in Figure 9–5. In this fracture the head fragment is pushed into valgus but does retain some soft tissue connection and therefore theoretically a blood supply. However, it must be emphasized that the vascularity of the head fragment is tenuous at best and if internal fixation is undertaken, it should be done with great care using limited dissection and fixation. A deltopectoral approach is used and the head fragment gently rotated into a normal alignment. Nonabsorbable sutures are placed in the tuberosity fragment and the space under the head and between the tuberosities is filled with cancellous bone graft. Fixation is

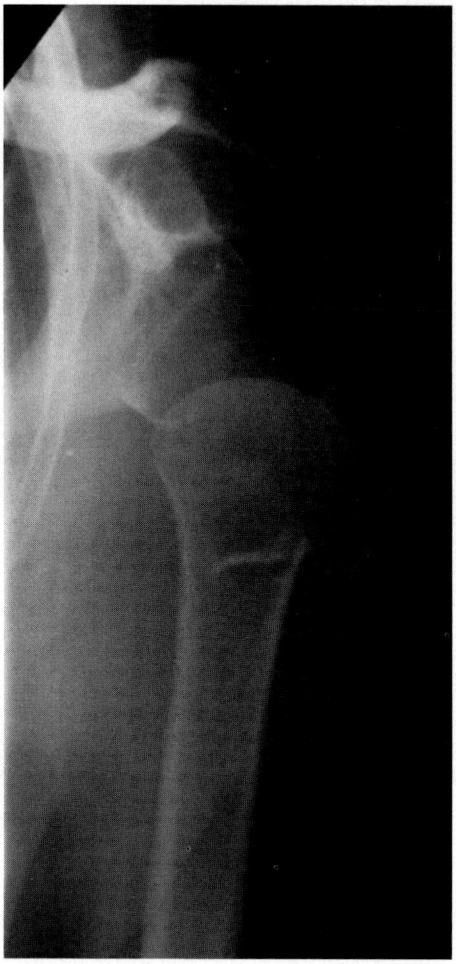

Figure 9–5. An impacted valgus four part fracture. Despite the radiological appearance, it is difficult to believe that the head is viable.

achieved using bone sutures or wires, although screws are occasionally used. The use of plates is not recommended. If there is any doubt as to the vascular supply of the humeral head in this fracture, a hemiarthroplasty should be used.

Alternative Methods of Management

The two principle alternatives in the management of the elderly four part proximal humeral fracture are hemiarthroplasty and nonoperative management. These have already been discussed. There is no place for internal fixation of the classical four part fracture in the elderly patient. The situation in younger patients has also been described. Classical four part fractures are extremely rare and it is unlikely that internal fixation is going to provide a good alternative to hemiarthroplasty.

Complications

The usual complications that follow hemiarthroplasty of the humeral head are joint stiffness and mild discomfort. Stiffness is best avoided by adhering to an active physiotherapy regime. However, in the elderly patient shoulder stiffness is common and essentially untreatable. Mild discomfort is usually tolerated by the patient, but

Type of Management	Advantages	Disadvantages	Comments
Nonoperative management	None	Poor results; avascular necrosis; pain	Only useful in the very elderly debilitated patient with a poor prognosis
Internal fixation	Proximal humerus reconstruction	Difficult surgery; uncommon fractures	Applicable only in the four part impacted valgus fracture in the young patient
Hemiarthroplasty	Straightforward technique; good pain relief; reasonable results	Poor shoulder mobility in elderly patients	Method of choice for most patients with four part fractures

if it becomes intolerable it can be treated by analgesics and nonsteroidal antiinflammatory drugs. Infection and dislocation are unusual, and fractures below the prosthesis can usually be treated by a Sarmiento brace.

The principle complication of attempting to internally fix the humeral head in a four part fracture is avascular necrosis. This should be treated by hemiarthroplasty as soon as the condition becomes clear. If the surgeon waits until the shoulder is stiff, the results of hemiarthroplasty will be poor.

Suggested Readings

Bengnér U, Johnell O, Redlund-Johnell I: Changes in the incidence of fracture in the upper end of the humerus during a 30 year period: study of 2125 fractures. Clin Orthop 1988; 231:179–182.

Flatow EL, Ulrich C: Humerus. Butterworth Heinemann, Oxford, 1996.

Gerber C, Schmeeberger A, Uinh T-S: The arterial vascularisation of the humeral head. An anatomical study. J Bone Joint Surg (Am) 1991; 72A:1486–1494.

Jakob RP, Miniaci A, Anson PS, Jarberg H, Osterwalder A, Ganz R: Four-part valgus impacted fractures of the proximal humerus. J Bone Joint Surg (Br) 1991; 73B:295–298.

Kelly IG: The Practice of Shoulder Surgery. Butterworth Heinemann, Oxford, 1993.

Neer CS: Displaced proximal humeral fractures. Parts I and II. J Bone Joint Surg (Am) 1970; 52A:1077–1103.

Stableforth PG: Four part fractures of the neck of the humerus. J Bone Joint Surg (Br) 1984; 66B:104–108.

Case 10

History and Physical Examination

An 18-year-old woman sustained multiple injuries as an unrestrained passenger in an automobile accident. She was extracted from the automobile, transported to the emergency department, and arrived 45 minutes after the accident. She was conscious and alert. Physical examination revealed that she had sustained a laceration that communicated with her right knee, a closed right femoral shaft fracture, and a closed fracture of the left humerus. Neurovascular examination of the leg distal to the open knee and fractured femur was within the limits of normal. Examination of the left upper extremity indicated that the peripheral pulses were intact, but the patient was unable to actively extend her left wrist and left metacarpal phalangeal joints. Sensation to pin prick was decreased over her entire hand and forearm and was absent in the distribution of the radial nerve over the dorsum of her first and second metacarpals. No other injuries were identified.

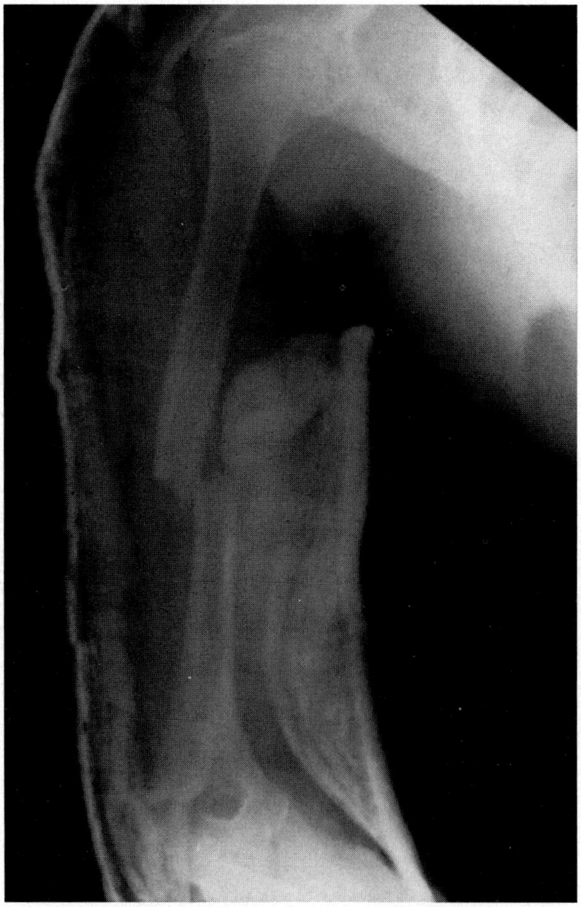

Figure 10–1. An anteroposterior radiograph of the arm indicating a middiaphyseal fracture of the humerus in acceptable alignment.

Radiologic Findings

Radiographs of the right knee, right femur, hip, pelvis, left humerus, shoulder, and elbow indicated an open knee joint with no fracture, a transverse midshaft femur fracture, and a transverse midiaphyseal humerus fracture (Fig. 10–1).

PEARL

- One of the few indications for fixation of a diaphyseal fracture of the humerus is multiple trauma. Fixation of the humerus allows greater use of the extremity than external immobilization; however, fixation is not strong enough to withstand the stresses of weight bearing.

Diagnosis

Open right knee, closed midshaft femur, and closed fracture of the humeral diaphysis with a radial nerve palsy. AO classification of the humerus fracture: 12–A3.2, or a simple transverse fracture of the diaphysis.

Surgical Management

The night of injury, the knee was debrided and irrigated, and the femur stabilized with a retrograde femoral nail. All wounds were closed over drains. The humerus was immobilized in a coaptation splint and sling (Fig. 10–1). The radial nerve palsy remained complete over the next 3 days. It became increasingly clear that the patient was having difficulty with self-care and transfers due to the external immobilization of the humerus. Because of these difficulties, it was decided to stabilize the humerus internally.

The patient was taken to the operating room where a general anesthetic was administered. She was turned to the prone position with the arm over an arm board. The arm was prepped and draped free. A straight posterior incision was made parallel with the long axis of the humerus. The triceps muscle was split, taking care to protect the radial nerve. The radial nerve was found interposed between the fracture fragments. The fracture was distracted, and the nerve, which was in continuity, was retracted from between the bone ends. The fracture was reduced anatomically, and stabilized with a broad dynamic compression plate (Fig. 10–2).

Postoperative Management

Postoperatively, passive range of motion exercises of the wrist and metacarpal phalangeal joints were initiated to prevent contracture secondary to the radial nerve palsy. At 7 days when incisional pain permitted, active range of motion exercises of the elbow and shoulder were initiated. Weight bearing on the extremity was not permitted, but the patient was allowed to use the extremity for personal care and transfers. Radial nerve function returned completely by 6 months following injury. Healing proceeded uneventfully, and at 6 months the fracture was clearly healed with cortical bridging of the fracture (Fig. 10–3).

Discussion

The two parameters that dictated management of the humeral fracture were the multiple trauma and the radial nerve palsy. In general, operative stabilization increases the incidence of complications of humeral shaft fractures. Therefore, the majority of humeral fractures are managed with closed methods (i.e., a coaptation splint followed at 1 to 2 weeks with a removable plastic cuff that allows elbow and shoulder motion). *Multiple trauma* is one of the relative indications for operative stabilization of humeral diaphyseal fractures. Operative stabilization with an intramedullary nail or plate and screws allows earlier motion of the elbow and shoulder without the encumbrance of an external splint. In patients with multiple long bone fractures, the additional freedom of motion often accelerates rehabilitation.

Radial nerve palsy is a common occurrence following fracture of the humeral diaphysis and usually resolves spontaneously. Relative indications for exploration of the radial nerve acutely are an open fracture, when the palsy follows a closed reduc-

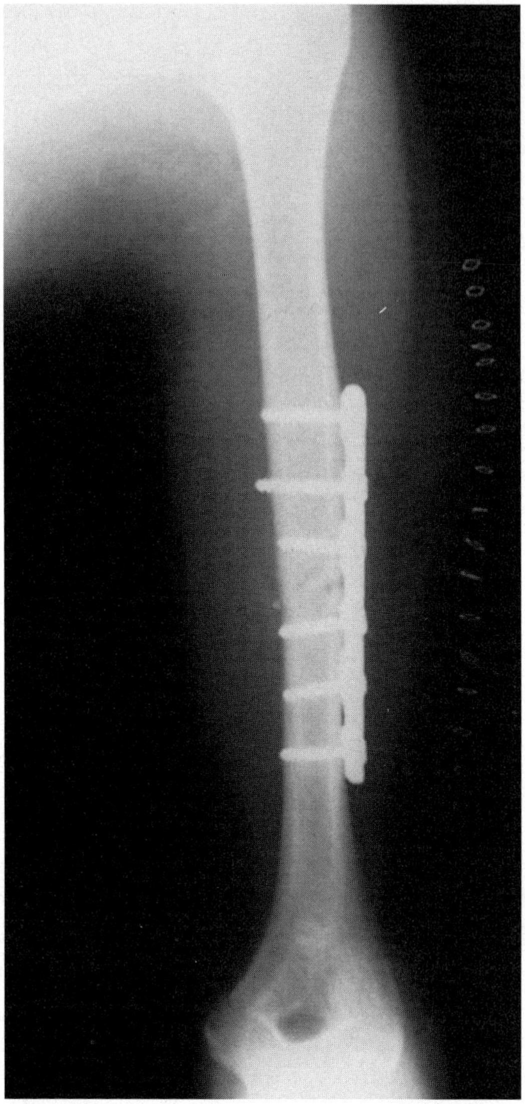

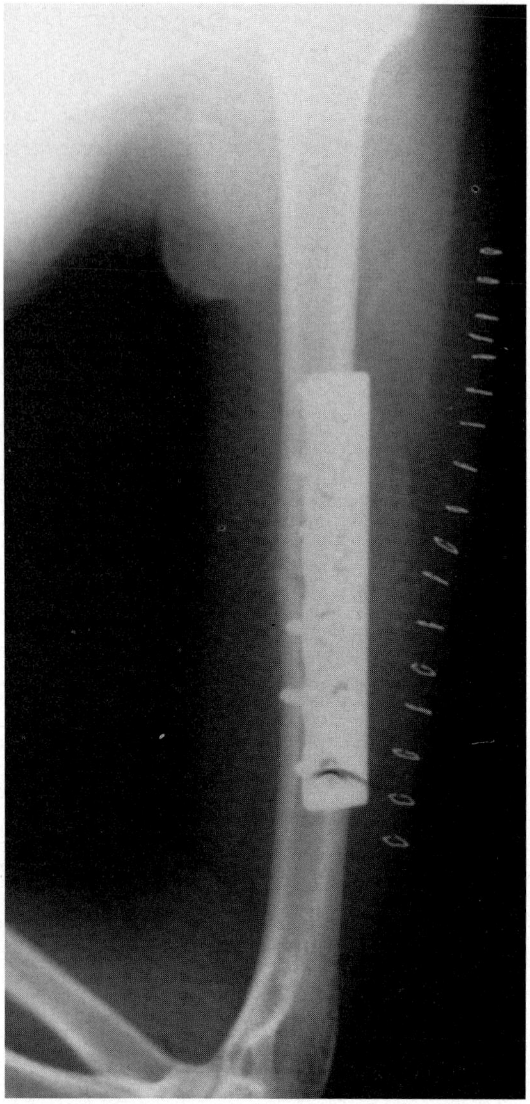

Figure 10–2. Anteroposterior (A) and lateral (B) radiographs of the humerus following reduction and fixation.

PEARL

- Following stable fixation, pain rapidly decreases and disappears. An overly aggressive regimen of physical therapy or overuse of the extremity prior to healing of the fracture will result in failure of fixation. The radiologic signs of healing are cortical and trabecular bridging of the fracture.

tion, and when the fracture is located in the distal third of the humerus and has a spiral pattern (i.e., a Holstein Lewis fracture).

Alternate Methods of Management

The alternative methods of management of this humeral fracture were closed with a splint, closed intramedullary nailing, and open with a plate and screws. The advantages of closed management are a high incidence of consolidation with a low incidence of complications. In this case, the disadvantage of closed management is the difficulty with rehabilitation. The advantages of closed intramedullary nailing are that rehabilitation can proceed more quickly and operative trauma is minimized, and therefore the risk of infection is low. The disadvantages of closed intramedullary nailing are that the radial nerve is not explored; the radial nerve may be trapped in the fracture site and injured during the procedure; and that compared to closed

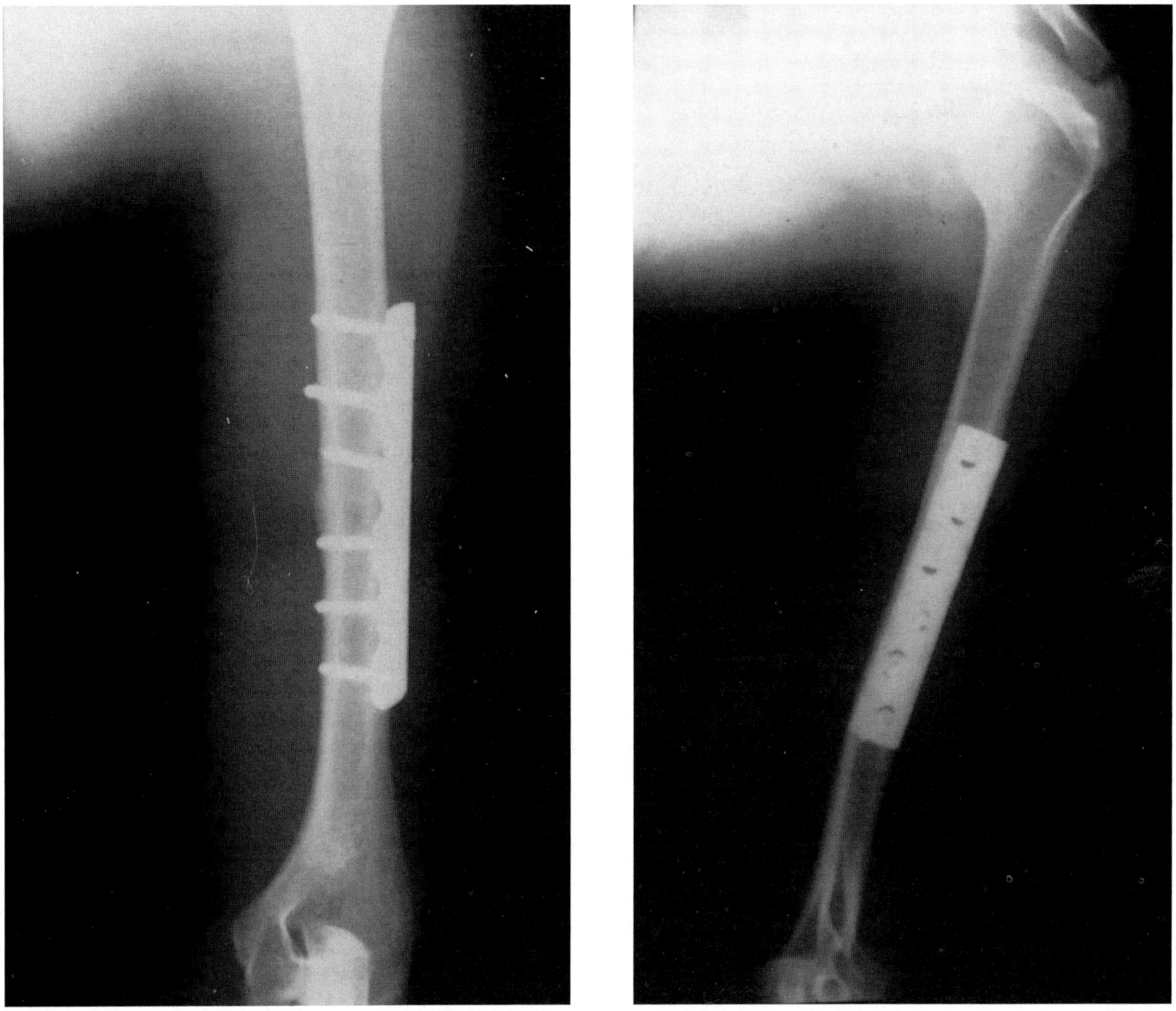

A B

Figure 10–3. Anteroposterior (A) and lateral (B) radiographs of the humerus 1 year after injury demonstrating healing of the fracture.

PEARL

- In most cases we will observe a radial nerve palsy associated with a humeral shaft fracture for 3 months. Clinically, if there is no return of function at 3 months, an EMG is obtained. If there is no EMG evidence of reinervation, the nerve is explored. If the EMG indicates that reinervation is occurring, conservative management is continued.

management there is an increased incidence of complications (i.e., nonunion and infection). The advantages of open stabilization with a plate and screws, in this case, are that the radial can be explored and repaired if it is not in continuity or it can be protected from further injury if it is in continuity. The disadvantage is that the extensive exposure increases the risk of infection and nonunion in comparison to closed management with an intramedullary nail or external splint.

Complications

The complications of open reduction and fixation of humeral shaft fractures are nonunion, malunion, and infection. Clinical signs of nonunion are pain at the fracture site, exacerbated by activity and motion. Radiologic signs of nonunion include failed fixation and a persistent radiolucent defect at the fracture site. Failure of fixation may be due to fracture or loosening of the implants. Management of humeral nonunions has a greater chance of success when shoulder and elbow motion has

Type of Management	Advantages	Disadvantages	Comments
Closed with external splint	No risk of infection, minimal risk of nonunion	Difficult rehabilitation	The most frequently used method of management of closed humeral
Closed with intramedullary nail	Minimal operative trauma, ease of postoperative rehabilitation	Potential for further injury to radial nerve	The potential for injury of the radial nerve is a relative contraindication
Open with plates and screws	Radial nerve is explored and protected or repaired; ease of postoperative rehabilitation	Extensive exposure increases the incidence of postoperative complications	The advantages of radial nerve exploration, and ease of postoperative rehabilitation outweigh the disadvantages

been preserved. Management consists of removal of the failed implants and stable fixation. Atrophic nonunions are decorticated with an osteotome and grafted with autogenous cancellous bone. It is not necessary to graft hypertrophic nonunions.

The amount of rotational and angular malalignment that is acceptable is debatable, because what is acceptable functionally may not be acceptable cosmetically. More angulation can be accepted in midshaft and proximal fractures than in fractures of the distal third. Up to 20 degrees of rotational malalignment is well tolerated if shoulder motion has been preserved. Up to 30 degrees of varus or valgus malalignment of middiaphyseal fractures is tolerated without los of function if full range of motion of the shoulder and elbow are present. However, this amount of angular malalignment causes a significant cosmetic deformity. Management of malunions consists of removal of implants, osteotomy, and revision fixation.

The clinical signs of infection following open reduction and internal fixation of a humeral fracture are redness, swelling, and culture positive drainage. Management consists of control of infection with decompression of abscesses and dressing changes. Systemic antibiotics are administered intravenously in the acute phase of infection and orally after the infection has been controlled. When the fracture has consolidated, all implants are removed and necrotic tissue is debrided. Systemic antibiotics based on sensitivities of the pathogenic organisms are administered for 4 to 6 weeks following debridement. Dead space is managed with antibiotic beads. The beads are explanted 3 weeks after implantation and the dead space filled with autogenous cancellous bone mixed with Tobramycin. When the infection cannot be controlled acutely, the fracture is aggressively debrided. Implants and necrotic bone are excised. Dead space is managed with beads and the fracture is stabilized with an external fixator.

Suggested Readings

Bostman O, Bakalim G, Vainionpaa S, Wilppula E, Patiala H, Rokkanen P: Radial palsy in shaft fracture of the humerus. Acta Orthop Scand 1986; 57(4):316–319.

Pollock FH, Drake D, Bovill EG, Day L, Trafton PG: Treatment of radial neuropathy associated with fractures of the humerus. J Bone Joint Surg 1981; 63A:239–243.

Rodriguez-Merchan EC: Compression plating versus Hackethal nailing in closed humeral shaft fractures failing nonoperative reduction. J Orthop Trauma 1995; 9(3):194–197.

Case 11

History and Physical Examination

A 22-year-old male sustained a gunshot wound to the left upper extremity 20 minutes prior to admission to the emergency department. On admission his pulse rate was 120 per minute and his blood pressures was 90/40 mm Hg. There was an open wound approximately 4 cm in diameter on the posterior lateral aspect of the middle third of the arm. Devitalized fragments of bone and soft tissue were present in the wound. Deformity and gross instability of the arm were obvious. A radial pulse was palpable at the wrist and the patient was able to extend the wrist, abduct the thumb from the palm, and abduct the fingers. Although the patient stated that his arm felt numb, he was able to distinguish sharp from dull in the ulnar, median and radial nerve distributions. There were no other injuries evident.

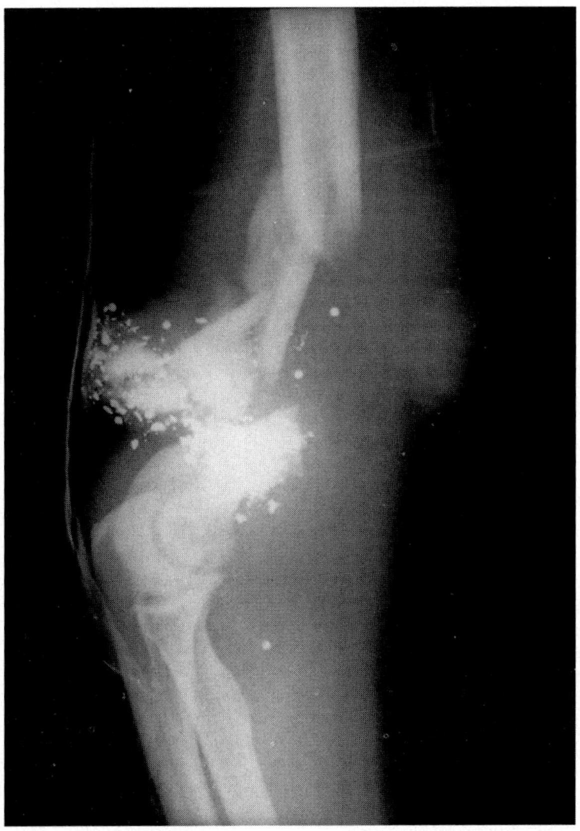

Figure 11–1. Radiograph obtained shortly after injury indicating a severely comminuted fracture of the distal metaphysis and diaphysis of the humerus.

Radiologic Findings

Radiographs of the arm indicated a comminuted fracture of the distal third of the humerus. The fracture extended into the joint, but the articular surface was minimally displaced. Retained metallic fragments were in the soft tissue and there appeared to be loss of metaphyseal and diaphyseal bone (Fig. 11–1).

Diagnosis

Grade III B fracture secondary to a high energy gunshot of the distal humerus. The fracture was grade III because of severe comminution. It was further classified as IIIB because of the bone loss and soft tissue defect. It was not IIIC because the neurovascular structures were intact as determined by physical examination. In addition to the open fracture, the patient was hypotensive and tachycardic, due to hypovolemia. The fracture was classified as an AO 13–C2.3 fracture.

Surgical Management

The wound was cultured and covered. Direct pressure was applied manually to the open wound to control bleeding. While the arm was being splinted, venous access was secured with a large bore needle, a specimen of blood was obtained for type and cross match, and a second generation cephalosporin was administered. Fluid management was initiated with rapid infusion of 2 liters of Ringer's lactate solution.

The patient was taken to the operating room where he was anesthetized. The arm was removed from the splint and carefully scrubbed and draped free. The arm was placed over the chest and the posterior lateral wound was extended proximally and

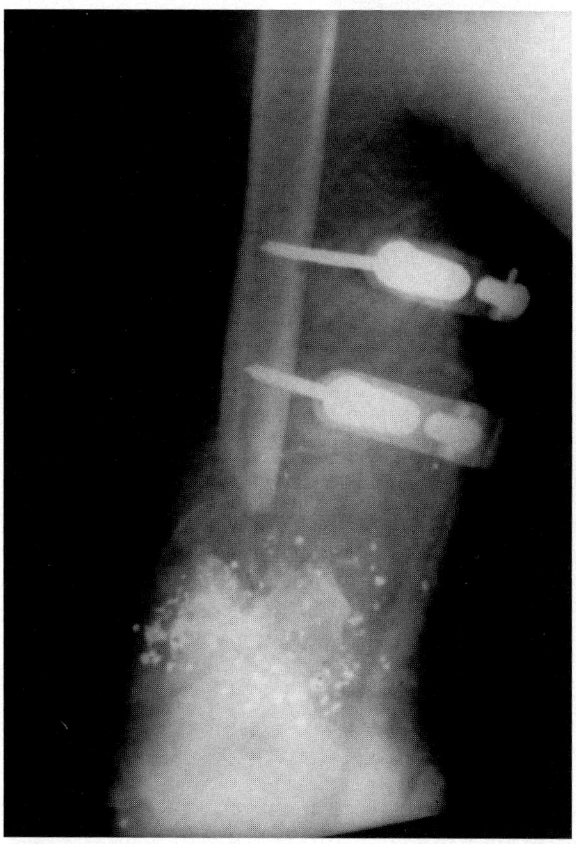

Figure 11–2. Intraoperative radiograph obtained the night of injury following external fixator application.

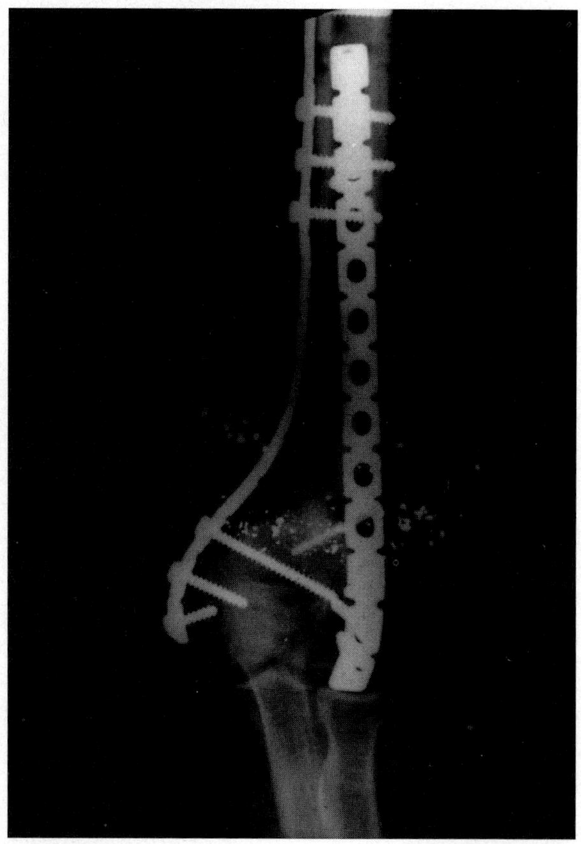

Figure 11–3. Intraoperative radiograph following removal of fixator and internal fixation with plates and screws. The olecranon has not been repaired and the defect not yet packed with antibiotic PMMA beads.

PEARLS

- The first step in the management of an open fracture is removal of devitalized tissue. Surgical exposure (i.e., extending the wound) aids in the identification of devitalized tissue.
- Injury of the radial nerve frequently complicates external fixator application to the humerus. To avoid radial nerve injury it is important to actually dissect through the muscle so that if the radial nerve is encountered, it is easily identified and can be protected.

distally 4 cm. Devitalized soft tissue and fragments of bone were removed, deep tissue was obtained for culture, and the wound was irrigated with 3 liters of normal saline.

The fracture was stabilized with an external fixator that bridged the elbow. Two pins were inserted in the humerus and two in the ulna. The humeral pins were inserted through one incision located on the lateral aspect of the arm. Instead of cutting down directly to the bone, the overlying muscle was carefully dissected to avoid inadvertent injury of the radial nerve. The ulnar pins were inserted percutaneously (Fig. 11–2). The incisions by which the wound had been extended were closed in a single layer, the wound was packed with antibiotic PMMA beads, and covered with an adhesive plastic drape.

Two days later, the wound was examined in the operating room, it was clean and no necrotic tissue was identified, and the decision was made to reduce and stabilize the fracture. The patient was positioned prone with the arm draped free. The skin was incised posteriorly from the olecranon proximally. Exposure of the fracture was facilitated with an osteotomy of the olecranon. The ulnar nerve was identified and protected, the olecranon was predrilled with a 3 mm drill bit, and then osteotomized with an oscillating saw. The osteotomy was V-shaped with the apex distal. The triceps tendon and muscle were retracted proximally and the radial nerve was identified and protected as it crossed the posterior aspect of the humerus. The ulnar nerve was protected and a plate was placed medially. A second plate was placed laterally (Fig. 11–3). The olecranon was repaired with a large fragment cancellous screw, washer, and tension band wire. The ulnar nerve was transposed anteriorly and held in place with a fascial sling. The wound was packed with antibiotic

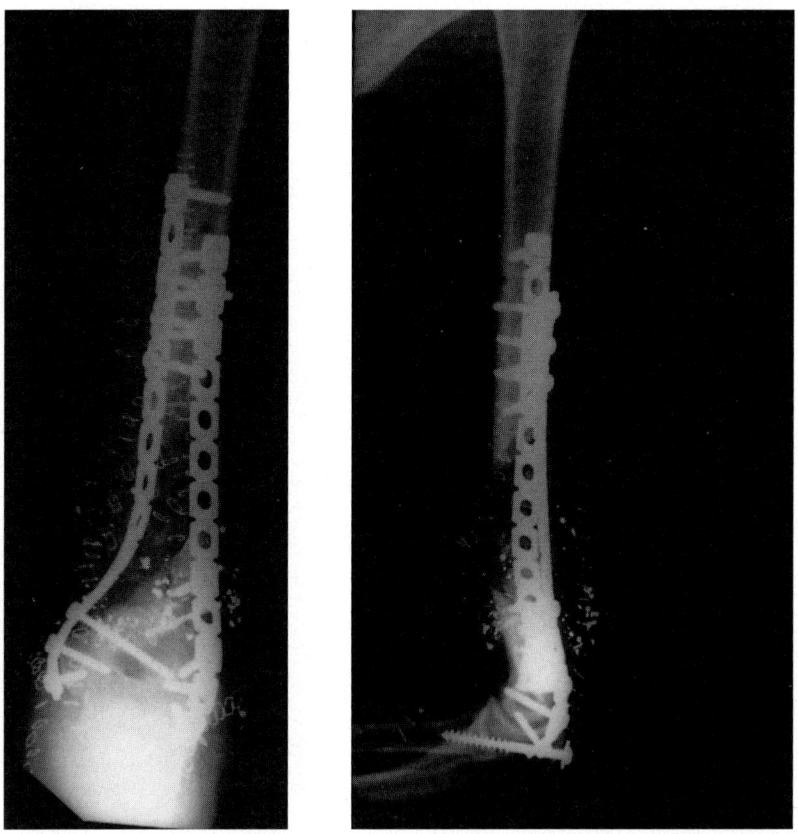
A B

Figure 11–4. Anteroposterior (A) and lateral (B) radiographs following bead removal, autogenous bone grafting, closure, and skin grafting.

PITFALL

- In most cases it is a mistake to immobilize the upper extremity in an attempt to protect tenuous fixation. Immobilization results in stiffness of the elbow and is not rigid enough to insure that the fixation will not fail. If the fixation fails and the elbow is stiff, bony healing of the nonunion is very difficult to achieve. On the other hand, if the fixation fails and the elbow is not stiff, the nonunion can be managed with revision fixation and bone grafting with a good chance of success. We have found that an acceptable compromise is to fabricate a removable splint that is worn by the patient except when performing range of motion exercises. The splint protects the fixation and reminds the patient to protect the arm. The therapy restores elbow motion.

PMMA beads. Because of swelling only part of the wound could be closed; the rest was covered with an impermeable plastic drape.

At 3 days after the open reduction and fixation, the patient was taken back to the operating room and the antibiotic PMMA beads were removed. Autogenous cancellous iliac crest graft mixed with 1.2 g of Tobramycin was used to fill the space that had been occupied by the beads. The graft was covered with soft tissue. Split thickness skin was used to cover the portion of the wound that could not be closed primarily because of skin loss (Fig. 11–4).

Postoperative Management

The elbow was splinted postoperatively and intravenous antibiotics were continued for 3 days. On the third day after the bone grafting, the patient was fit with a plastic splint with the elbow at 90 degrees. The splint was removed 3 times a day for gentle active range of motion.

The wound healed uneventfully. Sutures were removed at 2 weeks. Systemic antibiotics were continued an additional 3 weeks. Unresisted range of motion exercises were continued until 4 months post grafting when radiographs indicated incorporation of the bone graft (Fig. 11–5). At 4 months strengthening exercises were initiated. The final range of motion achieved was 10 to 135 degrees. The medial plate was removed 1 year postinjury because of irritation of the overlying soft tissue.

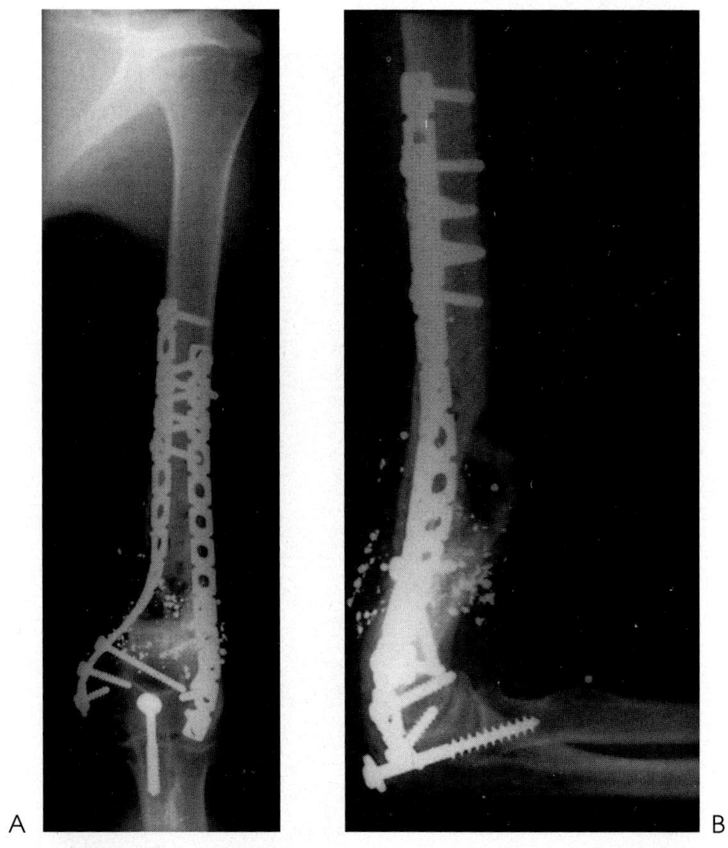

Figure 11–5. Anteroposterior (A) and lateral (B) radiographs 1 year after injury. The defect has healed.

Discussion

The primary objectives in the acute management were correction of hypovolemia due to blood loss, debridement of the wound, and stabilization of the fracture. It was recognized immediately that the patient was *hypovolemic.* The steps taken to correct the hypovolemia included obtaining venous access, administering a bolus of physiologic saline, preventing further blood loss by applying pressure to the wound, and typing and crossmatching the patient for eight units of blood for transfusion.

Debridement of the wound minimizes the chance of infection. The goal of debridement is removal of all devitalized bone and soft tissue. Fragments of bone without soft tissue attachments, skin edges that do not bleed, and muscle that does not contract when stimulated with electrocautery are removed. To identify devascularized tissue it is necessary to extend the wound, as opposed to simply working through it. When debridement of all questionably viable tissue will result in significant functional loss, as in this case, marginally viable tissue is left in situ, and the wound is reexamined in the operating room 24 to 48 hours after injury. By the time this "second look procedure" is performed, tissue that was initially marginally viable has declared itself (i.e., it is obviously viable or necrotic). Two other steps taken to minimize the chance of infection are obtaining material from the wound for culture and the "bead pouch technique." The wound is initially cultured in the emergency room and broad spectrum antibiotics are administered. The antibiotics are administered not to treat an infection, but to retard the conversion of a contaminated wound to an infected wound. In the operating room, devitalized tissue from the depths of the wound is obtained for culture. The results of these cultures are monitored and antibiotic therapy is adjusted accordingly.

Following debridement of the wound a significant dead space was present. This dead space was packed with PMMA-Tobramycin beads. The beads deliver antibiotics locally to the wound and fill the dead space, thus decreasing the amount of hematoma present. When the beads are removed, a space is left for autogenous bone grafting.

Stabilization of the fracture was achieved with an external fixator. The advantages of an external fixator are that it can be applied quickly and it stabilizes the fracture without leaving a foreign body in the wound.

The objectives of the subacute management were maintenance of motion, suppression of infection, and reconstruction of the humerus. *Motion was maintained* with physical therapy. Once motion is lost following a fracture of this severity it cannot be regained. Simple, nonresistive, range of motion exercises are continued until there is radiographic evidence of bone graft incorporation.

Infection is suppressed with local and systemic antibiotics. Initially, following fixation, the dead space is again packed with PMMA-Tobramycin beads. Three days following fixation the beads are removed and the defect grafted with autogenous cancellous bone. Grafting is not performed immediately because the autogenous cancellous bone (which is necrotic) may protect bacteria in the wound from host defense mechanisms and serve as medium for the bacteria. Grafting is done as atraumatically as possible through an incision adequate to remove the beads and insert the graft. Tobramycin is mixed with the bone graft because it is a broad spectrum antibiotic that does not decrease the healing potential of autogenous cancellous bone. In this case systemic antibiotics were continued for 3 weeks following reconstruction to further protect the bone graft. The rationale for 3 weeks of systemic antibiotics is that we assume that by this time the graft has vascularized and is therefore not as susceptible to infection.

Reconstruction of the humerus was achieved with plating and bone grafting. Autograft and plating were the methods selected to reconstruct the humerus because it is a simple procedure with little risk to the patient and postoperative management is simple.

Alternative Methods of Management

Alternatives to plating and bone grafting as a method of reconstruction of the humerus are free tissue transfer, distraction osteogenesis, and allograft. The best free tissue transfer is the fibula or iliac crest. Both can be transferred with overlying skin. As viable tissue is being transferred into the wound, this decreases the chance of flareup of infection. Consolidation of the ends of the transferred bone segment to the humerus can be prolonged. To decrease the incidence of nonunion at these sites, fixation must be stable (e.g., a plate) and the site grafted with autogenous cancellous bone.

Distraction osteogenesis can be accomplished with a small wire circular fixator or a large pin cantilever frame. Both fixators have the advantage of de novo bone formation. Both methods have the disadvantages of limited patient acceptance, loss of motion at the elbow and shoulder because of pain, and failures to obtain union at the docking site.

An intercalary allograft would be an ideal temporary method of management if the risk of infection were not so great following a severely contaminated open fracture. A segmental allograft of cortical bone will never fully incorporate and will eventually fail structurally.

Type of Management	Advantages	Disadvantages	Comments
Plating and autogenous bone grafting	Simple procedure with minimal risk	Prolonged postoperative course until graft incorporates; risk of infection until graft incorporates	Simplicity outweighs the disadvantages; probably most frequently used method
Free tissue transfer	Viable tissue in wound decreases chance of infection	Donor site morbidity; extensive procedure; prolonged consolidation of graft to humerus	Excellent alternative method of management
Distraction osteogenesis	No donor site morbidity	Complex postoperative management; difficult to maintain motion at elbow; limited patient tolerance; risk to neurovascular structures; failure of consolidation at docking site	Seldom performed on the upper extremity because of loss of motion and risk to neurovascular structures
Plating and allograft	No donor site morbidity; rapid recovery	Risk of infection; prolonged consolidation; eventual allograft failure	The risk of infection makes this a poor alternative method

Complications

Complications of an open humeral fracture with segmental bone loss are infection, nonunion, and loss of motion. Infection is managed conservatively with dressing changes or aggressively with surgical debridement, dead space management (antibiotic beads and autogenous bone graft), and antibiotic therapy. Nonunion is managed with removal of failed implants and internal fixation and bone grafting or application of a dynamic external fixator. Limited range of motion at the elbow and shoulder indicates a poor prognosis for consolidation. Loss of motion is managed conservatively with physical therapy. When conservative measures fail, adhesions between the humerus and triceps and brachialis can be excised. In cases in which a fracture has involved the distal articular surface of the humerus, it may be necessary to excise intraarticular adhesions.

Suggested Readings

Christian EP, Bosse MJ, Robb G: Reconstruction of large diaphyseal defects without free fibular transfer in Grade IIIB tibial fractures. J Bone Joint Surg 1989; 69A:19–27.

Eckman JB, Henry SL, Mangino PD, Seligson D: Wound and serum levels of tobramycin with the prophylactic use of tobramycin-impregnated polymethylmethacrylate beads in compound fractures. CORR 1988; 237:213–215.

Lindsey RW, Probe R, Miclau T, Alexander JW, Perren SM: The effects of antibiotic-impregnated autogenic cancellous bone graft on bone healing. CORR 1993; 291:303–312.

Vander Griend R, et al: Open reduction and internal fixation of humeral shaft fractures. Results using AO plating techniques. J Bone Joint Surg 1986; 68A:430–433.

Case 12

History and Physical Examination

A 14-year-old male presented to the emergency room after falling on his right elbow while skateboarding. Examination showed his right elbow to be swollen and deformed. Movement was impossible because of pain. There was no other injury and examination of the right arm showed no evidence of neurovascular damage. There was an abrasion over the olecranon, but the fracture was closed.

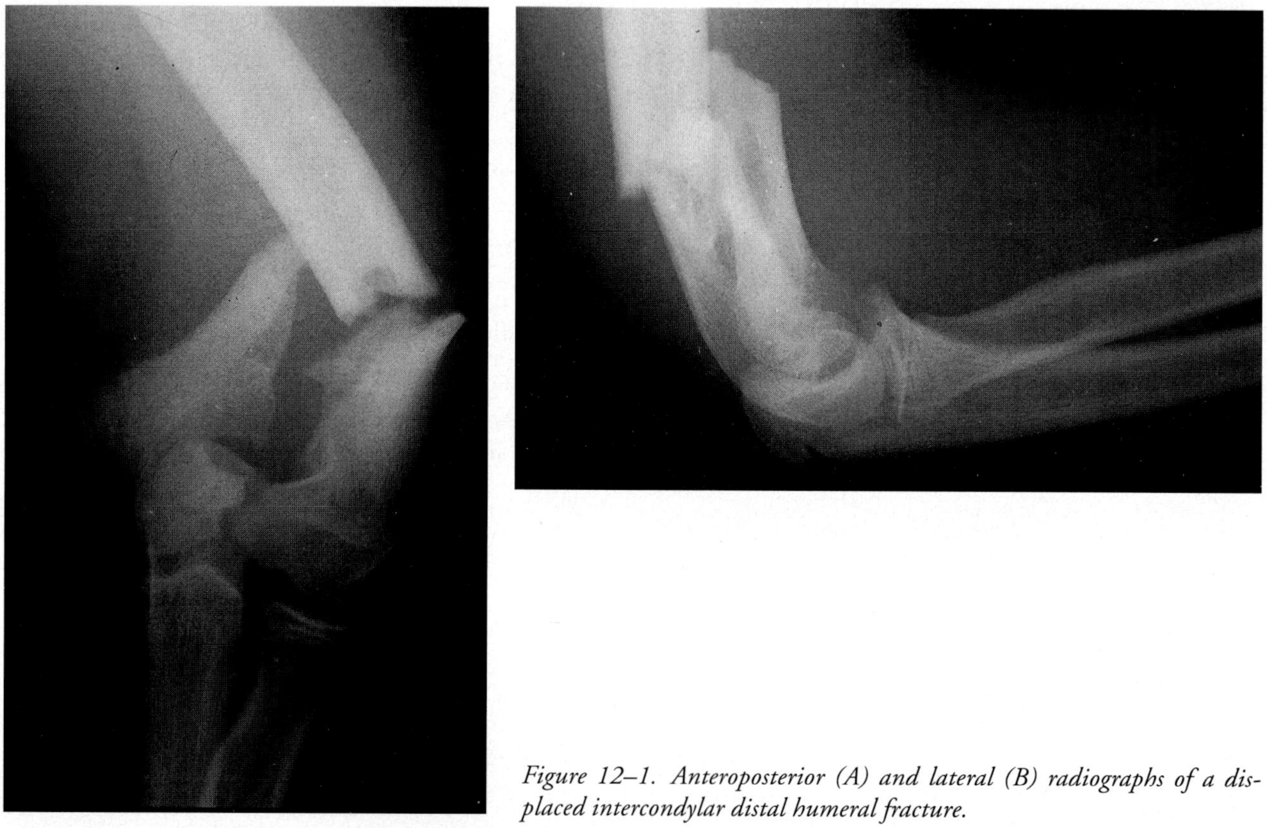

B

A

Figure 12–1. Anteroposterior (A) and lateral (B) radiographs of a displaced intercondylar distal humeral fracture.

Radiologic Findings

Anteroposterior and lateral radiographs of the right elbow showed a high T-shaped intercondylar fracture with displacement of the two columns (Fig. 12–1).

Diagnosis

A closed intercondylar fracture of the right distal humerus. AO classification: 13–C1.1.

Surgical Management

The patient was admitted to the orthopedic trauma unit and a temporary plaster slab was applied to the dorsum of the arm to minimize the risk of further bone and soft tissue damage and ease the discomfort. On the following day the patient was taken to the operating room where he was placed on his left side on an operating table with the right shoulder in abduction and the elbow in flexion. The upper arm was supported by a U-shaped padded splint.

After prepping and draping a midline incision was made over the lower third of the upper arm. It was curved to the lateral side of the olecranon to avoid damage to the ulnar nerve and then carried on over the crest of the proximal ulnar. The dissection was continued down to the triceps muscle, and medial and lateral skin flaps were raised.

An intraarticular olecranon osteotomy was then undertaken using a power saw to divide the bone to the level of the subchondral bone. A sharp osteotome was used to complete the osteotomy. A tongue of triceps was then elevated from the distal humerus, taking care not to detach the proximal olecranon fragment and mobilize the triceps muscle from the medial and lateral borders of the humerus. Care was also taken on the medial side to identify and protect the ulnar nerve. The triceps was turned upward and protected with a saline soaked swab.

Internal fixation was undertaken by reducing and fixing the two articular fragments with two interfragmentary screws. Plates were placed on the medial and lateral columns of the distal humerus. The olecranon osteotomy was fixed with a large

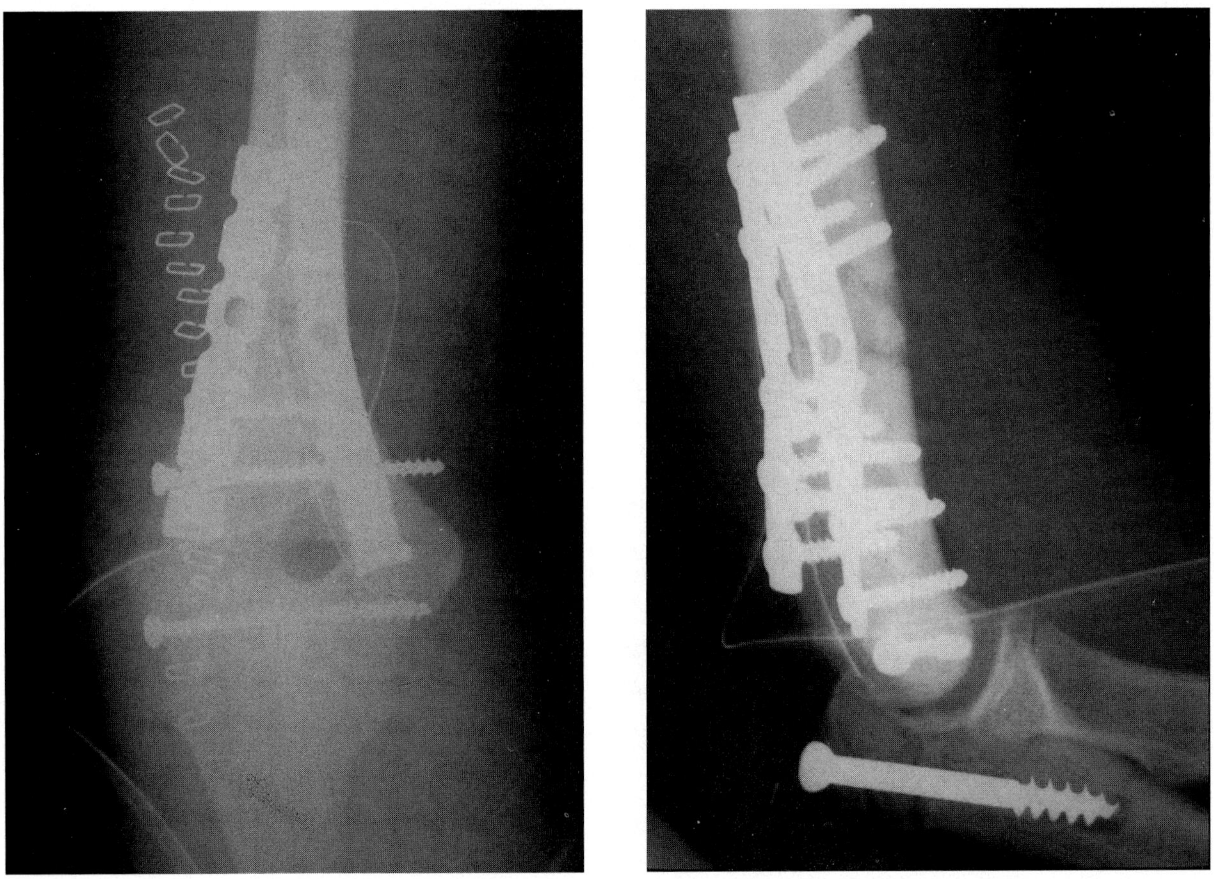

A B

Figure 12–2. Good fixation was achieved with two plates. Anteroposterior (A) and lateral views (B).

PITFALL

- The surgeon should be careful that the mobilized triceps is not too narrow to allow adequate exposure and reduction of the fracture.

PEARL

- Olecranon osteotomies are either intraarticular, as in this case, or extraarticular. In the latter a thinner piece of bone is removed from the proximal olecranon without disturbing the articular cartilage. This can be useful for straightforward intraarticular distal humeral fractures but rarely provides enough exposure for complex fractures.

fragment cancellous screw and the incision closed. Good fixation was achieved and postoperative radiographs were satisfactory (Fig. 12–2).

Postoperative Management

Postoperatively the arm was immobilized with a plaster back slab for 24 hours to allow the postoperative discomfort to settle. Subsequently, a program of active and passive physiotherapy was instituted and the patient regained elbow function very quickly. Four weeks after surgery he had flexion from 20 to 110 degrees. Unfortunately 7 weeks after surgery he was swinging on a rope and fell 10 feet, again landing on his right arm. He presented to the emergency department with a deformed right elbow but still with some function. Anteroposterior and lateral radiographs showed that he had bent both plates in the fall and that the one-third tubular plate on the medial column was broken (Fig. 12–3). Radiographs showed good evidence of new bone formation, but clearly union had not occurred in the area of the metaphysis although the intraarticular component appeared to have healed.

The patient was brought to the operating room and the original incision reopened. The osteotomy was taken down again and inspection of the distal humerus confirmed that the interarticular component of the fracture had united. The two plates were removed and the fracture was stabilized with a posterior dynamic compression plate that provided excellent stability.

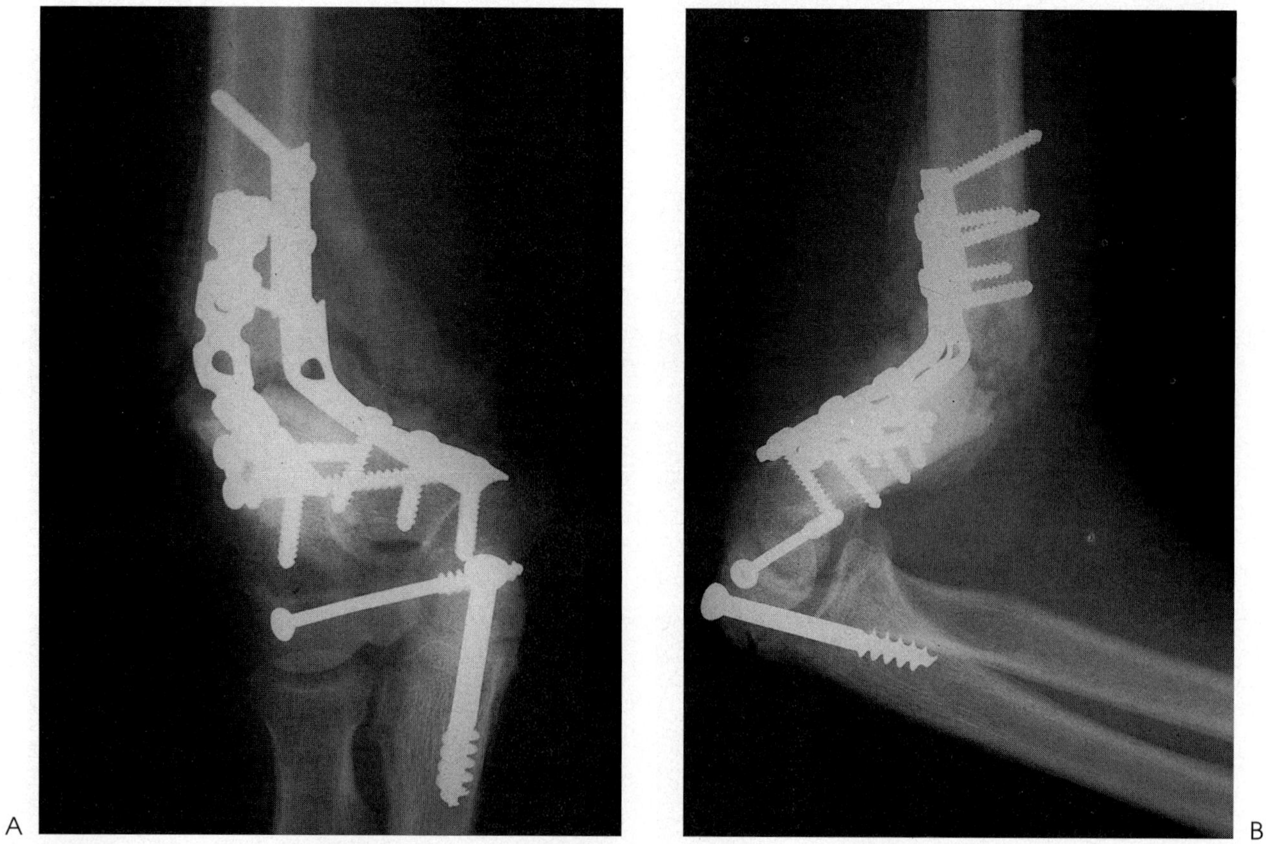

Figure 12–3. After a second fall both plates bend and the medial plate broke. Anteroposterior (A) and lateral (B) views.

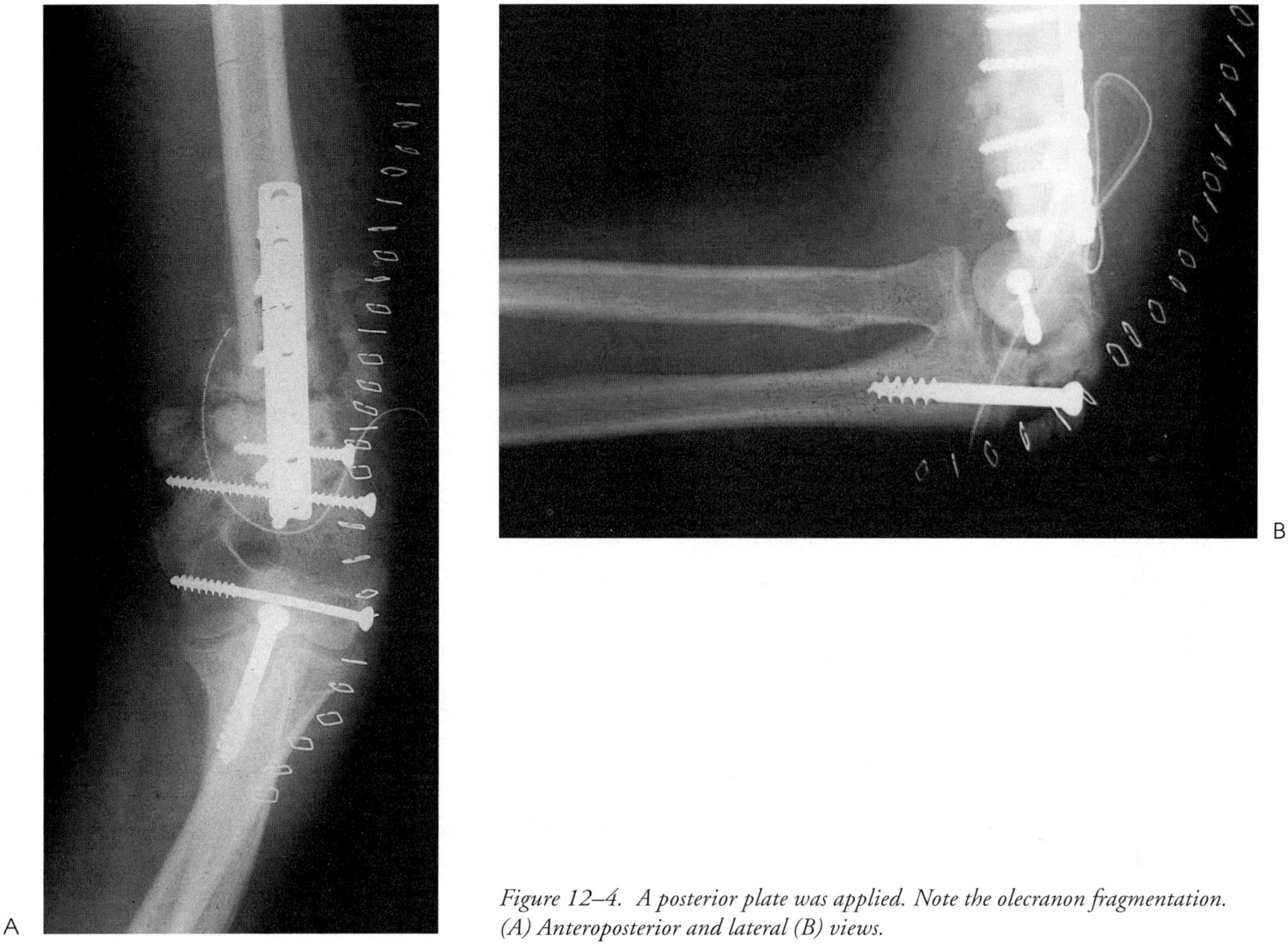

Figure 12–4. A posterior plate was applied. Note the olecranon fragmentation. (A) Anteroposterior and lateral (B) views.

The postoperative radiograph showed good position of the distal humerus but indicated some fragmentation of the olecranon (Fig. 12–4). Clinically, it was felt that the olecranon fixation was satisfactory and an early physiotherapy program was instituted. The humeral fracture healed well and the patient regained excellent function with flexion from 15 to 130 degrees 6 weeks after the second operation. Unfortunately, the olecranon did not unite and 12 weeks later the patient experienced elbow pain on lifting a heavy object. Radiographs indicated that the proximal olecranon had migrated proximally around the bone screw (Fig. 12–5). The patient was readmitted and taken to the operating room where the distal humeral plate was removed and the olecranon fixed with Kirschner wires and a figure of eight wire (Fig. 12–6). Six months later the patient was entirely asymptomatic with normal elbow movement and full function.

Discussion

The management of intraarticular distal humeral fractures highlights the problems of treating displaced intraarticular fractures in general. It is important to accurately reduce the articular fragments and fix them rigidly to facilitate early joint move-

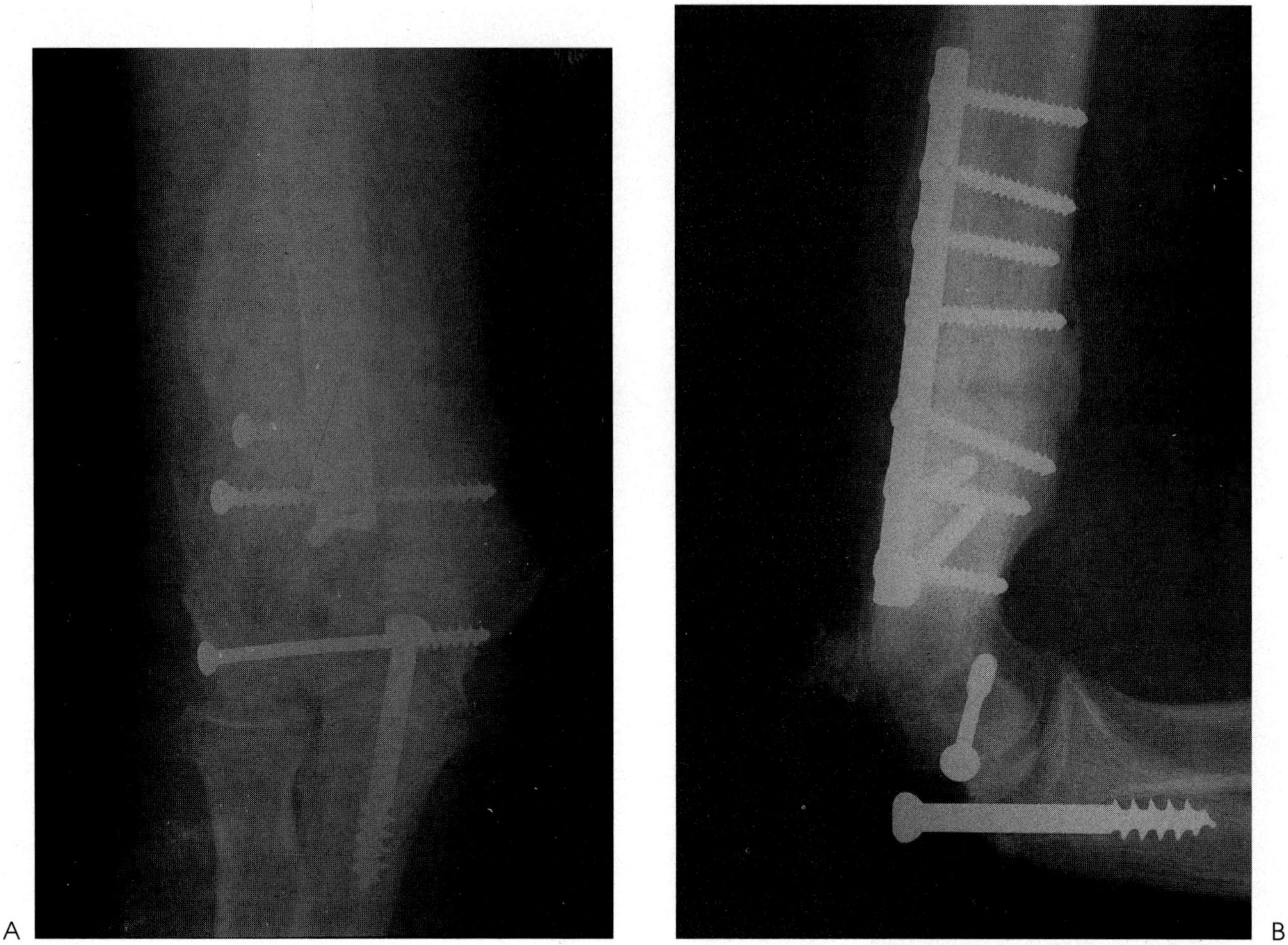

Figure 12–5. The olecranon has not united and the proximal part has been pulled proximally by triceps. Anteroposterior (A) and lateral (B) views.

ment. In fractures such as the one illustrated in this case, this is relatively straightforward because the bone is of good quality and the fragments are relatively large. One could reasonably predict a good outcome and indeed, despite the complications that occurred in his management, this was the case. Problems arise with more complex fractures where the bone fragments are smaller and the articular surface is comminuted. It is always difficult to internally fix osteoporotic bone and therefore fractures in the elderly can be difficult to treat.

A review of 160 consecutive distal humeral fractures treated in the Edinburgh orthopedic trauma unit over a 6-year period illustrates the problems found by orthopedic surgeons in treating distal humeral fractures. The average age of the overall group was 50.7 years. Sixty eight (42.5%) were extraarticular type A fractures, 47 (29.4%) were partial articular type B fractures, and the remaining 43 (28.1%) were complete articular type C fractures. Analysis of the various subgroups shows that the most common distal humeral fracture is the A2.3 transcondylar fracture that accounted for 14.4% of the whole group. The average age of the patients with this fracture was 70.3 years. The other relatively common fractures were the A1.2 medial epicondylar fracture (10%), the B1.2 simple trans-trochlear fracture (8.7%), the B3.1 capitellar fracture (8.1%), and the C1.2 simple complete articular fracture with marked displacement. These latter fractures occur in younger patients.

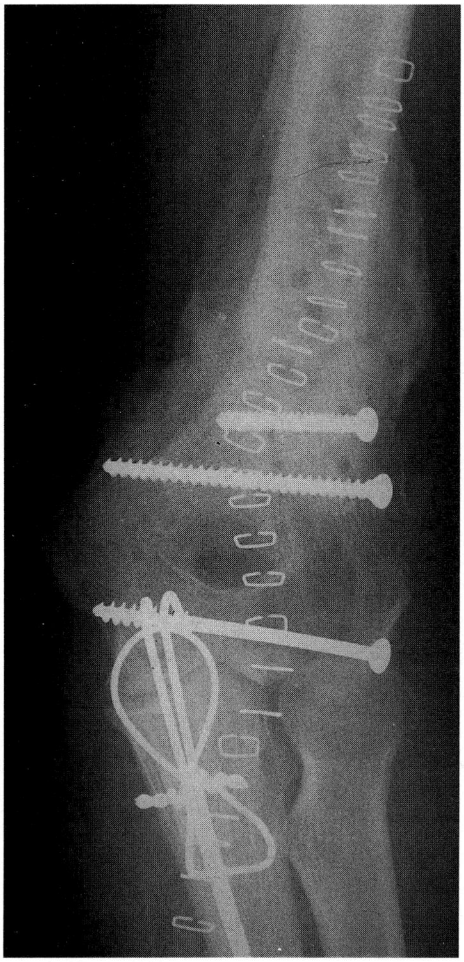

A

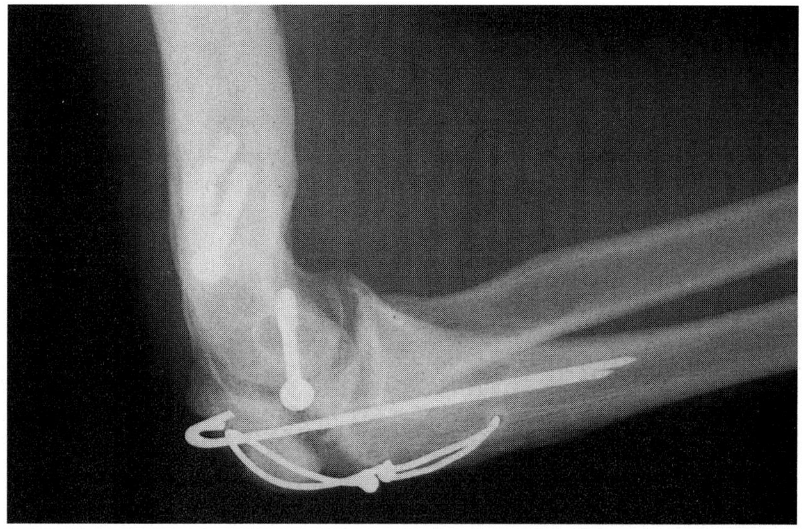

B

Figure 12–6. Refixation was successful. The osteotomy united and a good result was obtained. Anteroposterior (A) and lateral (B) views.

Analysis of the 43 patients who presented with type C complete articular fractures showed that the C1.1 fracture illustrated in this case tended to occur in young patients but that the more severe type C fractures occur in the elderly. The average age of the 11 patients who had type C3 fractures of the distal humerus was 67.4 years, with the average age of the C3.2 subgroup 75 years and the C3.3 subgroup 71.7 years. Thus, it is obvious that the most difficult fractures tend to present in the most difficult patients, and great care is required if good results are to be obtained.

The same surgical principles that were employed in this case should be applied to all fractures regardless of their degree of complexity. The articular surface should be reconstituted and held by one or more interfragmentary bone screws. The articular surface is then fixed to the medial and lateral columns using plates. If the distal fragments are small, the fixation can be supplemented by screws that pass up both columns.

In this case two complications occurred. One was unfortunate in that the patient fell again before the fracture had united. This is a problem that all surgeons will face from time to time and it should be treated by immediate refixation. It is usually ill advised to wait until union and then osteotomize and refix the fracture. The second complication was failure of the olecranon screw to hold the proximal olecranon fragment after revision surgery.

Olecranon osteotomies are usually reconstructed using a bone screw as in the first operation or Kirschner wires and a figure of eight wire as in the second procedure.

Biomechanically, the use of Kirschner wires and figure of eight wiring is preferable and it should be noted that bone screws are not actually designed to get good purchase on the endosteal surface of the intramedullary canal. In this case, however, the screw thread held but the head of the screw did not hold the proximal olecranon fragment adequately. Kirschner wires are probably the treatment of choice, but patients complain of discomfort over the ends of the wires, necessitating their removal.

Alternative Methods of Management

Internal fixation using screws and plates has become the accepted method of treating two column fractures of the distal humerus. In the fracture illustrated in this case there is really no sensible alternative management. In more severe fractures some surgeons still advocate nonoperative management using the "bag of bones" technique. There is, however, no place for this technique in today's climate and its use usually points to surgical inexperience rather than an unreconstructable fracture. In elderly patients osteoporotic bone fixation may indeed be difficult, but even if the columns are reconstructed an elbow arthroplasty can be used at a later date. This is often difficult if reduction of the columns has not been undertaken primarily. Primary arthroplasty may be preferred if the surgeon feels that the fracture is truly unreconstructable, but a hinged device will be required if the columns are significantly damaged and loosening is likely to be a major problem.

Type of Management	Advantages	Disadvantages	Comments
Nonoperative	None	Nonunion; malunion; pain; stiffness	The only place for nonoperative management is if the patient is so infirm that surgery is contraindicated.
Internal fixation with plates and screws	Rigid fixation; early joint movement	May be technically difficult	Method of choice
Internal fixation with Kirschner wires	Technically easier	Nonrigid fixation; early movement not possible; joint stiffness; malunion	Inferior method of management; frequently equates to nonoperative management

Complications

The major complications of distal humeral fracture fixation, particularly in the elderly, is failure to maintain the fracture position while permitting early elbow movement. Surgeons should use a meticulous technique during distal humeral reconstruction because reoperation is often very difficult. Posttraumatic osteoarthritis may be treated by arthroplasty and a tight anterior capsule may be treated by later anterior capsulectomy or capsulotomy. However, this is a difficult procedure that requires considerable patient cooperation with a difficult and time consuming physiotherapy regime after the surgery. Ulnar neuritis is best treated by anterior transposition of the ulnar nerve and olecranon nonunion should be treated by refixation and bone grafting where necessary.

Suggested Readings

Helfet DL, Schmeling BJ: Bicondylar fractures of the distal humerus in adults. Clin Orthop 1993; 292:26–36.

Holdsworth BJ, Mossad MM: Fractures of the adult distal humerus: elbow function after internal fixation. J Bone Joint Surg (Br) 1990; 72B:362–365.

Jupiter JB, Mehne DK: Trauma to the adult humerus and fractures of the distal humerus. In: Browner BD, Jupiter JB, Levine AM, Trafton PG: Skeletal Trauma. WB Saunders, Philadelphia, 1992.

Jupiter JB, Neff U, Hozach P, Allgöwer M: Inter-condylar fractures of the humerus. J Bone Joint Surg (Am) 1985; 67A:226–239.

Rommens PM: Fractures of the distal third of the humerus. In: Flatow EL, Ulrich C (eds): Humerus. Butterworth Heinemann, Oxford, 1996.

Schatzker J, Tile M: The Rationale of Operative Fracture Care. Springer Verlag, Berlin, 1987.

Case 13

History and Physical Examination

An 83-year-old woman fell on her outstretched hand, injuring her elbow. The onset of pain and swelling about the elbow was immediate. When the patient arrived in the emergency department, there was no obvious deformity present. Palpation of the epicondyles of the humerus and any attempt at flexion or extension of the elbow was painful. The neurovascular examination of the hand and forearm was within the limits of normal.

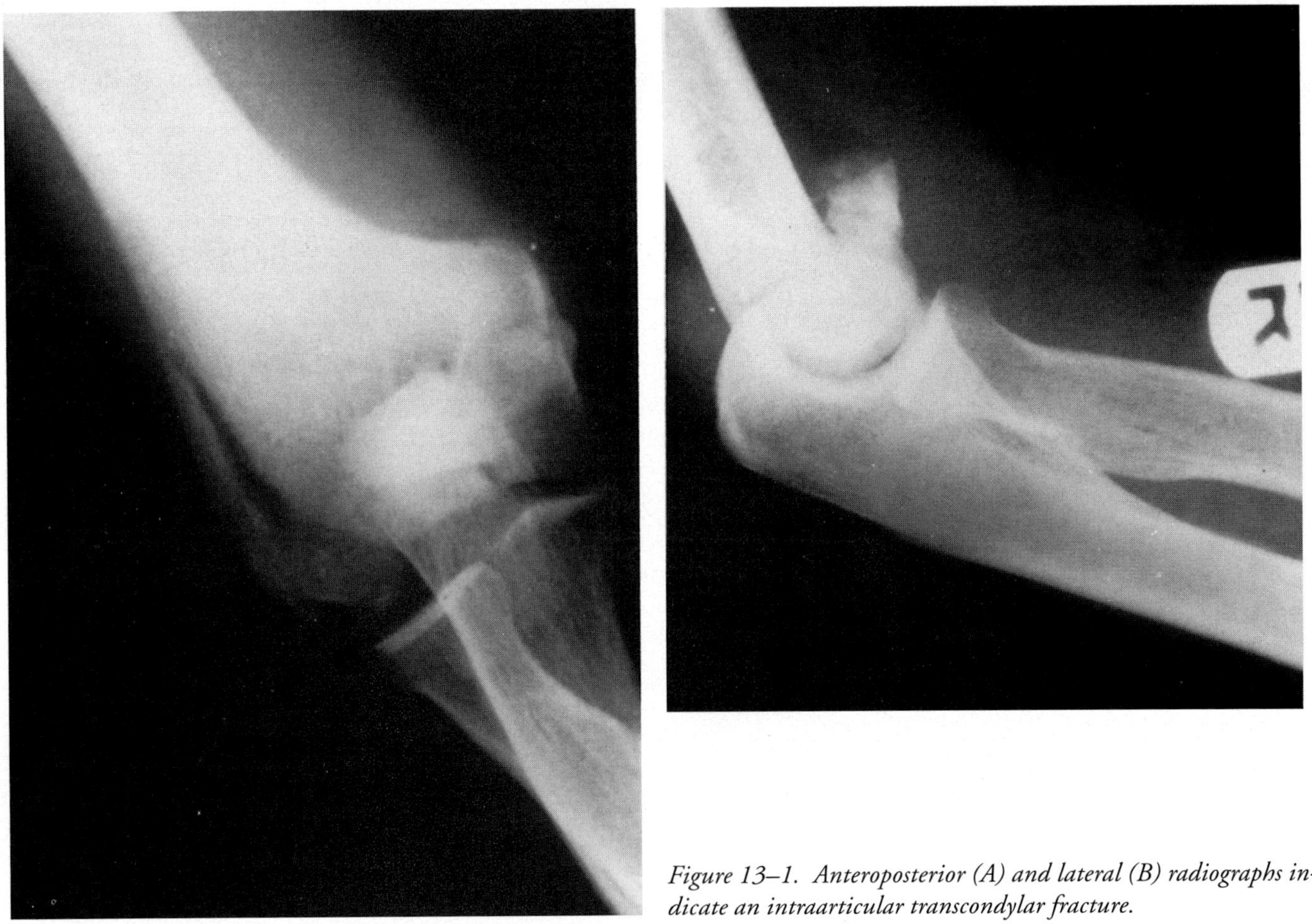

A B

Figure 13–1. Anteroposterior (A) and lateral (B) radiographs indicate an intraarticular transcondylar fracture.

Radiologic Findings

In most cases, plain radiographs are adequate for evaluating fractures of the distal humerus. Other studies such as tomograms or computerized axial tomograms are not necessary to evaluate the injury. In this case radiographs indicated that the fracture was transverse and intraarticular (Fig. 13–1).

Diagnosis

Transcondylar fracture with intraarticular extension and osteopenia. Comprehensive AO classification: 13–C3.1.

Surgical Management

One day after injury, under general anesthesia, the patient was positioned prone, with the arm abducted 90 degrees, the elbow flexed 90 degrees, and the forearm hanging over an armboard. The arm and forearm were scrubbed and a tourniquet inflated around the upper arm. The fracture was exposed through two incisions centered over the medial and lateral epicondyles. The periosteum was elevated from the posterior aspect of the humerus, and the fracture was reduced anatomically. Two 6.5 mm cancellous screws were inserted up the medial and lateral columns and across the fracture.

The technique of management is based on the fracture classification. Displaced fractures are managed with open reduction and internal fixation. Positioning the patient prone with the injured arm over an arm board and the elbow flexed 90 degrees with the forearm hanging free greatly facilitates reduction. Displaced simple transverse fractures are exposed via medial and lateral incisions, reduced and stabilized with one screw in the medial and the lateral column of the humerus. Even in osteopenic patients, the bone in the medial and lateral columns is dense enough to allow stable fixation. Screw placement is important; the screws should be centered in the columns. On the lateral side, the screw starts in the most distal portion of the capitellum, slightly posterior to the coronal midline, and is countersunk to avoid impingement on the radial head when the elbow is extended.

T-type fractures and fracture dislocations are exposed via the trans-olecranon approach. The olecranon is exposed through a straight posterior incision, the ulnar nerve is identified and protected, and the olecranon is predrilled and then osteotomized. The V-shaped osteotomy is centered over the deepest portion of the trochlear notch. The olecranon is then reflected proximally on the triceps tendon, exposing the fracture. The fragments of the distal humerus are reduced and stabilized with K wires and screws. Medially, the ulnar nerve is transposed and the cubital tunnel is used as an additional point of fixation. The reconstructed distal humerus is reduced to the metaphysis and stabilized with plates and screws or screws alone. The olecranon is reduced and stabilized with a 6.5 mm cancellous screw and washer and a tension band wire is added when the screw alone does not provide sufficient stability. The ulnar nerve is held in its transposed position with a flap of fascia raised from the flexor muscles and the wound is closed (Fig 13–2).

PEARL

- The key to the radiographic evaluation is whether there is intraarticular extension of the fracture between the trochlea and capitellum. This is important because it directs the surgical approach (i.e., transolecranon approach if an intraarticular fracture is present versus medial and lateral incisions if an intraarticular fracture is absent).

PITFALL

- The strength of fixation is limited by the small size of the distal fragment and the osteopenia that is frequently associated with transcondylar fractures. The temptation is to immobilize the elbow until the fracture has healed. The risk of extended immobilization is that the elbow will become stiff. If this occurs and the fracture does not heal, the prognosis for union is very poor. Therefore, postoperative management must include carefully supervised range of motion exercises several times a day. At all other times the arm is protected in a long arm splint.

Postoperative Management

Postoperatively, the patient's elbow was immobilized in a posterior splint at 90 degrees. Starting on postoperative day 3, the splint was removed 3 times a day for supervised, gentle, active, flexion exercises. At 6 weeks active extension exercises were initiated. At 8 weeks the splint was discontinued. Six months postinjury the fracture was healed clinically and radiographically. The final range of motion was 20 to 120 degrees.

The goals of postoperative management are to prevent failure of fixation and regain a functional range of motion. Flexion seems to put less stress across the fracture

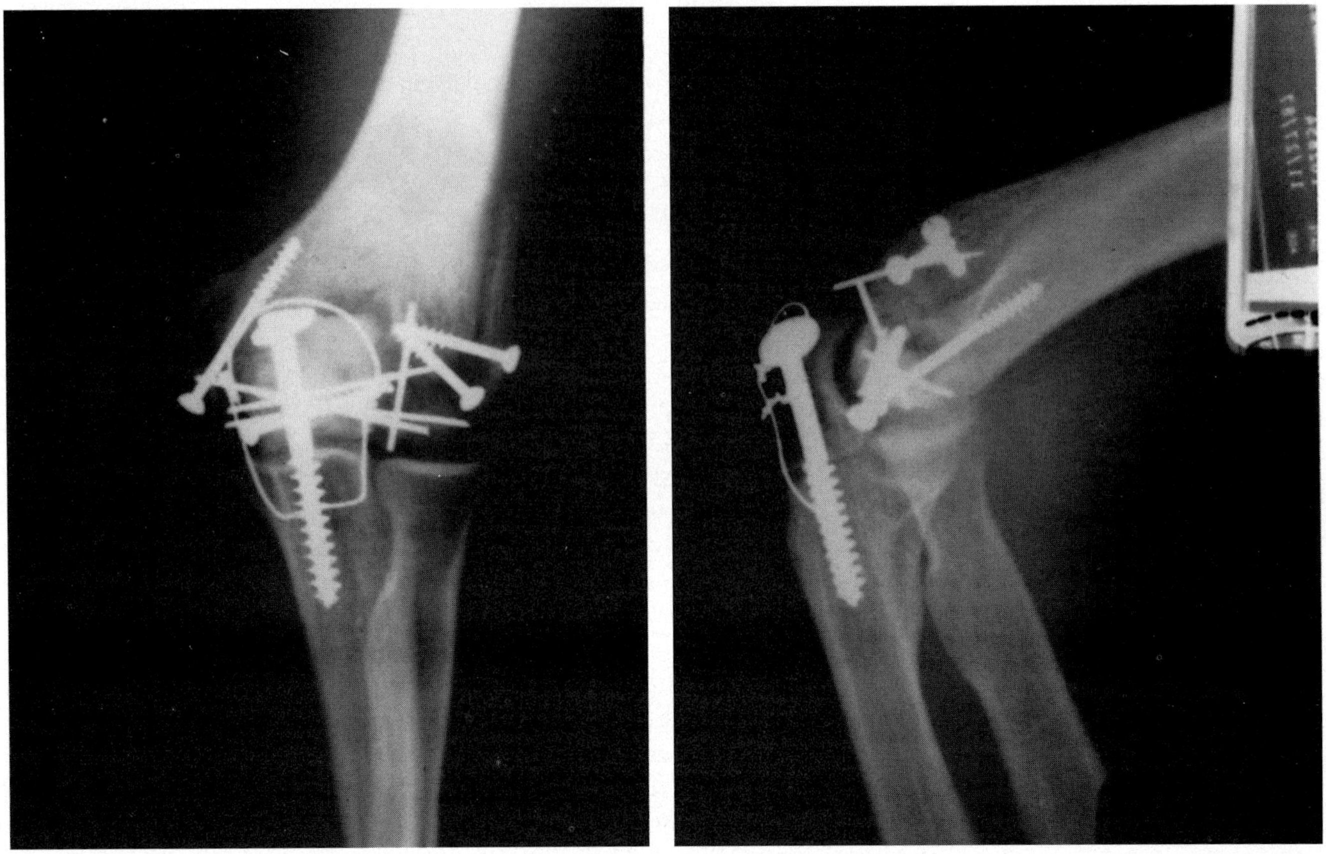

A B

Figure 13–2. Stable fixation was difficult to achieve because of the small size of the distal fragments. Anteroposterior (A) and lateral (B) views.

than extension, therefore extension exercises are not initiated until 5 to 6 weeks after surgery when some bony healing has occurred.

Discussion

Transcondylar fractures of the distal humerus are characterized by a unique transverse fracture at the level of the olecranon and coronoid fossae. This fracture is intracapsular and separates the medial and lateral epicondyles from the trochlea and capitellum. In addition to the primary transverse fracture, there may be intraarticular extension and anterior dislocation of the condyles from the olecranon.

Transcondylar fractures have been considered a subset of supracondylar fractures. Because of this, there is very little written specifically about them. Several older studies that purportedly cover transcondylar fractures do not. Two examples are studies authored by Ashurst (1910) and Chutro (1904). Ashurst authored one of the largest series (and perhaps most frequently referenced). He described eight "transverse diacondylar fractures" and classified them according to their displacement and angulation into extension or flexion type fractures. However, all eight of Ashurst's patients were skeletally immature and he was actually describing supracondylar fractures, not true transcondylar fractures. Writing in Portuguese, Chutro reported five cases of anterior fracture dislocation of the humeral condyles from the olecranon. He called this injury Posada's fracture. The title of Chutro's book and a review of the radiographs in his book indicate that his patients were children.

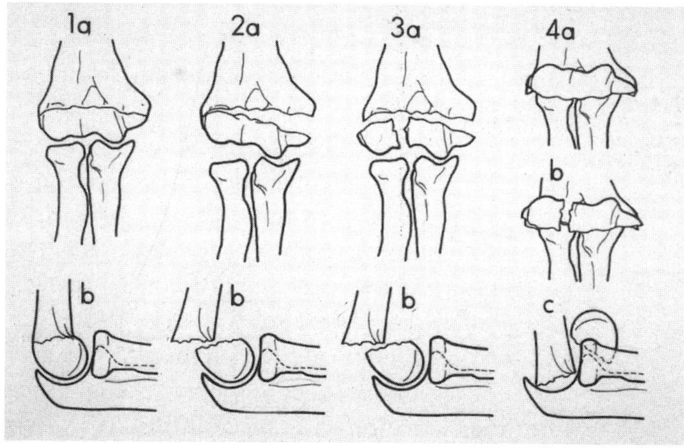

Figure 13–3. The system by which transcondylar fractures are classified.

The *classification* of transcondylar fractures is based on the presence of displacement, intraarticular extension (i.e., the presence of a fracture line between the trochlea and capitellum), and whether the humeral condyles are dislocated from the trochlear notch. In order of increasing complexity these fractures are classified as: undisplaced, simple displaced (as in this case report), T-type, and fracture dislocation of the humeral condyles from the trochlear notch (Fig. 13–3).

Alternative Methods of Management

Elbow arthroplasty is considered when comminution and osteopenia make open reduction impossible and the patient has low demands.

Fractures are managed without surgery when they are undisplaced or the patient is too debilitated for surgery. The two closed methods of management are immobilization, and early mobilization with the "bag of bones" technique. Immobilization is accomplished by casting or splinting the arm with the elbow flexed 90 degrees and the forearm in neutral rotation. At 6 weeks the cast is removed and gentle active range of motion is begun. The bag of bones technique consists of suspending the wrist by a collar and cuff with the elbow flexed over 90 degrees. As pain and swelling resolve, active flexion exercises are initiated. At 6 to 8 weeks, the collar and cuff are discarded and extension exercises are initiated. When used to manage a displaced fracture, the bag of bones technique is more likely to preserve motion than extended immobilization; however, the elbow may be unstable and require bracing.

Type of Management	Advantages	Disadvantages	Comments
Open reduction and internal fixation	Potentially can result in almost full recovery of function	Extremely difficult	Recovery of function outweighs difficulty of technique
Arthroplasty	Results in better function than closed treatment	Limited survival of implant in active patients	Limited indications in active patients
Closed management	Technically easy; no infection	Significant loss of function	The loss of function makes this a poor alternative method

Complications

Complications include loss of motion, loss of fixation and reduction, infection, and painful hardware.

Some loss of motion is inevitable following a transcondylar fracture. This is because the fracture involves the olecranon and coronoid fossae. Loss of motion becomes clinically significant when the patient cannot reach his mouth or the back of his head. Assuming that the reduction is adequate and that there are no implants impinging on the olecranon and coronoid fossae, capsular scarring and intraarticular adhesions are the most likely causes of loss of motion. When this is the case, patience and physical therapy are the method of management. In high demand patients who have not responded to conservative therapy, a capsular release, removal of adhesions from the olecranon and coronoid fossae, and distraction arthroplasty with an external fixator, is performed. Malreduction resulting in loss of motion is managed with an osteotomy and internal fixation. When impingement of a screw or other implant on the coronoid or olecranon fossae results in loss of motion, it is removed.

When fixation and reduction are lost, if possible, the fracture is rereduced and the fixation revised. When this is not possible, closed methods (i.e., splinting and bracing) are used or an elbow arthroplasty is performed.

Infection is managed conservatively with wound care and oral antibiotics until the fracture is healed. When the fracture is healed, the implants are removed, the area debrided of necrotic tissue, and culture specific systemic antibiotics are administered for 6 weeks.

Painful implants are managed by removing them after healing has occurred.

Suggested Readings

Ashurst APC: An anatomical and surgical study of fractures of the lower end of the humerus. The Samuel D Gross Prize Essay of the Philadelphia Academy of Surgery. Lea and Feiberger, Philadelphia, 1910.

Bryan RS: Fractures about the elbow in adults. AAOS Instructional Course Lectures 1981; 30:200–223.

Bryan RS, Morrey BF: Fractures of the distal humerus. In: Morrey BF: The Elbow and Its Disorders. WB Saunders, Philadelphia, 1985.

Cassebaum WH: Operative treatment of T and Y fractures of the lower end of the humerus. JAMA 1963; 184:553.

Chutro P: Fractures de la Extremidad Inferior del Humero en los Ninos. Theses J Peuser, Buenos Aires, 1904.

DeLee JC, Green DP, Wilkins KE: Fractures and dislocations of the elbow. In: Rockwood CA, Green DP: Fractures in adults, 2nd ed. JB Lippincott, Philadelphia, 1984.

Grantham SA, Tietjen R: Transcondylar fracture—dislocation of the elbow: a case report. J Bone Joint Surg 1976; 58A:1030–1031.

Hitzrot JM: Fractures at the lower end of the humerus in adults. Surg Clin North Am 1932; 12:291–304.

Nieman KMW: Transcondylar fractures of the distal humerus in adults. South Med J 1977; 70:915–918.

Perry CR, Gibson CT, Kowalski MF: Transcondylar fractures of the distal humerus. J Orthop Trauma 1989; 3(2):98–106.

Case 14

History and Physical Examination

A 42-year-old man was admitted to the emergency department having been the driver of a car involved in a traffic accident. Physical examination revealed a number of superficial skin abrasions on his arms and legs. The only injury was to his right elbow, which was deformed and painful. There was an area of soft tissue loss on the posteromedial aspect of the elbow joint measuring approximately 6 cm × 3 cm (Fig. 14–1). There was superficial contamination and obvious bone and articular cartilage damage, with bone fragments present in the wound. Examination of the neurovascular status of the arm showed no abnormality, with good peripheral circulation and no evidence of nerve damage. The right wrist and hand were apparently normal.

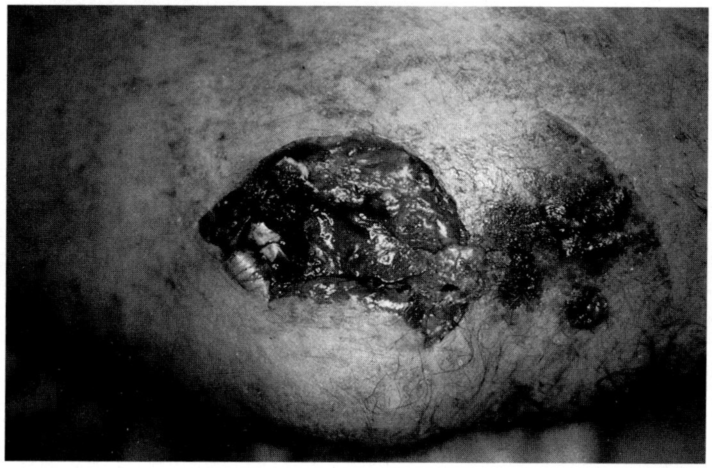

Figure 14–1. A preoperative view of the open wound. The area on the right of the wound looks as if it may be degloved; this was found to be the case at surgery.

Radiologic Findings

Anteroposterior and lateral radiographs showed an intraarticular distal humeral fracture (Fig. 14–2). The articular surface consists of three fragments. The radiographs give the impression that there is not enough bone to permit an anatomical reconstruction of the distal humeral metaphysis.

Diagnosis

Open distal humeral fracture, probably associated with metaphyseal bone loss, but with a reconstructable articular surface. The size of the wound, degree of contamination, and the extent of the associated soft tissue damage suggest that this is a Gustilo type III fracture, and the presence of significant metaphyseal bone loss means that it is in fact Gustilo IIIb in severity. AO classification: 13–C3.3 fracture.

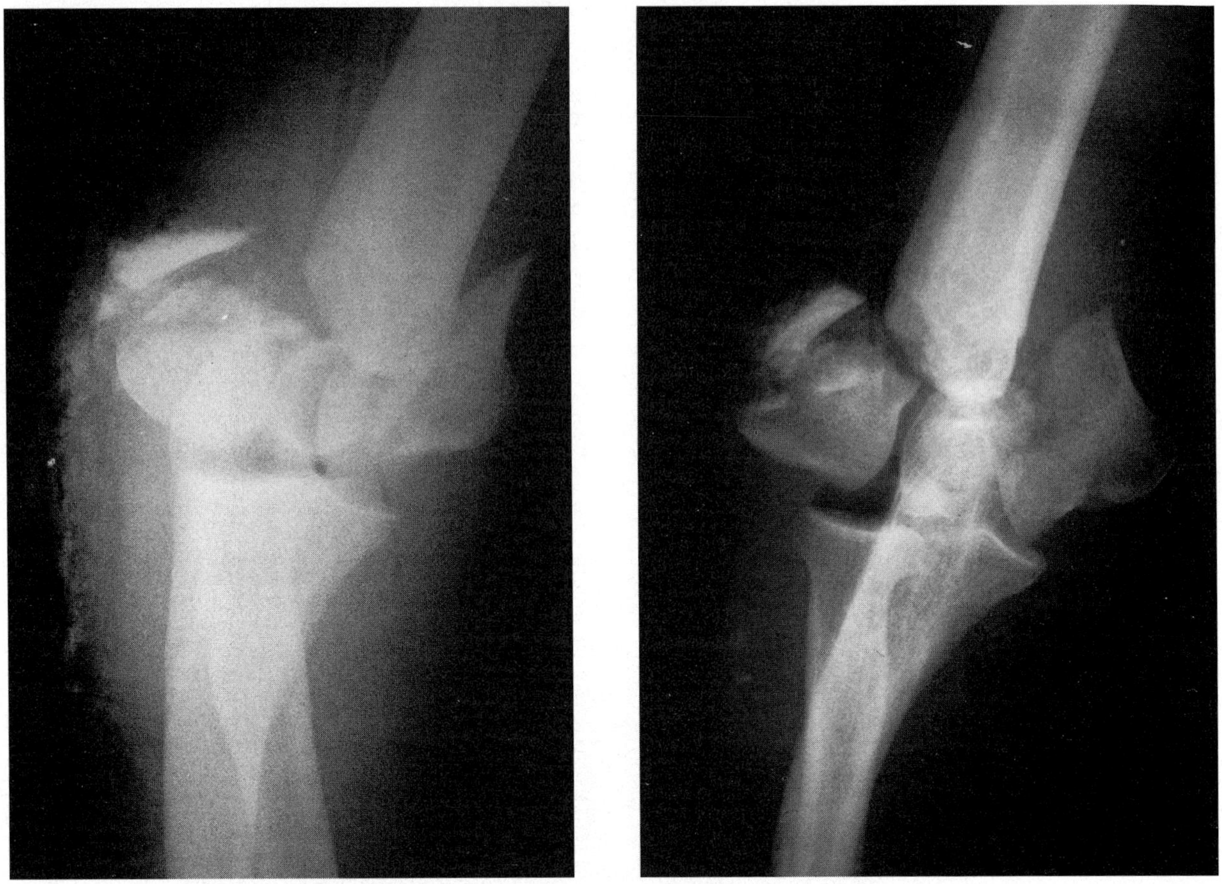

Figure 14–2. Anteroposterior (A) and lateral (B) radiographs of the distal humeral fracture.

PEARL

- This case highlights some of the deficiencies of modern classifications. Neither the Gustilo or AO classifications mentions bone loss, although the implication must be that bone loss constitutes extreme comminution and bone devascularization! The other problem is that of defining "simple" articular damage. This fracture had extensive intraarticular involvement but the fragments were comparatively large and relatively easy to fix.

Surgical Management

The patient was admitted to the trauma unit and taken to the operating room within 4 hours of the accident. The wound was cleaned and lavaged free of contaminating debris and the arm was prepped and draped. The patient was placed on his left side with the brachium supported in a U-shaped support extending from the axilla to the elbow. The contused wound edges were excised and careful digital palpation of the wound undertaken. It was confirmed that there was degloving above the open wound (Fig. 14–1) and the wound extensions were placed with this in mind. The wound was extended proximally through the degloved area toward the posterior midline of the upper arm. Distally it was extended over the subcutaneous border of the ulna. After the extensions had been made, the degloved skin was resected until dermal bleeding was encountered.

A thorough debridement was then performed, removing all contaminated and devitalized tissue. It was found that there was good periosteal cover over the distal humerus and little muscle damage was present. A standard posterior approach was made to the lower humeral diaphysis by undertaking an intraarticular olecranon osteotomy and turning the triceps upward. Care was taken to identify and protect the ulnar nerve.

It was then possible to reconstruct the distal humerus. It was noted that about 1 in of the humeral metaphysis was missing but that all the articular surface was

PITFALL

- It is important to resect all degloved skin and subcutaneous fat. It can often be difficult to decide on the margin of resection, but initially the surgeon should resect the soft tissues until dermal bleeding is encountered. If necessary, further resection can be undertaken at postprocedure examination, 24 to 48 hours following surgery.

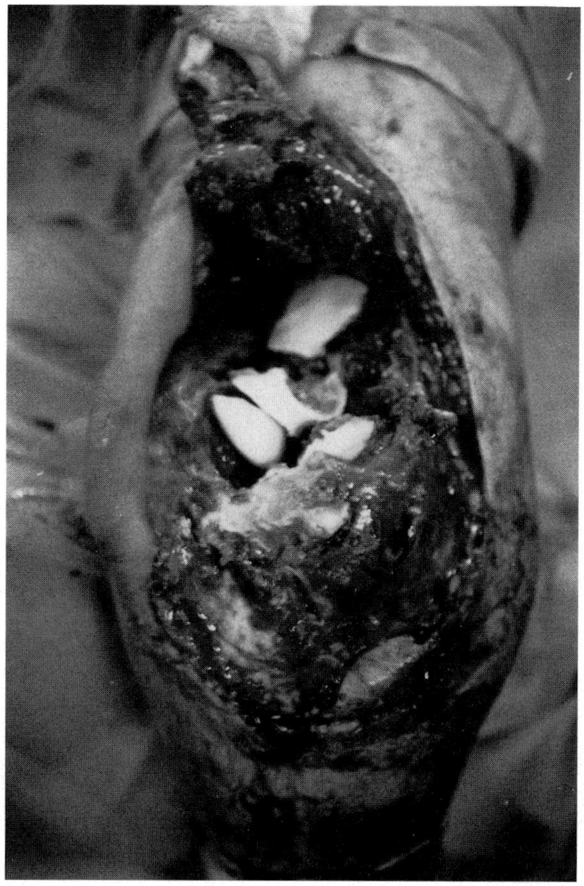

Figure 14–3. An intraoperative view of the bone damage. The articular fragments and the diaphysis are seen but the metaphyseal bone is missing.

present (Fig. 14–3). The articular surface was rebuilt from the three fragments using temporary Kirschner wire fixation, and subsequently an interfragmentary screw was inserted to secure all three fragments. The length of the remaining metaphyseal bone fragment and tension of the soft tissues were both used to assess the degree of bone loss and an appropriately shaped block of ilium was removed from the right side of the pelvis. The pelvic autograft was then transferred to the distal humerus and secured with three reconstruction plates. Two plates were placed on the medial and lateral columns but they failed to adequately secure the graft. Consequently a third plate was used to fix the graft to the humeral diaphysis. It was positioned away from the olecranon fossa so as not to obstruct elbow extension (Fig. 14–4). The olecranon was reconstructed with Kirschner wires and a figure of eight wire loop.

The wound was left open and dressed with antibiotic impregnated moist dressing. The patient was transferred to the ward but was returned to the operating room 48 hours later. On this occasion the wound was explored and no further debridement was required. The defect was closed with a local radial forearm flap; the donor site was covered by a split skin graft (Fig. 14–5).

Postoperative Management

Postoperatively a well padded long-arm cast was applied for 3 weeks until the soft tissues had healed. Passive and active physiotherapy was begun 3 weeks later, but the

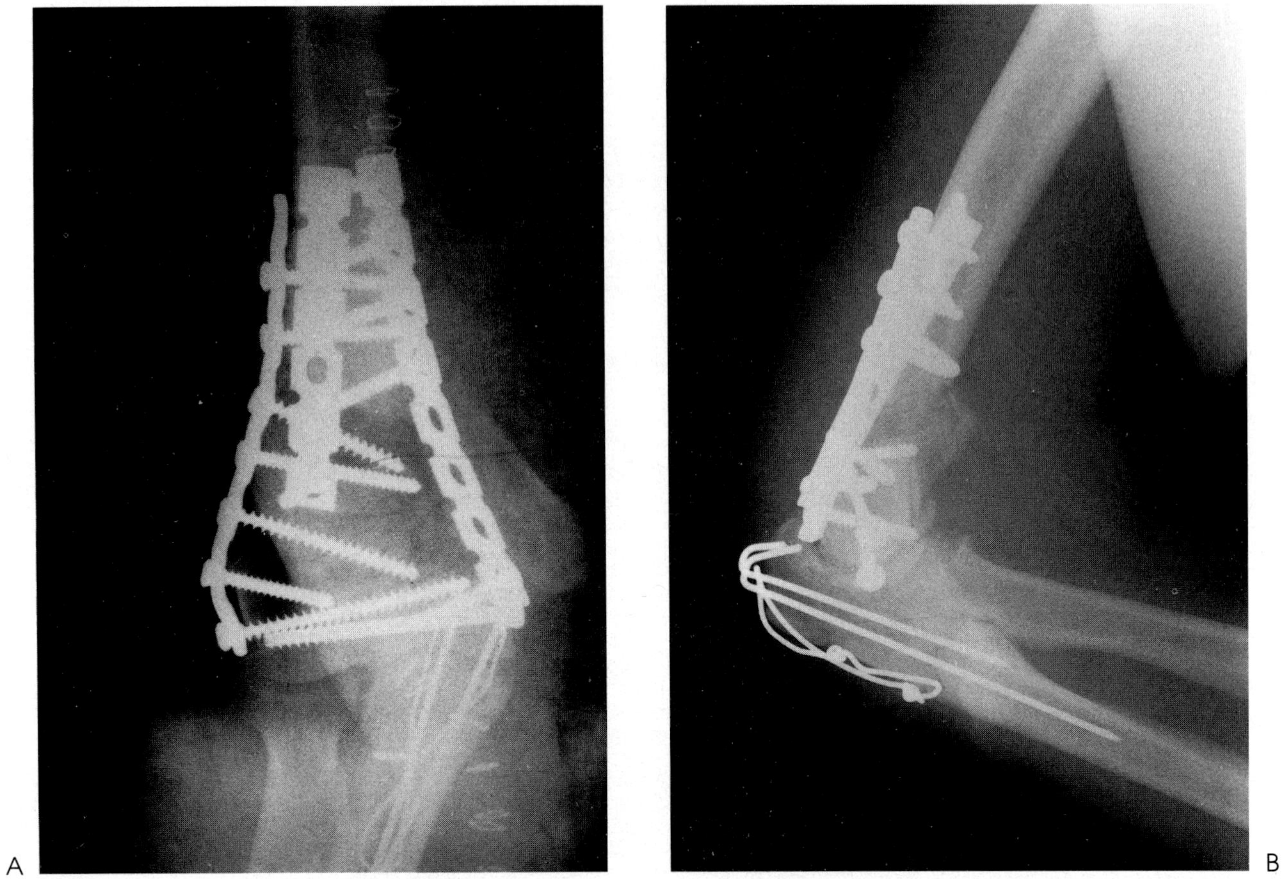

Figure 14–4. Postoperative anteroposterior (A) and lateral (B) radiographs.

PEARL

- Distal humeral reconstruction is very difficult to perform without an olecranon osteotomy. There is debate about whether the osteotomy should be extra- or intraarticular. Extraarticular olecranon osteotomies cause less damage but provide inferior exposure. On balance, intraarticular osteotomies are recommended for these difficult fractures.

fracture was supported in a functional brace for a further 6 weeks after which all bracing was discarded. At 1 year the results were excellent. Examination of the elbow showed flexion from 20 to 130 degrees, with good pronation and supination. The patient did not complain of pain, although he was somewhat troubled by the appearance of the donor flap site.

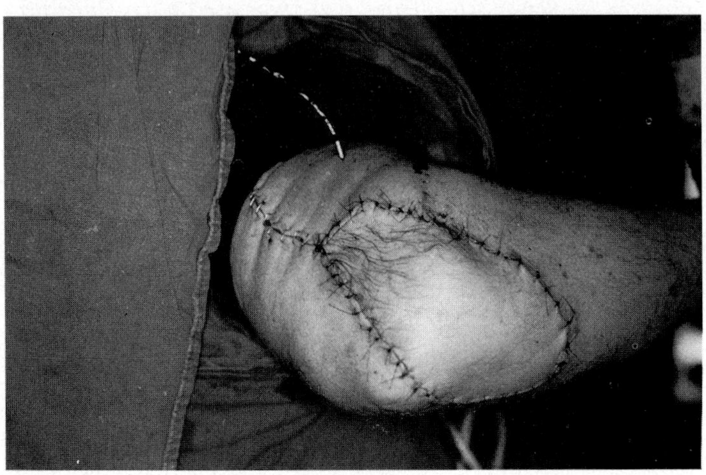

Figure 14–5. Soft tissue cover was achieved with a radial forearm flap.

Discussion

The association of open fractures with bone loss is comparatively rare. Usually all the bone is retained within the soft tissue envelope, although it may be extensively comminuted and devitalized. Thus most bone defects are postoperative rather than preoperative, the bone having been removed by the surgeon at the initial debridement. The missing bone segment may be intraarticular or extraarticular and the latter may be metaphyseal, as in this case, or diaphyseal. However, the treatment of metaphyseal and diaphyseal defects is similar.

The combination of metaphyseal bone loss with a potentially reconstructable articular surface is relatively uncommon because the high energy injuries responsible for the missing bone segments usually cause severe articular damage. Such a situation is most likely to occur in the elbow or knee and the treatment is similar for both joints. The key is an adequate initial debridement, rigid stabilization of the fracture, and early flap cover. If these basic tenets of treatment are followed, a good result can be expected.

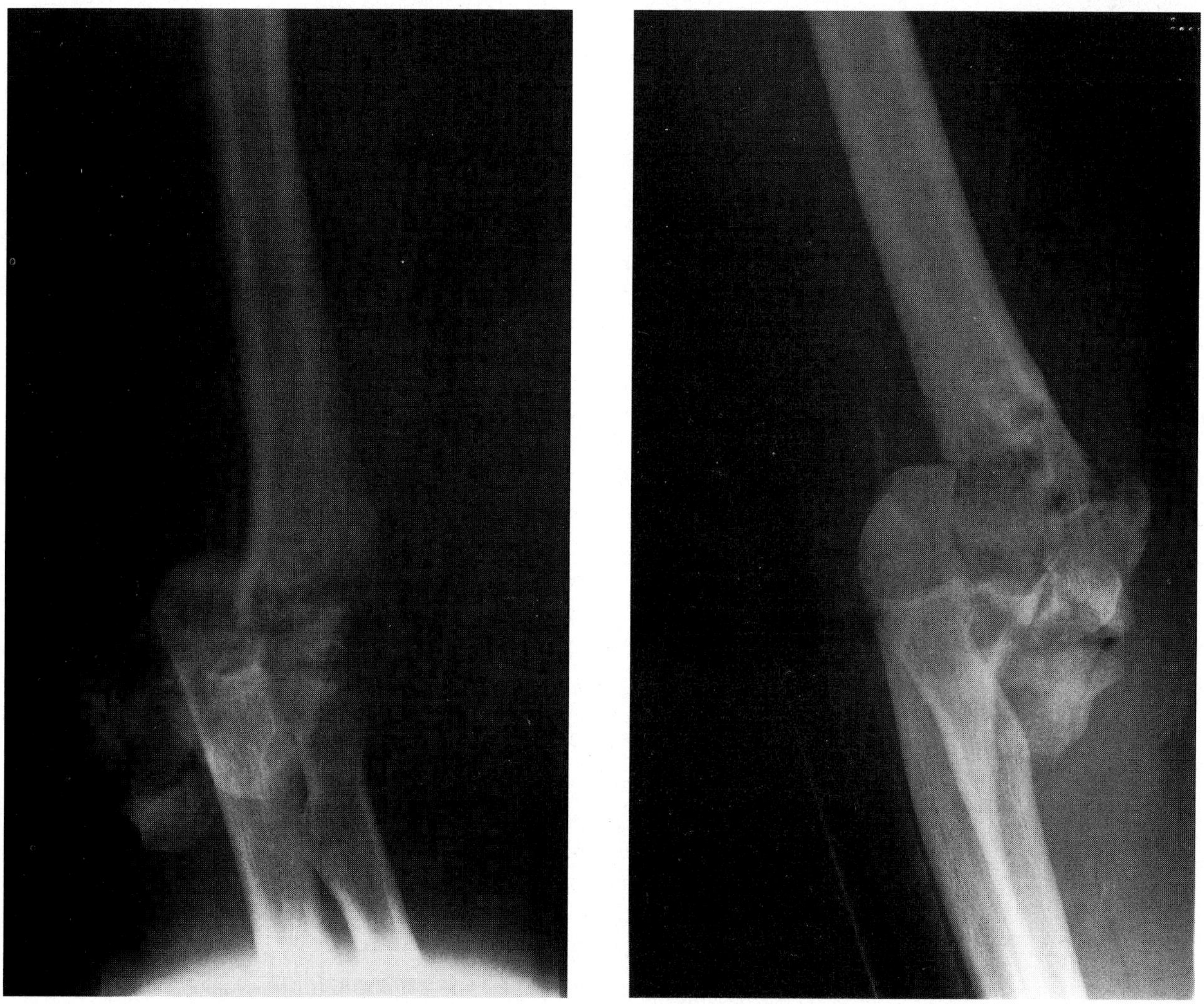

A B

Figure 14–6. Anteroposterior (A) and lateral (B) radiographs of a 13–C3.3 fracture with articular bone loss.

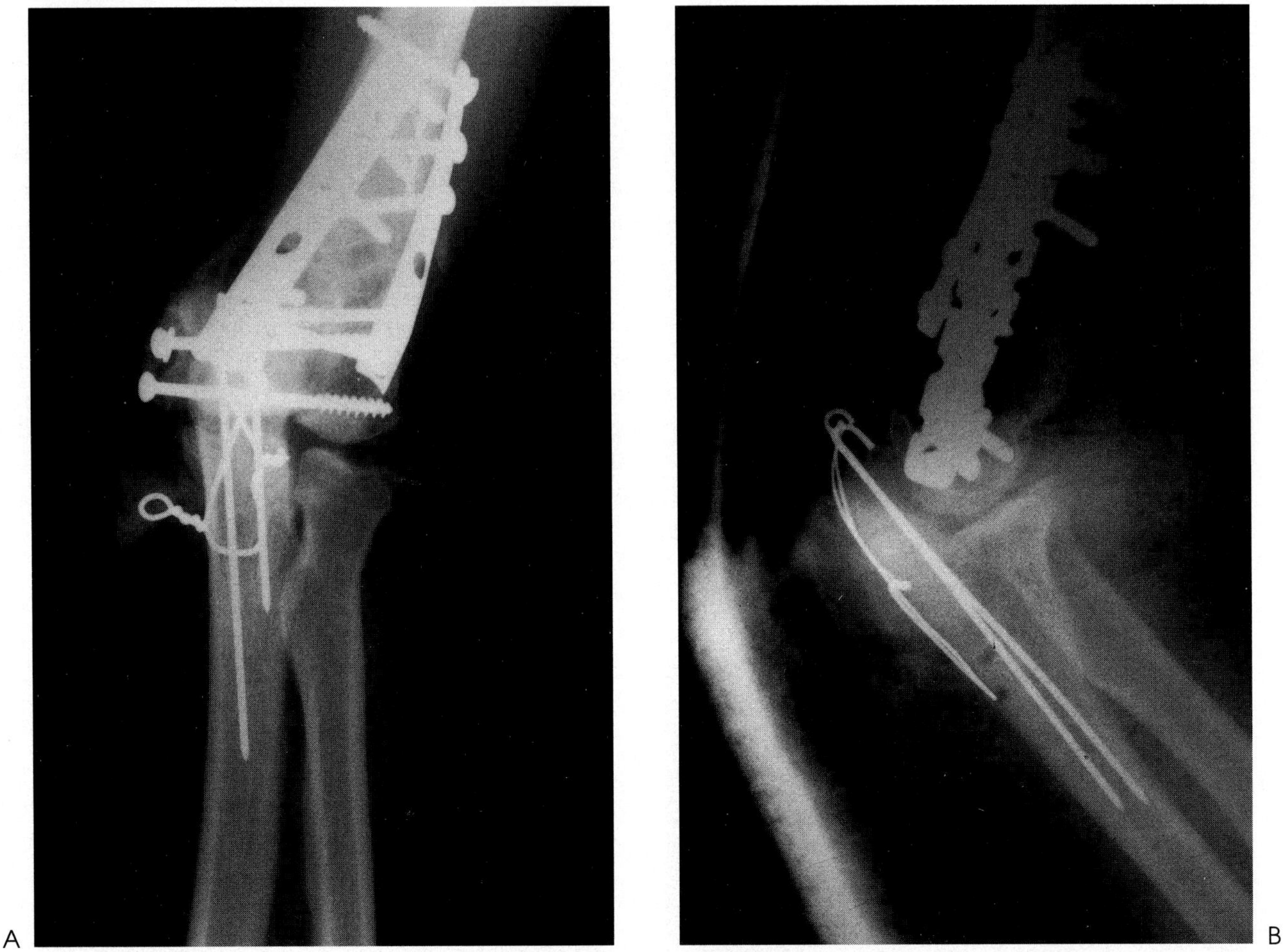

Figure 14–7. Anteroposterior (A) and lateral (B) radiographs taken 9 months after the injury.

In rare circumstances the missing bone segment may be intraarticular in location. Again, this is most likely to occur in the knee and elbow, although the medial malleolus may occasionally be at risk. An example of a patient with a missing intraarticular bone segment is shown in Figures 14–6 and 14–7. A 43-year-old female who jumped 50 feet from a building sustained multiple injuries including a closed head injury and a number of severe musculoskeletal injuries. The most severe fracture was an open fracture of the left distal humerus. There was a 5 cm skin incision on the posteromedial aspect of the joint. Anteroposterior and lateral radiographs showed an extremely comminuted distal humeral fracture (Fig. 14–6). This shows extensive bone destruction of the metaphysis and joint surface. Using the AO classification this is a 13–C3.3 fracture.

The surgical approach was the same as for the first patient. The articular surface was sought, but the only part that could be located was the capitellum. This was reduced to the humeral diaphysis and fixed with a one third tubular plate. Some remnant of the trochlea were found, but they were small and most were devitalized. They were therefore discarded. This left a large bone defect that required reconstruction. The left iliac crest was prepared and a tricortical block of bone harvested and shaped to fit the trochlear defect. The bone graft was oriented so that the crest of the ilium fitted into the olecranon and initially it was secured to the capitellum with two interfragmentary screws. Definitive fixation was subsequently provided by a bone plate. The olecranon was secured with Kirschner wires and figure of eight wiring and the wound was closed. Radiographs taken 8 months after surgery revealed good union of the graft with the adjacent bone (Fig. 14–7). The joint surface looked reasonable and the patient functioned well. Five years after the surgery she was pain free and able to play tennis, although she only had elbow flexion from 50 to 120 degrees.

Alternative Methods of Management

There are no good alternatives to the use of bone plates and screws in the reconstruction of the distal humerus. Nonoperative management would guarantee articular incongruity, posttraumatic osteoarthritis, and pain. It is likely that the use of Kirschner wires to reconstruct the joint surface would give a similar result. The obvious alternative method of management is to reconstruct the articular fragments and then shorten the arm by about 1 in by fixing the reconstructed articular fragment to the humeral metaphysis. There is as yet little data in the literature about the success of this type of approach, although it might be just as successful as the method chosen. It would be unlikely that secondary humeral lengthening would be required because the loss of 1 in of humeral length would be unlikely to give rise to significant symptoms. The fixation of a shortened metaphysis would be relatively straightforward, although the application of two plates might be technically difficult.

Theoretically, external skeletal fixation could have been used to stabilize the fracture, particularly if the metaphysis had been shortened. However, pin fixation in the distal metaphyseal fragment would have been difficult and it is likely that the fixa-

Type of Management	Advantages	Disadvantages	Comments
Nonoperative	None	Inadequate fixation; high infection rate; poor function; malunion; nonunion	There are no indications for nonoperative management in these types of fractures providing the patient is fit for surgery
Open reduction; internal fixation	Stable fixation; good alignment; ease of flap cover; early movement	Technically difficult	The optimal fixation method for these fractures
External fixation (nonbridging)	Probably none	Technically very difficult; neurovascular damage from pins or wires; interference with flap cover; pin sepsis	There is little information in the literature about the use of external fixation in this type of fracture
Intramedullary nailing	None	An almost impossible technique	It would be very difficult to use an intramedullary technique for this type of fracture.
Arthroplasty	Secondary joint replacement very useful for posttraumatic osteoarthritis	Primary arthroplasty very difficult in severe fractures	Secondary arthroplasty recommended for posttraumatic osteoarthritis

tion would have been suboptimal. If a small wire external fixator had been used, great care in wire placement would have been required to avoid the neurovascular structures in the area. Pin track sepsis and interference with flap cover would probably also occur. External fixation has no advantages over plate fixation in this fracture.

In the second patient the obvious alternative treatment is primary or secondary arthroplasty. Primary arthroplasty could be considered, but the destruction of the two columns of the distal humerus would mean that a hinged elbow replacement with long humeral and ulnar stems would be required. In a young person the prognosis for this would be poor and any salvage surgery, should the prosthesis fail, would be difficult if not impossible. Thus, it is preferable to treat the fracture by internal fixation and bone grafting and reserve arthroplasty for a secondary procedure if necessary.

The alternative plastic surgery treatment for the first patient would have been to use a free latissimus dorsi or rectus abdominis flap. The surgery would have been more complex but the donor site cosmesis might have been more acceptable to the patient.

Complications

The most likely complications associated with these types of severe open fracture are infection and joint stiffness. Infection can be minimized by an adequate initial debridement, repeat debridement within 48 hours, and early flap cover. The literature suggests that flap cover should be performed within 5 days to lessen the chance of infection, but ideally the flap should be applied within 2 or 3 days and the most convenient time to do this is at the follow-up procedure. If infection occurs, it may lead to nonunion, osteoarthritis, joint stiffness, and even to amputation if untreated. Treatment requires early debridement and appropriate soft tissue cover with secondary bone grafting as needed.

Secondary osteoarthritis in the elbow is not uncommon and can often be successfully treated by nonsteroidal antiinflammatory drugs; but if the symptoms are severe, consideration should be given to elbow arthroplasty.

Suggested Readings

Court-Brown CM, McQueen MM, Quaba AA (eds): Management of Open Fractures. Martin Dunitz, London, 1996.

Flatow EL, Ulrich C (eds): Humerus. Butterworth Heinemann, Oxford, 1996.

Helfet DL, Schmeling GJ: Bicondylar intraarticular fractures of the distal humerus in adults. Clin Orthop 1993; 292:26–36.

Jupiter JB, Neff U, Hozach P, Allgöwer M: Intercondylar fractures of the humerus. J Bone Joint Surg (Am) 1985; 67A:226–239.

Müller ME, Allgöwer M, Schneider R, Willenegger H: Manual of Internal Fixation, 3rd ed. Springer Verlag, Berlin, 1991.

Södergard J, Sandelin J, Böstman Ö: Postoperative complications of distal humeral fractures. Acta Orthop Scand 1992; 63:85–89.

Case 15

History and Physical Examination

A 16-year-old male was admitted to the emergency department following an accident. He had been attempting a cartwheel when his right elbow gave way underneath him. On admission the right elbow was very painful. The patient held the elbow at 90 degrees of flexion and no movement was possible. Examination showed no evidence of distal neurovascular deficit.

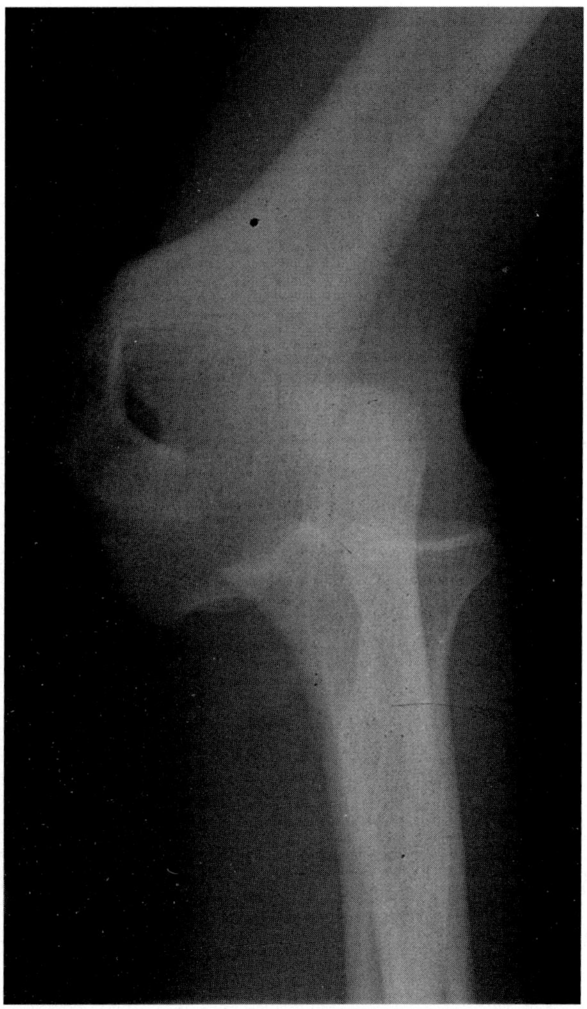

A

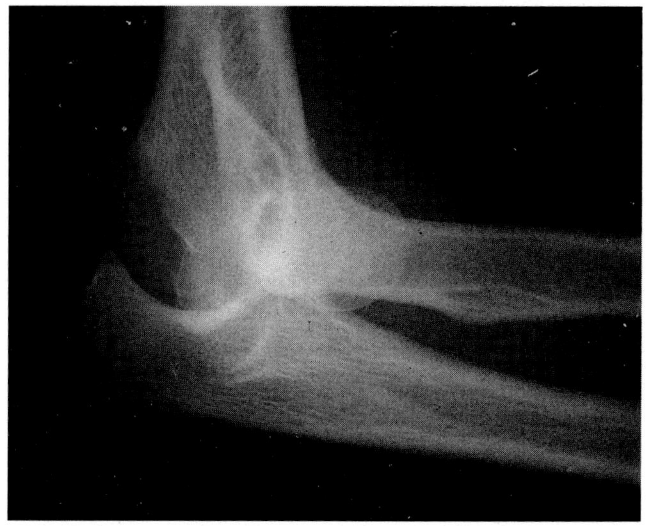

B

Figure 15–1. Anteroposterior (A) and lateral (B) radiographs showing a dislocated elbow with a fracture of the medial epicondyle.

Radiologic Findings

Anteroposterior and lateral radiographs showed a dislocation of the elbow, with the proximal forearm lying lateral to the distal humerus (Fig. 15–1). Close inspection of the anteroposterior radiograph showed a radio-opaque area in the distal humerus and the lateral radiograph showed a foreshortened medial epicondyle, suggesting the presence of an intraarticular bone fragment.

Diagnosis

An elbow dislocation associated with a medial epicondylar fracture.

Surgical Management

The patient was admitted to the orthopedic unit and taken to the operating room. Initially a gentle manipulation was undertaken and fluoroscopy used to determine whether there was a piece of bone within the joint. The fluoroscopic image confirmed the presence of the medial epicondyle within the joint and that the joint was subluxed (Fig. 15–2).

Accordingly, the right arm was prepped and draped for surgery and a curved incision made along the medial side of the elbow joint just above the medial epicondyle. The ulnar nerve was visualized and seen to be intact. The anterior capsule and me-

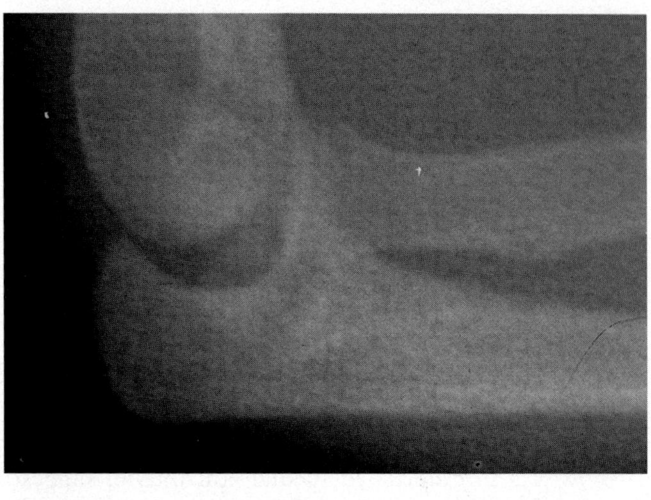

Figure 15–2. Fluoroscopy indicated the intraarticular bone fragment.

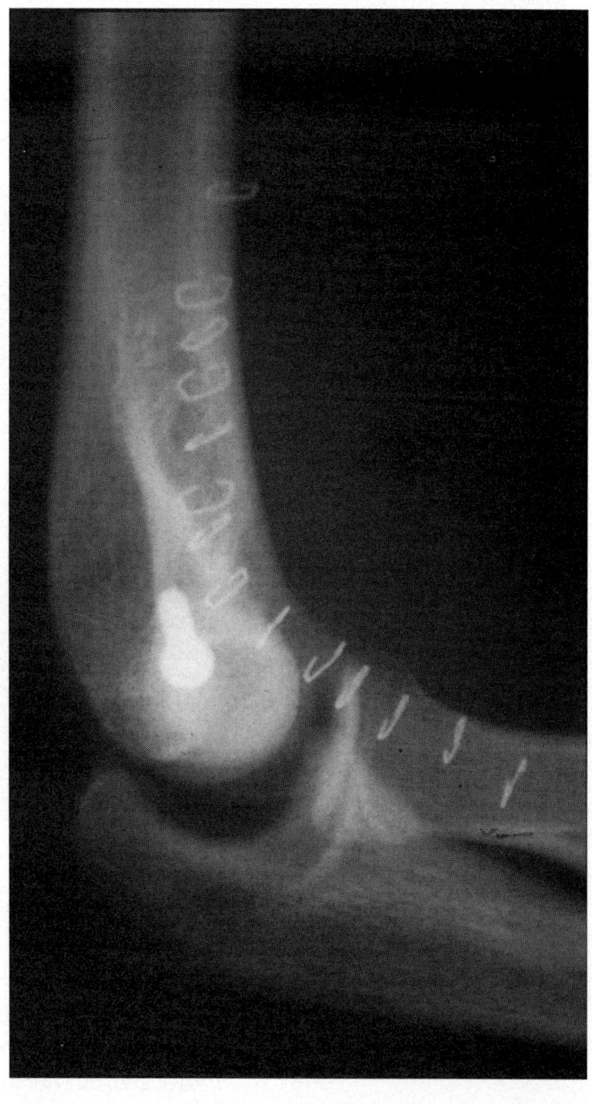

Figure 15–3. A lateral radiograph showing apparent subluxation.

PEARL

- Under anesthesia a lateral radiograph of an elbow associated with significant soft tissue damage may show an apparent subluxation. This is due to tissue laxity and the temporary paralysis of the local muscle. If the joint remains subluxed with the patient awake, the surgeon should be aware of the possibility of a loose body.

dial collateral ligament had been divided and the medial epicondyle with the attached flexor muscle mass was seen to be within the joint. The joint was extremely unstable when a valgus force was applied.

The joint was inspected, but there was no evidence of any other intraarticular bone fragments. The joint was thoroughly lavaged and the medial epicondyle was reduced and fixed with one small fragment bone screw. The anterior capsule was repaired with absorbable sutures and the skin closed. The elbow was noted to be more stable, although it still opened slightly when a valgus force was applied. A postoperative radiograph suggested persistent subluxation (Fig. 15–3) but this was thought to be due to the deficient anterior capsule and the patient was returned to the ward.

Postoperative Management

A plaster back slab was applied postoperatively and further radiographs were obtained the following morning. These showed that the joint was well reduced (Fig. 15–4). The back slab was maintained for 1 week to rest the elbow and then a functional brace was applied with a single lateral hinge. This permitted elbow flexion extension but minimized the valgus force across the joint. The functional brace was retained for 2 weeks and then a gradual physiotherapy regime was introduced. Six months after the injury the patient had full flexion and rotation and had lost only 10 degrees of active extension. He had virtually normal function.

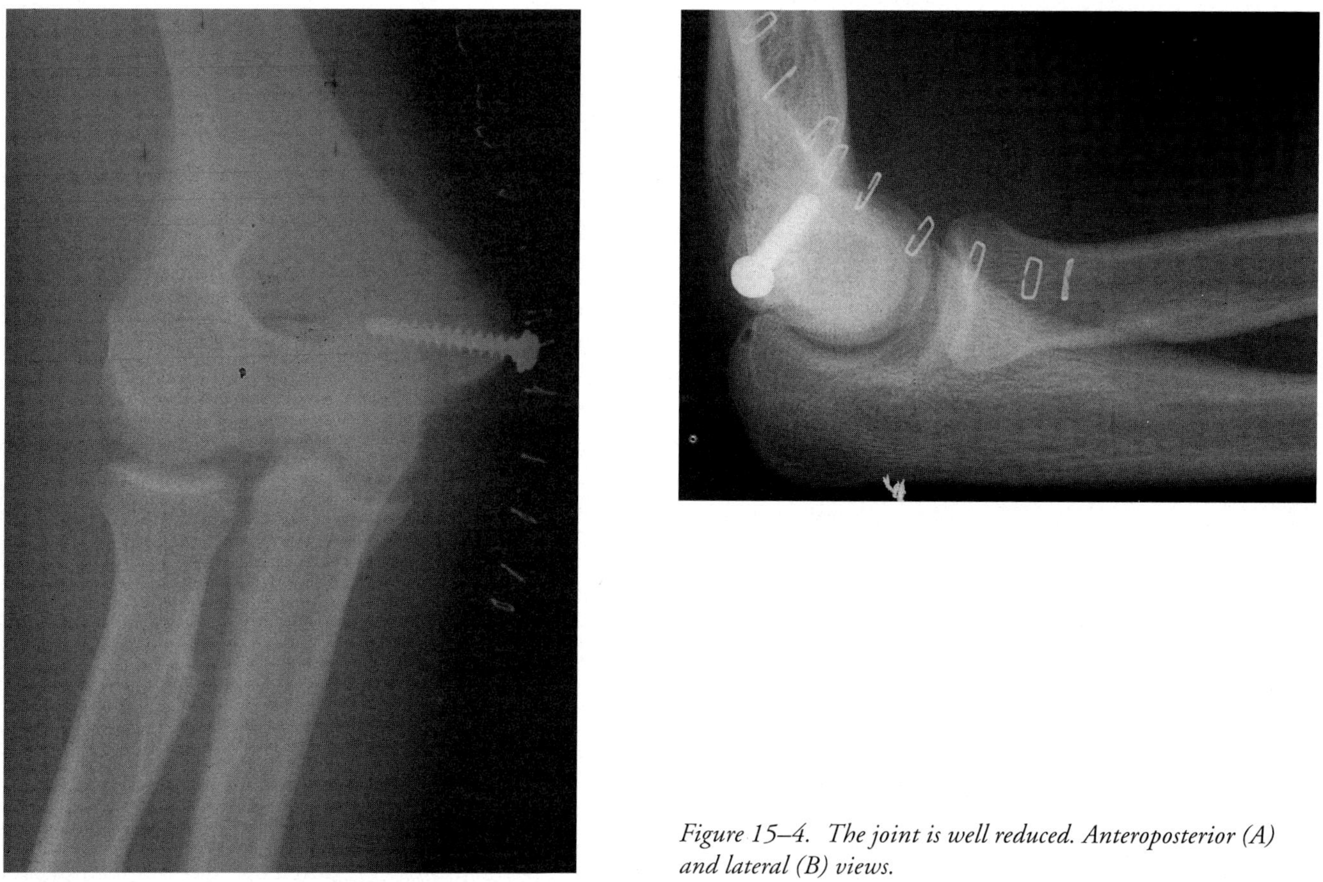

A B

Figure 15–4. The joint is well reduced. Anteroposterior (A) and lateral (B) views.

Discussion

The soft tissue damage associated with an apparently simple elbow dislocation is often inadequately appreciated by orthopaedic surgeons. It is impossible to dislocate the normal elbow without some soft tissue damage being present. The extent of the damage will often define the prognosis and may well dictate treatment in some circumstances. Josefsson et al. (1987) analyzed the instability that followed elbow dislocation in 31 cases. They showed that there was medial instability in all cases, but lateral instability was only present in eight cases. Nine of the elbows that they examined could be re-dislocated under general anesthesia. Their most common finding at surgical exploration was that the muscular origin of the flexor muscles was partially or totally avulsed from the medial epicondyle or ruptured in the tendinomuscular substance. This had occurred in 19 of their 31 patients, and they noted that the medial collateral ligament had been ruptured or avulsed in all cases. The authors explored the lateral side of the elbow in 18 cases and found that the lateral collateral ligament had been avulsed in all cases and that in 14 of the 18 cases there was significant local muscle damage. The anterior capsule and brachialis muscle were damaged in all patients. They further noted that eight of the nine patients who had elbows that were re-dislocated under anesthesia had significant medial and lateral damage. There has been considerable debate about whether the extensive soft tissue damage associated with elbow dislocation should be repaired. Superficially, this seems an attractive concept on the grounds that the elbow joint would regain stability earlier and joint movement would be facilitated. However, remarkably little evidence exists that this is the case. Josefsson and his coworkers extended their earlier work on elbow instability and compared surgical and nonsurgical treatment of ligamentous injury after dislocation. They found no evidence that surgery helped the patient and even in those patients with elbows that were re-dislocatable under anesthesia they could not demonstrate any advantage in repairing the soft tissue injury. Their work has confirmed the findings of other orthopaedic surgeons.

Operative intervention for closed elbow dislocation would seem to have few indications. The case illustrated here is an example of a bony block to elbow reduction. This usually occurs because a medial epicondylar fragment has been pulled into the joint or a fragment of the head of the radius or a large osteochondral fragment has become displaced into an intraarticular location. Other indications for operative exploration and repair of soft tissues are persistent instability of the elbow such that the reduced position cannot be maintained in a cast or significant fracture of the coronoid process or olecranon. In these instances it is important to internally fix the associated fracture.

Osborne and Cotterill (1966) described the phenomenon of recurrent dislocation of the elbow. They suggested that in this condition the posterolateral ligament and capsule fail to reattach properly after dislocation. This creates a soft tissue defect into which the radial head can dislocate. They suggested that if there had been osteocondylar damage or damage to the medial soft tissue structures, the tendency to repeatedly dislocate was higher. This condition is rare but if it is encountered, surgical stabilization is advocated. The operation of choice is application of the lateral structures supplemented by a repair of the medial tissues if these are lax.

Alternative Methods of Management

It has been suggested that the intraarticular medial epicondylar fragment could be removed by arthroscopic means. This is almost certainly true, but there would seem to be little benefit from this procedure. If stability is to be gained, the epicondylar

PITFALL

- If Kirschner wire fixation is to be used, the wires should be passed under direct vision because of the proximity of the ulnar nerve.

fragment should be reattached with a screw. Kirschner wire fixation might well be used in children; in adults rigid screw fixation is preferable. Repair of the anterior capsule is not mandatory but does seem sensible if the joint is open to allow epicondylar reattachment. Care must be taken not to overtighten the anterior capsule and thereby interfere with later joint extension.

Type of Management	Advantages	Disadvantages	Comments
Epicondyle fixation and cast management	Regain stability; early soft tissue motion; good joint congruity	Ulnar nerve damage	This is the method of choice for elbow dislocations associated with a fracture of the medial epicondyle
Epicondylar fixation and repair of soft tissues	Regain stability; early soft tissue motion; good joint congruity	Ulnar nerve damage	Would appear to have no advantage over traditional cast management unless the elbow is very unstable

Complications

The phenomenon of recurrent dislocation has already been described. This is a rare complication and unlikely to be encountered by most surgeons. More common complications of elbow dislocation include joint stiffness, myositis ossificans, and occasional neurovascular dysfunction.

The most likely problem encountered by surgeons is joint stiffness. With an adequate physiotherapy regime it is unusual to find significant stiffness unless there has been a coexisting fracture with the dislocation. The patient may not regain full extension, but the deficit rarely provides a functional problem. Anterior capsulotomy or capsulectomy can be undertaken if there is a significant block to extension.

The treatment of myositis ossificans has been detailed in the case dealing with Monteggio fracture dislocation. The ideal method of management is to wait until the heterotopic ossification is mature and then excise it using prophylactic indomethicin, which should be given for at least 6 weeks.

Suggested Readings

Dürig M, Müller W, Rüedi T, Gauer EF: The operative treatment of elbow dislocation in the adult. J Bone Joint Surg (Am) 1979; 61A:239–244.

Habernek H, Ortner F: The influence of anatomic factors in elbow joint dislocation. Clin Orthop 1992; 274:226–230.

Josefsson PO, Gentz CF, Johnell O, Wenderberg B: Surgical versus nonsurgical treatment of ligamentous injuries following dislocations of the elbow joint. Clin Orthop 1987; 214:165–169.

Josefsson PO, Johnell O, Gentz CF: Long term sequelae of simple dislocation of the elbow. J Bone Joint Surg (Am) 1984; 66A:927–930.

Josefsson PO, Johnell O, Wendeberg B: Ligamentous injuries in dislocations of the elbow joint. Clin Orthop 1987; 221:221–225.

Osborne G, Cotterill P: Recurrent dislocation of the elbow. J Bone Joint Surg (Br) 1966; 48B:340–346.

Case 16

History and Physical Examination

A 46-year-old man was admitted to the emergency department having been found lying by the side of a road. He had been struck by a car. Examination showed the patient to be drunk, confused, and irritable, with a Glasgow Coma Scale of 12. Neurological examination failed to show any sign of a serious head injury and a subsequent computerized axial tomography (CAT) scan of the head did not indicate significant intracranial damage.

There was an open fracture dislocation of the left elbow associated with a 15 cm soft tissue wound on the lateral side of the joint. An adequate neurological examination of the arm was not possible because of the patient's condition, but he did not appear to have normal movement in the left arm. On admission to the emergency department, the radial pulse could not be palpated although there was capillary return in the fingers.

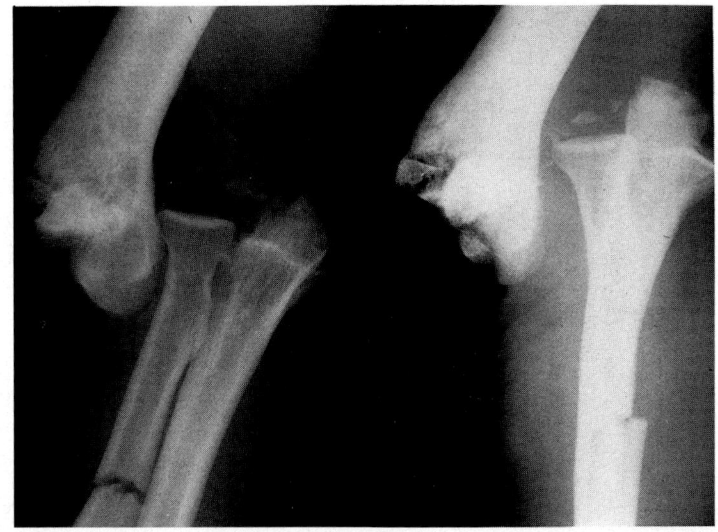

Figure 16–1. Anteroposterior (A) and lateral (B) radiographs of a severe open fracture of the distal humerus associated with elbow dislocation and a fracture of the radial diaphysis.

Radiologic Findings

Anteroposterior and lateral radiographs of the left elbow showed a fracture dislocation of the elbow (Fig. 16–1). There was a coronal fracture of the capitellum and an avulsion fracture of the olecranon. There was also a minimally displaced transverse fracture of the proximal radial diaphysis. There was considerable displacement of the elbow joint suggesting gross soft tissue damage and instability.

Diagnosis

Gustilo type III fracture of the distal humerus associated with dislocation of the elbow and significant soft tissue damage. It can be difficult to distinguish between Gustilo IIIa and IIIb fractures preoperatively, but the absence of a radial pulse also raised the possibility of this being a Gustilo IIIc fracture.

Surgical Management

It was obviously important to reduce the dislocation and see if the radial pulse returned. The patient did not require sedation for this maneuver. Fortunately, elbow reduction completely revascularized the arm and the radial pulse became palpable. The patient was subsequently taken to the operating room and the wound cleaned and lavaged. The arm was then prepped and draped and the lateral soft tissue defect was extended proximally and distally to facilitate exposure of the joint. The soft tissue damage was noted to be severe. There was complete disruption of the triceps mechanism and both the medial and lateral collateral ligaments had been transected. Examination of the joint capsule showed that only the lateral portion remained intact.

The radial diaphyseal fracture was plated using a 6-hole dynamic compression plate and the posterior interosseous nerve was inspected and found to be intact. The capitellar fracture was reduced and fixed using three cancellous screws. A careful inspection was made of the ulnar and median nerves and both were noted to be damaged but intact. The triceps mechanism and both collateral ligaments were repaired and the olecranon was reattached using Kirschner wires and a figure of eight wire (Fig. 16–2). The joint was stabilized by a transarticular external fixator with half pins placed in the humeral and ulnar diaphyses (Fig. 16–3). The wound was left open and dressed with a moist antiseptic dressing.

PEARLS

- The Gustilo classification applies particularly to diaphyseal fractures. In intraarticular fractures there is often much less periosteal and muscle damage than in a diaphyseal fracture of equivalent severity. Its use in these fractures is debatable.
- Care must be exercised in placing the humeral external fixation pins. They must be placed away from the area of the radial nerve. To avoid nerve damage, an open insertion technique should be used and the bone exposed before pin insertion.

PITFALL

- When a patient is drunk and may also have a closed head injury it is important to try to assess the degree of intoxication and the extent of the head injury. The distinction between the two is sometimes difficult and the Glasgow Coma Scale may be inaccurate if the patient is drunk. Not only might there be medical problems if the wrong condition is treated but there may also be significant medico-legal implications. If possible, a blood alcohol level should be obtained.

Postoperative Management

On the day following surgery it was possible to examine the neurological state of the left arm. There were complete ulnar and radial nerve palsies, but median nerve function was normal. Because surgery had indicated that the nerves were intact it was concluded that the patient had either a neuropraxia or axonotmesis of both the radial and ulnar nerves and no further action was taken. The patient was returned to the operating room 2 days after admission and inspection indicated that there was no residual contamination or further muscle damage. The soft tissues were closed at that time.

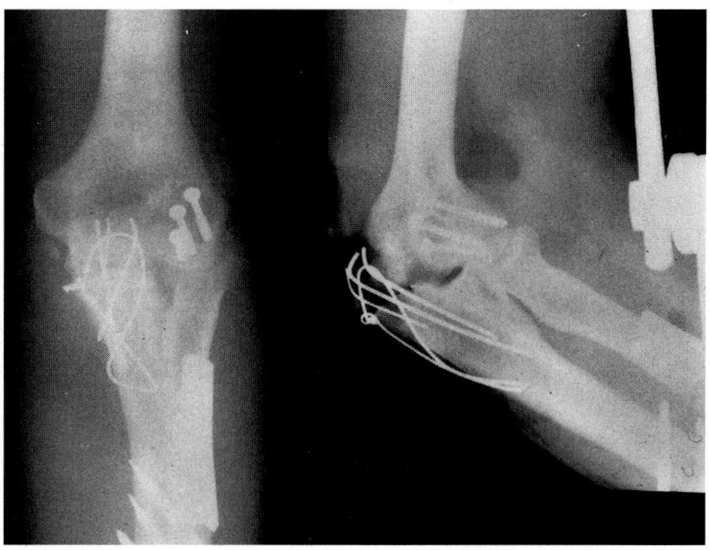

A B

Figure 16–2. Anteroposterior (A) and lateral (B) postoperative radiographs showing the articular reconstruction, the radial plating, and the position of the fixator pins.

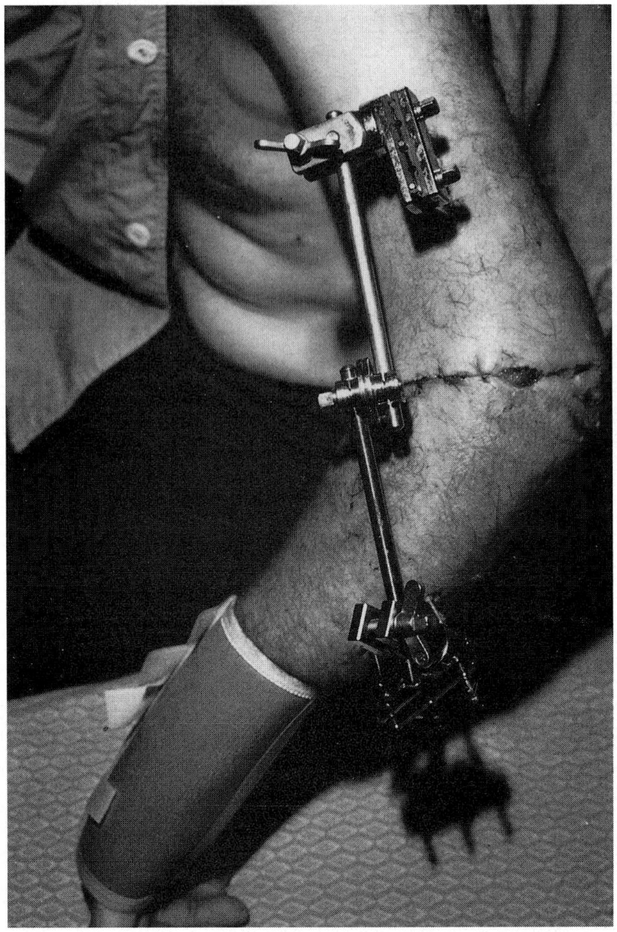

Figure 16–3. The transarticular external fixator. Note the size of the skin wound. A simple wrist splint was used to compensate for the posterior interosseous nerve palsy.

The external fixation device was maintained for 2 weeks and following its removal an elbow mobilizer was used to help regain elbow motion. The elbow mobilizer was maintained for 2 weeks and then a physiotherapy regime of passive and active elbow motion was started. Nerve conduction studies were undertaken 4 weeks after the injury and showed no evidence of voluntary activity in the radial

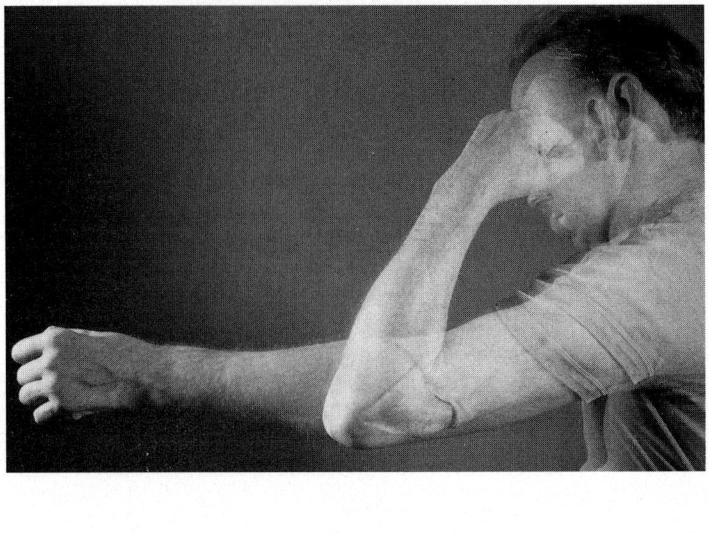

Figure 16–4. The final result showing that good movement was obtained.

or ulnar nerves. The study was reported to be suggestive of radial and ulnar axonotmesis.

Five months after the accident there was no evidence of return of radial or ulnar nerve function; however, electromyographic studies did suggest some reinnervation of the proximal forearm musculature, and full function in both radial and ulnar nerves was reestablished about 18 months after the injury. Final elbow function was good with flexion from 15 to 140 degrees, and full rotation was obtained (Fig. 16–4).

Discussion

Open fractures of the distal humerus occur with about the same frequency as open fractures of the humeral diaphysis. Court-Brown et al. (1996) analyzed 1000 consecutive open fractures presenting to the Edinburgh orthopaedic trauma unit over a 6 year period and found that 17 (1.7%) involved the distal humerus. However, the majority of these were extraarticular. The average age of the patients who presented with open distal humeral fractures was 44 years, and over 70% had sustained their injury in a traffic accident or a simple fall. Most of the soft tissue injuries were fairly minor, with eight (47.1%) of the patients having Gustilo type I fractures, seven (41.2%) had type II fractures, and the remaining two (11.8%) Gustilo type III in severity. Thus the type of open fracture illustrated here is relatively unusual.

The management of open intraarticular fractures has received little attention in recent years. However, the general principles of treatment are the same as for extraarticular fractures. These involve a thorough debridement with removal of all devitalized and contaminated tissue, rigid stabilization of the fracture, and early joint mobilization. In this case the soft tissues were closed secondarily, but flap cover may often be required because it is important to have good quality soft tissue over the elbow joint. The only real difference between intra- and extraarticular fractures is that many of the soft tissues around the joint have a stabilizing role and consequently should be repaired. It is interesting to note that there is little evidence that surgical repair of damaged collateral ligaments in closed elbow dislocations is worthwhile. However, the severe soft tissue damage associated with this type of injury should be repaired to improve joint stability and facilitate early joint movement.

There has been a move away from transarticular external fixation in the management of juxta- and intraarticular fractures with surgeons preferring periarticular external fixators that permit joint movement. However, this case represents a good indication for spanning a joint with an external fixator. Obviously the soft tissue repair will need to be protected for a period, but the alternative use of a plaster cast would prevent the surgeon from examining the damaged soft tissues. A transarticular frame supports the joint with minimal damage.

Alternative Methods of Management

There are no adequate alternatives to the method of management used in this case. Nonoperative management utilizing either plaster management or traction followed by the use of a cast would be ill advised. It would guarantee an incongruous joint, posttraumatic osteoarthritis, pain, and stiffness. The risk of infection would also be much higher. Kirschner wire fixation of the intraarticular fragments would also provide inadequate fracture fixation and early movement would be impossible because a postoperative cast would be required.

Type of Management	Advantages	Disadvantages	Comments
Nonoperative	None	Instability; pain; joint stiffness; osteoarthritis	No indication if facilities for surgery exist
Internal fixation and soft tissue repair	Early motion; stable joint; good range of motion	Technically difficult	Would need postoperative cast stabilization if external fixator not used
Transarticular external fixation	Good stability; soft tissue access; patient comfort	Radial nerve damage	Best method if combined with appropriate internal fixation

Complications

The main complications that follow this type of severe intraarticular injury are joint stiffness and posttraumatic osteoarthritis. The former is minimized by early joint movement and the latter by good reconstructive surgery. However, no matter how good the surgery and the postoperative rehabilitation regime, the severity of the soft tissue injury and the damage to the articular cartilage means that these complications occur fairly frequently.

Joint stiffness is difficult to treat. Usually the patient complains of poor extension and an inability to reach forward easily. The loss of up to 30 degrees of extension is rarely accompanied by a serious functional deformity and the patient should be advised of this before any form of surgical intervention is undertaken. However, if the deformity is severe, the surgeon may undertake an anterior capsulotomy or capsulectomy. This operation is straightforward, provided the surgeon is careful to avoid damaging the local neurovascular structures. However, the postoperative regime can be exacting if a good result is to be achieved. The patient should be made aware of this before treatment. Postoperative osteoarthritis initially will be treated by the use of nonsteroidal antiinflammatory medication and local physiotherapy measures. However, if these are unsuccessful, consideration should be given to elbow arthroplasty.

In this case the patient had a neuropraxia of both the ulnar and radial nerves. His neural signs resolved, although he took over a year to return to normal. Unfortunately, not all nerve damage resolves and the surgeon may be faced with reconstructive surgery involving muscle transfer, nerve grafting, and joint stabilization.

Suggested Readings

Aitken GK, Rorabeck CH: Distal humeral fractures in the adult. Clin Orthop 1986; 207:191–197.

Court-Brown CM, McQueen MM, Quaba AA (eds): Management of Open Fractures. Martin Dunitz, London, 1996.

Flatow EL, Ulrich C (eds): Humerus. Butterworth Heinemann, Oxford, 1996.

Josefsson PO, Gentz CF, Johnell O, Wendeberg B: Surgical versus non-surgical treatment of ligamentous injuries following dislocations of the elbow joint. J Bone Joint Surg 1987; 69A:605–608.

Jupiter JB, Mehne DK: Trauma to the adult elbow and fractures of the distal humerus. In: Browner BD, Jupiter JB, Levine AM, Trafton PG (eds): Musculoskeletal Trauma. WB Saunders, Philadelphia, 1992.

Simpson LA, Richards RR: Internal fixation of a capitellar fracture using Herbert screws. Clin Orthop 1986; 209:166–169.

Case 17

History and Physical Examination

A 32-year-old woman slipped and fell, injuring her right arm. She immediately experienced severe pain and deformity of the right elbow. She arrived at the emergency department 30 minutes later, where the physical examination revealed no injury other than that to the elbow. Obvious varus deformity of the elbow and shortening of the arm were present. The elbow was fixed at 30 degrees, and attempted flexion and extension were extremely painful. Despite the onset of swelling, the epicondyles were palpable and their normal relationship to the olecranon was absent. The neurovascular examination of the wrist and hand was within the limits of normal. Pain was not present with palpation of the distal radioulnar joint.

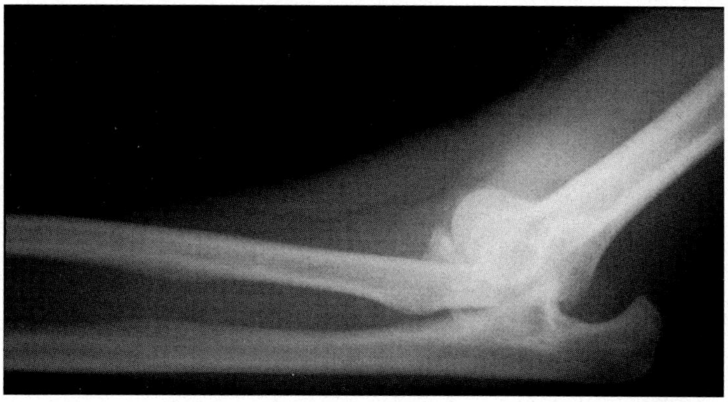

Figure 17–1. Lateral radiograph of elbow indicating a posterior dislocation and fracture of the radial head.

Radiologic Findings

Anteroposterior, lateral, and oblique radiographs of the elbow indicated a posterior lateral dislocation of the elbow with a displaced radial head fracture (Fig. 17–1). A fracture of the coronoid process or the epicondyles was not evident. Anteroposterior and lateral radiographs of the wrist and forearm were within the limits of normal.

Diagnosis

Posterior dislocation of the elbow with a displaced intraarticular fracture of the radial head. (There was no evidence on physical examination or radiographically of radioulnar diastasis, distal radioulnar joint disruption, bony avulsion of the ligaments, or fracture of the coronoid process.)

Surgical Management

The patient was sedated in the emergency department and 10 cc of 2% lidocaine was injected into the elbow. Reduction was performed by applying traction in line with the long axis of the forearm. Countertraction was applied to the humerus. The elbow relocated with an audible clunk. The elbow was flexed to 90 degrees and splinted.

PEARLS

- It is important to determine whether there is an associated wrist injury. A fractured radial head in combination with an injury of the distal radial ulnar joint indicates a possible radioulnar diastasis (e.g., Essex-Lopresti injury). The Essex-Lopresti injury can occur in association with an elbow dislocation and together these injuries have a far worse prognosis than either does singly.
- The stability of the elbow to varus and valgus stresses is determined with the elbow flexed to 30 degrees. This prevents an increase in stability that occurs when the olecranon engages the olecranon fossa.

PITFALL

- When evaluating an elbow dislocation, it is key to obtain good radiographs of the radial head and neck to determine whether a fracture is present. Displacing a previously undisplaced radial head or neck fracture during reduction of a dislocated elbow potentially compromises the final result and necessitates one of the following: radial head fixation, radial head replacement, medial collateral ligament repair, or external fixation. When an undisplaced or minimally displaced radial head or neck fracture is present, reduction should be performed with adequate local or general anesthesia. The reduction is monitored fluoroscopically to minimize the chance of displacing the radial head fracture.

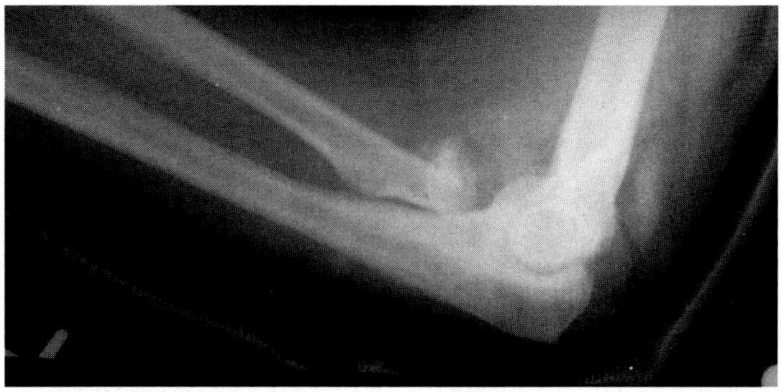

Figure 17–2. Lateral radiograph following closed reduction. The radial head is fractured

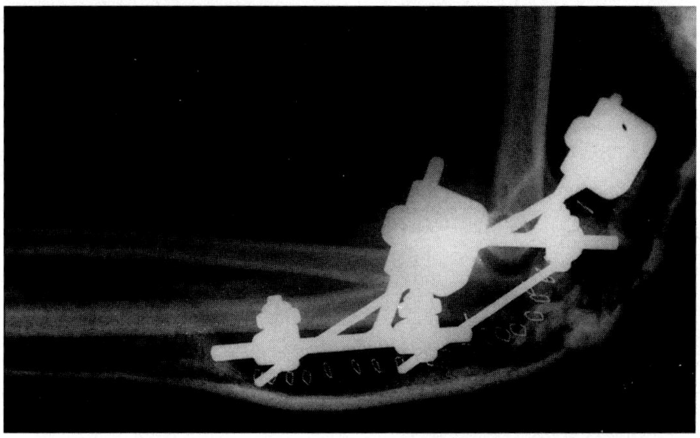

Figure 17–3. Lateral radiograph following resection of the radial head and application of a dynamic external fixator. At this point the elbow is immobilized in a posterior splint.

Reduction was confirmed by the physical examination (i.e., prior to reduction, flexion was not possible because of pain, whereas postreduction, gentle passive flexion was relatively painless and the normal relationship of the epicondyles to the olecranon was reestablished). Radiographs indicated a concentric reduction of the humeroulnar articulation and persistent displacement of the radial head fracture (Fig. 17–2).

The anconeus approach was used to expose the radial head in hopes of being able to reduce the fracture and stabilize it. The extensive comminution and compression of the articular surface made anatomic reduction and fixation impossible. The radial head was excised. When the elbow was not fully extended, it was extremely unstable to valgus stress.

An external fixator was applied across the elbow. The proximal fixator pin was driven from the medial epicondyle through the lateral epicondyle along the axis of rotation of the elbow. Two pins were placed in the ulna. The fixator allowed flexion and extension of the elbow and forearm rotation while preventing a change in varus or valgus alignment and medial or lateral displacement (Fig. 17–3).

Postoperative Management

Postoperatively, the elbow was splinted at 90 degrees for 1 week. At 1 week, when incisional pain had subsided, active and passive range of motion was initiated. The range of motion slowly increased, and 6 weeks after surgery the patient was able to extend her elbow to 30 degrees and flex it to 120 degrees. The fixator was removed

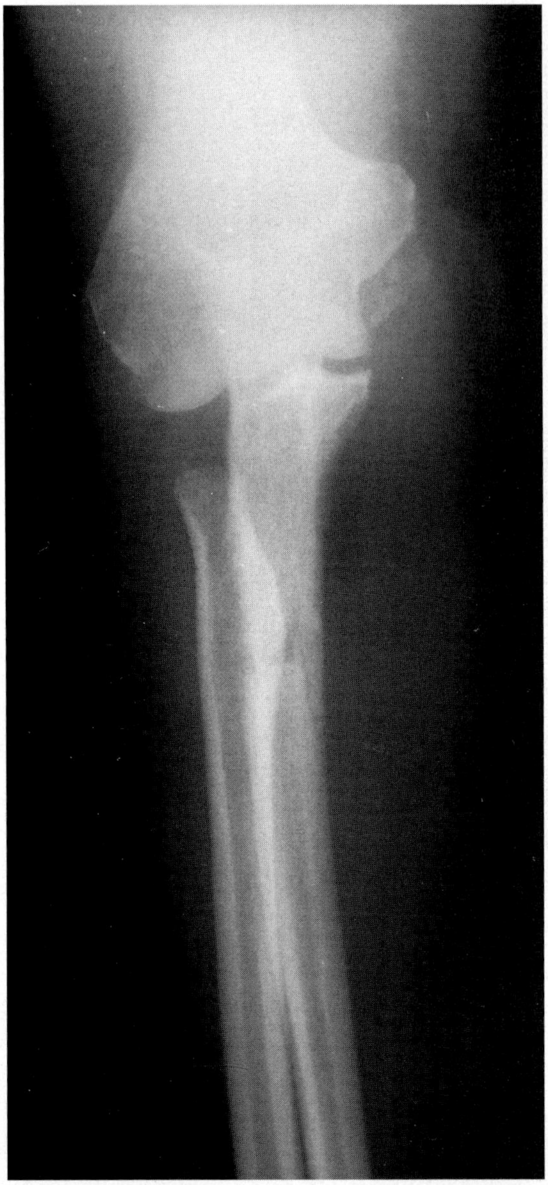

A

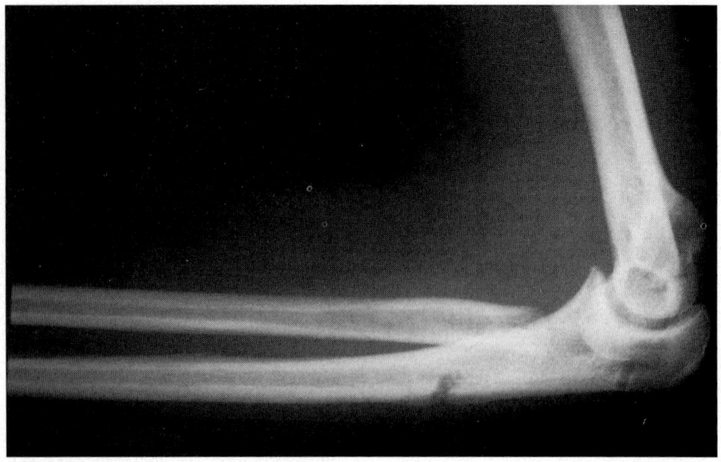

B

Figure 17–4. Anteroposterior (A) and lateral (B) radiographs of the elbow following fixator removal. The varus/valgus alignment and relationship of the olecranon to the distal humerus has been restored.

under general anesthesia at 6 weeks. The elbow was stable to a gentle valgus stress (Fig. 17–4). A hinged elbow brace was worn by the patient for the next 4 weeks. The range of motion at 6 months was 135 to 10 degrees of flexion and extension and 60 to 90 degrees of supination and pronation (Fig. 17–5).

Discussion

Elbow dislocations are classified according to the position of the olecranon and radial head in relation to the distal humerus as posterior, lateral, medial, anterior, and divergent. The majority of elbow dislocations are posterior. Lateral and medial dislocations are rare, and anterior and divergent dislocations are extremely rare. A fall on the outstretched upper extremity accounts for the vast majority of posterior

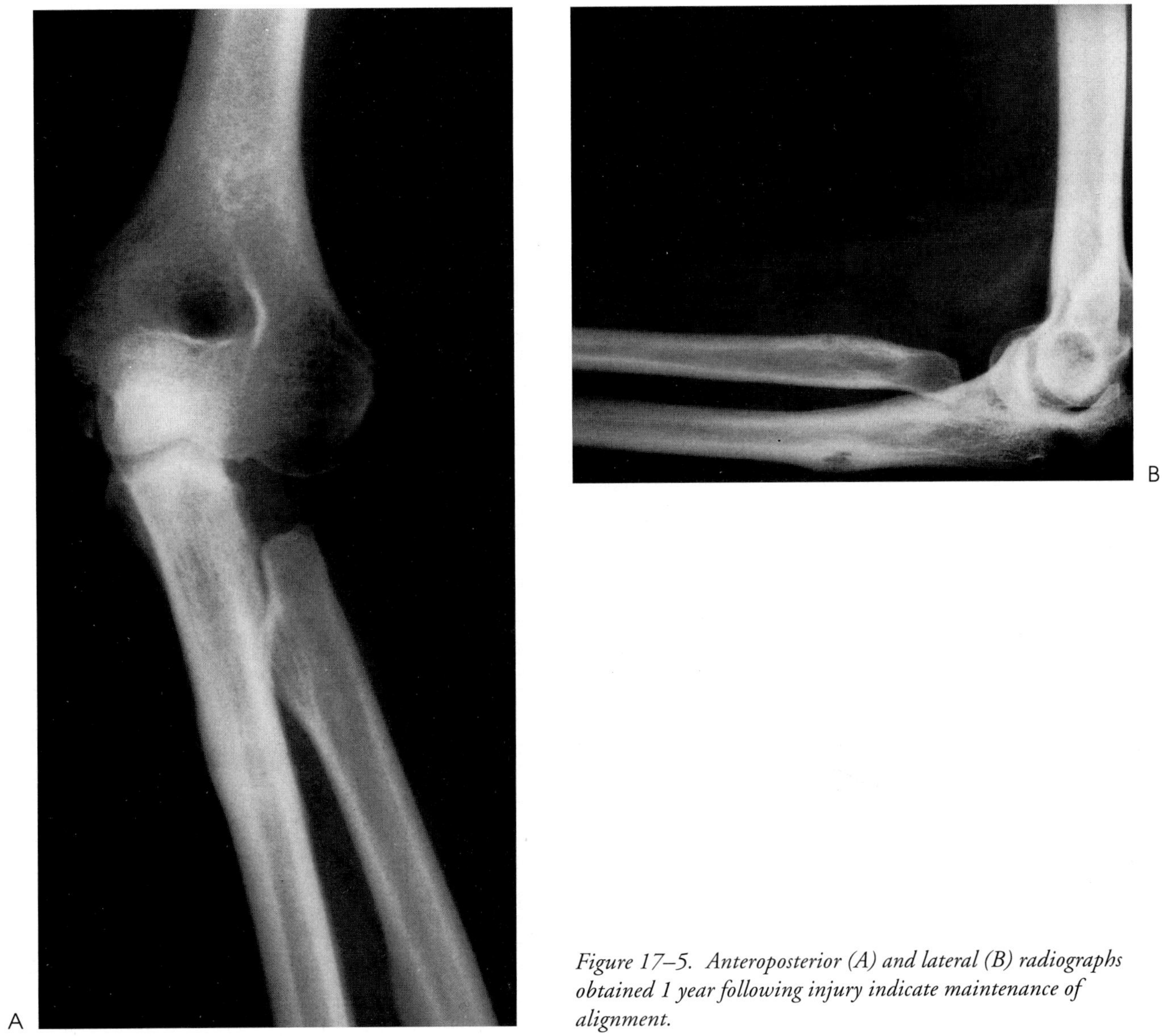

Figure 17–5. Anteroposterior (A) and lateral (B) radiographs obtained 1 year following injury indicate maintenance of alignment.

elbow dislocations. The mechanism of injury is either hyperextension or the ulna is driven posteriorly, as the coronoid impacts the distal humerus the coronoid usually fractures. Fractures of the radial head and neck complicate approximately 10% of posterior dislocations of the elbow. Other fractures frequently associated with posterior dislocations are avulsion fractures of the epicondyles, compression fractures of the capitellum, and fractures of the coronoid process. These associated fractures are all important because they indicate which structures have been damaged (e.g., the medial collateral ligament has been avulsed with a portion of the medial epicondyle) and because fragments of bone can become trapped between the articular surfaces during reduction, preventing a concentric reduction. An associated fracture of the radial head or neck is particularly troublesome because reduction and fixation are seldom possible, yet the radial head cannot be removed without the risk of valgus instability of the elbow.

Alternative Methods of Treatment

The goal of management of a posterior elbow dislocation with a radial head fracture is a stable joint with a functional range of motion. The radial head functions as the fulcrum against which the medial collateral ligament works. If the fractured radial head is simply removed following dislocation, valgus malalignment of the elbow is likely to occur, leading to laxity of the medial collateral ligament when it heals. A lax medial collateral ligament and absent radial head result in a chronically unstable elbow (Figs. 17–6 and 17–7). Prevention of valgus deformity by immobilization with pins across the elbow, a bridging external fixator, or a cast may result in unacceptable loss of joint motion. Because of these considerations, potential methods of management of a posterior elbow dislocation with a radial head fracture are to retain the radial head by reducing it and internally stabilizing it; replace the radial head with a prosthesis, which will resist valgus stresses applied to the elbow; repair the medial collateral ligament; or remove the radial head and prevent valgus stresses with a fixator that allows protected motion (dynamic external fixator) at the elbow. The radial head not only acts as a restraint to valgus

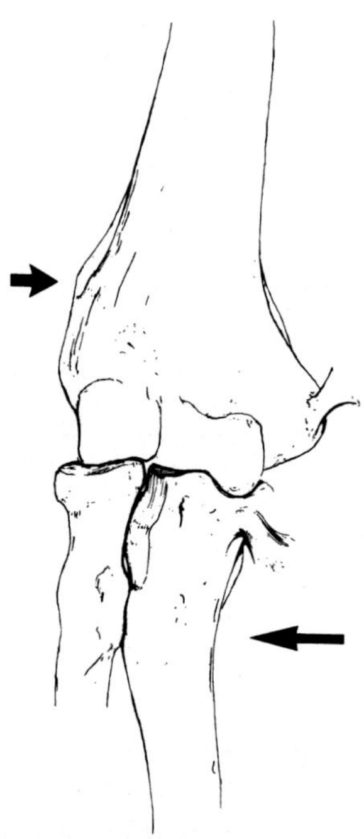

Figure 17–6. Schematic drawing of the elbow following radial head excision and stretching or tearing of the medial collateral ligament. When a valgus stress is applied, the elbow shortens laterally because the radial head is not present to act as a fulcrum; it opens medially because the medial collateral ligament is attenuated. The result is valgus instability.

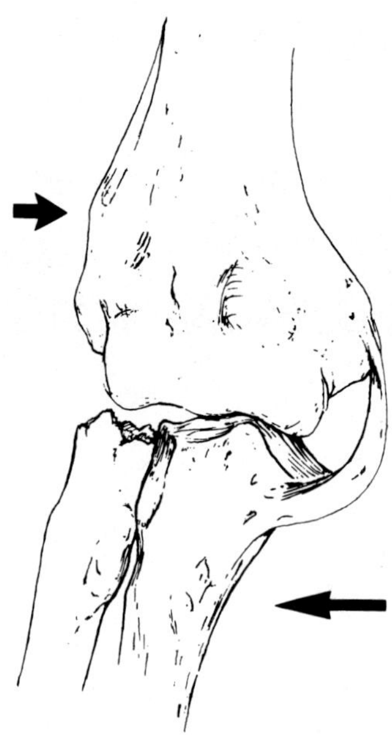

Figure 17–7. Schematic drawing of the elbow following rupture of the medial collateral ligament without fracture of the radial head. The radial head minimizes valgus instability by preventing lateral shortening.

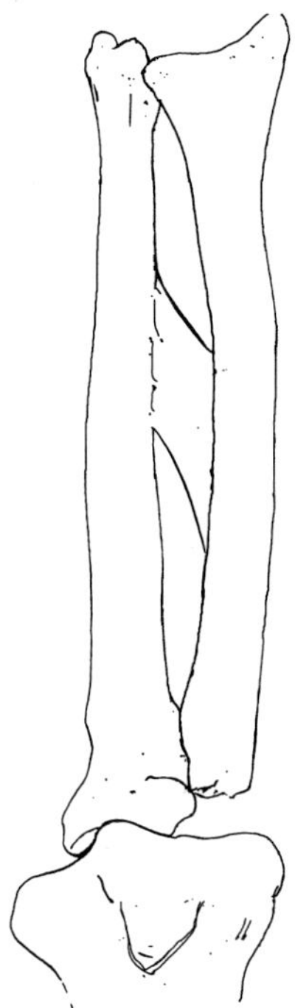

Figure 17–8. Schematic drawing of the forearm following isolated excision of the radial head. The intact interosseous membrane prevents proximal migration of the radius.

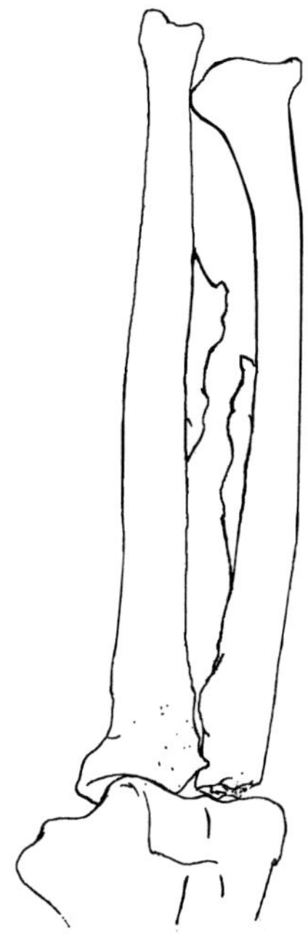

Figure 17–9. When the radial head is excised and the interosseous membrane is torn, there is no block to proximal migration of the radius.

stresses if the medial collateral ligament is intact, but also prevents proximal migration of the radius when the interosseous membrane is torn (Figs. 17–8 and 17–9). This is particularly important in the management of radioulnar dissociation with an associated radial head fracture. When this occurs, every effort must be made to retain or replace the radial head.

Type of Management	Advantages	Disdvantages	Comments
Open reduction and internal fixation (ORIF)	Restores normal anatomy	Anatomic reduction is difficult to achieve; loss of reduction can occur	Technically very difficult
Replacement with silastic prosthesis	Technically very easy	Does not provide adequate resistance to valgus stress; can fragment and cause synovitis	Titanium prosthesis may give better long term results than silastic
Repair medial collateral ligament	Restores normal anatomy	Difficult to achieve a solid repair; elbow must be immobilized postoperatively resulting in loss of motion	Difficult to achieve a repair that is strong enough to resist valgus stresses
Dynamic external fixation	Allows early motion; technically easy	Limited patient acceptance	Limited patient acceptance for wearing a fixator

Complications

The complications of an elbow dislocation with an associated radial head fracture are instability and loss of motion. In cases in which a silastic radial head prosthesis has been used, synovitis and fracture of the prosthesis can occur.

Instability of the elbow is the most disabling complication of elbow dislocation. The method of management of the unstable elbow is determined by the time from the original injury, the patient's demands, and the presence of posttraumatic arthritis. Instability identified within the first 6 weeks after injury is managed with delayed primary repair of the medial collateral ligament and application of a dynamic external fixator. Late instability is managed with ligamentous reconstruction using free tendon grafts (e.g., palmaris longus). In cases of late instability complicated by painful posttraumatic arthritis, an elbow fusion or facial arthroplasty is performed.

Loss of motion can be secondary to heterotopic ossification or scarring of the capsule and pericapsular structures. Inability to flex the elbow to greater than 90 degrees is disabling in that the patient cannot reach his mouth or perform tasks such as buttoning his shirt. Loss of terminal extension is less disabling than loss of flexion. Management consists of aggressive physical therapy. If therapy is not successful, resection of heterotopic bone and capsulectomy is performed.

Synovitis and fracture of a radial head prosthesis are managed with synovectomy and removal of the prosthesis.

Suggested Readings

Hotchkiss RN, Weiland AJ: Valgus stability of the elbow. J Orthop Res 1987; 5:372–377.

King JW, Evans DC, Kellam JF: Open reduction and internal fixation of radial head fractures. J Ortho Trauma 1991; 5(1):21–28.

Morrey BF: Post-traumatic contracture of the elbow. J Bone Joint Surg 1990; 72A(4):601–618.

Morrey BF, Askew RP, Miller JH: Silastic prosthetic replacement for radial head. J Bone Joint Surg 1981;63A:454–458.

Perry CR, Tessier JE: Open reduction and internal fixation of radial head fractures associated with olecranon fracture or dislocation. J Orthop Trauma 1987; 1(1):36–42.

Case 18

History and Physical Examination

A 42-year-old woman fell on her outstretched hand. She experienced immediate onset of pain in the ipsilateral elbow and came to the emergency department. On physical examination the patient had pain to palpation over the lateral aspect of the elbow. She held the elbow flexed to 90 degrees and in neutral rotation. Any attempted motion of the elbow was extremely painful. The remainder of the physical examination was within the limits of normal. Specifically, there was no tenderness to palpation at the wrist or on the medial side of the elbow. The relationship of the condyles to the tip of the olecranon appeared normal and the neurovascular examination of the hand was normal. The elbow was aspirated, injected with 5 cc of 2% lidocaine, and reexamined. After the elbow had been anesthetized, the arc of forearm rotation was from 30 degrees of supination to neutral. There was a block to pronation past neutral.

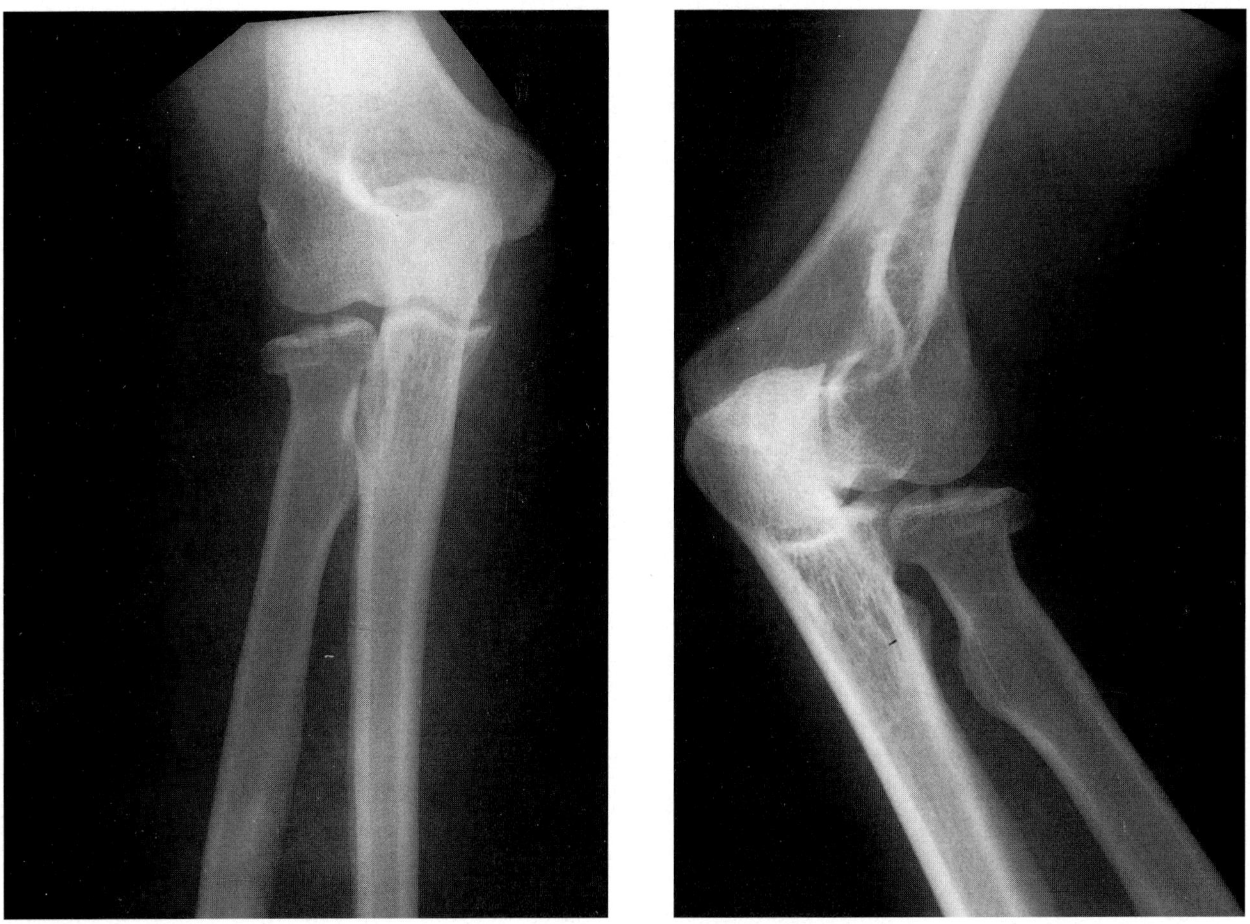

A B

Figure 18–1. Anteroposterior (A) and oblique (B) radiographs of the elbow indicating an isolated fracture of the radial head. The fracture appears to only involve the lateral portion of the head. There is no other pathology evident.

PEARLS

- Radial head fractures are often a relatively minor part of a more extensive injury (e.g., elbow dislocation or radioulnar diastasis). These injuries must be ruled out prior to determining the optimum method of management. In most cases, a physical examination will rule out other injuries. When there is doubt, stress radiographs with the patient anesthetized are obtained.

- The primary indication for surgery in the management of a displaced radial head fracture is whether a block to forearm rotation is present. This cannot be determined until the elbow has been anesthetized. To anesthetize the elbow by an intraarticular injection it is necessary to first aspirate the elbow. If the elbow is not aspirated, the intraarticular injection of the anesthetic agent is extremely painful.

PITFALL

- Associated injuries to the interrosseus (i.e., the triangular fibro cartilage and interrosseus membrane) must be identified. Failure to diagnose and treat this associated injury may result in instability of the distal radioulnar joint.

Radiologic Findings

Anteroposterior, lateral, and oblique radiographs of the elbow and wrist indicated an isolated fracture of the anterolateral third of the radial head. The fracture was displaced 2 mm and impacted (Fig. 18–1). No other pathology was evident.

Diagnosis

Displaced isolated radial head fracture with a block to forearm rotation. When classified according to the system originally described by Speed and modified by Mason, this is a type 2 fracture because it is displaced and involves approximately one third of the radial head, with the remainder of the articular surface of the radius intact. When classified according to the AO system, this is a B2 articular fracture of the radius because it is intraarticular, displaced, involves only part of the articular surface, and there are no associated injuries (e.g., fracture of the olecranon, dislocation of the elbow, etc.).

Surgical Management

The upper extremity was splinted with the elbow at 90 degrees and the forearm in neutral rotation.

The day following injury, the patient was taken to the operating room where an anesthetic was administered. She was positioned supine on the operating table with the arm draped free over the chest. A straight posterior incision was made starting 8 cm distal to the olecranon and extending 2 cm proximal to the tip of the olecranon. A skin flap superficial to the fascia was raised laterally, allowing the identification of the interval between the anconeus muscle and the extensor carpi ulnaris. The fascia was incised over this interval from the ulna to the capitellum. As the anconeus was elevated from distal to proximal the joint capsule of the elbow was encountered. The anconeus was elevated off the capsule to its origin from the capitellum. The radial head and fracture were palpable through the capsule. A T-shaped incision, with the vertical part of the T extending distally, was made through the capsule. The transverse limb of the T was located over the radial neck and parallel to the articular surface of the radial head. Exposure of the fracture was facilitated by external rotation of the forearm. A single large anterolateral fragment was identified, reduced anatomically, and held in place with a countersunk lag screw. The wound was closed by repairing the capsule, suturing the anconeus, and closing the subcutaneous tissue and skin over a drain. The elbow was splinted at 90 degrees.

Postoperative Management

The second postoperative day the splint was replaced with a sling and gentle passive flexion-extension and forearm rotation were initiated. At six weeks the fracture appeared to have healed radiographically, the sling was discontinued, and resistive exercises were initiated (Fig. 18–2). The final range of motion at 12 months was flexion-extension from 150 to 0 degrees, and supination pronation from 80 to 80 degrees. There were no radiologic signs of osteoarthritis or avascular necrosis (Fig. 18–3).

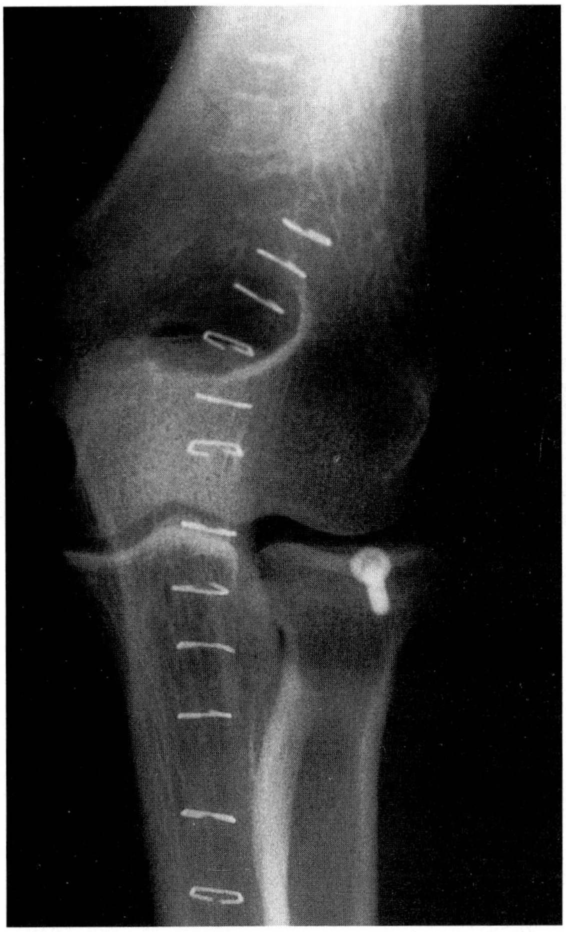

A

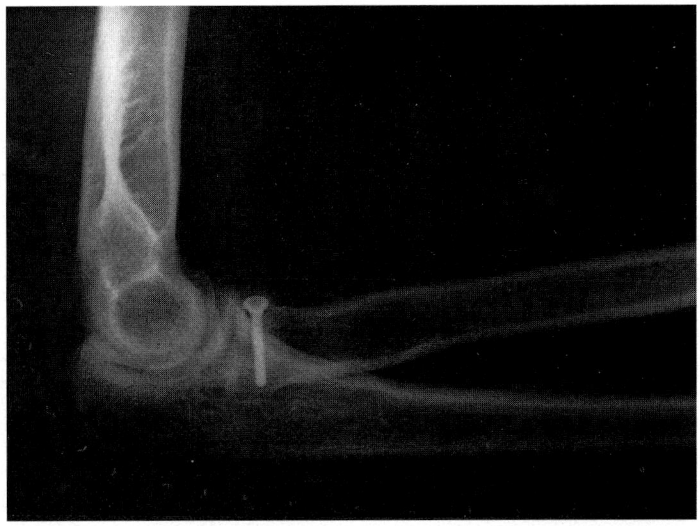

B

Figure 18–2. Anteroposterior (A) and lateral (B) radiographs obtained following reduction and fixation of the fracture with a single screw. The screw has been countersunk.

PEARL

- It is key to countersink the head of the screw. The screw is inserted from anterolateral to medial posterior and does not engage the lesser sigmoid notch of the ulna; therefore, the risk of causing osteoarthritis is minimal. However, if the screw is not countersunk, its head will irritate the lateral joint capsule.

Discussion

Isolated radial head fractures are caused by the capitellum impacting the radial head. This most often occurs during a fall on the outstretched hand with the elbow extended. The entire radial head may be fractured, but frequently, as in this case, the injury is limited to the anterolateral third of the head. When a valgus stress in addition to the primary axial load is applied to the elbow, the fracture is more likely to involve only the anterolateral third of the head. The architecture of the proximal radius also increases the risk of fracture of the anterolateral third of the head. The center of the radial head is lateral to the center of the radial neck; thus the lateral border of the radial head is less well supported by underlying bone than the remainder of the radial head, and more susceptible to fracture.

Alternative Methods of Management

The goals of management are to restore elbow motion, minimize the incidence of posttraumatic arthritis, and minimize the incidence of radial shortening. Alternatives to open reduction in the management of radial head fractures are excision of the entire radial head, excision of the radial head with prosthetic replacement, and excision of the fracture fragment. Excision of the radial head with or without prosthetic replacement is the most frequently utilized method of management of radial

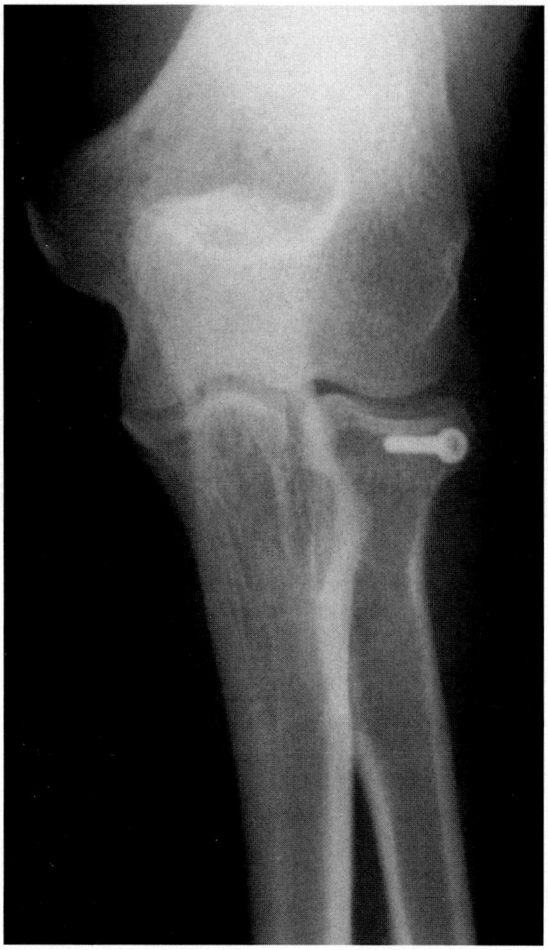

A

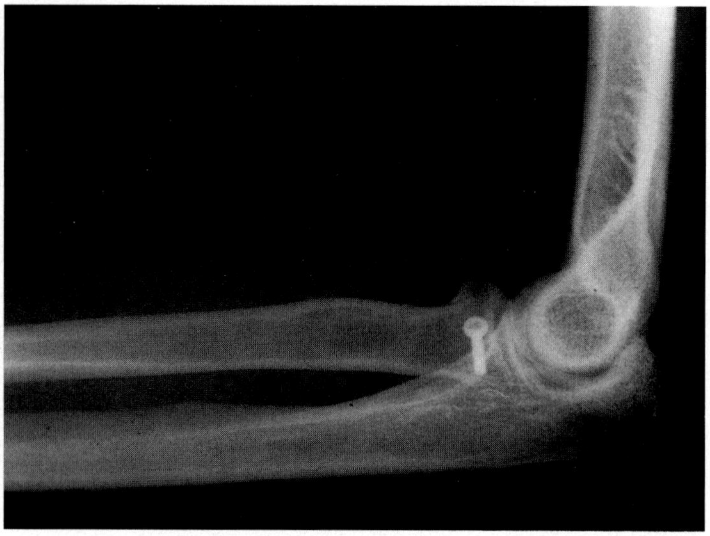

B

Figure 18–3. Anteroposterior (A) and lateral (B) radiographs obtained at 12 months following injury. The fracture has healed without signs of arthritis or avascular necrosis.

Type of Management	Advantages	Disadvantages	Comments
Excision of radial head	Simple procedure; early motion	May result in radial shortening	Probably most frequently used as an alternative to fixation
Excision with prosthetic replacement	Simple procedure; early motion; may minimize radial shortening	Silastic synovitis; prosthesis breakage	Often the radial head prosthesis is removed at one year to minimize synovitis and breakage
Excision of the fragment	Simple procedure; early motion	Painful forearm rotation	Invariably results in irritation of the lateral capsule; not a good alternative
Open reduction and internal fixation	Restoration of anatomy	Complex procedure, not always possible	If reduction is stable and anatomic, yields the most complete recovery

head fractures. The complication unique to this method of radial head excision is shortening of the radius in relation to the ulna. This can occur even without a well defined injury to the interosseous complex (i.e., the triangular fibrocartilage complex, the interosseous membrane, and the interosseous membrane). Shortening is due to gradual stretching of the interosseous complex as the muscles of the hand and wrist contract and to ulnar migration of the proximal radius, resulting in incompetence of the interosseous ligament and membrane.

Complications

The complications of radial head fracture are arthritis resulting in elbow pain, shortening of the radius with pain at the wrist, and synovitis following silastic prosthesis insertion. Arthritis and elbow pain are due to damage of the articular cartilage at the time of radial head fracture or inaccurate reduction of the radial head fracture. Management of arthritis is either conservative or operative. Conservative management consists of nonsteroidal antiinflammatories and occasionally intraarticular injections of steroids. Operative management of arthritis following radial head fracture is excision of the radial head. If the original injury was an isolated radial head fracture and not an elbow dislocation or radioulnar diastasis, ligamentous stability of the elbow and forearm is not an issue and the radial head can be excised with minimal risk of elbow instability or radial shortening. Implantation of a silastic prosthesis is not recommended because it exposes the patient to the risk of synovitis.

Pain at the wrist is due to proximal migration of the radius. It occurs following excision of the radial head and injury to the interosseous membrane and triangular fibrocartilage. If caught very early when the radius can still be brought out to length with traction, proximal migration can be managed with insertion of a radial head prosthesis. A titanium prosthesis will resist compression more effectively than a silastic prosthesis. Usually reduction of the radius is not possible. When this is the case, the distal radio ulnar joint is fused and a 1 cm segment of the distal ulna is removed to allow forearm rotation. This procedure should not be performed following a radioulnar diastasis because the ulna and entire forearm will shorten.

Suggested Readings

Geel CW, Palmer AK, Ruedi T, Leutenegger AF: Internal fixation of proximal radial head fractures. J Orthop Trauma 1990; 4(3):270–274.

Mason ML: Some observations on fractures of the head of the radius with a review of one hundred cases. Br J Surg 1954; 42:123–132.

Pankovich AM: Anconeus approach to the elbow joint and the proximal part of the radius and ulna. J Bone Joint Surg 1978; 60A:124–126.

Perry CR, Tessier JE: Open reduction and internal fixation of radial head fractures associated with olecranon fracture or dislocation. J Orthop Trauma 1987; 1(1):36–42.

Case 19

History and Physical Examination

A 34-year-old man fell from a horse and injured his forearm and elbow. The patient arrived in the emergency department 30 minutes after injury. There was obvious deformity at the elbow as well as abrasions of the skin overlying the posterior surface of the elbow and dorsum of the forearm. The neurovascular examination of the hand was within the limits of normal.

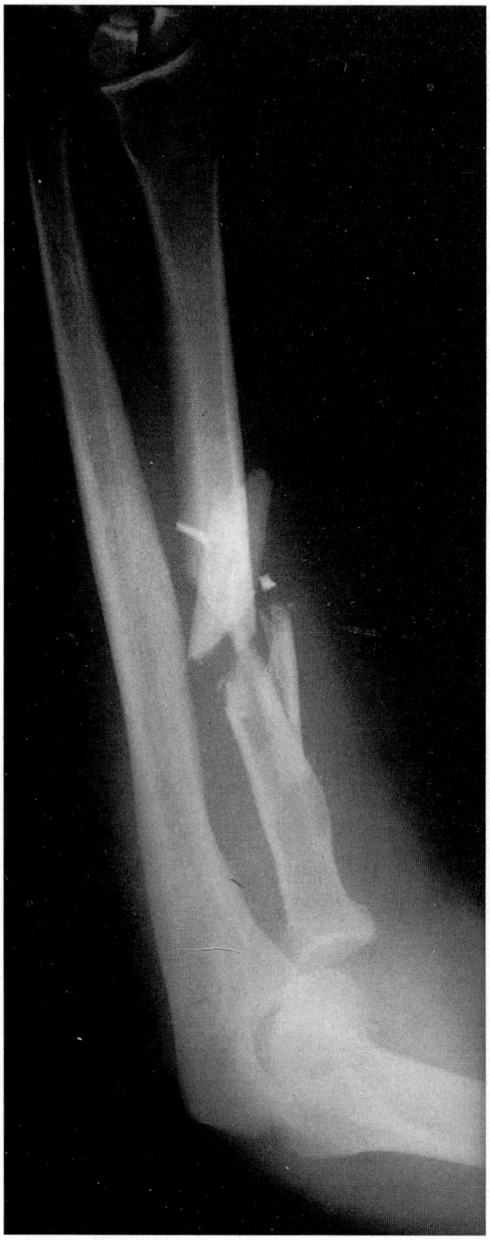

A

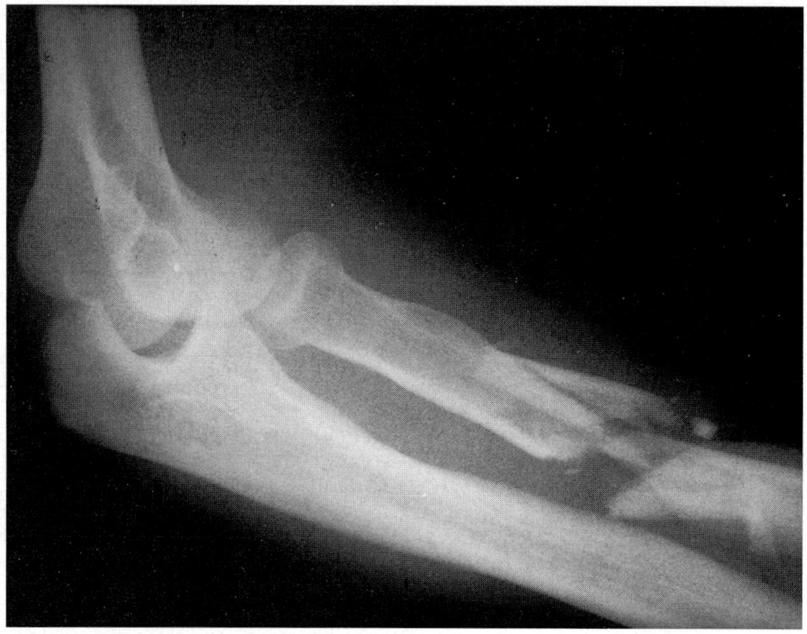

B

Figure 19–1. Lateral radiographs of the forearm (A) and elbow (B) indicating a comminuted fracture of the proximal radial diaphysis, dislocation of the radial head, and subluxation of the humeroulnar articulation. The distal radioulnar joint also appears subluxed, indicating radioulnar dissociation.

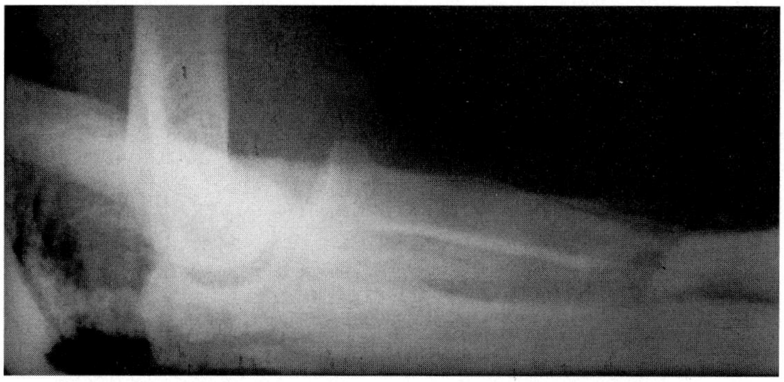

Figure 19–2. Lateral radiograph of elbow obtained after attempted closed reduction. Persistent dislocation of the radial head is evident; the humeroulnar articulation is reduced.

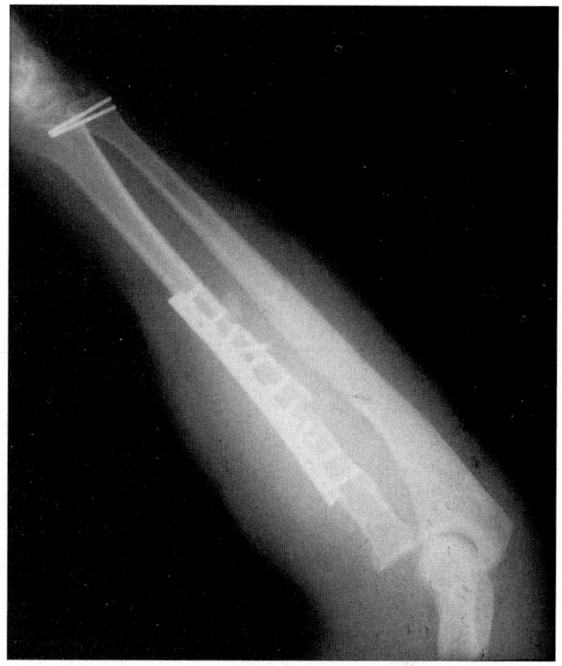

Figure 19–3. Lateral radiograph of elbow obtained after reduction and fixation of the radial fracture and distal radioulnar articulation. Persistent anterior dislocation of the radial head is evident.

PEARL

- The elbow must be reduced emergently to minimize swelling and its sequelae (i.e., compartment syndrome and neurovascular compromise). However, applying traction through an injured forearm is risky. The patient must be sedated or anesthetized and, if more than gentle traction is required, an open reduction should be performed. Fluoroscopy is helpful when attempting a closed reduction.

Radiologic Findings

Radiographs indicated a fracture of the proximal third of the radius, radioulnar diastasis with subluxation of the distal radioulnar joint, and anterolateral dislocation of the radial head. In addition, the humeroulnar articulation was subluxed (Fig. 19–1).

Diagnosis

Radioulnar dissociation, with subluxation of the humeroulnar articulation and fracture of the proximal radius. (This injury complex is the Essex-Lopresti injury with an associated subluxation of the humeroulnar articulation.)

Surgical Management

The patient was sedated and a gentle closed reduction of the forearm was attempted with longitudinal traction. Although the normal relationship of the humeroulnar articulation was restored and the radial fracture aligned, the anterolateral dislocation of the radial head was not reduced. The forearm and elbow were splinted with the elbow at 90 degrees and the forearm in neutral rotation (Fig. 19–2).

Because the dislocation of the proximal radius could not be reduced, the patient was taken to the operating room. An anesthetic was administered and the arm was prepped and draped free on a hand table. Henry's anterior approach was used to expose the proximal radius fracture. This approach achieves exposure of the proximal radius via the interval between the brachioradialis and the biceps proximally

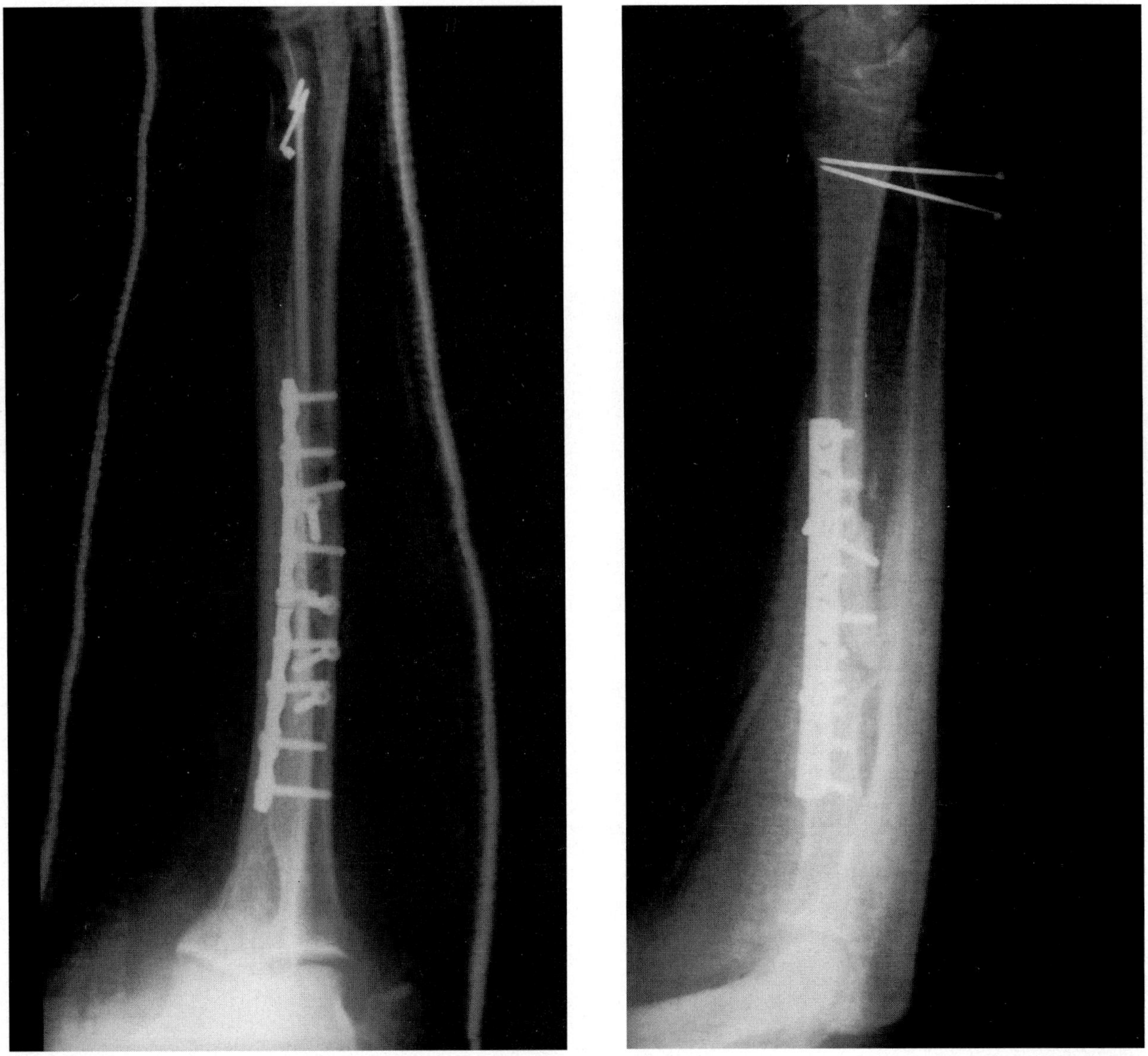

A B

Figure 19–4. Anteroposterior (A) and lateral (B) radiographs obtained after open reduction of the radial head. The elbow is splinted.

and the brachioradialis and pronator teres distally. The fracture was reduced and stabilized with a dynamic compression plate. The distal radioulnar joint was extremely unstable. It was reduced under fluoroscopy and stabilized with Kirschner wires, with the forearm in neutral rotation. Intraoperative radiographs indicated persistent dislocation of the radial head (Fig. 19–3). The anconeus approach was used to expose the radial head. To do this the hand table was removed and the arm positioned over the patient's chest. An incision was made that extended from 5 cm proximal to the elbow joint along the posterior aspect of the arm along the dorsal border of the ulna, distal to the elbow 10 cm. The anconeus was identified, elevated subperiosteally, and retracted proximally, exposing the lateral aspect of the joint capsule. The radial head was buttonholed through the capsule. The capsule was incised, allowing reduction of the radial head. The reduction was stable, with the elbow flexed to 90 degrees in neutral rotation. Closure was not possible because of swelling. The wound was packed and the arm was immobilized in a "sugar tong" splint (Fig. 19–4).

Postoperative Management

The patient was observed for compartment syndrome. The dressing was changed on the second postoperative day with the patient sedated. One week after injury the open wound was skin grafted. The elbow was immobilized in a posterior plastic splint. At 2 weeks the splint was removed daily for active flexion exercises. Extension past 90 degrees was not allowed. The Kirschner wire stabilizing the distal radioulnar joint was removed at 6 weeks and forearm rotation exercises were initiated. At 8 weeks unrestricted range of motion exercises were initiated (Fig. 19–5).

At 6 months the elbow was properly aligned, but flexion and extension were limited to 100 to 70 degrees, and supination and pronation were limited to 0 and 30

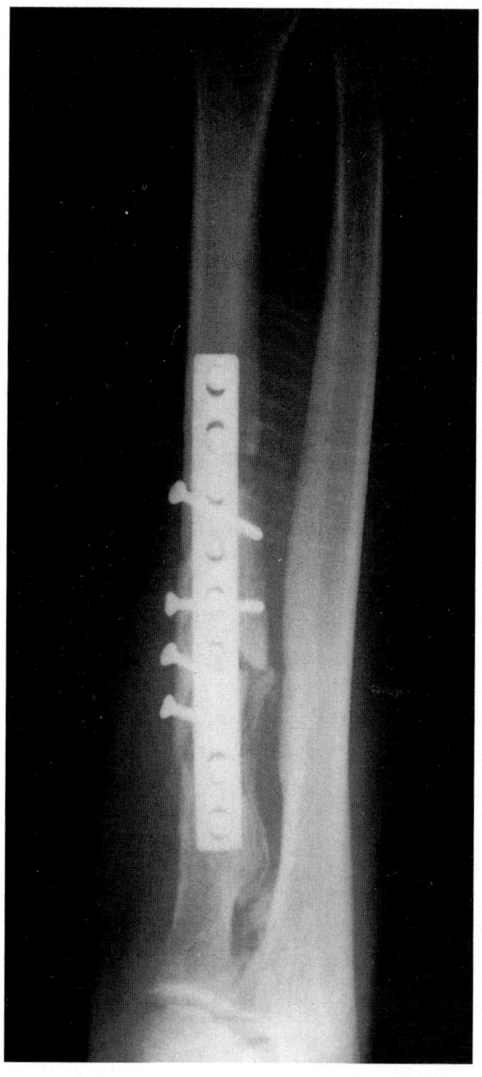
A

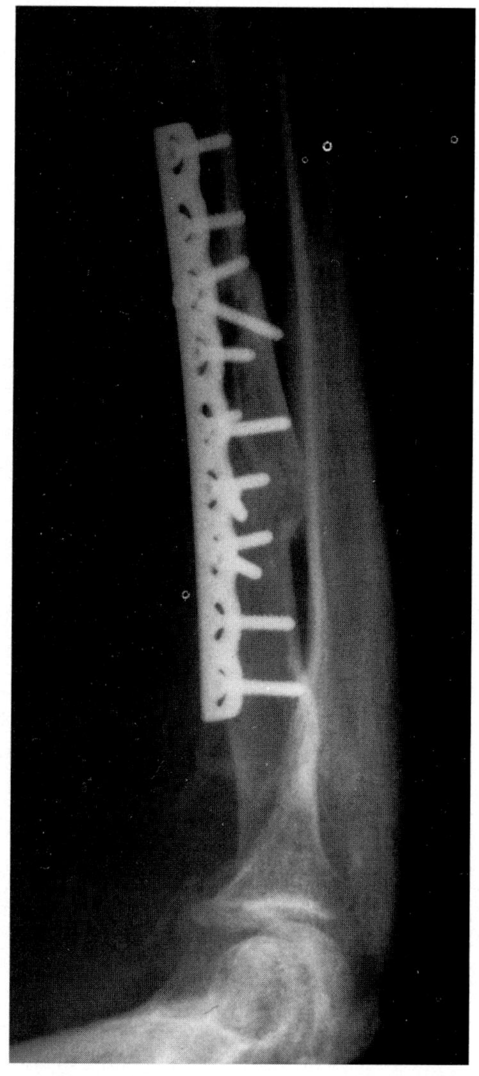
B

Figure 19–5. Anteroposterior (A) and lateral (B) radiographs obtained 6 months after injury. The radial fracture is healed, but heterotopic ossification is present.

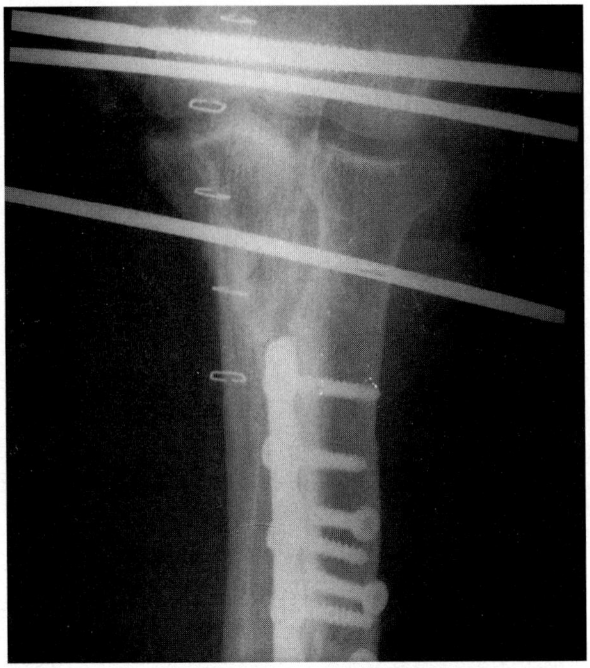

Figure 19–6. Anteroposterior radiograph of the elbow following soft tissue release, excision of heterotopic bone, and application of a dynamic external fixator.

degrees. Loss of motion of the elbow was managed initially with physical therapy. At 1 year the patient continued to have significant limitation of motion. Most bothersome was the inability to flex the elbow more than 100 degrees. A soft tissue release and excision of heterotopic bone was performed through a lateral approach. A dynamic external fixator was applied to prevent elbow dislocation postoperatively and allow early motion (Fig. 19–6). Postoperatively the elbow was irradiated to minimize heterotopic ossification. Six months following release of the elbow the range of motion was 120 to 20 degrees of flexion and extension of the elbow and 60 to 60 degrees of forearm supination and pronation (Fig. 19–7).

Discussion

Radioulnar dissociation is a devastating injury. In this case it was further complicated by fracture of the proximal radial diaphysis and subluxation of the humeroulnar articulation. The degree of radial instability is indicated by the dislocation of the radial head following stabilization of the fractured radius and the distal radioulnar articulation. It was necessary to stabilize the radial fracture to prevent displacement and nonunion or malunion with subluxation of the proximal and distal radioulnar articulations. Stabilization of the distal radioulnar articulation was necessary because of marked instability.

The anconeus approach was used to expose the radial head when persistent dislocation of the radial head was noted intraoperatively. The use of a second surgical exposure is somewhat controversial. The proximal radius had already been exposed via Henry's approach, and theoretically the radial head could have been reduced through this approach. Practically, however, the anatomy was distorted and the exposure was very difficult due to swelling. To reduce the risk of injury to the surrounding neurovascular structures, and in particular to the radial nerve, the anconeus approach was used to expose the radial head.

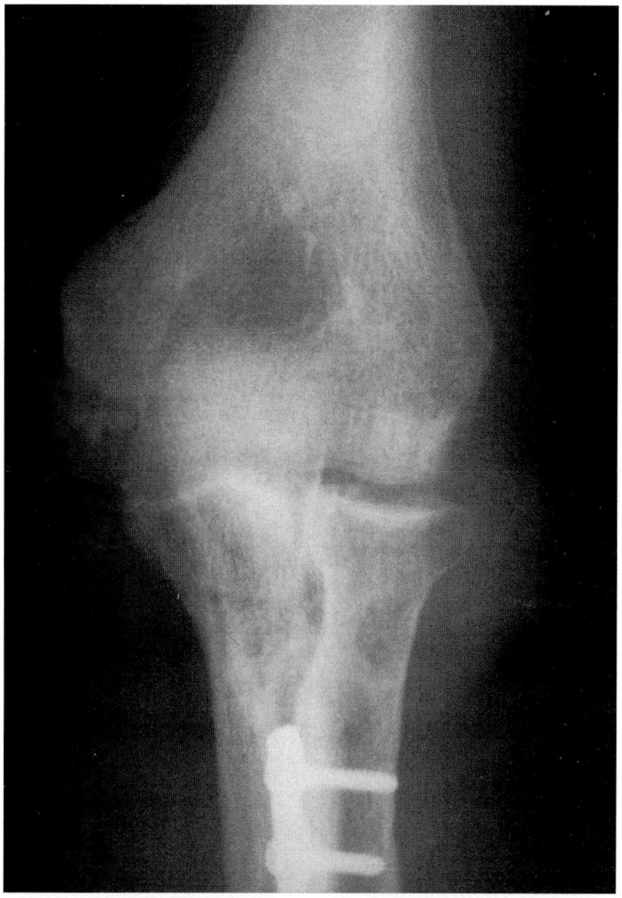

A

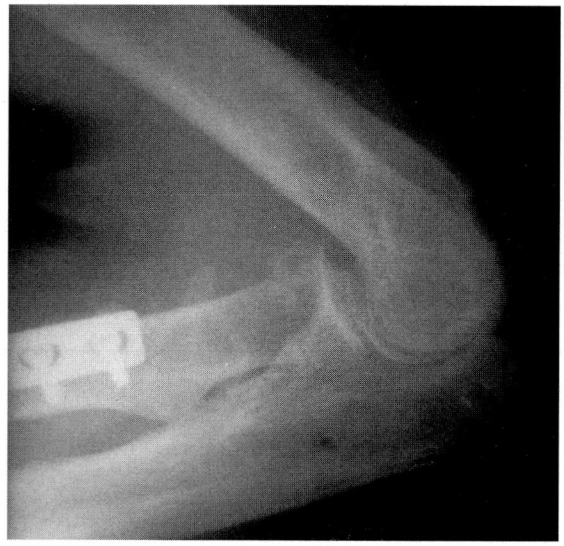

C

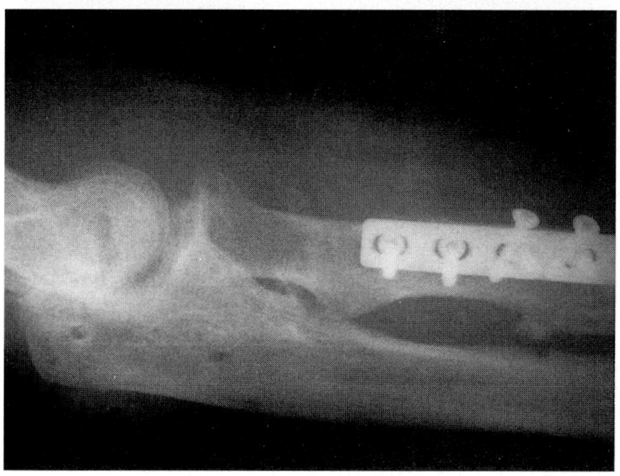

B

Figure 19–7 (A–C). Anteroposterior and lateral radiographs indicating the final range of motion of the elbow.

Alternative Methods of Management

There are no alternatives to open reduction and internal fixation in this case. Failure to stabilize the fracture of the radius along with the distal radioulnar articulation would have resulted in loss of reduction. Failure to immobilize the elbow would have resulted in dislocation of the radial head, the humeroulnar articulation, or both.

Complications

The complications unique to this injury are loss of motion and chronic instability of the elbow or wrist. Loss of forearm rotation, flexion, and extension of the elbow can be due to scarring or heterotopic ossification. Loss of motion is managed initially with therapy. If therapy is not successful in restoring a functional range of motion, surgical release of scar tissue or excision of heterotopic bone is performed.

Instability of the elbow or wrist is often more disabling than loss of motion because it is painful. Instability of the elbow is managed with reconstruction of the ligaments and application of a dynamic external fixator. Numerous techniques to repair the medial collateral (e.g., using palmaris longus) and annular ligaments (e.g., using triceps tendon) have been described. Repair of the triangular fibrocartilage complex distally is more difficult. Fusion of the distal radioulnar joint and excision of a segment of the ulna may add to instability of the radioulnar syndesmosis and should only be performed as a last resort.

Suggested Readings

Edwards GS, Jupiter JB: Radial head fractures with acute distal radioulnar dislocation: Essex Lopresti revisited. CORR 1988; 234:61–69.

Essex-Lopresti P: Fractures of the radial head with distal radio-ulnar dislocation: report of two cases. J Bone Joint Surg 1951; 33B(2):244–247.

Jupiter et al: The floating radius in bipolar fracture—dislocation of the forearm. J Orthop Trauma 1994; 8(2):99–106.

Trousdale RT, Amadio PC, Cooney WP, Morrey BF: Radioulnar dissociation: a review of twenty cases. J Bone Joint Surg 1992; 74A(10):1486–1497.

Case 20

History and Physical Examination

A 38-year-old woman was a front seat passenger in a traffic accident. She was not wearing a seat belt at the time of the accident and her car was not fitted with air bags. She was thrown forward and had damaged both her arms. Examination in the emergency department showed that both elbows were painful and deformed. There was some superficial skin damage on the right elbow but no evidence of an open wound and obvious soft tissue damage. Careful neurological examination showed no abnormality in either arm and both radial pulses were normal. There was good capillary return in each hand.

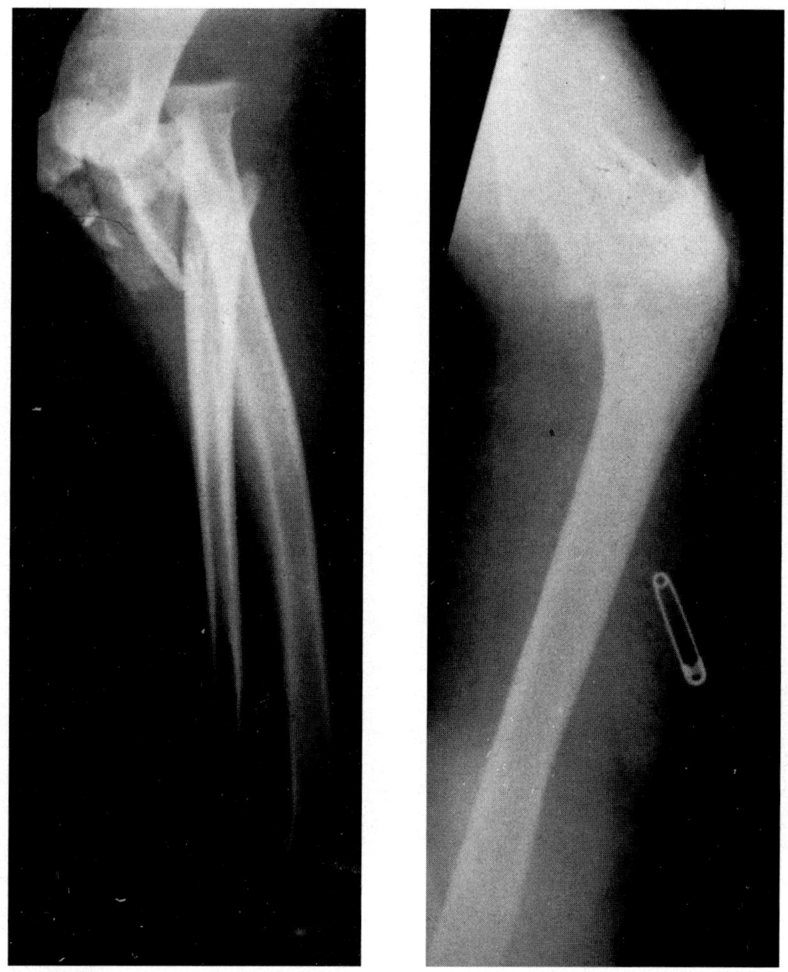

A B

Figure 20–1. Anteroposterior (A) and lateral (B) radiographs of a comminuted proximal ulna fracture associated with a radial head dislocation.

Radiologic Findings

Anteroposterior and lateral radiographs of the right elbow showed a comminuted proximal ulnar fracture with a dislocation of the radial head (Fig. 20–1). She also had a fracture of the left distal humerus.

PEARL

- Elbow dislocations can be associated with a high incidence of neurovascular injuries. Damage to the brachial artery necessitating vein grafting has been reported even in simple dislocations, and the incidence of vascular damage increases in high energy injuries where there is extensive bone damage. There may also be damage to the median ulna and radial nerves. Where possible, it is important to define the neurovascular status of the arm preoperatively.

Diagnosis

A closed fracture dislocation of the elbow with extensive comminution of the proximal ulnar and dislocation of the radial head. AO classification: 21–B1.3.

Surgical Management

Initially, plaster back slabs were applied to both elbows to minimize discomfort and reduce the risk of further soft tissue damage. The patient was then admitted to the orthopaedic trauma unit. She was taken to the operating room on the following day and both fractures were stabilized. The right proximal forearm fracture was approached posteriorly. To facilitate this, the patient was placed on her side with her right upper arm supported in a gutter splint. This allowed the arm to hang down. Care was taken to pad the splint to prevent neural compression.

A posterior skin incision was made, curving it laterally around the olecranon to prevent damage to the ulna nerve. Standard AO techniques were used to reconstruct the proximal ulna. Transfixion screws were used to fix two of the larger bone frag-

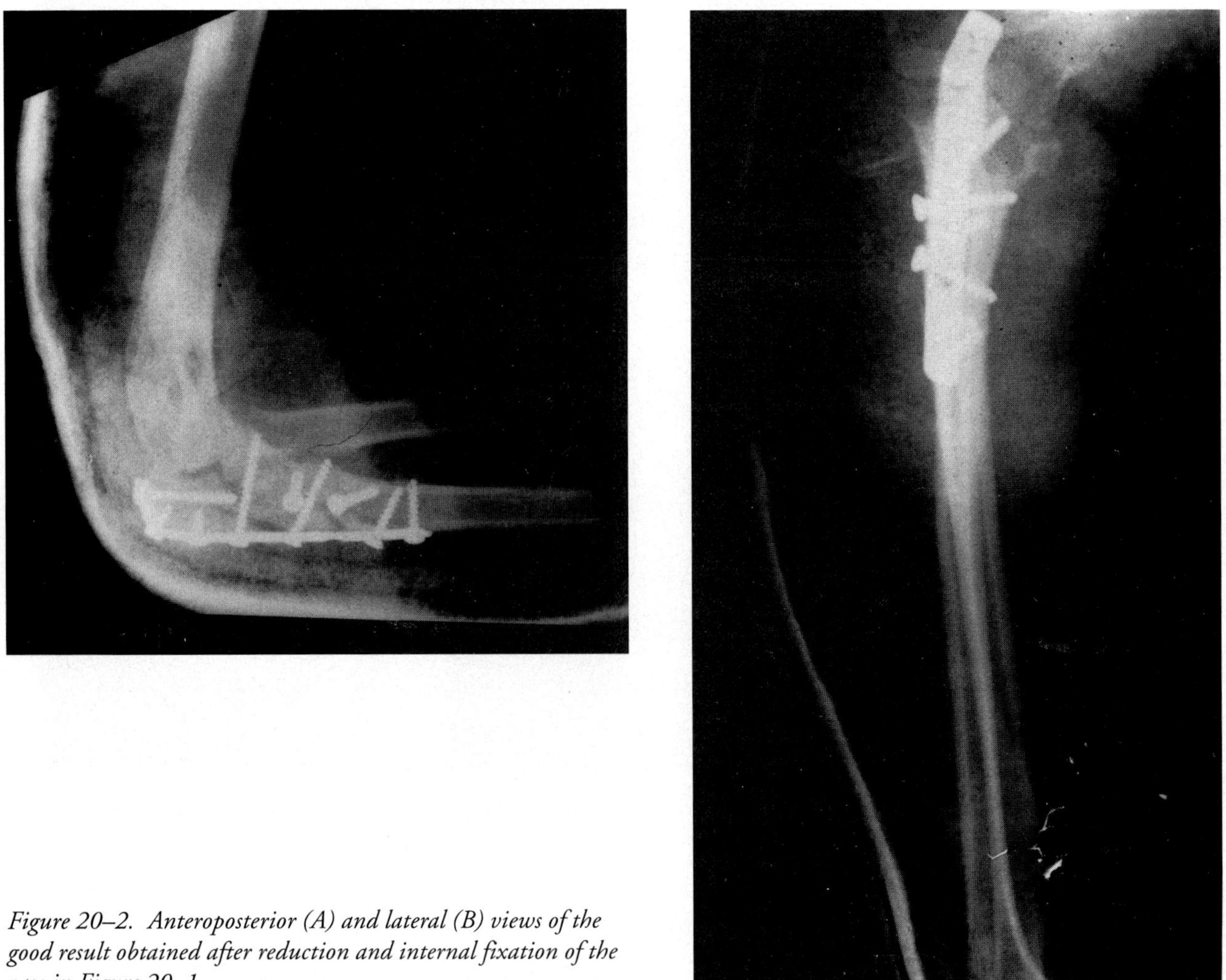

A

B

Figure 20–2. Anteroposterior (A) and lateral (B) views of the good result obtained after reduction and internal fixation of the case in Figure 20–1.

PITFALL

- Radiographs of juxtaarticular fractures usually fail to indicate the true extent of any comminution. Surgeons should be aware of this when planning their procedure.

ments and a posterior plate was applied. Improved fixation was obtained by curving the plate proximally to allow a screw to be placed in the axis of the ulna and by placing a screw in the coronoid process. The radial head was noted to be undamaged and was relocated; the annular ligament was intact. After wound closure a plaster back slab was applied. Postoperative radiographs were satisfactory (Fig. 20–2).

Postoperative Management

It was thought that the degree of comminution mitigated against immediate postoperative elbow movement. A cast was therefore maintained for 4 weeks and following its removal a physiotherapy program was instituted. The fracture position was maintained until union. The patient regained good function and 1 year after the injury had flexion from 15 to 130 degrees with full rotation. She complained of some discomfort over the ulnar plate 14 months after the accident, so the plate and screws were removed.

Discussion

This case represents one injury in a spectrum of injuries in which comminuted proximal ulnar fractures are associated with damage to the radial side of the elbow joint. In this case the radiocapitellar damage took the form of a simple dislocation. However, the damage to the radial side of the joint may be more severe. Figure 20–3 shows a lateral radiograph of a closed comminuted proximal ulnar fracture associ-

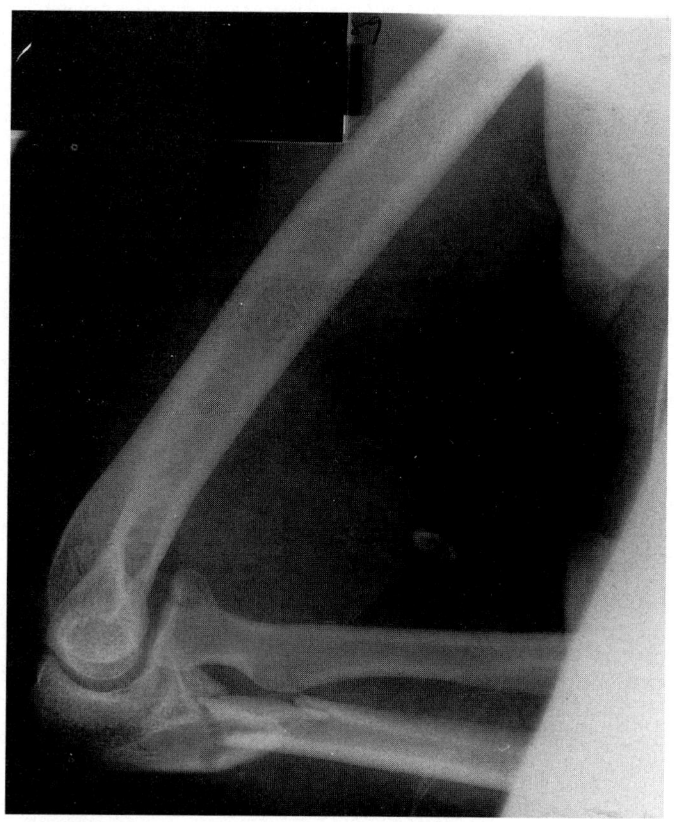

Figure 20–3. A lateral radiograph of a comminuted proximal ulna fracture associated with a radial head fracture.

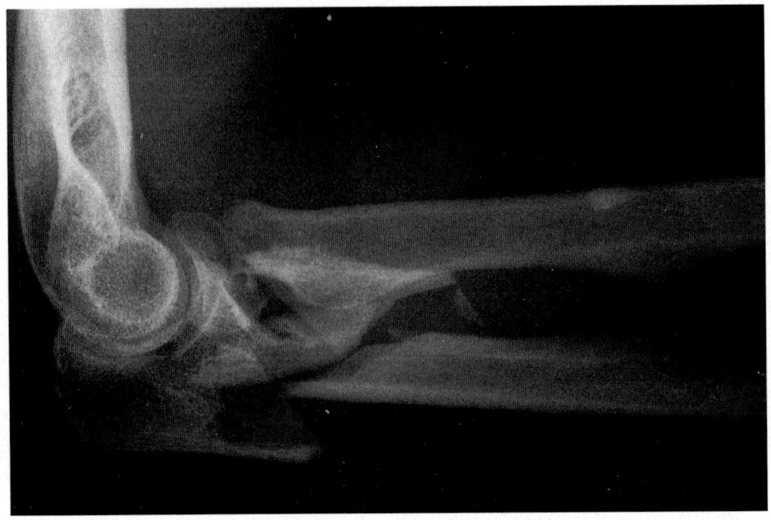

Figure 20–4. A lateral radiograph of a comminuted proximal ulna fracture associated with a radial neck fracture.

ated with a medially displaced radial head fracture involving about one quarter of the head (AO classification 21–C2.1). This fracture occurred as an isolated injury in a 48-year-old female who fell on her right elbow. The undisplaced nature of the radial head fracture suggests that the annular ligament is intact and this was confirmed at surgery. The treatment was the same as undertaken for the case shown in Figures 20–1 and 20–2.

The next variant of this type of fracture is one in which a radial neck fracture occurs in association with the proximal ulnar fracture. Figure 20–4 shows such a fracture. This was a 58-year-old woman who injured her elbow in a simple fall. There is extensive comminution of the ulnar metaphysis with a slightly angulated radial neck fracture (AO classification 21–B3.3). An adequate anteroposterior X ray could not be obtained because of pain. In this case Kirschner wires were used to aid proximal ulnar reconstruction and a posteromedial plate was applied. Radiographs taken after proximal ulnar reconstruction (Fig. 20–5) showed that the radial neck had reduced to an acceptable position and fixation was considered unnecessary because the radial head appeared stable. A supporting cast was used for 3 weeks followed by the use of a functional brace, which was maintained for an additional 5 weeks. The plate and screws were removed 6 months after the injury and the final results at 1 year were good (Fig. 20–6). The patient had flexion from 10 to 135 degrees, with slight loss of pronation. The final radiographs showed good maintenance of the elbow joint and excellent radial head alignment.

The extent of the surgery required on the radial side of the joint depends on the extent and type of the damage. In the case of a pure dislocation of the radial head it is important to repair the soft tissue, particularly the annular ligament, to enhance stability. Should there be a displaced, but reconstructable, radial head fracture, it is important that it be reconstructed. If the radial head is composed of two or three fragments, it can usually be internally fixed using Herbert screws or countersunk small cannulated bone screws, followed by meticulous annular ligament reconstruction. Failure to reduce an internally fixed reconstructable radial head fracture will increase the likelihood of late pain and decreased elbow mobility. If the radial head cannot be reconstructed, it should be excised; there is some debate about the use of a prosthetic radial head under these circumstances.

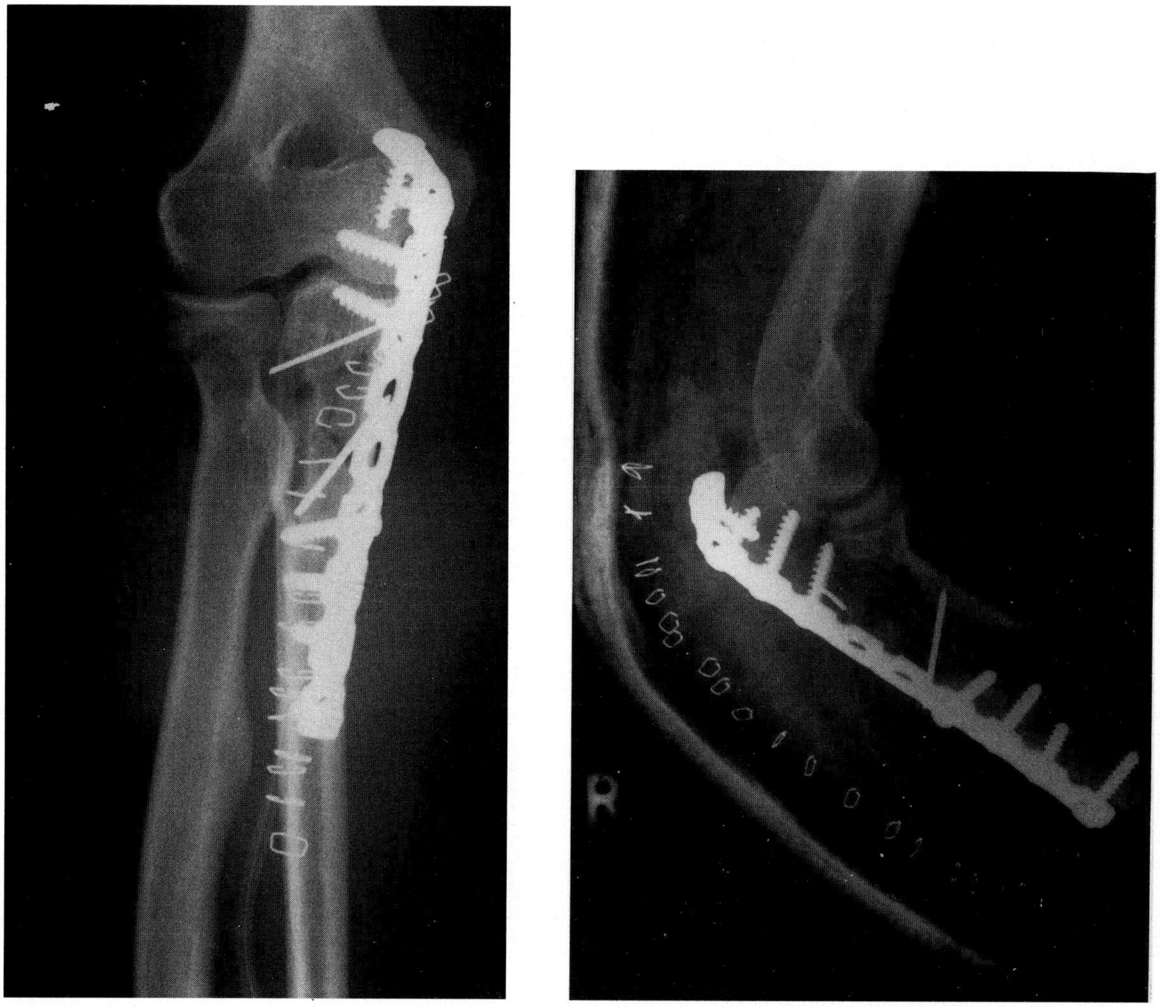

A B

Figure 20–5. Anteroposterior (A) and lateral (B) radiographs after fixation. The radial head fracture was stable and did not require fixation.

The treatment of radial neck fractures depends on the degree of displacement and the stability of the radial head fragment. If the radial head is undisplaced or only minimally displaced and stable, nonoperative management is indicated. Internal fixation might theoretically allow earlier joint movement, but it is technically difficult and the amount of soft tissue dissection tends to outweigh the benefits of fixation. It is also unlikely that fixation of the radial neck fracture will confer sufficient stability to allow the patient to mobilize postoperatively without a protective brace. Nonoperative management should not equate with patient neglect and serial radiographs should be taken over the next 2 to 3 weeks to check that the position of the radial head remains adequate. If the radial head displaces, internal fixation, prosthetic replacement or resection must be considered.

Internal fixation of a displaced radial head can be difficult. The most common operation is the application of a small T plate to the radial neck and head, but it is not an easy procedure and many surgeons would either remove the radial head or use a prosthetic replacement if removal resulted in instability. There is debate about the usefulness of prosthetic radial head replacement in the management of both iso-

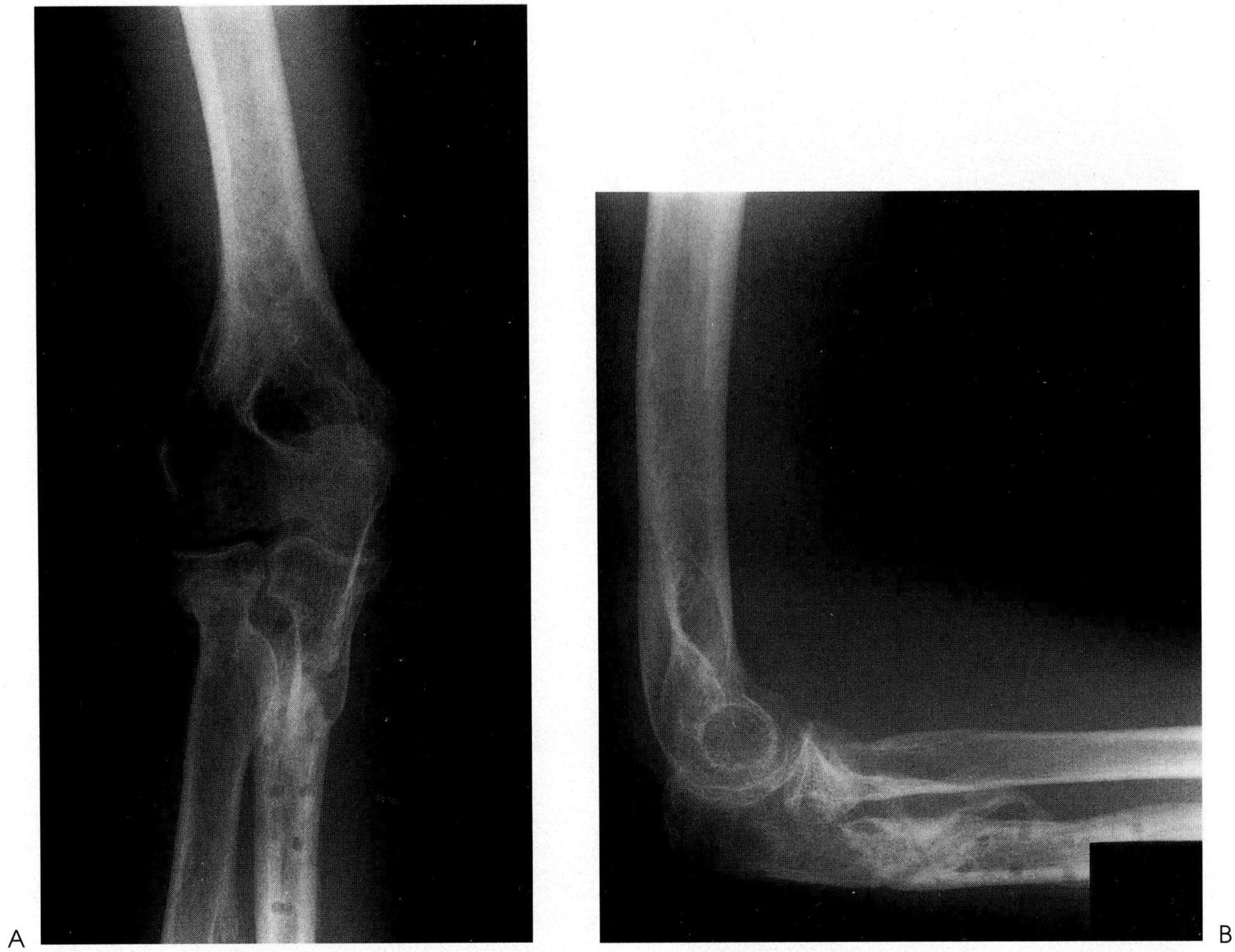

Figure 20–6. Anteroposterior (A) and lateral (B) views of the excellent final result obtained in the patient in Figure 20–5.

lated radial head fractures and when the radial head fracture occurs with elbow dislocation, distal radioulnar dislocation, the Essex-Lopesti lesion, or a significant proximal ulnar fracture. There is some evidence that posterior dislocation of the elbow in association with an unreconstructable radial head fracture is best treated by radial head replacement. However, there is little evidence for or against radial head replacement in the presence of a comminuted proximal ulnar fracture. It seems reasonable to use prosthetic head replacement in elbows that remain unstable after ulnar fixation. This will occur if there is significant ligamentous damage associated with the fracture. If the elbow is stable after fixation, there is no need for prosthetic head replacement.

Alternative Methods of Management

Most fractures of the proximal ulna will be treated by internal fixation using plates and bone screws. These fractures may be very comminuted and if some of the fragments are too small for screw fixation but still retain a vascular supply, they can be fixed using interfragmentary wiring techniques. If small fragments have no blood supply, they should be discarded and the resulting defect packed with corticocancellous bone graft.

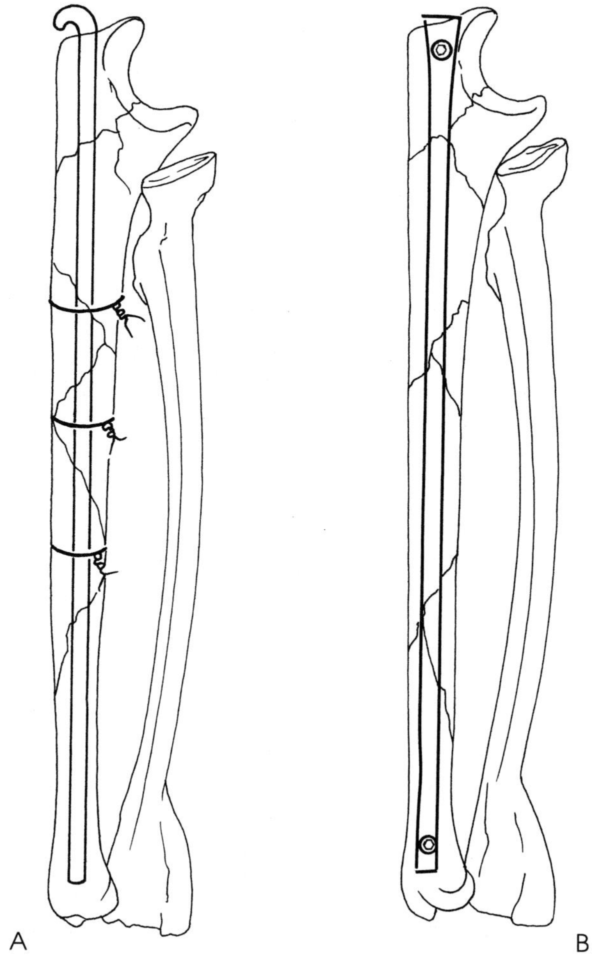

Figure 20–7. (A) Diagrammatic representation of the use of a Rush nail and cerclage wiring in the treatment of a comminuted fracture of the ulna. (B) The use of a locked intramedullary nail.

Occasionally, the ulna will be fractured over a considerable amount of its length. This usually occurs in older patients with osteoporotic bone in which plate fixation is less reliable. Under these circumstances an intramedullary device can be placed into the ulna through the olecranon fragment. It should run the whole length of the ulna into the distal metaphysis. Conventionally, the comminuted diaphyseal fragments are reconstructed using cerclage wiring techniques (Fig. 20–7). If this method is chosen, care must be taken not to devascularize the bone fragments during the wiring process. Until recently the use of Rush pins was advocated for this technique, but the recent introduction of interlocking intramedullary ulna nails has improved the fixation of comminuted ulna fractures; if these nails are available, and the size of the proximal olecranon fragment permits their use, they should be used. Both techniques are illustrated in Figure 20–7. It is probable that cerclage wires will be required to reduce the fragments of the ulna no matter which type of nail is applied, although the use of an interlocking intramedullary nail may minimize the requirement for cerclage wiring.

One other alternative is the use of distraction external fixation to regain ulnar length and radial head reduction. However, interfragmentary screws would still be required to reduce the interarticular olecranon fracture. In addition, the small size of the olecranon fragment would make external fixation difficult and the frame would be unlikely to maintain fracture reduction for a prolonged period.

The additional problem of securing external fixator pins in the olecranon fragment would probably result in troublesome pin sepsis. Transarticular external fixation should not be used for this type of fracture because elbow stiffness will almost certainly result. This type of treatment should be reserved for the occasional salvageable fracture that has extensive comminution in the distal humerus and proximal forearm.

Type of Management	Advantages	Disadvantages	Comments
Nonoperative	None	Inability to control fracture position; malunion; osteoarthritis; pain; elbow instability	Only useful in patients who are either too old or infirm for surgery; poor results are to be expected
Open reduction and internal fixation	Accurate fracture reduction; early joint motion; improved elbow function; less pain	Theoretically higher risk of infection; difficult surgery	Treatment of choice; allows for earliest possible joint motion and good results can often be achieved
External fixation	None unless there is distal humeral damage associated with proximal forearm damage (floating elbow); bridging external fixation would then be useful	Nonbridging fixation very difficult; poor stability because of size of olecranon fragment; sepsis	Very difficult technique and difficult to justify its use in a nonbridging form
Intramedullary nailing	Useful in proximal ulnar fractures associated with diaphyseal comminution particularly in elderly patients; new interlocking ulnar nails may extend the use of this technique	Fixation is not rigid; requires postoperative cast	Useful but rarely required technique

Complications

Ulnar fractures tend to be either high energy injuries in younger patients or lower energy fractures in older patients. The complications most likely to be encountered are difficulties in reconstructing the ulna using intrafragmentary screws and plates, in which case the technique of intramedullary fixation and cerclage wiring should be considered.

Postoperative complications are likely to be infection, joint stiffness, and osteoarthritis. The incidence of infection can be minimized by preoperative attention to detail. It should be remembered that the ulna is subcutaneous and thus even superficial wound infection may be potentially dangerous. The skin and subcutaneous tissue should be handled carefully and the wound never closed under tension. It is advisable to operate as soon as possible before significant elbow swelling occurs.

If superficial infection occurs, it should be treated with antibiotics and rest. Deep infection must be treated with debridement, appropriate soft tissue cover, and local and systemic antibiotics, with removal of the hardware after union has occurred.

Nonunion of these metaphyseal fractures is rare; if it occurs, it will lead to considerable joint stiffness. Nonunion should be treated by rigid internal fixation and bone grafting. A much more likely complication is joint stiffness because these intraarticular fractures are associated with considerable soft tissue damage. It is important to strive for early joint mobility. As previously discussed, this may prove difficult even with well fixed fractures. However, supplementary functional bracing may permit early joint movement. Physiotherapy is the best method for avoiding joint stiffness, but if stiffness occurs, surgical management may be considered. The two options are the use of a distraction external fixator to encourage elbow motion and anterior capsulectomy to allow more extension. Both are difficult techniques that demand attention to detail, good patient cooperation, and a strict rehabilitation regime.

Posttraumatic osteoarthritis needs to be carefully assessed. A relatively high percentage of these fractures will develop some signs of osteoarthritis and mild symptoms can be treated by antiinflammatory medication. However, a few patients will require more than merely symptomatic treatment. Many patients will accept a degree of disability and discomfort. If patients have intolerable pain or significant reduction in movement, elbow arthroplasty should be considered.

Suggested Readings

Broberg MA, Morrey BF: Results of treatment of fracture-dislocation of the elbow. Clin Orthop 1987; 216:109–119.

Essex-Lopresti P: Fractures of the radial head with distal radio-ulnar dislocation. J Bone Joint Surg (Br) 1951; 33B:244–247.

Harrington IJ, Tountas AA: Replacement of the radial head in the treatment of unstable elbow fractures. Injury 1981; 12:405–409.

Jupiter JB, Mehne DK: Trauma to the adult elbow and fractures of the distal humerus. In: Browner BD, Jupiter JB, Levine AM, Trafton PG (eds): Skeletal Trauma, pp 1126–1173. WB Saunders, Philadelphia, 1992.

Regan W, Morrey B: Fractures of the coronoid process of the ulna. J Bone Joint Surg (Am) 1989; 71A:1348–1354.

Swanson AB, Jaeger SH, LaRochell D: Comminuted fractures of the radial head. The role of silicon implant replacement arthroplasty. J Bone Joint Surg 1981; 63A:1039–1049.

Case 21

History and Physical Examination

A 37-year-old woman who had been the driver of an automobile involved in a head-on collision was brought to the emergency department. She had not been unconscious at any time and her Glasgow Coma Scale was 14 on admission. She was hemodynamically stable, but tender over the sternum and left costal margin. Chest X ray demonstrated a fracture of the left tenth rib without any associated pulmonary contusion and abdominal ultrasound revealed a right renal contusion.

The majority of the patient's injuries were musculoskeletal and left-sided. She had a Gustilo IIIA fracture of her left tibia and combined diaphyseal and subcapital fractures of her left femur. Examination of the left arm showed a closed fracture of the distal third of the humeral diaphysis. There was also deformity of the left elbow with significant pain on attempted movement of the joint. There was no evidence of any neurovascular deficit in the left arm.

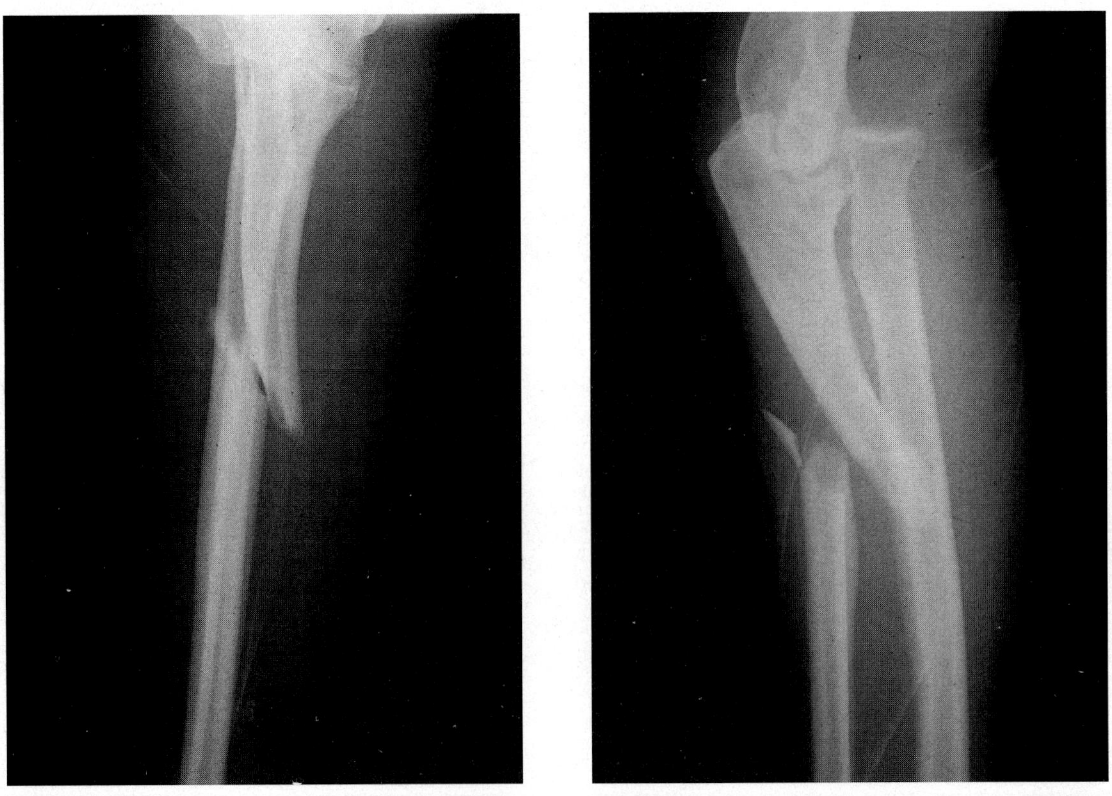

A B

Figure 21–1. Anteroposterior (A) and lateral (B) radiographs showing an anterior Monteggia fracture dislocation.

Radiologic Findings

Anteroposterior and lateral radiographs of the elbow showed anterior displacement of the proximal radius and a spiral fracture of the ulnar diaphysis with minor comminution (Fig. 21–1). The humeral diaphyseal fracture was noted to be a transverse fracture in the middle third of the humeral diaphysis.

Diagnosis

Multiple injuries with a closed anterior Monteggia fracture dislocation of the left arm.

Surgical Management

After resuscitation and investigation of her potential pulmonary and intraabdominal injuries, she was taken to the operating room. The left femoral fracture was stabilized using a reamed, interlocked, intramedullary nail, with cancellous screws placed behind the proximal end of the nail to stabilize the femoral neck fracture. The open tibial fracture was treated by wound debridement and intramedullary nailing and the left humeral diaphyseal fracture was stabilized with an AO dynamic compression plate. During this procedure the radial nerve was examined in the spiral groove of the humerus and was seen to be undamaged.

The Monteggia fracture dislocation was treated by closed reduction of the radial head and open reduction and internal fixation of the ulnar diaphyseal fracture using intrafragmentary screws and a small fragment AO six hole dynamic compression plate (Fig. 21–2). After reduction and fixation of the ulnar diaphyseal fracture the

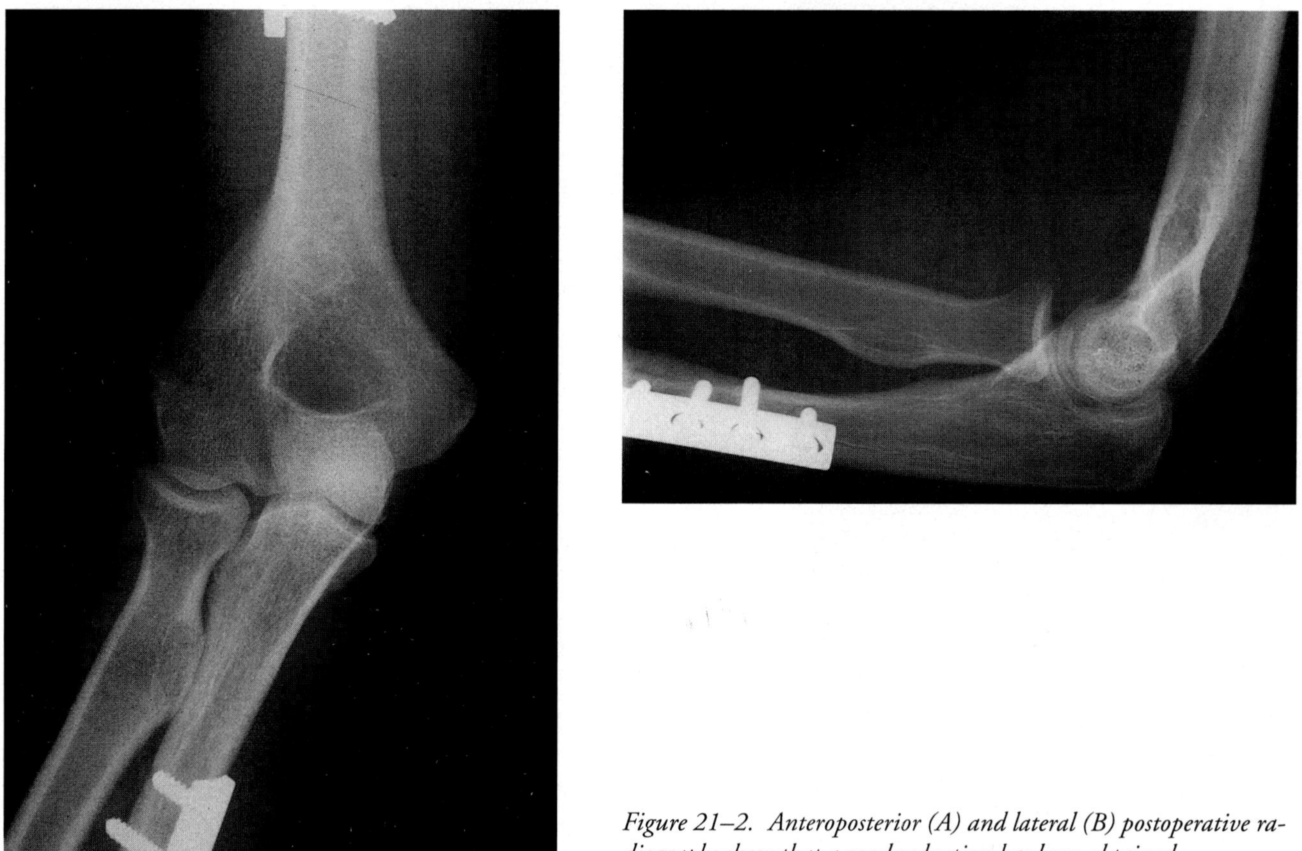

A

B

Figure 21–2. Anteroposterior (A) and lateral (B) postoperative radiographs show that a good reduction has been obtained.

elbow was freely mobile and check X rays showed that the radial head was reduced. Postoperatively a plaster back slab was applied to the left arm for 48 hours to facilitate nursing in the immediate postoperative period. On the day after surgery it was noted that the patient had a wrist drop with an inability to extend the wrist or fingers of the left hand, but sensory examination showed no abnormality. Because there was no damage to the radial nerve during humeral plating, the nerve was not explored.

Postoperative Management

After 48 hours elbow motion was encouraged and a physiotherapy regime instituted. However, the elbow proved difficult to mobilize and the patient had impaired movement. Check radiographs of the elbow taken 3 weeks after surgery showed the elbow joint to be congruous and no other abnormality was seen. By this time there was some return of function in the extensor musculature of the forearm.

Seven weeks after surgery there was good return of muscle function in the forearm and hand, but the elbow remained stiff despite intensive physiotherapy. Check

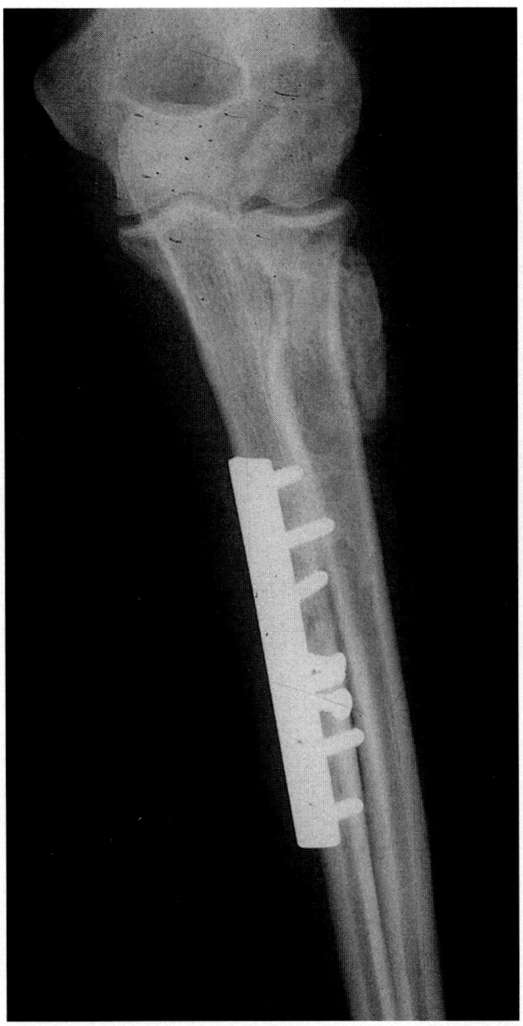

A

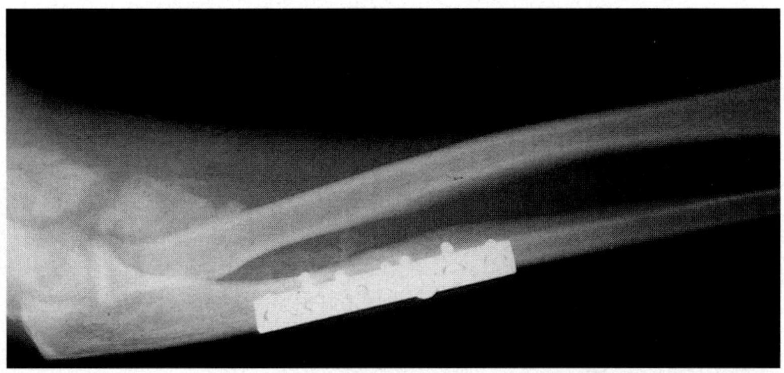

B

Figure 21–3. Seven weeks after the accident anteroposterior (A) and lateral (B) radiographs show signs of heterotopic new bone formation. This is evident anterior to the elbow joint and between the radius and ulna.

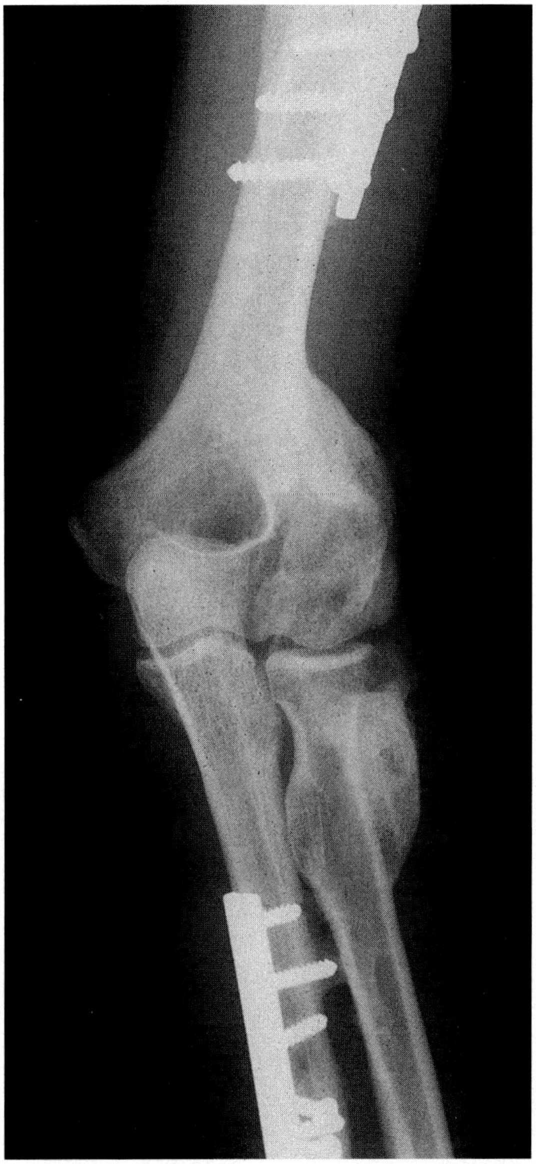

A

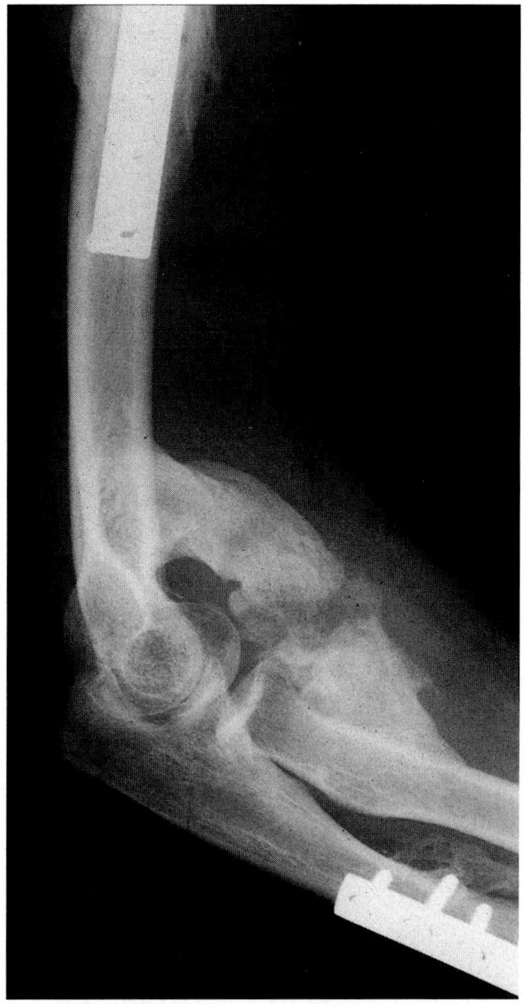

B

Figure 21–4. The heterotopic has reformed after the initial excision. There is dense bone anterior to the joint and around the head of the radius. Anteroposterior (A) and lateral views (B) .

radiographs at this time showed significant early myositis ossificans in the soft tissues anterior to the elbow joint (Fig. 21–3). It was decided to allow the heterotopic bone to mature and continue the physiotherapy regime. The patient was readmitted to the hospital 6 months after the accident for excision of the heterotopic bone. By that time she had regained normal neurological function in the left arm.

At surgery the elbow was approached anteriorly and sharp dissection used to elevate the soft tissues from the heterotopic bone mass. It was estimated that about 90% of the heterotopic bone was removed at surgery, and 5 days after surgery she had flexion from 25 to 105 degrees, with about 30 degrees of supination and pronation. Unfortunately, her wrist drop had returned and she had no function in the wrist or finger extensors.

Once again a physiotherapy regime was instituted and the elbow stiffened again. Two months after the excision of the heterotopic bone the patient was complaining of deteriorating elbow function. As before, there were signs of increasing heterotopic bone on the radiographs (Fig. 21–4). By this time the extensor muscles were once again recovering their function.

A second operation to excise the heterotopic bone from the anterior aspect of the left elbow was undertaken approximately 6 months after the initial procedure and 1 year after the accident. By this time the neurological function of the left arm was again normal. The elbow was opened anteriorly using the same incision and on this occasion a substantial amount of scar tissue was encountered in the wound. It was noted that the lateral cutaneous nerve of the forearm had been pulled to the medial side of the arm by scar tissues. Again bone was excised and about 120 degrees of passive flexion was achieved with the patient anesthetized. Postoperatively the patient again had a wrist drop.

On this occasion the patient was given indomethacin for 6 weeks after the bone excision; 1 year after the second bone excision procedure the patient had maintained reasonable elbow motion with full extension, 120 degrees of flexion, and about 75 degrees of pronation and supination. The neurological status of the arm had returned to normal and there was full extensor power in the wrist and fingers.

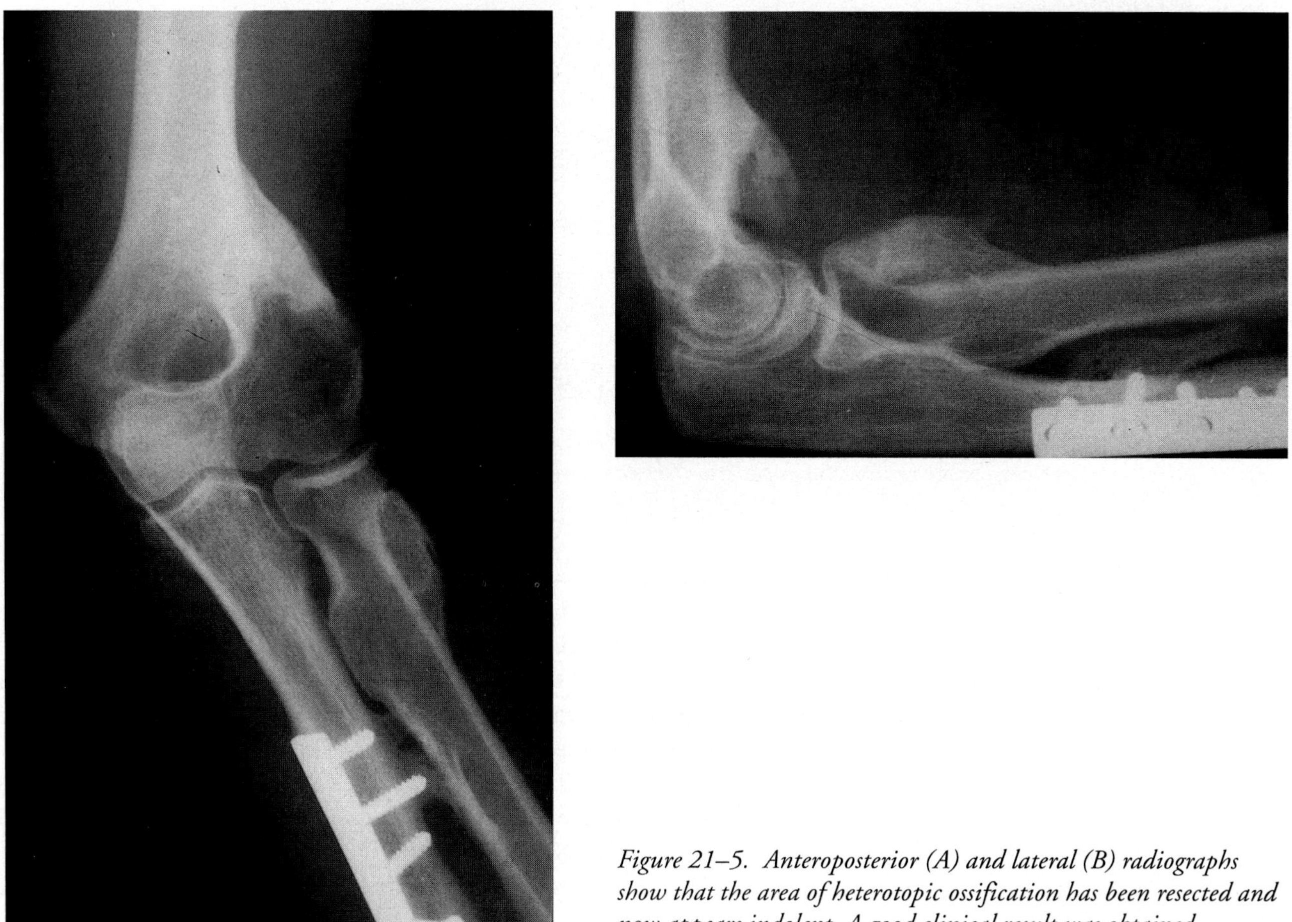

A

B

Figure 21–5. Anteroposterior (A) and lateral (B) radiographs show that the area of heterotopic ossification has been resected and now appears indolent. A good clinical result was obtained.

PEARLS

- As with the Galeazzi fracture dislocation at the distal end of the forearm, the Monteggia lesion exemplifies the importance of imaging the joints above and below any diaphyseal fracture. This is an aphorism that is often quoted but not always heeded!
- Accurate neurological examination is important. In this case there was a neuropraxia of the posterior interosseous rather than the radial nerve. The prognosis is good and no surgical intervention is required.

PITFALL

- Always obtain an adequate lateral radiograph. An anterior or posterior Monteggia lesion may be difficult to see on an anteroposterior radiograph.

Radiographs still showed some evidence of heterotopic bone (Fig. 21–5), but it was clear that the ossific process had ceased.

Discussion

The Monteggia fracture dislocation was first described in 1814 by Giovani Monteggia of Milan. Interestingly, he actually described an anterior dislocation of the radial head in association with an ulnar diaphyseal fracture, as shown in this case. The term Monteggia lesion was used by Bado (1967), who pointed out that anterior dislocation of the radial head was the most common form of the Monteggia lesion, comprising about 60% of cases. Posterior or posterolateral radial head dislocation occurred in about 15% of cases and a lateral or anterolateral dislocation combined with a metaphyseal ulnar fracture was seen in about 20%. Bado pointed out that the remaining 5% of cases presented with an anterior dislocation of the radial head associated with fractures of both the proximal ulnar and radius.

The treatment of the Monteggia lesion is straightforward. It is important to stabilize the ulnar fracture and accurately reduce the head of the radius. However, the radial head dislocation is not infrequently missed initially and is often detected at a later stage when the patient complains of elbow pain and stiffness. It was suggested by Boyd and Boals (1969) that up to 24% of Monteggia lesions are missed, although it is likely that currently, with increased awareness and improved radiological techniques, this figure is an overestimate of the problem. However, little doubt exists that the condition is sometimes missed at the initial examination because surgeons and radiologists tend to focus on the obvious ulnar fracture and overlook the radial head dislocation. Even if the elbow is included in a radiograph centered on the middle third of the ulnar, the bony overlap of an anterior or posterior Monteggia lesion may be missed.

In this case the patient presented with an apparent radial nerve palsy after the initial ulnar plating and reduction of the radial head had been performed. There was confusion because of the presence of the humeral diaphyseal fracture; it was initially thought that the postoperative paralysis of the extensor musculature of the forearm might be related to radial nerve damage secondary to the humeral diaphyseal fracture. However, the clue to the true nature of the neurological lesion lay in the presence of normal sensation in the distribution of the superficial branch of the radial nerve.

Damage to the motor branch of the radial nerve (the posterior interosseous nerve) is well recorded after Monteggia fracture dislocation. Jessing (1975) documented 14 patients with Monteggia lesions; six presented with neurological abnormalities in the distribution of the posterior interosseous nerve. All six patients had Bado type I anterior Monteggia lesions. No posterior or lateral Monteggia lesion presented with damage to the posterior interosseous nerve. Bruce et al. (1974) reviewed 35 patients with Monteggia lesions and noted that six (17%) had nerve palsies. Only one had a pure interosseous nerve lesion and three patients apparently had a complete radial nerve palsy. Two patients had involvement of the posterior interosseous nerve as well as the median nerve, with the ulnar nerve also involved in one case. All patients in both series had spontaneous resolution of their nerve palsies and in no case was surgical exploration required or undertaken.

In this case the patient obviously had a posttraumatic neuropraxia of the posterior interosseous nerve that recurred after each surgical intervention, suggesting that despite an apparent return to normality after each operation the nerve remained sensitive to traction, presumably because of permanent intraneural damage. This phenomenon of persistent susceptibility to handling or stretching following earlier nerve damage is well known.

The other major problem encountered in this patient was myositis ossificans or the formation of heterotopic bone anterior to the elbow joint. In Boyd and Boals' paper in 1969 they quote Watson-Jones' belief that the incidence of heterotopic ossification increased after open reduction of the elbow, although other authors at the time disputed this. Bruce et al. (1974) documented two cases of radioulnar synostosis following nonoperative management of a Monteggia lesion with at least one of the synostoses occurring in a Bado type I lesion with anterior dislocation of the radial head. Although this patient did not develop a synostosis, radiographs indicated heterotopic bone in the appropriate location.

Myositis ossificans often occurs around the elbow and is associated with damage to the brachialis muscle. It is of course unlikely that the brachialis muscle would have been significantly damaged by the Monteggia lesion in this case, but the combination of a humeral diaphyseal fracture and a Monteggia lesion would presumably have resulted in increased muscle damage and a higher chance of heterotopic bone formation. Thomson and Garcia (1967) studied myositis ossificans after elbow injuries reviewing 41 patients who had developed heterotopic bone around the elbow. They concluded that the overall incidence of myositis ossificans after elbow injuries was 3%, but that it was five times more common after a fracture dislocation than after a pure elbow dislocation. In younger patients the incidence was less and there was a tendency to absorb the heterotopic bone before it become mature. This group also demonstrated the best results after treatment. They also stated that the condition usually developed between 3 and 4 weeks after the fracture dislocation, and they urged that early diagnosis and definitive fracture treatment be carried out within 24 hours. Thomson and Garcia also suggested that passive movement should not be used during convalescence and were pessimistic about the results of surgical excision of mature myositis ossificans.

There is no doubt that the treatment of myositis ossificans is difficult. The accepted method of treatment is to cease active motion and immobilize the elbow in the position of function. The heterotopic bone is excised when it is mature. Unfortunately, there is no good definition of when the bone is mature, but it is usually accepted that excision be delayed for a year. The obvious problem with this therapeutic philosophy is that there will be secondary soft tissue contracture present at the time of bone excision and, as Thomson and Garcia predicted, the results may often be poor if the tight anterior capsule is not also released. If this occurs, good results have been reported (Roberts and Pankratz, 1979).

In recent years there has been interest in the prevention of heterotopic bone reformation after excision. The two suggested methods for preventing the formation of further heterotopic bone are radiotherapy and indomethacin administration. Unfortunately, no evidence exists regarding the use of these treatment modalities in the management of elbow heterotopic ossification because all of the work has been carried out in the hip either following arthroplasty or the operative treatment of acetabular fractures. However, there is evidence that preoperative and postoperative irradiation is useful in reducing heterotopic ossification after hip arthroplasty. Researchers have used different doses of radiation and demonstrated that doses of between 800 and 2000 centigray are effective, provided the radiation is given preoperatively or within 4 days of surgery.

Moed and his coworkers (1994) have investigated the use of indomethacin in the management of heterotopic ossification after acetabular fracture surgery and have documented that its use can significantly decrease the amount of heterotopic ossification around the hip. They also demonstrated that the reduction in heterotopic ossification was associated with improved functional results. Their recommended dose was 25 mg of indomethacin given three times a day. This regime should be instituted 24 hours after surgery and continued for 6 weeks postoperatively. If there are radiographic signs of heterotopic ossification at 6 weeks, the indomethacin regime should be continued for an additional 6 weeks. This regime was used in this case with success, but of course it is difficult to know what factors caused the second operation to be more successful than the first. However, it seems reasonable to use this indomethacin regime unless there is a medical contraindication to the use of nonsteroidal antiinflammatory drugs.

Alternative Methods of Management

Most surgeons would treat a Monteggia lesion in the manner illustrated here using an ulna dynamic compression plate and closed reduction of the radial head. The fracture pattern is usually fairly simple because Monteggia lesions are usually caused by low velocity injuries, commonly a simple fall or a direct blow to the forearm. The plating is straightforward and, provided AO technical guidelines are followed, the results should be good. The older literature contains many references to nonoperative management, but there is no current indication for this method of management. Internal fixation of the ulnar is the best method of realigning the ulnar diaphysis and securing the reduction of the radial head. Surgeons have used Rush pins or other thin intramedullary nails, but the fixation is less rigid and complications are likely to be greater than when using rigid fixation. There are no reports of the use of locked intramedullary nails in the management of a Monteggia lesion, although there is no reason why they should not be used, provided the diaphyseal fracture is accurately reduced.

After fixation of the ulnar it is important to check the congruency of the radiocapitellar joint using radiographs. If the joint is not reduced, it is probable that there is soft tissue interposition and an open reduction is required. If there is a significant fracture of the radial head, the surgeon will have to choose between internal fixation or resection; the former is preferred if possible.

Type of Management	Advantages	Disadvantages	Comments
Internal fixation of ulna; closed reduction of radial head	Stable fixation; congruent joint; early elbow motion	None	The procedure of choice
Internal fixation of ulna; open reduction of radial head	Stable fixation; congruent joint; early elbow motion	Possibly an increased risk of heterotopic ossification around the elbow	May be necessary if the radial head is irreducible
Nonoperative management	None	Ulnar malunion; unstable radial head	No advantage over internal fixation

Complications

The patient illustrated in this case presented with two of the complications associated with a Monteggia lesion: posterior interosseous neuropraxia and heterotopic ossification. However, the most common complication associated with Monteggia fracture dislocations is probably a failure to correctly diagnose the fracture. Surgeons are then faced with the problem of treating a late radial head dislocation associated with an ulnar malunion. Treatment will depend on the time of presentation, but frequently the Monteggia lesion is not diagnosed until 4 or 6 weeks after the accident. At this time the optimal treatment is rigid fixation of the ulna of the radial head excision.

Other complications can occur and infection or nonunion of the ulnar fracture may follow inappropriate surgery. However, these are easily treated using techniques described elsewhere in this book.

Suggested Readings

Bado JL: The Monteggia lesion. Clin Orthop 1967; 50:71–76.

Boyd HB, Boals JC: The Monteggia lesion. A review of 159 cases. Clin Orthop 1969; 66:94–100.

Bruce HE, Harvey JP, Wilson JC: Monteggia fractures. J Bone Joint Surg (Am) 1974; 56A:1563–1576.

Jessing P: Monteggia lesions and their complicating nerve damage. Acta Orthop Scand 1975; 46:601–609.

Moed BR, Karges DE: Prophylactic indomethacin for the prevention of heterotopic ossification after acetabular fracture in high risk patients. J Orthop Trauma 1994; 8:34–39.

Roberts JB, Pankratz DG: Surgical treatment of heterotopic ossification at the elbow. J Bone Joint Surg (Am) 1979; 61A:760–763.

Thomson HC, Garcia A: Myositis Ossificans: aftermath of elbow injuries. Clin Orthop 1967; 50:129–134.

Case 22

History and Physical Examination

The forearm and hand of a 24-year-old baker were caught in a machine that kneads dough. He was able to turn the machine off and extract his hand and forearm from the machine. He arrived in the emergency department approximately 20 minutes after injury. On physical examination, the forearm was deformed. A 2 cm laceration was present over the radial border of the mid forearm. The skin edges of the laceration were clean and gross contamination was not present. The skin and soft tissues of the forearm did not appear to be avulsed or degloved. Pain was not elicited by palpation of the wrist, elbow, or hand. The neurovascular examination of the hand was within the limits of normal. There were no injuries other than to the forearm.

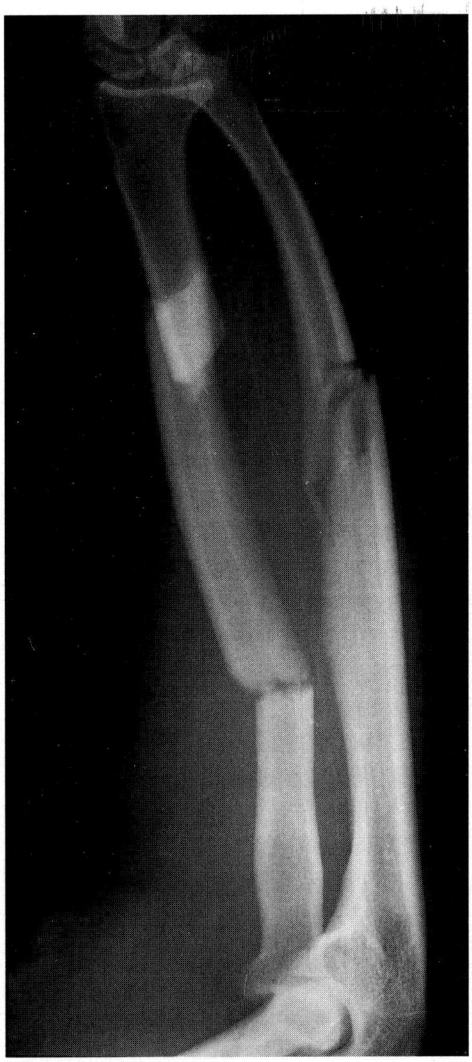

Figure 22–1. Radiograph of the forearm indicating a comminuted fracture of the ulna and a segmental fracture of the radius. There are no signs of injury to the wrist or elbow.

Radiologic Findings

Radiographs indicated a segmental fracture of the radius and a fracture of the ulna. All three fractures were oblique, displaced, and not significantly comminuted. There were no radiographic signs of injury to the elbow or wrist (Fig. 22–1).

Diagnosis

Open fracture of both bones of the forearm, with the radius fracture being segmental. This injury is classified as a C2 type fracture. Because the radius fracture was segmental, the open injury is classified as grade 3. AO classification: 22–C32.

Surgical Management

The wound was cultured, irrigated, and covered with a sterile dressing. The arm was immobilized in a long arm splint. A second generation cephalosporin was administered intravenously.

The patient was taken to the operating room where a general anesthetic was administered. The arm was prepped and draped on a hand table. The wound on the radial border of the forearm was extended proximally and distally and explored. The

A

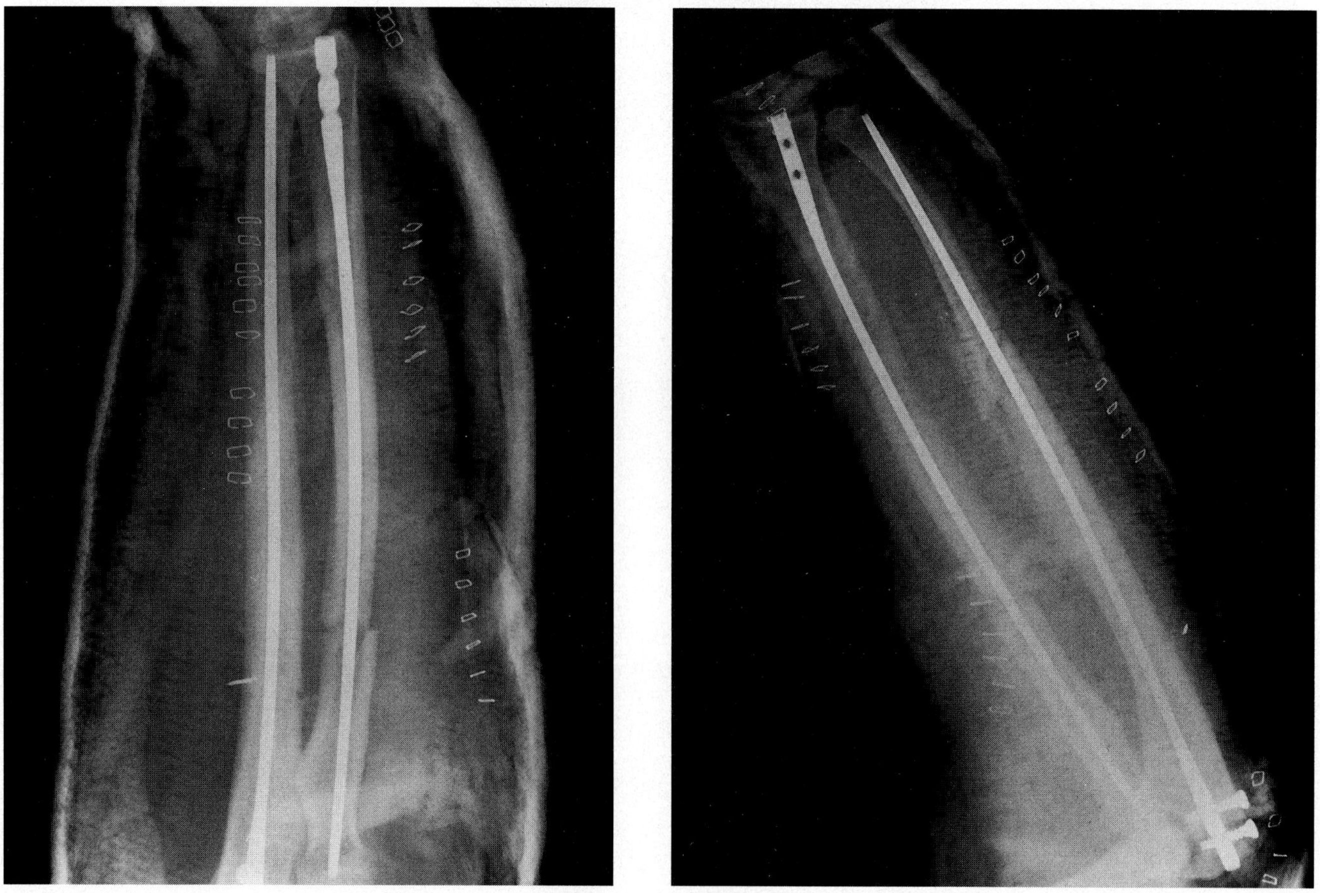

B

Figure 22–2. Anteroposterior (A) and oblique (B) radiographs of the forearm following intramedullary nailing.

PEARL

- The key to achieving an adequate debridement and determining the extent of injury is to extend the open wound by incising the soft tissue. It is important to design the incisions in such a way that additional soft tissue is not devitalized (e.g., skin flaps should not be raised; the incision should be a continuation of the laceration).

wound extended through the extensor muscles and communicated with the proximal fracture of the radius. Minimal nonviable tissue was found. The fracture hematoma was irrigated from the wound. A specimen of hematoma was sent for culture.

Next, the fractures were reduced and stabilized with intramedullary nails. The insertion portal for the radial nail was just ulnar to Lister's tubercle, at the level of the wrist joint. The insertion site was exposed through a 2 cm long incision, and care was taken to avoid injury of the surrounding tendons. The insertion portal for the ulnar nail was the olecranon. The radial and ulnar nails were driven to the level of the fracture. The fracture was manipulated and reduced with the aid of fluoroscopy. The nail was driven across the fracture. The proximal radial fracture was reduced through the open wound. The ulnar nail was locked at the insertion site to prevent it from backing out of the bone. The radial nail was not locked distally because of the risk of in-

A 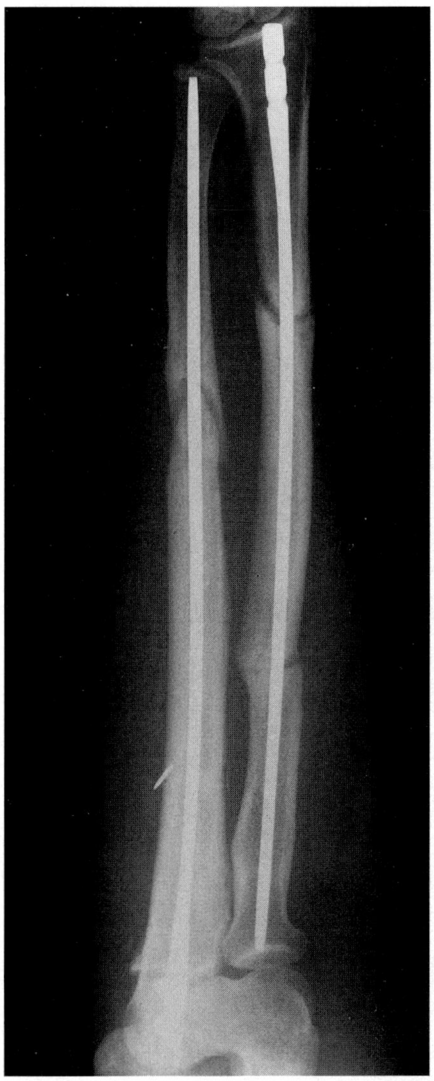 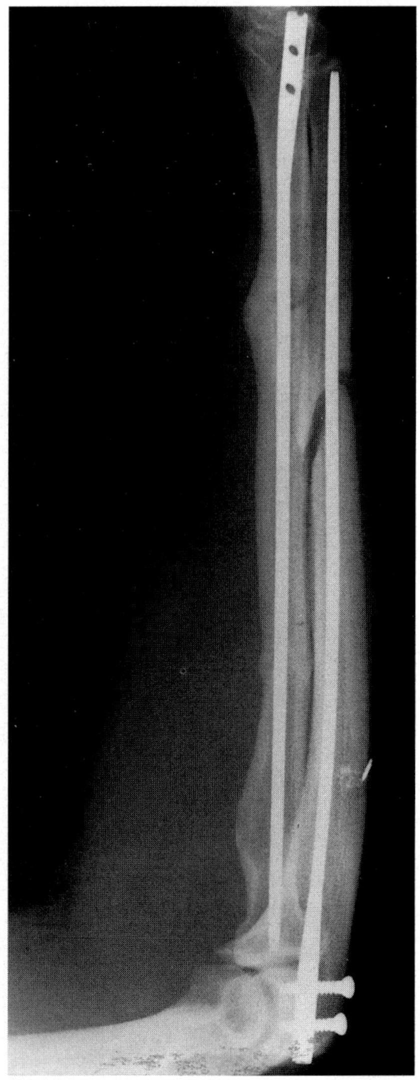 B

Figure 22–3. Anteroposterior (A) and lateral (B) radiographs of the forearm at 6 months following injury. The proximal radial fracture is healed, the distal radial fracture appears to be healing (in particular dorsally), and the ulnar fracture appears as though it will not heal.

PEARL

- Preoperatively, the patient did not have a compartment syndrome; however, the additional trauma of surgery can lead to elevated pressures and a compartment syndrome. Therefore, postoperatively the patient must be closely monitored. The first sign of impending compartment syndrome is an increase in pain at rest. This is followed by severe pain with gentle passive stretch of the muscles involved, and paresthesias of the nerves traversing the involved compartment. If it is not possible to monitor the patient clinically, either because a nerve block was used for anesthesia or because the patient is obtunded, intracompartmental pressures must be measured at regular intervals for the first 24 hours.

jury to the superficial radial nerve. An unsuccessful attempt was made to lock the radial nail proximally. The incisions through which the nails had been inserted were closed. The surgical extensions of the laceration were closed in a single layer and the laceration was loosely approximated with a single simple suture. A bulky compression dressing with a plaster splint was applied to the forearm (Fig. 22–2).

Postoperative Management

Postoperatively the arm was elevated and the patient was placed on bedrest for 48 hours. In the first 12 hours the forearm was carefully monitored for compartment syndrome.

At 48 hours the patient was allowed out of bed with the arm in a sling. Gentle range of motion of the shoulder, elbow, wrist, and hand was begun. Intravenous antibiotics were continued for a total of 48 hours from the time of injury. The cultures from the emergency department and operating room were sterile. The patient was discharged on the third day after injury. Consolidation of both fractures of the ra-

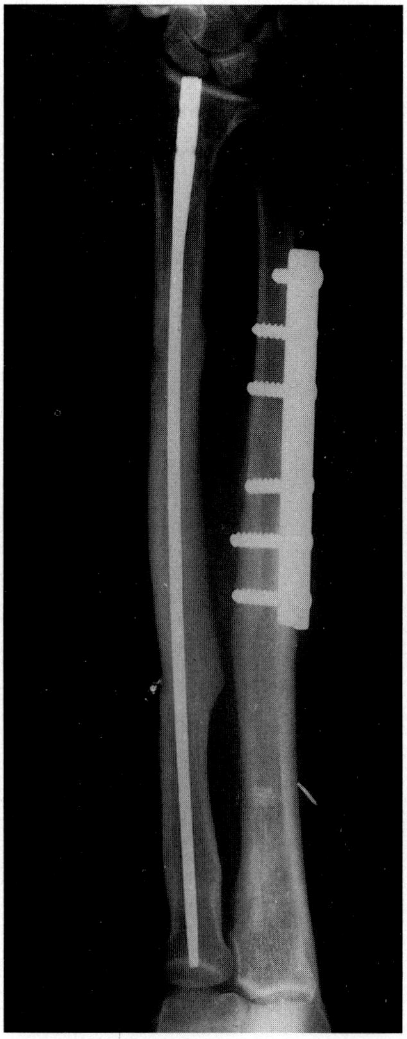

Figure 22–4. Radiograph 6 months following plating and bone grafting of the ulna. Both the radius and ulna appear solidly healed.

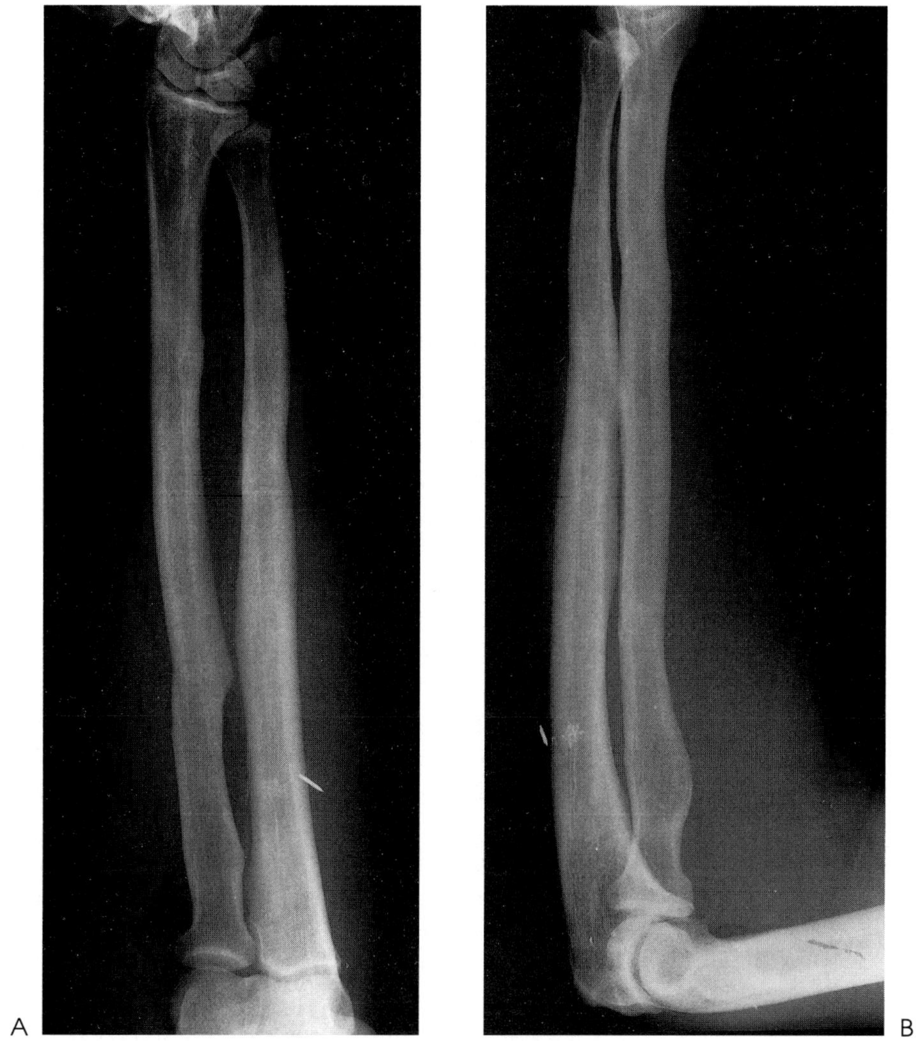

Figure 22–5. Anteroposterior (A) and lateral (B) radiographs following removal of the internal fixation devices. All fractures are solidly healed.

dius proceeded as expected. The ulnar fracture did not heal (Fig. 22–3). At 6 months the ulnar nail and locking screws were removed. The ulna was exposed along its subcutaneous border. The area around the nonunion was decorticated with an osteotome and grafted with autogenous bone harvested from the iliac crest. The ulnar nonunion consolidated (Fig. 22–4). The plate, screws, and radial nail were eventually removed because of local irritation (Fig. 22–5). Final flexion and extension of the elbow was 135 to 0 degrees. Forearm rotation was 80 degrees of supination to 80 degrees of pronation.

Discussion

The primary goals of the acute management are to determine the extent of injury (e.g., whether there is an extensive soft tissue injury), debride the soft tissue injury, and open fracture, and stabilize the fractures. In this case the soft tissue injury was limited and an extensive debridement was not required.

This patient had a potential to develop a compartment syndrome because of the high energy injury he had sustained. Compartment syndrome was ruled out clinically in the emergency department because none of the cardinal physical signs were present (i.e., more pain than expected at rest, pain with gentle passive stretch of muscles, paresthesias, and palpably tense compartments). If any of these signs had been present, compartment pressures would have been measured and, if elevated, a fasciotomy would have been performed.

Alternative Methods of Management

Alternative methods of fracture stabilization are intramedullary nails; plates and screws; a combination of intramedullary nail for the radius and plates and screws for the ulna; and external fixation. Closed management with immobilization is not an acceptable alternative for this injury because instability of the fracture would lead to loss of reduction and nonunion or malunion. Intramedullary nails were used because the fracture of the radius was segmental. Plating of the segmental radial fracture would have required an extensive exposure and may have further compromised the blood supply of the segmental fragment. Stabilization with intramedullary nails has the advantage of minimizing the surgical exposure and thus minimizing devitalization of the bone at the fracture site and the chance of iatrogenic nerve injury. On the other hand, the use of nails has several disadvantages. First, if the patient develops osteomyelitis as a sequelae of his open fracture, the presence of the nail may lead to infection of the entire medullary canal. Second, while the radial fracture is segmental, the ulnar fracture is not, and nailing may be more time consuming than exposing the fracture, which is subcutaneous, and plating it. Finally, the medullary canal of the radius and ulna vary widely in diameter from patient to patient. Either nail may become incarcerated if the canal has a smaller diameter than that of the nail.

Stabilization with plates and screws has the advantage of achieving immediate rigid stabilization; however, this method requires an extensive exposure and leads to

Type of Management	Advantages	Disadvantages	Comments
Intramedullary nailing	Limited surgical exposure	Technically difficult; may lead to intramedullary osteomyelitis	Intramedullary nailing of the ulna is probably not necessary
Plates and screws	Rigid fixation	Requires an extensive surgical exposure to stabilize radial fracture	Probably the most commonly used method of management
Plate on the ulna, nail in the radius	Combines the advantages of nailing and plating	Nailing the radius may be technically difficult	Probably the optimum method of management
External fixation	Foreign body not left in wound	Limited patient acceptance; technically difficult to apply pins to proximal fragments of radius	Advantages do not outweigh disadvantages of limited patient acceptance and technical difficulty

devitalization of the bone at the fracture site. Exposure of the proximal radial fracture carries with it a significant risk of iatrogenic injury of the posterior interosseous nerve. Because this fracture was open, the chance of infection is increased by leaving a foreign body, such as a plate, in the wound.

Stabilization with an external fixator has the advantage of not leaving a foreign body in the wound. The disadvantages of external fixation are that it is poorly tolerated by most patients and that, in this case, it would be extremely difficult technically to apply the external fixator to the proximal and intercalary fragments of the radius.

Complications

Complications of this injury are nonunion, infection, and malunion. Nonunion is most likely to occur at one of the fractures of the radius. In this case it occurred at the ulnar fracture. Nonunion can be managed conservatively until the hardware fails. Once the hardware has failed, operative management is indicated. Conservative management of the nonunion consists of a protective splint extending from the elbow to the wrist. It is important that the splint does not prevent forearm rotation or elbow flexion and extension (i.e., a long arm cast is inappropriate because it will result in loss of motion). The application of pulsed electromagnetic fields may stimulate fracture consolidation. Operative management of the nonunion consists of rigid fixation and autogenous bone grafting. Decorticating or "fish scaling" the bone around the nonunion site may stimulate an acute response to injury (i.e., the reinjury phenomena) and aids in incorporation of the autogenous graft.

Infection is managed conservatively until the fracture has healed. When consolidation has occurred, the implants are removed and infected or necrotic tissue excised. Dead space is managed by packing with antibiotic beads and delayed autogenous bone grafting. Antibiotics are administered systemically for 4 to 6 weeks.

Malunion may result in loss of motion or cosmetic deformity. If malunion is symptomatic, the bones are osteotomized and the deformity is corrected. The osteotomy is plated and grafted with autogenous bone.

Suggested Readings

Jones JA: Immediate internal fixation of high-energy open forearm fractures. J Orthop Trauma 1991; 5(3):272–279.

Morgan WJ, Breen TF: Complex fractures of the forearm. Hand Clinics 1994; 10(3):375–390.

Case 23

History and Physical Examination

A 14-year-old male was admitted to the emergency department after falling from a rope swing in his yard. He had fallen about 6 feet and landed on his outstretched arm. Following the injury his left distal forearm was painful and deformed. Examination of his hand showed no neurovascular impairment and, in particular, he had no objective evidence of median nerve damage, although examination of the muscle function in the hand and forearm was difficult because of discomfort. There was no other injury.

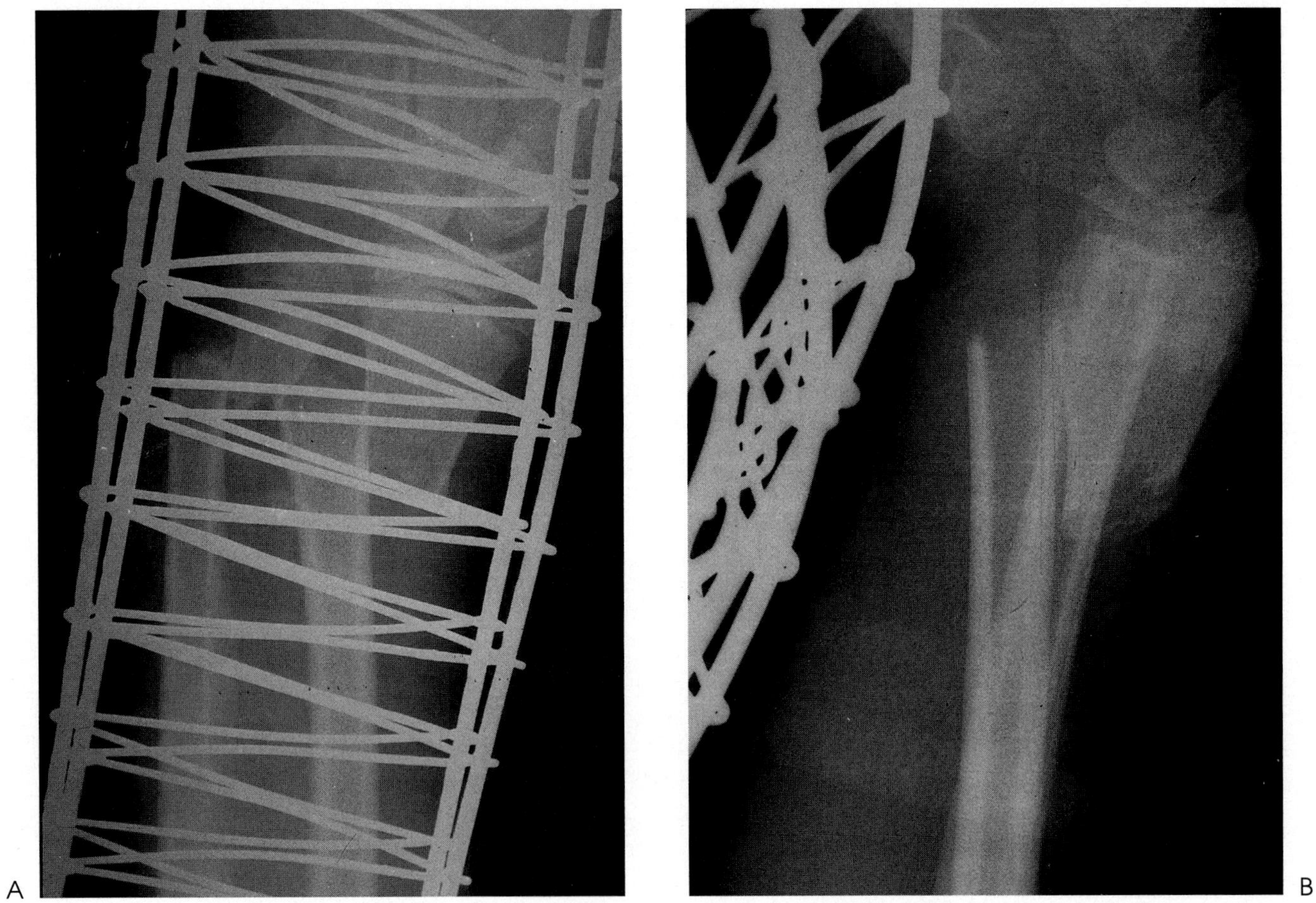

Figure 23–1. A distal forearm fracture in an adolescent. Anteroposterior (A) and lateral (B) views.

Radiologic Findings

Anteroposterior and lateral radiographs showed displaced fractures of the distal radius and ulna (Fig. 23–1). Both fractures were transverse and both distal fragments had been displaced dorsoradially by more than the circumference of the bone.

Diagnosis

Displaced transverse fractures of the distal radius and ulna. AO classification: 22–A3.3.

Surgical Management

The patient was treated in the emergency department by a closed manipulation of the fracture under an axillary nerve block. The postreduction radiographs showed slight dorsal angulation, but the overall alignment was considered acceptable (Fig. 23–2). The patient was admitted to the orthopedic trauma unit after a supportive plaster back slab had been applied to the reduced fracture.

The patient entered the orthopaedic ward at about 10:00 PM and required no analgesia overnight. The nurses maintained an hourly assessment of the circulation in his hand and no abnormality was detected. The axillary block gave excellent anesthesia for about 8 hours but the effect started to wear off the following morning, leaving the patient in great pain. He was unable to actively move his fingers and passive movement was extremely painful. He also had dysesthesia in the distribution of the median nerve and examination showed diminished sensation in the median nerve distribution.

A

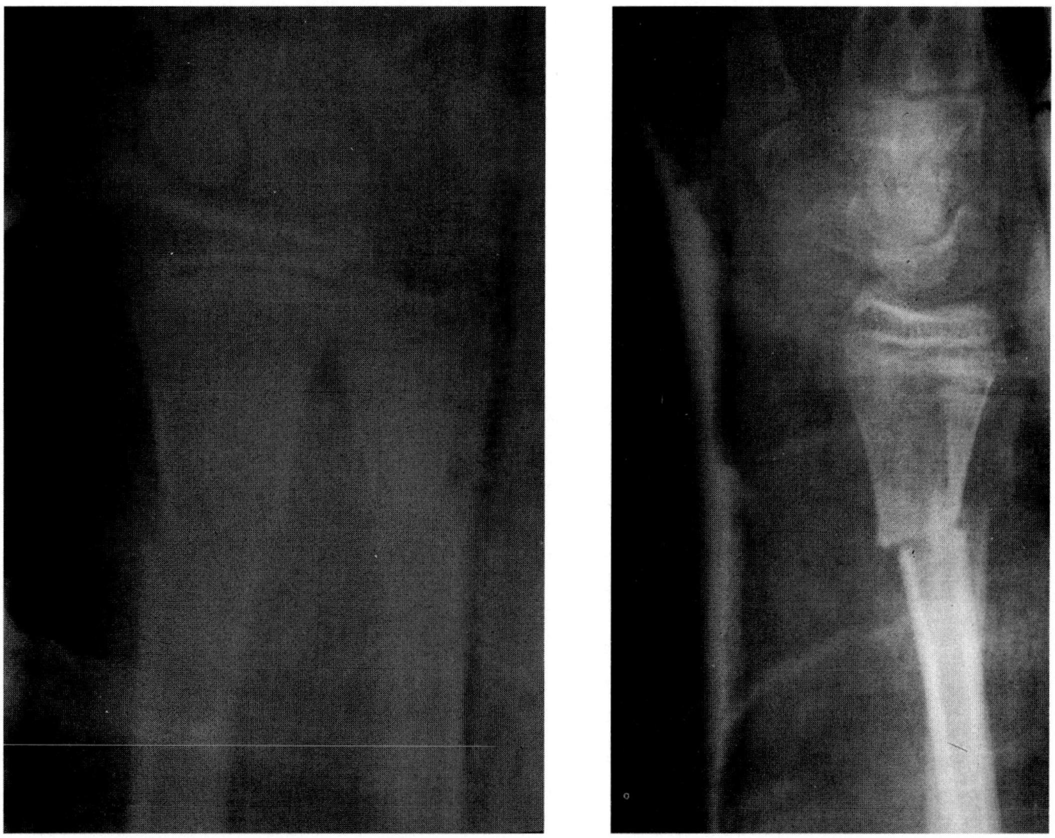

B

Figure 23–2. An acceptable, but not perfect, reduction was obtained. Anteroposterior (A) and lateral (B) views.

PEARL

- A volar compartment decompression is adequate. Once the volar compartment pressure has been reduced, the extensor compartment is flaccid and the pressure is low. If there is doubt about the extensor compartment, the pressure can easily be measured.

A diagnosis of a compartment syndrome of the forearm was made and the patient prepared for surgery. Under general anesthetic a slit catheter was inserted into the flexor compartment of the forearm and a pressure of 85 mm Hg was recorded. The blood pressure prior to anesthesia had been 95/70 mm Hg. (The relationship between the compartment pressure and the diastolic blood pressure has been discussed in the section describing the management of compartment syndrome in closed tibial fractures.) The pressure study confirmed the clinical findings of a compartment syndrome and a flexor compartment fasciotomy was performed. The forearm was decompressed through a longitudinal incision from just below the elbow to the wrist; the carpal tunnel was opened at the same time. Wide separation of the skin edges was noted.

The distal radial and ulnar fractures were reduced and plated using dynamic compression plates. The volar fasciotomy wound was left open and dressings applied. Following fracture fixation a slit catheter was placed into the extensor compartment and the pressure noted as 6 mm Hg.

Postoperative Management

Within 4 hours of surgery it became obvious that the pain of muscle ischemia had been relieved. The patient's fingers were held in flexion, but examination showed that he did have active finger extension. However, there was no change in the area and severity of the median nerve dysesthesia.

The patient was returned to the operating room 48 hours after the fasciotomy and the muscles of the flexor compartment were examined. All were normal and the fasciotomy wound was partially closed. The remaining deficit was slowly closed over the next few days with a banding technique. The neurological symptoms persisted for about 7 weeks. There was a gradual recovery over this time, with lessening of the dysesthesic symptoms and return of full sensation. The fracture united and 4 months after the injury the patient had full painless movement of the wrist and hand with no residual neurological sequelae (Fig. 23–3).

Discussion

Most surgeons associate forearm compartment syndrome in children with supracondylar fractures of the distal humerus. However, there is no doubt that other forearm fractures in young people are associated with this complication. There are not very many references in the literature dealing with this problem and it is probable that compartment syndrome complicating distal forearm fractures in adolescents is more common than many surgeons realize. However, compartment syndrome has been reported to complicate most types of distal forearm fracture. It is important to remember that the intracompartmental pressure only rises after the fracture is reduced. The act of reduction increases the tension in the damaged muscle and starts the cycle of events that causes compartment syndrome.

This case raises a number of important points. The fracture itself is fairly straightforward to treat and many such fractures will be successfully treated by manipulation and the application of a cast. The initial impression is that this is a simple transverse fracture of both forearm bones and that after fracture reduction there will be few, if any, problems. However, it is important to remember that this is usually a high energy injury and this particular fracture configuration in young adults is asso-

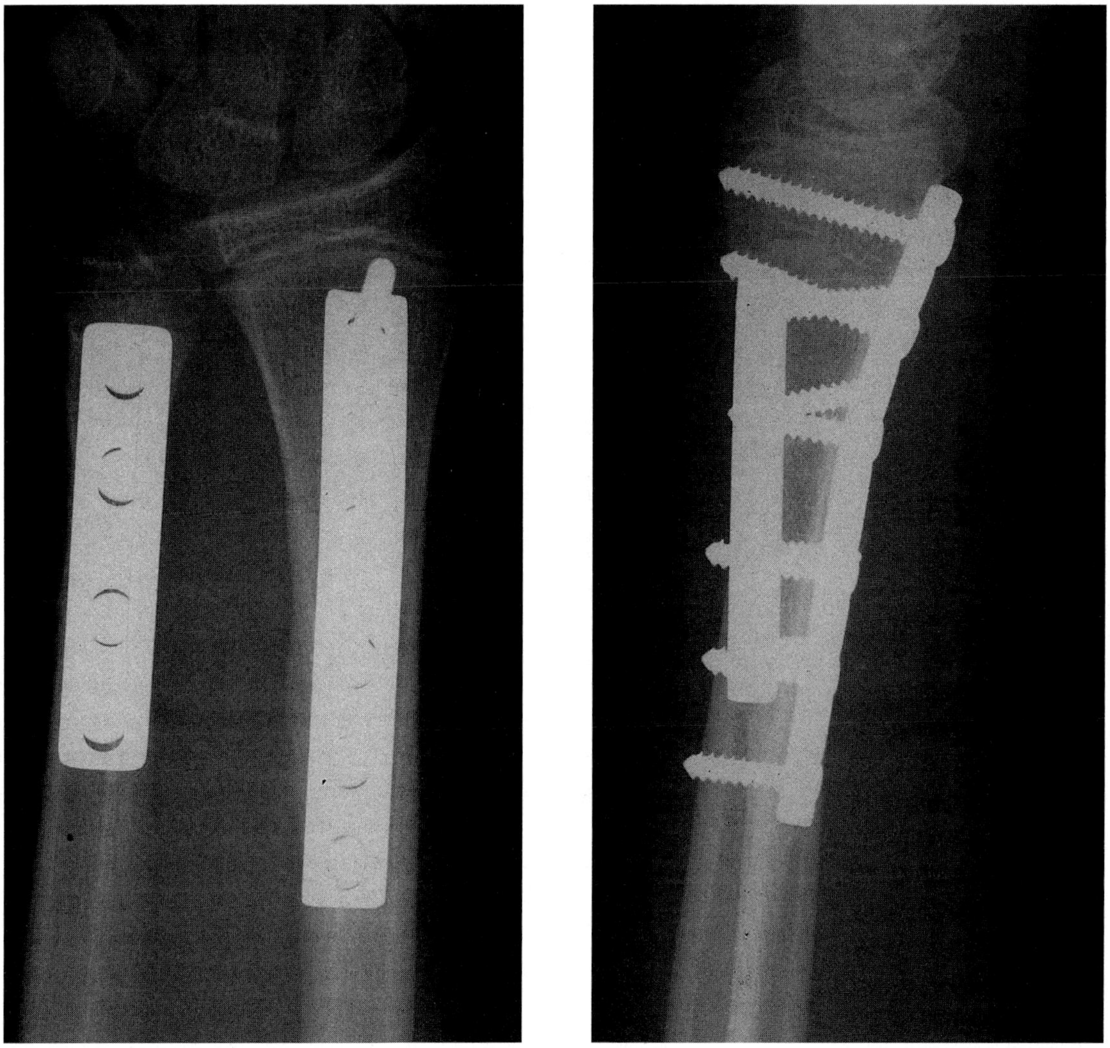

A B

Figure 23–3. Anteroposterior (A) and lateral (B) radiographs showing a good radiological result after union.

ciated with a relatively high incidence of either direct median nerve damage or flexor compartment syndrome. Therefore it is important that all such fractures are admitted to the hospital for 24 to 48 hours until the surgeon is sure that there is neither neurological sequelae or a compartment syndrome. If the surgeon adopts a policy of discharging these patients after manipulation in the emergency department, a compartment syndrome will eventually occur in the patient at home.

The second obvious problem is the choice of an axillary block for the initial manipulative procedure. Surgeons and anesthetists should be very careful about the type of anesthetic that is used for fractures associated with compartment syndrome. If analgesia is prolonged for 6 to 10 hours, then a compartment syndrome may be missed with obvious sequelae. Compartment syndromes are particularly common in tibial diaphyseal fractures and in distal forearm fractures and these two groups of patients not uncommonly receive nerve blocks for anesthesia or analgesia. There is no reason why nerve blocks should not be used, but if they are, compartment pressure monitoring should also be used. It is safer to use general anes-

PEARL

- It is important that the anesthesiologists and the orthopaedic surgeons agree on a protocol for these patients to avoid missed compartment syndromes.

PITFALL

- Most surgeons would probably treat the fracture nonoperatively if there was no evidence of a compartment syndrome. However, the fracture should be fixed if a fasciotomy is performed, because the requirement for fasciotomy destabilizes the fracture and increases the incidence of complications such as infection, malunion, and nonunion.

thesia and retain the ability to examine the limb following fracture reduction and fixation.

The third important lesson to be learned from this case is that urgent forearm decompression is required to avoid prolonged neurological symptoms. Even a delay of 8 hours may result in neurological symptoms that may take a considerable time to resolve. It is obviously important to distinguish between median nerve damage and flexor compartment syndrome. In the initial stages both may have a similar presentation, but median nerve damage merely requires a carpal tunnel decompression while flexor compartment syndrome requires a full fasciotomy. Compartment pressure monitoring can be used to distinguish between the two conditions; if the surgeon has any doubt, it is always safer to perform a volar fasciotomy and carpal tunnel decompression.

Alternative Methods of Management

If distal radial and ulnar fractures are not associated with compartment syndrome, most surgeons would probably elect to use an above elbow cast to treat the fracture. Because these patients are young and have excellent periosteum, rapid union can be expected and the patient will regain good function. If a compartment syndrome occurs, plate fixation is ideal because the patient can then be treated without a cast.

Alternative methods of management include plate fixation of only one of the two fractures or the use of Kirschner wires. If the radius is plated and the ulna merely reduced, a supplementary cast must be applied. This prevents adequate examination of the soft tissues and also prevents early wrist movement. The fixation provided by Kirschner wires is poor and again a supplementary cast is necessary. Usually the plates can be placed so that they do not need to cross the epiphysis and therefore that is no clinical indication for the use of Kirschner wires. Theoretically, Rush pins or other similar thin intramedullary nails could be placed into the distal radius to secure fixation; the same arguments apply and there seems to be little advantage to be gained using this technique.

Type of Management	Advantages	Disadvantages	Comments
Cast/traction	Straightforward technique	Poor fracture stability; malunion; infection	Not indicated if a fasciotomy is required
Plating	Good stability; early joint motion	Theoretical increase in the incidence of infection	Method of choice if a fasciotomy is required
Kirschner wires	Straightforward technique	Poor stability; malunion	No advantage over plating
Rush pins	Easy technique	Poor stability; malunion	No advantage over plating

Complications

The major complications resulting from failure to perform a timely fasciotomy are persistent neurological sequelae, irreversible muscle damage with secondary joint contractures, and impaired forearm function. Compartment syndromes rarely remain untreated today, but, if so, the end result may well be irreversible joint dys-

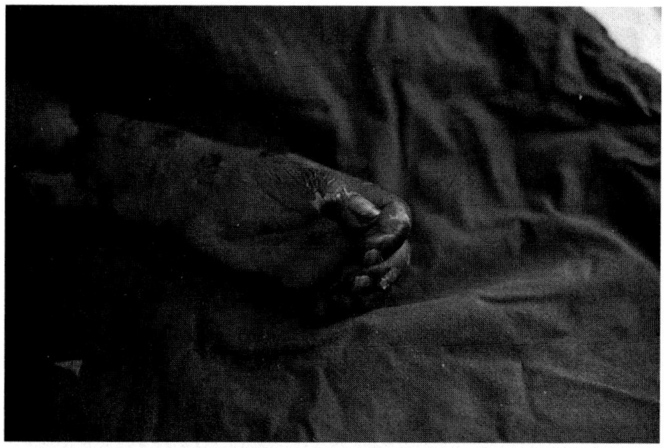

Figure 23–4. The late presentation of missed compartment syndrome of the forearm includes digital gangrene, contractures, and marked impairment of function.

function, muscle paralysis, and gangrene of the fingers, resulting in amputation (Fig. 23–4).

Suggested Readings

Eaton RG, Green WT: Volkmann's ischaemia. Clin Orthop 1975; 113:58–64.

Hernandez J, Peterson HA: Fractures of the distal radial physis complicated by compartment syndrome and premature physeal closure. J Paediatr Orthop 1986; 6:627–630.

Matson FA, Veitch RG: Compartment syndrome in children. J Paediatr Orthop 1981; 1:33–41.

McQuillan WM, Nolan B: Ischaemia complicating injury. J Bone Joint Surg (Br) 1968; 50B:482–492.

Royle SG: Compartment syndrome following forearm fracture in children. Injury 1990; 21:73–76.

Stockley I, Harvey IA, Getty CJM: Acute volar compartment syndrome of the forearm secondary to fracture of the distal radius. Injury 1988; 19:101–104.

Case 24

History and Physical Examination

A 62-year-old female was brought to the emergency department after slipping on the ice and falling onto her right arm. She had a painful right wrist that showed the classic dinner fork deformity suggestive of an extraarticular distal radial fracture or Colles' fracture. There was no other injury.

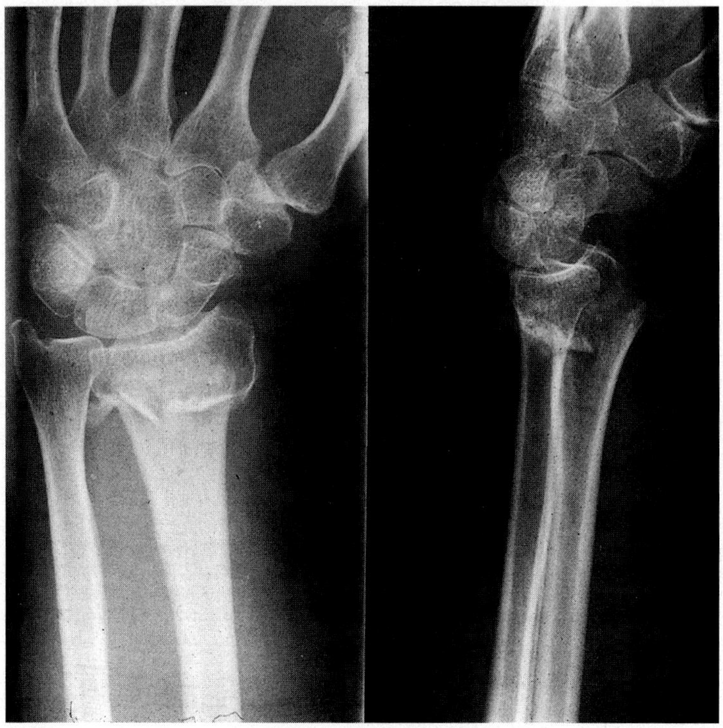

Figure 24–1. A classical extraarticular distal radial Colles' fracture.

Radiologic Findings

Anteroposterior and lateral radiographs showed an extraarticular distal radial fracture associated with dorsal angulation, dorsal displacement, and radial shortening (Fig. 24–1). The radiographs also show evidence of comminution on the dorsum and ulnar side of the distal radius.

Diagnosis

Extraarticular distal radial fracture. The eponym *Colles' fracture* is in widespread use for this fracture type. AO classification: 23–A2.2.

Surgical Management

The patient was treated by manipulation under general anesthesia in the emergency department. Check radiographs showed that a better reduction had been achieved, although residual dorsal angulation was present. The radial length had been im-

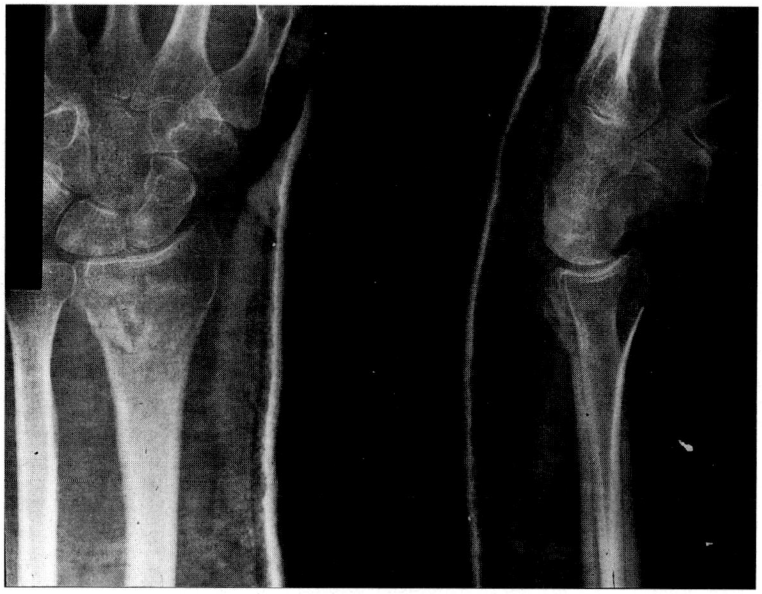

Figure 24–2. The fracture has been manipulated and a reasonable reduction achieved. Note that there is still dorsal angulation.

proved. A plaster back slab was applied and the patient was discharged home with instructions to maintain finger movement and return if there were signs that the supportive cast and bandages were too tight (Fig. 24–2). Further radiographs were taken 6 days later. These showed that position of the fracture had significantly worsened. There was also evidence of carpal malalignment (Fig. 24–3).

The patient was admitted to the orthopaedic unit and taken to the operating room. The arm was prepped and draped and a periarticular joint sparing external fixator applied (Fig. 24–4). This configuration of external fixator is relatively easy to apply, although the use of fluoroscopy is essential. Two external fixator pins are inserted into the distal radial metaphyseal fragment. To do this, the surgeon must palpate Lister's tubercle on the distal radius. A 2 cm transverse incision is centered on Lister's tubercle and the tendon of extensor pollicis longus is identified. Blunt dis-

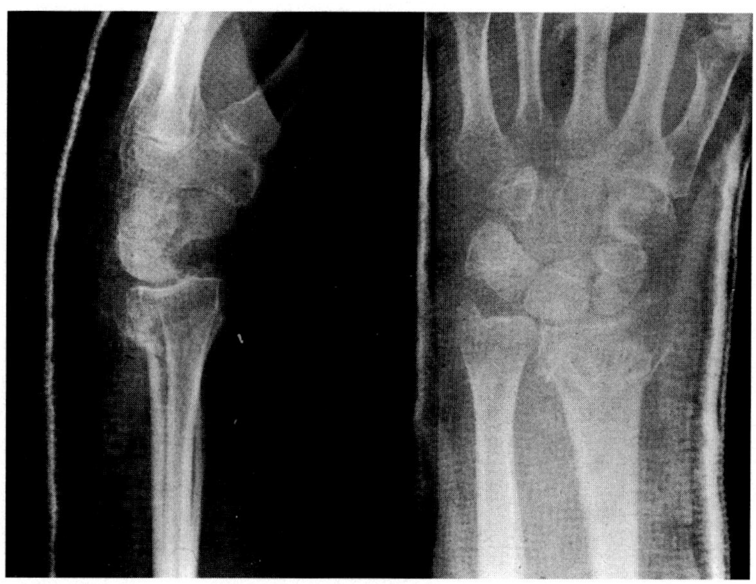

Figure 24–3. Ten days later the fracture has displaced further. There is carpal malalignment and the dorsal comminution is obvious.

PEARL

- When applying a periarticular frame the extensor pollicis longus tendon must be visualized. Failure to do this may result in tendon damage.

PITFALL

- Never insert external fixator pins through stab incisions especially in an area that has tendons, nerves, and large blood vessels. It is always wise to make an incision and then use blunt dissection to expose the bone. In the distal radius the superficial radial nerve should be exposed to prevent damage.

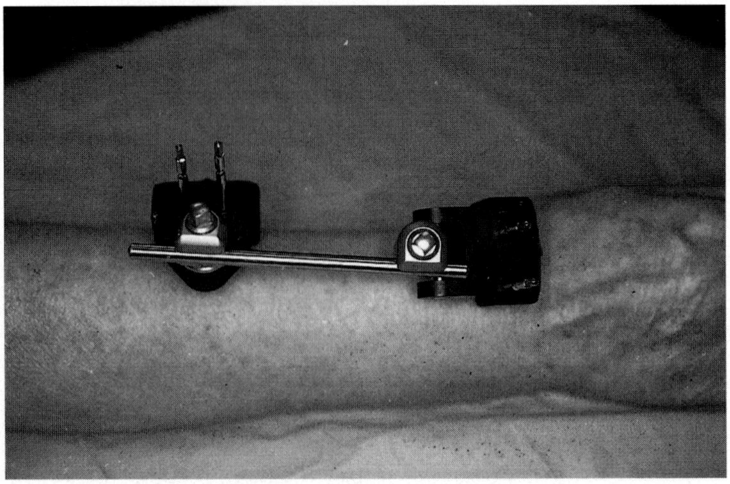

Figure 24–4. A periarticular external wrist fixator. There are two pins in the radial diaphysis and two in the distal radius. The patient is allowed immediate movement.

section is used to expose the bone on each side of the tendon and two external fixator pins are inserted adjacent to the tendon. The angle of the pins is determined by fluoroscopy. The surgeon rotates the wrist to a lateral view and then, using the fluoroscope, angles an external fixator pin so that it is parallel to the articular surface of the distal radius and lies just proximal to the joint surface adjacent to the subchondral bone. It is recommended that a pin tract be drilled prior to insertion of the external fixator pin because this facilitates pin insertion. A second external fixator pin is then inserted parallel to the first and the position carefully checked with fluoroscopy. Both pins should engage the volar cortex (Fig. 24–5).

An incision is then made over the radial diaphysis about 6 to 8 cm proximal to the wrist joint. Two external pins are inserted using an open technique, being careful to avoid the superficial branch of the radial nerve. A periarticular external fixator is then applied with a clamp placed around each pair of half pins. The two clamps are connected by a radiolucent bar and dressings and bandaging are applied (Fig. 24–4).

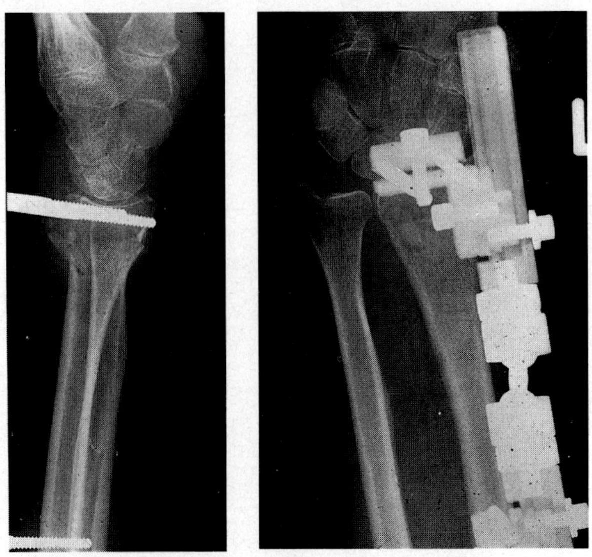

Figure 24–5. Note the two parallel pins in the subchondral bone. Distally they just engage the volar cortex.

PITFALL

- After manipulation, the wrist should be placed in slight volar flexion and ulnar deviation. The Cotton Loder position of extreme volar flexion should never be used because it is painful and may result in a median neuropathy.

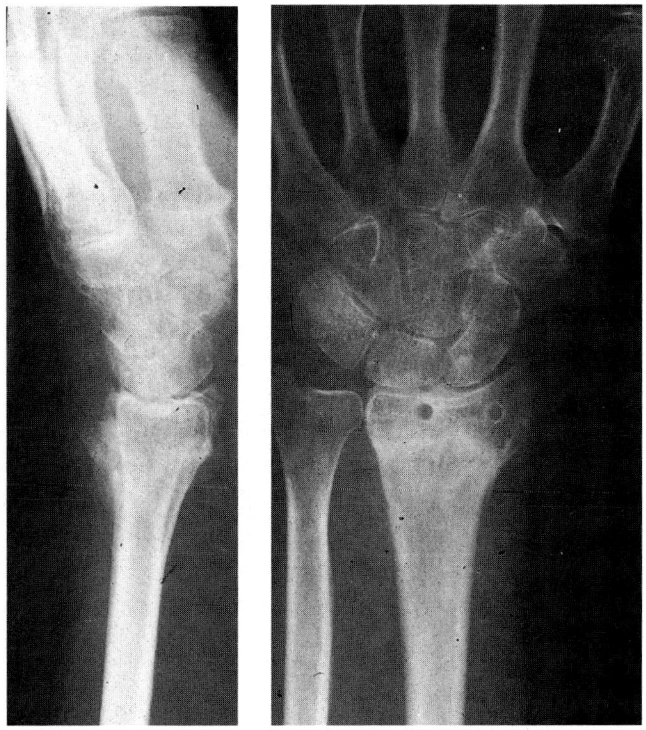

Figure 24–6. The result at 3 months. There is good alignment.

Postoperative Management

The patient was encouraged to mobilize the wrist on the first postoperative day after the immediate discomfort had settled. An active physiotherapy program was instituted and she had good joint mobility by about 3 weeks. The fixator was maintained for 6 weeks and then removed in the out-patient department without anesthetic. A physiotherapy program was maintained for an additional 6 weeks and radiographs at 3 months showed a good result (Fig. 26–6). At 1 year she had excellent wrist movement and complained of only a minor loss of grip strength.

Discussion

Extraarticular distal radial fractures are extremely common. They frequently occur in middle-aged or elderly females, usually as a result of a fall or other low energy injuries. Their management is different from the high energy intraarticular distal radial fracture that frequently occurs in younger patients after a traffic accident.

The traditional method of management is a closed manipulation of the distal radius under general anesthesia, regional anesthesia, or a local anesthetic block. The fracture is usually easy to reduce and a dorsal plater slab is applied with the wrist in slight volar flexion and ulnar deviation.

A proportion of these fractures are unstable and will re-displace within a few days. The re-displacement is frequently blamed on an inappropriate cast, but in fact it occurs because of dorsal metaphyseal comminution and the resulting lack of a dorsal bone buttress. There have been many articles written about the effectiveness of different casts and braces and the position in which the forearm and wrist should be placed to prevent re-displacement, but there is no evidence that any cast or brace is superior to others and it is recommended that surgeons use a simple dorsal back slab

PITFALL

- If transarticular external fixation is used, it is important not to distract the fracture during the application of the fixator. Distraction may lead to reflex sympathetic dystrophy.

after the initial manipulation. Traditionally, a re-displaced distal radial fracture is remanipulated within 10 to 12 days of the initial injury and a further cast applied. However, there is no evidence that this method of management is effective and McQueen and Caspers (1988) clearly showed that re-manipulation was a pointless procedure in older patients.

Surgeons faced with an unstable re-displaced distal radial fracture should not undertake a re-manipulation merely because they feel they should do something and this is an easy option. It is rarely successful and the surgeon must determine whether or not the patient needs surgical treatment. A number of patients will be demented or dependent on caregivers for much of their normal function and these patients should probably be left with a distal radial malunion. In the unlikely event that the surgeon feels that he or she has made the wrong decision, the option of a secondary distal radial osteotomy still exists.

If the patient is in good health, the surgeon must choose between several different methods of stabilizing the distal radius to avoid a malunion. In recent years many surgeons have turned to external skeletal fixation. Currently, there are three main methods of external fixation in the distal radius: static transarticular external fixation, dynamic transarticular external fixation, and periarticular external fixation.

In static transarticular external fixation two pins are usually placed in the distal radius and two in the second metacarpal. An external fixator is then placed across the wrist joint, with the distal radius reduced by manipulation. Dynamic transarticular external fixation is identical to this, but the external fixator has a hinge or ball joint built into it that, if centered appropriately over the wrist joint, should theoretically permit early wrist movement. The third method—periarticular external fixation—has already been described.

Transarticular external fixation is a superficially attractive concept. It is easy to apply and well tolerated by patients. However, studies indicate that its use does not lead to results that are substantially better than plaster management. A prospective study carried out by McQueen et al. (1996) showed that static external fixation was associated with a 43% incidence of malunion and dynamic external fixation with a 37% incidence. The functional results of both dynamic and static external fixation were no better than cast management and the results of static and dynamic external fixation were virtually identical. McQueen further analyzed her data and demonstrated the importance of the association between distal radial fracture malunion and subsequent carpal malalignment, as seen in this case. She showed that carpal malalignment was associated with increased carpal pain and loss of grip strength. This conclusion led to the adoption of periarticular joint sparing external fixation and there is no doubt that in extraarticular distal radial fractures this is now the preferred treatment option.

A comparison between transarticular and periarticular external fixation shows that periarticular external fixation will restore the normal volar angulation of the distal radius. This cannot be done with transarticular external fixation because the volar carpal ligaments are shorter than the dorsal carpal ligaments, and direct traction at best merely reduces the angle of the distal radius so that there is no dorsal angulation. However, it appears that it is necessary to reestablish volar angulation to guarantee that carpal alignment is restored and that the best results will be obtained if the carpus has been realigned. Periarticular external fixation results in improved radiological and functional results and its use is to be encouraged. Its main indication is extraarticular distal radial fractures that cannot be controlled by the use of a forearm cast. However, this method can also be used for undisplaced distal radial intraarticular fractures whose distal radius is split into two fragments.

Alternative Methods of Management

Once a surgeon has decided that the patient requires operative reduction and fixation of the extraarticular distal radial fracture, he or she can use a number of internal fixation techniques rather than external skeletal fixation. Many surgeons have used different types of wiring techniques to stabilize distal radial fractures. The simplest pinning technique involves reducing the fracture and passing one or more Kirschner wires through the distal fragment into the distal radial diaphysis. If good stabilization is achieved, some surgeons suggest that the patient may be able to manage without a cast. Unfortunately, Kirschner wires are flexible and the bone is usually osteoporotic. Thus, despite the use of two or three pins, the distal fragment often dorsally angulates and shortens.

Several modifications to this technique have been introduced. The most popular is intrafocal pinning in which, after fracture reduction, the surgeon places dorsal pins through the fracture site that then penetrate the volar cortex. This technique was introduced by Kapandji in 1976. The principle is that the distal fragments abut onto the pins, preventing dorsal angulation. If three pins are used, no cast is required. The first pin is placed laterally between the tendons of extensor carpi radialis and extensor pollicis brevis, the second pin is inserted posterolaterally close to Lister's tubercle, and the third is inserted posteromedially between the tendons of the extensor digitorum and extensor carpi ulnaris. The technique can be complicated by pin migration and nerve and tendon damage; for this reason surgeons often use threaded pins. Recently, an expanded conical nut, called an Arum pin, has been introduced. These nuts are inserted onto the threaded K-wire and placed into the fracture. As they are pushed into the fracture, the fracture reduces, improving the fracture position. Intrafocal pinning is reported to have good results with a low complication rate.

A number of other internal fixation techniques have been described for extraarticular distal radial fractures. Py introduced the concept of isoelastic pinning in which two flexible pins are passed through the distal fragment into the intramedullary canal of the radius after fracture reduction. However, this method provides poor fixation and, if employed, is probably more useful in younger, better quality bone.

An alternative technique is to insert a flexible intramedullary pin into the intramedullary canal of the proximal radius and push the pin up into the radial styloid of the reduced distal radial fragment. There is little information about the usefulness of this technique, but it is unlikely to provide good fracture stability in unstable distal radial fractures.

Of all the various pinning techniques, the Kapandji intrafocal pinning is the most popular. However, none of these techniques has been submitted to a rigorous clinical trial or compared with external fixation. It is unlikely that any pinning technique can reliably regain volar tilt and therefore it is probable that a high incidence of carpal instability and associated symptoms will result.

Plating is very popular for volar displaced extraarticular distal radial fractures. The anatomy of the volar aspect of the radius is ideal for the application of a buttress plate. Unfortunately, the overall shape of the dorsum of the distal radius is very different and a plate cannot be placed under any muscle to protect adjacent tendons from damage. Recently, a number of plates specifically designed for the distal radius have been introduced. The screw heads are recessed and the plates are thin, designed to minimize interference with tendon function. This would appear to be a somewhat naive concept and it is likely that dorsal plating of the distal radius will probably continue to be a difficult technique associated with interference of extensor tendon function. It may have a place in intraarticular fractures in younger patients, but it is likely that the less invasive techniques of external fixation and intrafocal pinning will prove better in older patients.

The most common bone substitute to be used in osteoporotic bone is polymethylmethacrylate bone cement. The use of bone cement in osteoporotic bone has been discussed in the section dealing with supracondylar fractures in elderly patients. It has been successfully used in the distal radius, but surgeons should be careful to insert it into the metaphyseal bone defect and then reconstruct the posterior metaphyseal bone surface. If bone cement is allowed to protrude through the posterior surface of the distal radius, it will not become covered in bone and will weaken the distal radius. Bone cement may provide immediate stability, but it will loosen inside the osteoporotic distal radius and eventually merely acts as a space filling material inside a weakened distal radius. Thus its use cannot be recommended under normal circumstances, although surgeons may find it occasionally useful in debilitated patients with a poor prognosis. Other bone substitutes have recently become available. An example is the Norian SRS hydroxyapatite bone substitute that can be injected into the defect in the distal radial metaphysis under fluoroscopic control.

Type of Management	Advantages	Disadvantages	Comments
Transarticular external fixation	Easy technique; reasonable function obtained in elderly	Malunion; carpal instability; cannot restore volar angulation	Better than plaster management but worse than periarticular external fixation
Periarticular fixation	Excellent results; straightforward technique; restores distal radial alignment	Needs fluoroscopy	Best results gained with this method
Percutaneous dorsal pinning	Straightforward technique	Pin damage to soft tissues; malunion; cannot restore volar angulation	If pinning is to be used, intrafocal pinning is preferable
Intrafocal pinning	Better fracture reduction	More difficult technique; soft tissue damage; probably will not restore volar alignment	Improvement on percutaneous pinning but probably not as good as periarticular external fixation
Intramedullary flexible pinning	Straightforward technique	Few results available; poor fixation	No advantage over other methods
Plating	None	Open surgery; tendon damage; osteoporotic bone infection	No indication for this technique in elderly patients
Bone substitutes	Reduce splintage or external fixation time	Learning curve	Probably a useful technique, but more results are required
Re-manipulation	Easy	Malunion; carpal instability; poor results	Not of any proven use in fit elderly patients

Early results with this show promise and, although it is unlikely that this type of bone substitute will allow surgeons to abandon supportive casts or external fixation, it may reduce the time such treatments require.

There is no real evidence that elderly patients with extraarticular distal radial fractures benefit from the use of bone graft to supplement the fracture fixation. The use of a bone block and supplementary Kirschner wire as primary treatment for an unstable distal radial fracture was examined by McQueen et al. (1996). They showed that the technique conferred no real advantage to the patient when compared with transarticular external fixation, and the open operation that was required to insert the graft certainly constituted a more major surgical procedure than external fixation. Bone grafting is not without morbidity and its routine use in the elderly patient is not justified.

Complications

The most common complication of the treatment of distal radial fractures is malunion. The definition of what constitutes a malunion varies, but if 10 degrees of dorsal angulation is used, then about 80% of patients who have a re-manipulation and 35 to 40% of those who have a transarticular external fixation will have a malunion. In some patients the principal problem will be cosmetic; in others the complaint will be pain and/or loss of function; some patients will be asymptomatic. Treatment will obviously depend on the degree of symptomatology, but if the malunion is considered unacceptable, the treatment is distal radial osteotomy and bone graft. The surgeon must be careful to analyze exactly what shape of bone graft is required to correct the malalignment. A transverse skin incision overlying the old fracture should be used. The tendons are separated and sharp dissection used to expose the distal radius. The bone is cut with a power saw and the distal radial fragment gently angulated forward using a flat dissector placed in the osteotomy. Two Kirschner wires can be inserted into the distal fragment to assist with opening the osteotomy as the bone graft is inserted. A triangular block of corticocancellous bone is taken from the ipsilateral iliac crest and held in the distal radius with a Kirschner wire placed through the radial styloid and across the osteotomy. A cast should be used for 6 weeks. The wire is then removed and a physiotherapy program started.

Radial shortening is very difficult to treat by interpositional bone grafting. The surgeon can either lengthen the radius or shorten the ulna to correct the distal radioulnar alignment. The latter procedure is much easier and is recommended. The easiest method of ulnar shortening is to expose the distal ulnar diaphysis, remove the desired length or cortex, and then use a small external fixator with a compression facility to close the osteotomy that can then be plated. Other complications of distal radial fracture are less common. Probably the most troublesome is reflex sympathetic dystrophy that is unquestionably associated with the use of a transarticular external fixator. This is best treated by aggressive physiotherapy, although guanethidine blocks may be helpful. Unfortunately the diagnosis is often delayed and the recovery is slow. Carpal tunnel syndrome should be treated by carpal tunnel decompression if it persists beyond 2 to 3 weeks. If the carpal tunnel syndrome is associated with a distal radial malunion, this should be corrected at the time of carpal tunnel decompression.

Extensor pollicis longus rupture is a well recognized complication of distal radial fractures. It should be treated by extensor indicis transfer. Any other tendon damage will probably have been caused by ill-judged attempts at percutaneous external fixator pin insertion and will need to be appropriately treated.

The last troublesome problem following distal radial fracture is wrist pain. This not infrequently follows a malunion and may arise from damage to the distal radioulnar joint, a malaligned prominent distal ulnar or carpal malalignment. The best treatment is the correction of any distal radial deformity, but consideration can be given to resection of the distal ulna for distal ulnar pain in the elderly or excision of the distal radioulnar joint if there is distal radioulnar joint pain.

The last factor the surgeon may consider is why the patient fell in the first place. In many incidences this is obvious and little can be done except to investigate the degree of osteoporosis if it is indicated. In other patients the fall may be symptomatic of failing health and an inability to cope in one's environment. A number of elderly patients have falls as a result of impaired consciousness because of the inappropriate use of antidepressants, sedatives, or other drugs, and this should be investigated.

Suggested Readings

Cooney WP, Dobyns JH, Linscheid RL: Complications of Colles' fractures. J Bone Joint Surg 1980; 62A:613–619.

Fernandez DL, Jupiter JB: Fractures of the Distal Radius. Springer Verlag, Berlin, 1997.

McQueen MM, Caspers J: Colles' fracture: does the anatomical result affect the final function. J Bone Joint Surg (Br) 1988; 70B:649–651.

McQueen MM, Hajducka C, Court-Brown CM: Redisplaced unstable fractures of the distal radius. J Bone Joint Surg (Br) 1996; 78B:404–409.

McQueen MM: Redisplaced unstable fractures of the distal radius. J Bone Joint Surg (Br) 1998; 80B:665–669.

Pennig D, Gausepohl T: External fixation of the wrist. Injury 1996; 27:1–15.

Taleisnik J, Watson HK: Midcarpal instability caused by malunited fractures of the distal radius. J Bone Joint Surg (Am) 1984; 9:350–357.

Section 2

Lower Extremity

Case 1

History and Physical Examination

A 24-year-old man was injured when the motorcycle he was riding collided at high speed with a guardrail. He was brought to the emergency department 15 minutes after the accident. On initial physical examination, the patient was conscious and oriented, yet agitated and in severe pain. He was noted to be tachycardic with a blood pressure of 100/40. He was bleeding actively from a laceration in his groin, and his right leg was externally rotated. On further examination it was noted that the laceration extended from the groin posteriorly and included the rectum. Diagnostic peritoneal lavage was negative for significant blood. The patient's chest was clear and his neurologic examination was within the limits of normal. The neurovascular examination of both lower extremities was within the limits of normal.

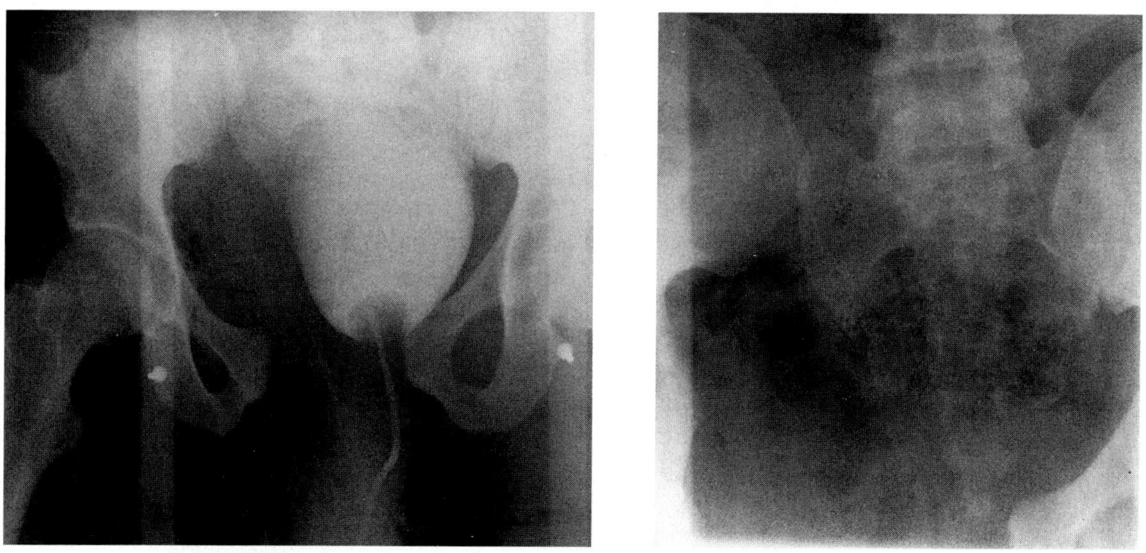

A B

Figure 1–1. Anteroposterior radiographs of the pelvis indicating a wide pubic diastasis (A) and dislocated right sacroiliac joint (B).

Radiologic Findings

A radiograph of the pelvis in the anteroposterior projection indicated the presence of a diastasis of the pubic symphysis and dislocation of the right sacroiliac joint (Fig. 1–1). A retrograde cystogram indicated that the urethra was ruptured but the bladder was intact.

Diagnosis

Hypovolemia secondary to an open dislocation of the right hemipelvis, or a Malgaigne dislocation. There was an associated disruption of the urethra.

PEARL

- The incidence of death following open pelvic fracture is decreased significantly by performing a colostomy. Colostomy should be performed as soon after injury as possible—ideally the day of injury.

Surgical Management

The patient's pulse and blood pressure responded to the rapid infusion of fluids and packed red blood cells. The laceration was gently packed with gauze roles and the patient was taken emergently to the operating room.

A general anesthetic was administered. The legs were abducted and slightly flexed, opening the laceration. A large "bump" was placed under the sacrum; the thighs, perineum, and lower abdomen were prepped. Very little devitalized tissue was found in the wound; however, stool was found in the rectum and wound. Bleeding was brisk and not localized. The wound was irrigated. A large potential space anterior to the sacrum was packed with gauze roles. An external fixator was applied, with two pins in either iliac crest, the pelvis was closed by compressing the iliac crests together, and the fixator was tightened. Despite these maneuvers, brisk bleeding continued, and the patient's blood pressure remained extremely labile. The anesthetized patient was taken to the angiography suite, where an angiogram indicated bleeding from branches of the internal iliac artery (Fig. 1–2). These branches were embolized. The bleeding slowed and the patient's blood pressure stabilized.

The patient's condition stabilized. Eighteen hours after injury he was taken back to the operating room where a general anesthetic was administered. His dressings were changed and his laceration was repacked. A diverting colostomy and cystostomy were performed.

The packing was changed daily under intravenous sedation. One week after injury, the patient was taken back to the operating room for definitive stabilization of his dislocation. The frame of the external fixator was removed, leaving the pins seated in the ilium. The iliac crests and lower abdomen were scrubbed and draped. An incision, which included the incisions for the pins, was made along the crest of the right ilium. The iliacus muscle was elevated from the inner surface of the ilium back to the joint. A Cobb elevator was used to elevate the periosteum and tissue from the anterior surface of the sacrum. The joint was debrided of fragments of

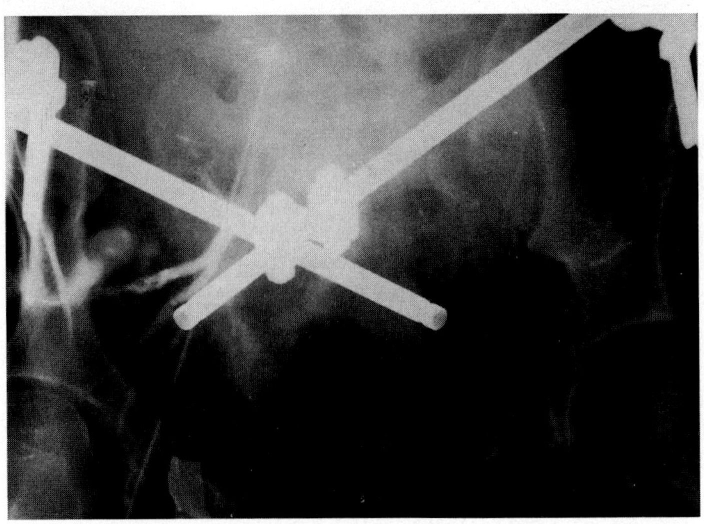

Figure 1–2. Anteroposterior radiograph during embolization of bleeders.

PEARL

- Hypovolemia secondary to hemorrhage is the most common cause of death following a displaced pelvic fracture. It is managed by aggressive fluid and blood replacement, decreasing the potential space in the pelvis into which bleeding can occur, and, if necessary, embolization. In this case because the pelvic fracture was open, reducing the pelvis and stabilizing it with an external fixator did not tamponade the bleeding vessels and embolization was necessary.

bone cartilage and soft tissue. Specimens were sent for culture. The sacroiliac joint was reduced under direct vision by manipulating the right hemipelvis. This was accomplished by an unscrubbed assistant who applied traction and internal rotation to the right leg under the drapes. Reduction was fine tuned by manipulating the pins in the right ilium. When reduction had been achieved, two large fragment reconstruction plates were applied anteriorly across the joint. The wound was closed over a large suction drain, and an external fixator frame was applied anteriorly using the in-situ pins. Final reduction of the symphysis was monitored fluoroscopically and achieved with medial and lateral compression, prior to tightening of the external fixator (Fig. 1–3).

Postoperative Management

The patient was taken out of bed into a recliner on the first day after definitive stabilization of his pelvis. On the third day physical therapy for weight bearing as tolerated on the left side was started. Daily packing of the wound anterior to the sacrum continued. The wound rapidly decreased in size and by 3 weeks had closed. The intraoperative cultures were negative; nevertheless, an aminoglycoside, second generation cephalosporin, and metronidazole were continued a total of 6 weeks. At 8 weeks weight bearing as tolerated was initiated on the right leg. Radiographs indicated that there was no change in alignment after weight bearing. At 12 weeks postdefinitive fixation of the pelvis, the external fixator was removed in the office (Fig. 1–4).

Discussion

Mortality following an open pelvic fracture has been reported to be as high as 50%. Acutely, death is most frequently due to hypovolemia. Subacutely, death most frequently results from sepsis. Hypovolemia is due to bleeding from the presacral

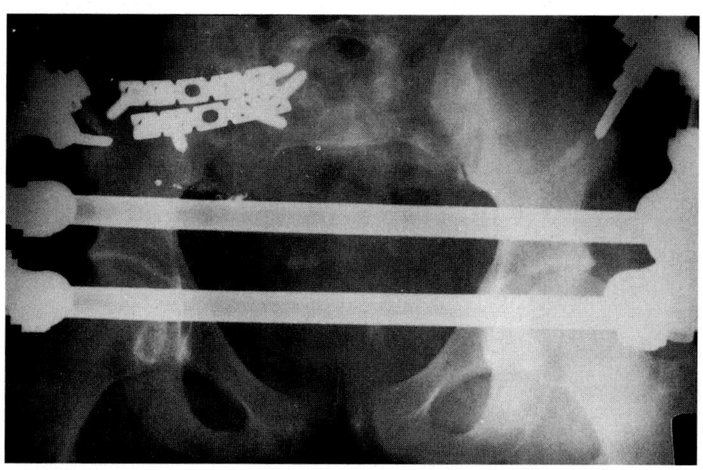

Figure 1–3. Anteroposterior radiograph following open reduction and internal fixation of the sacroiliac joint and reapplication of an external fixator.

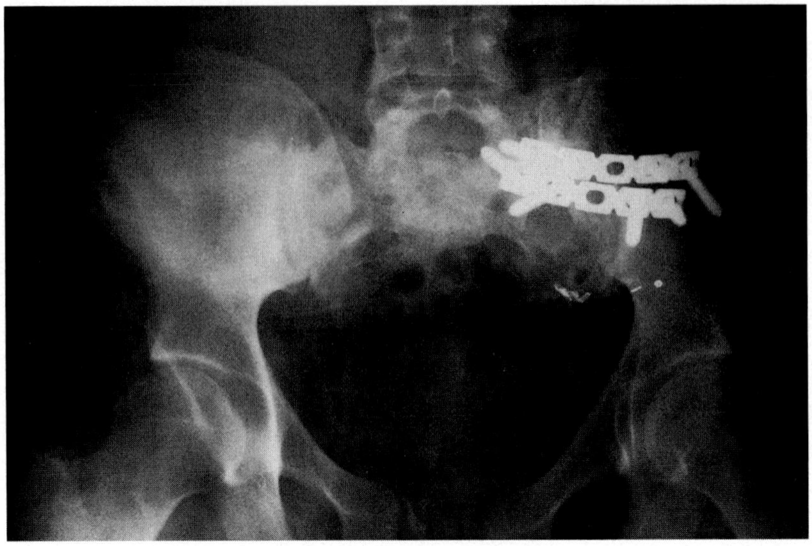

Figure 1–4. Anteroposterior radiograph of the pelvis following fixator removal.

veins, an artery, or the fracture itself. The first step in controlling hemorrhage is to reduce the fracture and thus decrease the volume of the pelvis into which bleeding can occur. Temporary pelvic compression is often noted to be accomplished by inflating a military anti-shock trousers (MAST) suit. More definitive management involves stabilization and closure of the pelvis with an external fixator. When applying the fixator, it is important to keep in mind that the objective is to decrease the volume of the pelvis. Attempts to reduce the pelvis anatomically or stabilize it with only an anterior frame are not warranted and will only prolong the procedure with no hope for success.

Alternative Methods of Management

Alternatives to an anterior external fixator and anterior plating of the sacroiliac joint are plating the symphysis pubis, an anterior external fixator alone, fixation of the sacroiliac joint with plates applied posteriorly, or percutaneous fixation of the sacroiliac joint with screws.

Stabilization of the symphysis with an anterior external fixator is a time tested method. Anterior external fixation as opposed to open reduction and plating is particularly applicable in this case because the diastasis was contaminated due to the open fracture and ruptured urethra. The disadvantage of anterior fixation is that reduction of the symphysis is accomplished with the aid of fluoroscopy and may not be anatomic.

Plating of the symphysis pubis has the advantage of direct visualization. This aids reduction and the surgeon can be certain that the ureter is not caught in the symphysis. However, in this contaminated case, plating exposes the patient to a greater risk of infection than an external fixator does.

Anterior plating of the sacroiliac joint is a relatively simple procedure in a thin patient. The anterior exposure of the sacroiliac joint in a large patient can be troublesome because of difficulty retracting the iliacus muscle and abdominal contents medially. The fifth lumbar nerve root lies on the sacrum 2 to 3 cm medial to the sacroiliac joint. It is at risk during the anterior exposure and limits medial fixation to a single screw per plate. Anterior exposure of the sacroiliac joint is the only method of stabilization that facilitates debridement and anatomic reduction while visualizing the joint.

Closed reduction and stabilization of the pelvis with an anterior fixator alone is theoretically possible. Both Slattis and Mears described complex pyramidal frames designed to stabilize pelvic fracture dislocations that were unstable anteriorly and posteriorly. Practically, these frames are difficult to apply, and because the lever arm is so great posterior stability is not always adequate to maintain reduction and allow patient mobilization.

Posterior plates are applied through a single transverse incision centered over the posterior iliac crests or through two longitudinal incisions. A specially designed "double cobra" plate was associated with an unacceptably high incidence of wound slough and infection. In addition, this method does not allow direct visualization of the sacroiliac joint. Reduction is achieved with the aid of fluoroscopy. Recently, we have utilized a method in which 7 mm screws inserted between the table of the ilium are used with Steffe plates to stabilize the sacroiliac joint. Exposure is via a midline incision centered over the spinous processes of the sacrum (Fig. 1–5).

Percutaneous screws can be used to stabilize the sacroiliac joint in conjunction with an anterior external fixator or anterior plate. Screw insertion is technically difficult, but the risk of infection is low because of the limited surgical trauma. The major disadvantage of this method is that accurate reduction of the joint can be extremely difficult to achieve when the sacrum and ilium are as displaced as they were in this case.

Type of Management	Advantages	Disadvantages	Comments
Anterior external fixator to stabilize symphysis	Decreased risk of infection of symphysis	Symphysis not visualized; reduction may not be anatomic; limited patient acceptance	Time tested method; reduction does not have to be perfect
Plate to stabilize symphysis	Better tolerated by patient than external fixator	Exposes patient to greater risk of infection if wound is contaminated	Risk of infection is too great
Anterior fixator to stabilize anterior and posterior pelvis	Procedure is closed, minimizing operative trauma and risk of infection	Limited stability posteriorly; extremely difficult to apply frame correctly	Limited posterior stability makes this the least desirable choice
Anterior plating of SI joint	Simple exposure in thin patient	Difficult in heavy patients; L5 nerve root at risk	Excellent method of stabilization in thin patients
Posterior plating of SI joint using Steffe plates	Technically simple procedure	Risk of wound slough	Extremely stable method of fixation
Percutaneus screws to stabilize SI joint	Limited operative trauma	Technically difficult; accurate reduction may be difficult to achieve	Good alternative to anterior plating of SI joint

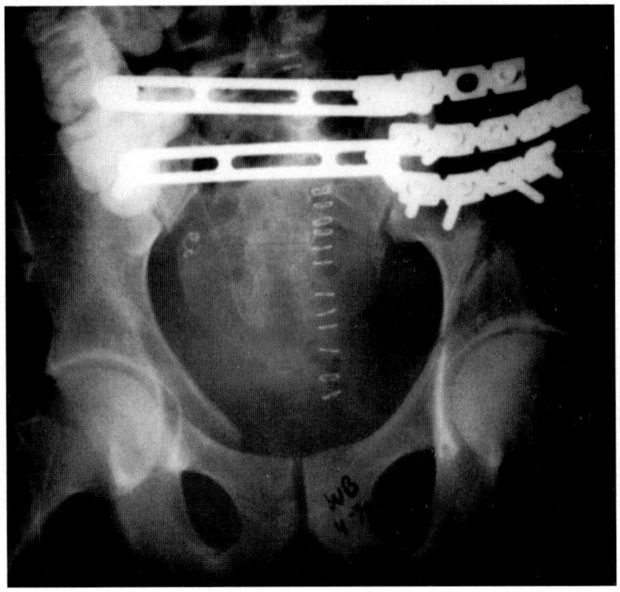

Figure 1–5. Anteroposterior radiograph of a pelvis in which a posterior plate has been used to stabilize a dislocated sacroiliac joint. A fracture of the ilium has also been plated.

Complications

Acute and subacute complications of an open pelvic fracture include hemorrhage and sepsis. Chronic complications include instability and arthritis, infection, and nerve damage. The acute complications of hemorrhage and sepsis have been covered previously. Clinically significant instability and arthritis are almost always posterior. Anterior instability is rarely a problem. Many patients have a large diastasis of the symphysis pubis and are completely asymptomatic. Instability of the sacroiliac joint is often extremely painful. Confirmation that pain is originating from the sacroiliac joint is obtained by injection of the joint with a long-acting anesthetic. Once the diagnosis of instability and arthritis has been confirmed, the management is conservative, with injections of steroids and oral nonsteroidal antiinflammatory medication or operative with fusion of the sacroiliac joint.

Infection of the pelvis is managed with control of the infection until the fractures and dislocations have healed. The infected areas are debrided and appropriate antibiotics are administered. Dead space is almost always present, necessitating the use of antibiotic beads. Frequently, soft tissue coverage is a problem, and soft tissue transfer may be required.

Injury to the lumbosacral plexus is often associated with displaced sacroiliac dislocations. Initial management is conservative. If symptoms do not resolve, decompression can be attempted, but the chance of success is very low.

Suggested Readings

Bucholz RW: The pathological anatomy of Malgaigne fracture—dislocations of the pelvis. J Bone Joint Surg 1981; 63A:400–404.

Ganz R, Krushell RJ, Jakob RP, Kuffer J: The antishock pelvic clamp. CORR 1991; 267:71–78.

Hanson PB, Milne JC, Chapman MW: Open fractures of the pelvis. Review of 43 cases. J Bone Joint Surg 1991; 73B:325–329.

Maull KI, Sachatello CR, Ernst CB: The deep perineal laceration—an injury frequently associated with open pelvic fractures: a need for aggressive surgical management. A report of 12 cases and review of the literature. J Trauma 1977; 17(9): 685–696.

Panetta T, Sclafani SJ, Goldstein AS, Phillips TF, Shaftan GW: Percutaneous transcatheter embolization for massive bleeding from pelvic fractures. J Trauma 1985; 25:1021–1029.

Simpson LA, Waddell JP, Leighton RK, Kellam JF, Tile M: Anterior approach to stabilization of the disrupted sacroiliac joint. J Trauma 1987; 27:1332–1339.

Case 2

History and Physical Examination

An 86-year-old woman was admitted to the emergency department. She had fallen while attempting to go to the toilet in her home where she lived alone. On admission it was obvious that her left leg was shortened and externally rotated. Examination showed her to be mentally alert and oriented. Her physical health was good, and normally she was able to move about inside her house but did not do her own shopping, relying on neighbors and friends to do this for her. She had good family support. Her medical history consisted of having a mastectomy for breast carcinoma 20 years earlier and her only medication was a mild diuretic.

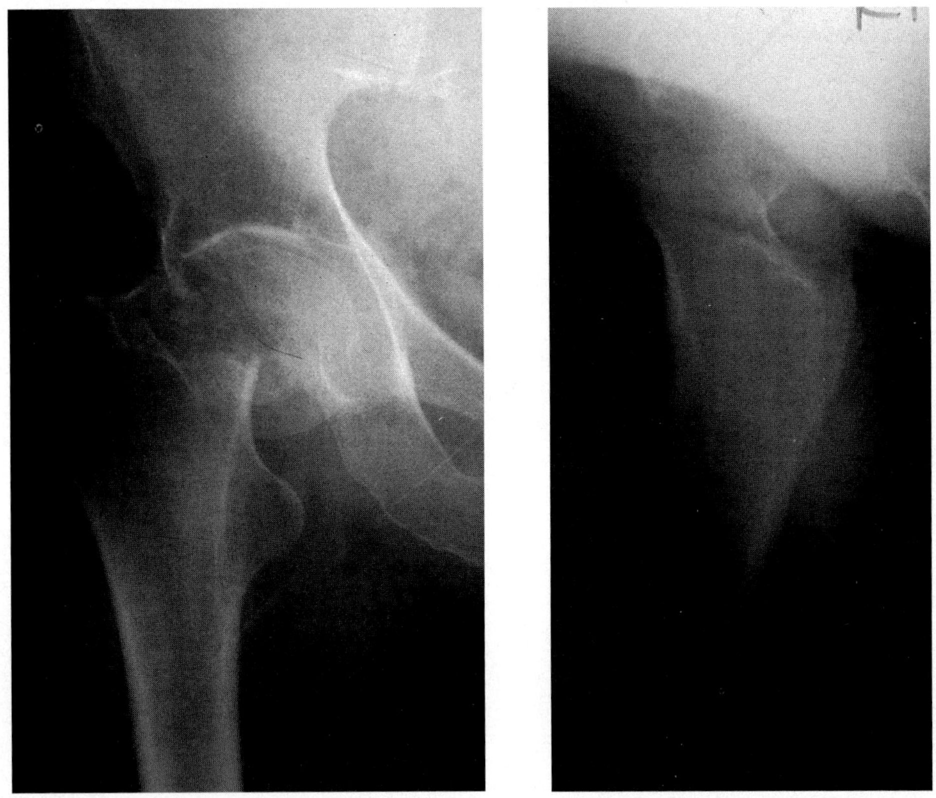

A B

Figure 2–1. A displaced subcapital fracture in an elderly patient.

Radiologic Findings

Anteroposterior and lateral radiographs showed a displaced subcapital fracture (Fig. 2–1). The femoral head is in varus and external rotation. AO classification: 31–B3.1 fracture.

Diagnosis

Displaced subcapital fracture.

PEARL

- Surgeons debate whether hemiarthroplasty prostheses should be cemented. Cement fixation decreases the incidence of stem loosening, but makes the implant more difficult to remove if there is acetabular erosion and pain. This problem can be circumvented by using a cemented or cementless press fit stem and an interchangeable head. Such a device is illustrated in Figure 2-3.

Surgical Management

The patient was admitted to the orthopaedic trauma unit and put on the operating list for a hemiarthroplasty. She had been admitted in the middle of the afternoon and her surgery was scheduled for the following morning. She was the fifth patient to be admitted with a proximal femoral fracture in a 24 hour period. Unfortunately, two multiply injured patients were also admitted to the unit that day and her surgery was eventually delayed for 3 days. During this time she was fasted on two occasions and surgery had to be cancelled because of lack of operating time.

She was eventually taken to the operating room where an Austin Moore hemiarthroplasty prosthesis was inserted laterally. The approach to the hip joint was through a midlateral skin incision that was centered over the greater trochanter. The fascia and gluteal muscles were incised and the soft tissues elevated from the front of the proximal femur using sharp dissection. The femoral head was then removed and the leg externally rotated; this allowed the femoral neck to be trimmed back with a saw. After determining the size of the acetabulum, surgeons inserted an appropriate Austin Moore hemiarthroplasty prosthesis. The hip was then reduced and the wound closed.

Postoperative Management

The patient was mobilized to be fully weight bearing on the day after surgery. However, she was noted to be confused and acting inappropriately. Her urine was strong smelling and a provisional diagnosis of a urinary tract infection was made. She was consequently started on broad spectrum antibiotics, with a sample sent for bacterio-

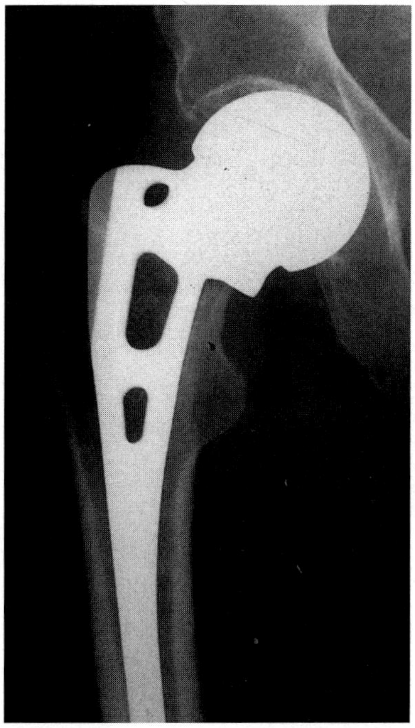

Figure 2–2. An Austin Moore hemiarthroplasty prosthesis.

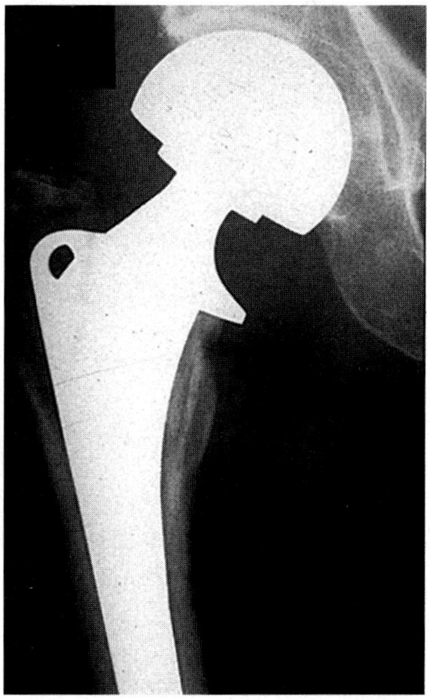

Figure 2–3. The use of a hemiarthroplasty prosthesis with a cementless stem and an interchangeable head. A 44 mm head was used.

PITFALL

- The elderly must be mobilized to be fully weight bearing. Partial weight bearing and non-weight bearing are impossible for frail elderly patients. Such a postoperative regime confines them to a bed or wheelchair.

logical analysis. Her confusion cleared within two days but her mobilization was slow and she required a walking frame with one nurse or physiotherapist to assist her. It was considered that she was not fit to return home, and she was consequently discharged to a nursing home for a period of rehabilitation. She returned home 6 weeks after surgery, but died of apparently unrelated causes 6 months later.

Discussion

Intracapsular fractures of the proximal femur are the most common fractures admitted to most orthopaedic trauma units. Reports from around the world have indicated that the incidence of these fractures is rising. Not only is the "at risk" geriatric population rising, but the incidence of proximal femoral fractures is increasing faster than can be calculated merely from this population. Estimates have indicated that the number of proximal femoral fractures presenting to orthopaedic trauma units may double in the next 30 years.

Elderly patients are fitter than in previous generations and may well live into their ninth or tenth decades. Many patients over 80 will be medically fit and live independently. Despite considerable advances in various branches of medical science, little progress has been made in preventing or curing osteoporosis and preventing dementia. Thus orthopaedic surgeons are facing an epidemic of very elderly patients who are profoundly osteoporotic and may well be demented, and consequently dependent on the social service system of the country in which they live. The average age of patients presenting with proximal femoral fractures in most series is about 80 years, but it is going to rise over the next few decades; unless osteoporosis can be successfully prevented or treated, future surgeons are going to have to treat very

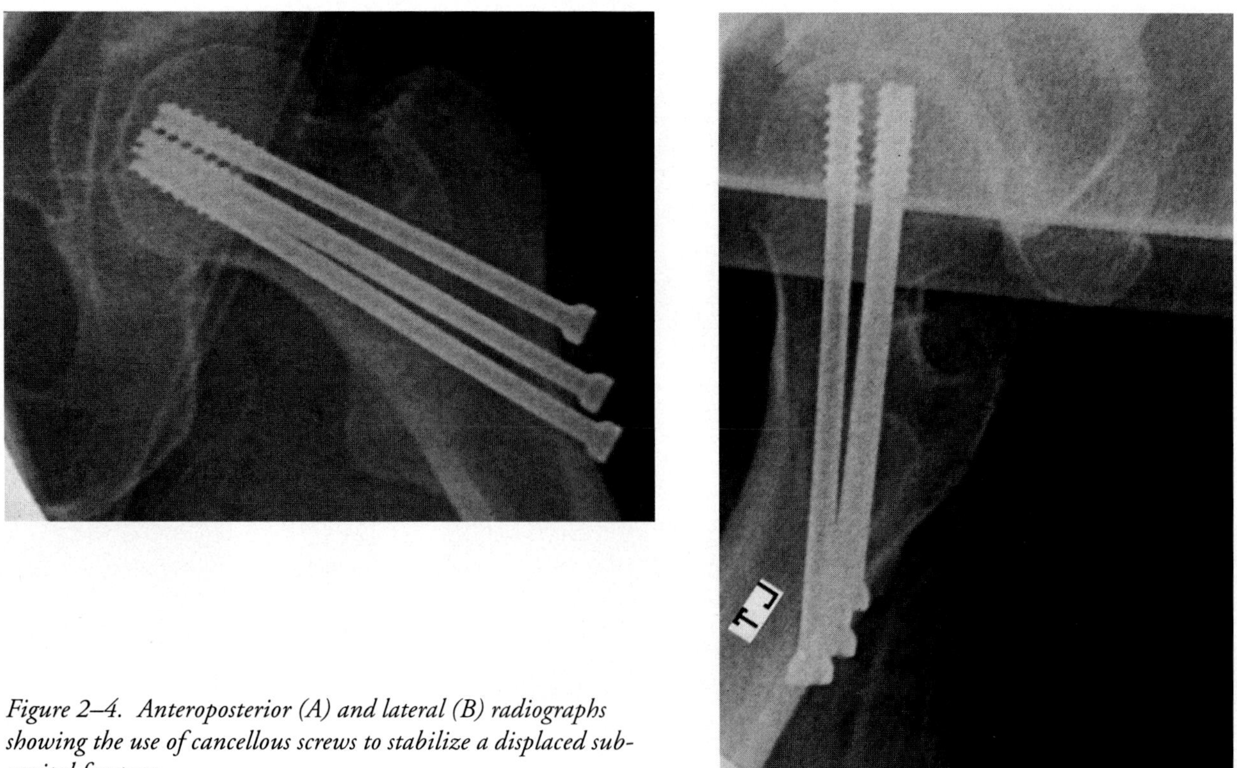

A

B

Figure 2–4. Anteroposterior (A) and lateral (B) radiographs showing the use of cancellous screws to stabilize a displaced subcapital fracture.

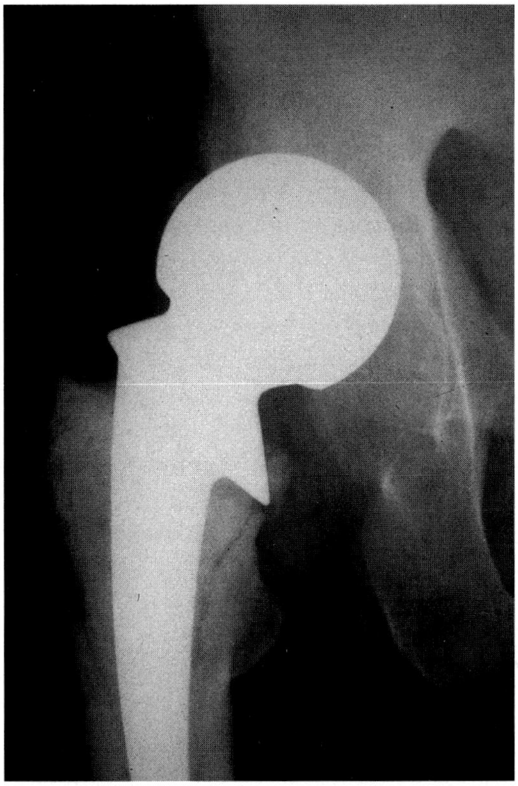

Figure 2–5. Significant acetabular erosion after the use of a hemiarthroplasty prosthesis in an elderly patient.

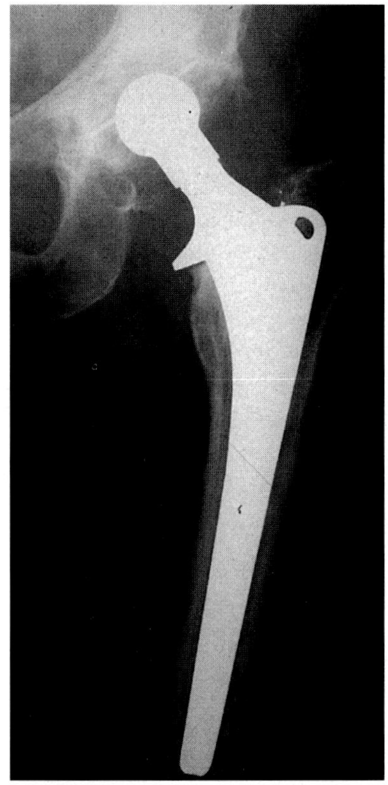

Figure 2–6. The hemiarthroplasty prosthesis illustrated in Figure 2–3 has been converted into a total hip replacement. This is also a useful primary procedure.

large numbers of very elderly patients whose bone is profoundly osteoporotic and may be impossible to fix.

A review of the epidemiological data of 2383 patients admitted to the orthopaedic trauma unit in Edinburgh, Scotland, indicates the problems of managing this group. The average age of the patients was 80 years, with 86.7% of the patients over 70 years and 61% over 80 years of age. About 37% showed objective evidence of a confusional state on admission, and over 15% were considered to be clinically depressed. The mortality was significant, with 8.2% of patients dying during the acute in-patient period, 13.3% dying within 1 month, and 24% dying within 4 months of their fall.

There are two current debates about the treatment of displaced subcapital femoral fractures. Should these fractures be internally fixed or replaced? If they are replaced, should the surgeon use a fixed head hemiarthroplasty prosthesis, a bipolar prosthesis that may be capable of revision to a total hip replacement, or a primary total hip replacement?

It is obvious that the ideal outcome for a subcapital fracture in an elderly patient would be for the femoral neck fracture to unite without any evidence of avascular necrosis or late segmental collapse and a low incidence of postoperative complications. When analyzing the literature to see if results can come close to this ideal, it is important to realize that virtually all results come from mixed series of patients

PEARL

- The Austin Moore prosthesis is one of the oldest hemiarthroplasty prostheses. It is, however, debatable whether modern implants are demonstrably better. If the prosthesis is inserted carefully with a tight fit between the stem and the intramedullary canal, the results are as good as those obtained with modern implants.

of different ages. Investigators have reported healing complications in between 30 and 70% of patients who present with subcapital fractures that are subsequently internally fixed (Fig. 2–4). In a series of 2418 patients in Sweden, Holmberg et al. (1987) documented that 37% of patients had complications after internal fixation of femoral neck fractures, and 70% who developed complications after primary, treatment required further surgery. Barnes et al. (1976) undertook an important study of 1503 subcapital fractures, all of which were treated by reduction and internal fixation. Overall, about 33% of the displaced fractures did not unite and about 27% developed late segmental collapse, although this was asymptomatic in about a quarter of these patients. However, as the age increased, so did the incidence of nonunion and almost 50% of displaced fractures failed to unite in patients over 84 years of age. In general, the rate of union was better in active patients compared with those who were handicapped or bedridden at the time of fracture. The rate of union, but not the incidence of late segmental collapse, was improved by the use of more modern fixation techniques utilizing either a sliding screw system or multiple screws. These large series can be criticized because many patients were fixed using implants that are now outdated, but even with modern multiple pinning techniques surgeons report healing complications in 35 to 40% of patients over 80 years of age.

The main theoretical advantage of joint replacement using a hemiarthroplasty, bipolar prosthesis, or a total hip replacement is that the surgery is definitive—once the head is removed, there can be no nonunion or late segmental collapse necessitating secondary surgery in this group of somewhat frail patients. However, the use of prostheses is not without its complications. The hemiarthroplasty became popular because of the problems encountered in attempting to internally fix displaced subcapital fractures. The Austin Moore prosthesis was the first hemiarthroplasty to gain widespread acceptance and, despite the introduction of a number of newer procedures, is still in widespread use. The main complaints about its use are hip pain that may be associated with femoral stem loosening or acetabular erosion (Fig. 2–5). Infection and dislocation may also occur and can be very difficult to treat in this age group. The literature suggests that the overall complication rate following fixed head hemiarthroplasty is between 25 and 40%, with Whittaker et al. (1972) reporting a 32% incidence of stem loosening and a 24% incidence of acetabular erosion.

These results caused surgeons to examine the use of bipolar prostheses. Such devices permit acetabular movement at the interface between the metal head and the acetabulum as well as between the smaller and larger prosthetic head. They also have the advantage of being able to be converted into a total hip replacement. Initial experience with their use was gratifying, with surgeons reporting lower complication rates, but over the last few years a number of prospective trials comparing the two different types of device have indicated that there appears to be very little difference between them. They have the same problems as fixed head hemiarthroplasty, with patients complaining of hip pain.

The third type of prosthetic replacement is the total hip replacement (Fig. 2–6). Again this is a superficially attractive operation in that elective hip replacements carried out for osteoarthritis and rheumatoid arthritis are extremely successful, with low complication rates and high patient acceptance. Unfortunately, the emergency hip fracture patient is different from the elective arthritis patients for a number of reasons. The arthritic patient has often lost a considerable amount of hip movement and at hip replacement surgery the arthritic hip is stiffer than the relatively normal joint found in the fracture patient. The elective arthritic patient also tends to be more medically fit than the emergency fracture patient. These two factors lead to several problems. The dislocation rate following hip arthroplasty for fracture is reported to be as high as 20%, presumably because of the presence of normal soft tissues around the joint. Fortunately, many patients only have one dislocation in the postoperative period, but some experience recurrent dislocation that necessitates revision surgery. The other problem occasionally encountered by surgeons is that the intramedullary pressure may rise to considerable levels during the insertion of a cemented hip arthroplasty. This may cause the release of marrow and fat emboli that may escape into the pulmonary circulation or the systemic circulation through a patent foramen ovale. In elderly patients who are medically unfit this may result in profound hypotension or even death, particularly if the patient is hypovolemic at the time of surgery.

All available methods of treating subcapital femoral fractures are associated with significant problems. Unfortunately, the morbidity of secondary hip surgery carried out because of problems after the initial procedure is high. This was detailed by Keating et al. (1993), who showed that 3.7% of 1,094 consecutive hip fractures required revision surgery within 3 months of the initial procedure. In 39 displaced subcapital fractures revised for recurrent dislocation, infection, or femoral shaft fracture, 19 (48%) ultimately had an excision arthroplasty and the overall mortality was 36% at 1 year. It is accepted that mortality is bound to be fairly high in elderly patients who have a subcapital fracture. Barnes et al. (1976) showed that 21% of women and 37% of men over the age of 84 years died within a month of surgery. It is likely that these figures will fall as the general health of the elderly population improves and geriatric physicians, rather than orthopaedic surgeons, assume responsibility for medical management of the patients.

This case highlights a number of problems that are commonly encountered in elderly patients who present with proximal femoral fractures. There is no doubt that an operative delay of more than 2 days is associated with an increased mortality and if, as in this case, the patient has to fast on more than one occasion, this can lead to hypovolemia and worsen an already precarious mental and physical condition. Unfortunately, orthopaedic trauma units around the world are often pressed for operating time and elderly patients not infrequently have their surgery cancelled to make way for younger, multiply injured patients. If elderly patients have a prolonged delay before surgery, their medical condition must be carefully monitored.

Despite much clinical research, it is still difficult to formulate a protocol for the surgical management of displaced subcapital fractures in the elderly. The high complication rate of internal fixation suggests that joint replacement is a better technique in patients who are over 85 years of age. When deciding which joint replacement technique is applicable, the overall physical and mental state of the patient must be considered. Between 25 and 30% of these patients will be demented and a number of others will have reduced life expectancy because of neoplasia or other serious illnesses. In these patients it is reasonable to consider the use of a hemiarthroplasty. However, when the patient is fit and active and may well live for several years, hemiarthroplasty is an inappropriate operation and a total hip replacement should be undertaken if possible. The surgeon should strive to undertake a definitive procedure and ideally it should be performed by an experienced surgeon.

Alternative Methods of Management

There have been a number of proponents of nonoperative management over the years. However, the only indication for nonoperative management is when the patient is moribund on admission usually because the proximal femoral fracture has been associated with a massive cerebrovascular accident. There is every justification for allowing these patients to die with dignity. Otherwise, nonoperative management merely confines the patient to bed for a prolonged period and this can have major physical and psychological consequences. Surgeons have used functional braces to little effect and internal fixation or a joint replacement procedure is indicated for all proximal femoral fractures.

Type of Management	Advantages	Disadvantages	Comments
Multiple screw fixation	Best result if the operation is successful	Nonunion; avascular necrosis; segmental collapse	This gives the best result if the operation works, but there is a very high complication rate in the elderly
Hemiarthroplasty	Straightforward surgery	Pain; acetabular migration; femoral loosening	High complication rate; useful in demented or dependent patients
Bipolar procedures	Straightforward surgery	Pain; acetabular migration; loosening	High complication rate; useful in demented or dependent patients
Total hip replacement	Good results, particularly in ambulant patients	High dislocation rate	Probably the method of choice in ambulant fit patients
Nonoperative	None	Prolonged bed rest; high mortality; poor results	Only suitable for patients who are too ill for anesthesia

Complications

Several complications have been discussed as well as the importance of trying to avoid complications that necessitate further surgery. However, there are many complications associated with the treatment of proximal femoral fractures. If multiple screw fixation is chosen, the usual complications are nonunion and late segmental collapse. If the patient is symptomatic—and that will largely depend on the functional status—the surgeon will normally undertake a hemiarthroplasty or hip replacement.

If an arthroplasty is used, the complications that the surgeon will encounter are infection, dislocation, loosening, and hip pain. The infection rate in elderly patients is between 4 and 5%, which is much higher than in elective arthroplasty. Unfortunately, it is extremely difficult to eradicate infection in this group of patients and exchange arthroplasty will almost certainly fail. Excision arthroplasty is frequently performed, but the prognosis following this procedure is dreadful and many patients will die within a short period. In the elderly debilitated patient the surgeon may choose to treat the infection symptomatically and at least leave patients with a hip joint for the remaining few months of their life.

Dislocation is treated by reduction; in the case of a primary dislocation of a total hip replacement, one reduction may be all that is required before the joint may be stable. However, a number of patients will present with current dislocation that necessitates revision surgery. Hemiarthroplasty dislocation is associated with a very poor prognosis probably because of the debilitated state of the patients who present with this complication.

The most common complication of hemiarthroplasty or bipolar arthroplasty is hip pain. There may be radiological signs of prosthetic loosening or acetabular erosion (Fig. 2–5), but the pain may merely follow the articulation of metal head on normal articular cartilage in an elderly patient who was probably too active to have had a hemiarthroplasty originally. The treatment is conversion to a total hip replacement.

Suggested Readings

Barnes JT, Brown JT, Garden RS, Nicoll EA: Subcapital fractures of the femur; a prospective review. J Bone Joint Surg (Br) 1976; 58B:2–24.

Bateman JE (ed): Bipolar femoral prosthesis. Clin Orthop 1990; 251.

Holmberg SH, Kalén R, Thorngren KG: Treatment and outcome of femoral neck fractures: an analysis of 2418 patients admitted from their homes. Clin Orthop 1987; 218:42–52.

Keating JF, Robinson CM, Court-Brown CM, McQueen MM, Christie J: The effect of complications after hip fracture on rehabilitation. J Bone Joint Surg (Br) 1993; 75B:976.

Swiotkowski MF: Intracapsular hip fractures. In Browner BD, Jupiter JB, Levine AM, Trafton PG (eds): Skeletal Trauma, pp 1369–1442. WB Saunders, Philadelphia, 1992.

Whittaker RP, Abeshaus MM, Scholl HW, Chung MK: Fifteen years experience with metallic endoprosthetic replacement of the femoral head for femoral neck fractures. J Trauma 1972; 12:799–806.

Case 3

History and Physical Examination

A 66-year-old man fell down the steps leading to his house. He experienced the immediate onset of left hip pain and was unable to stand or crawl. A neighbor found him approximately 15 minutes after injury. He was brought to the emergency department via ambulance, arriving approximately 45 minutes from the time of injury. Evaluation in the emergency department revealed that the left leg was shortened and externally rotated. Gentle palpation of the knee, thigh, and iliac crests was painless. However, there was pain with palpation of the greater trochanter and with gentle internal and external rotation of the extremity. The neurovascular examination of the leg and foot was within the limits of normal. In addition to the hip injury the patient had sustained a laceration of the forehead but had not lost consciousness. There were no other injuries. The patient saw an internist at yearly intervals and had no significant medical problems.

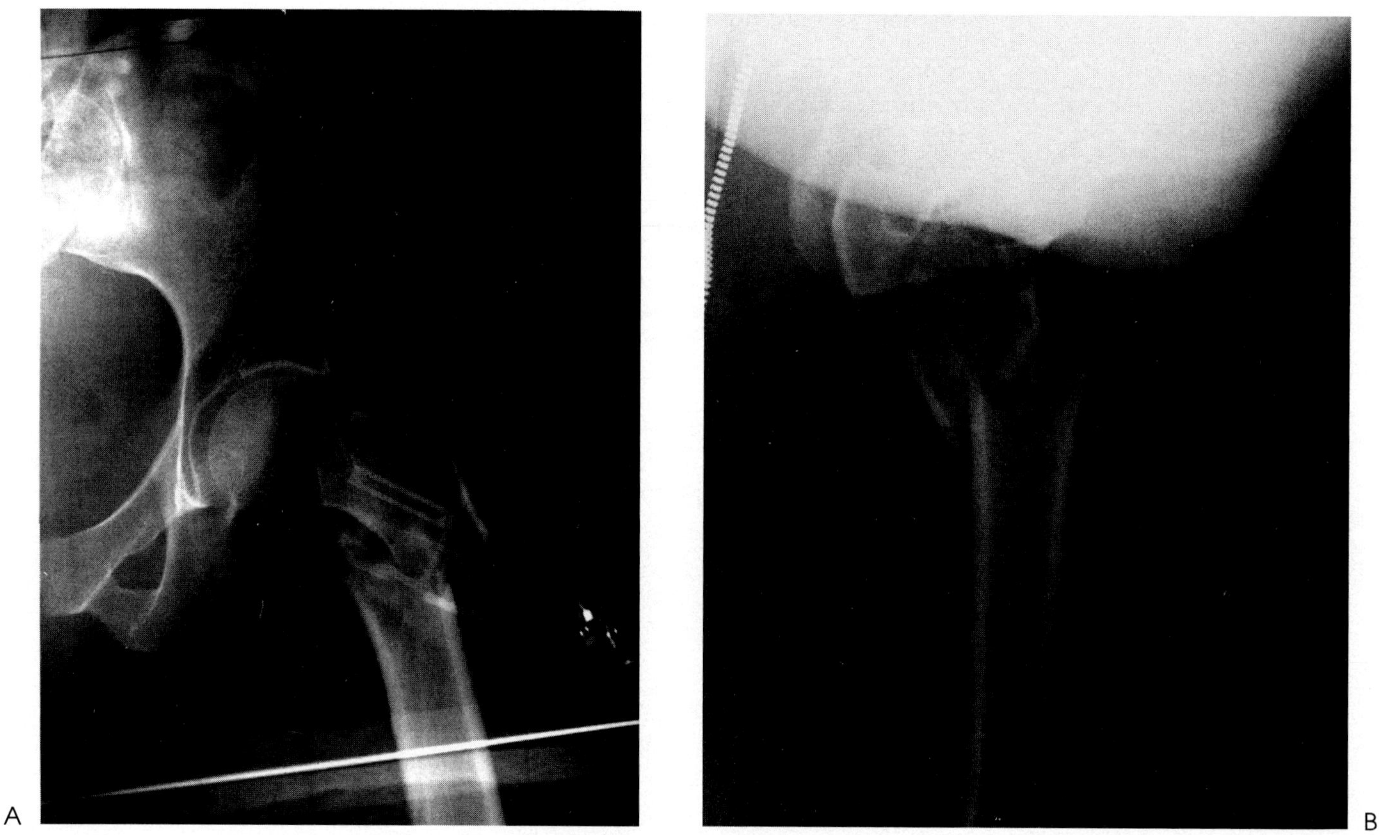

Figure 3–1. Anteroposterior (A) and lateral (B) radiographs of the hip indicating a reverse obliquity intertrochanteric fracture of the femur.

Radiologic Findings

Radiographs of the left hip, femur, knee, and pelvis were obtained and indicated a displaced two part peritrochanteric fracture of the left hip. The plane of the fracture was parallel to that of the femoral neck. The bone appeared relatively dense with preservation of the primary tension trabeculae in the contralateral proximal femur (Fig. 3–1).

PITFALL

- The pitfall to avoid is failure to recognize this subtype of peritrochanteric fracture. Reverse obliquity fractures may collapse with unacceptable shortening if managed with a conventional 135 degree side plate and compression screw.

Diagnosis

Reverse obliquity peritrochanteric fracture of the proximal femur. According to the Comprehensive Classification of Fractures of long bones, this is a 31–A3.1 fracture.

Surgical Management

The patient was placed in 10 pounds of skin traction with the knee flexed approximately 20 degrees over a pillow. The next day he was taken to the operating room and a general anesthetic administered. He was moved to a fracture table and placed in the lateral position with the injured side up. Traction was applied and the fracture was reduced with the aid of fluoroscopy by rotating the extremity.

The fracture was stabilized with an antegrade intramedullary reconstruction type nail inserted via a gluteus maximus splitting approach. The piriformis fossae was identified and a short rigid 2.5 mm guidewire was driven into the proximal femur from the piriformis fossa to the level of the lesser trochanter. Care was taken to ensure that the guidewire was parallel to and centered over the medullary canal of the femur in both anteroposterior and lateral planes. The proximal femur was overreamed with a cannulated rigid reamer. A long guidewire was inserted down the

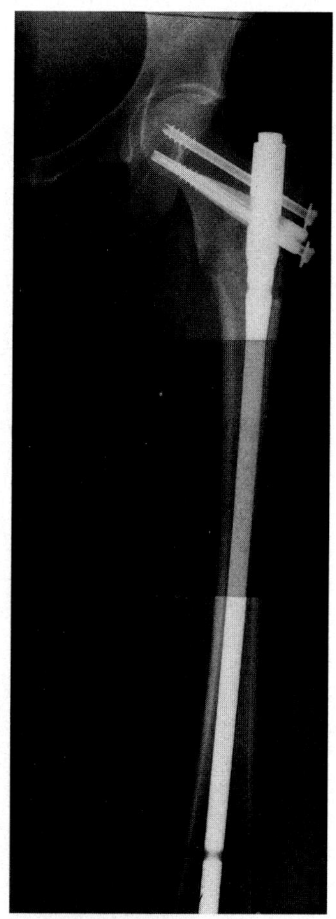

Figure 3–2. Anteroposterior radiograph following stabilization of the fracture with a long reconstruction nail and cannulated screws.

PEARLS

- When using a reconstruction type nail for proximal femur fractures, it is key to place the proximal fixation component (in this case the spiral blade) accurately in the neck of the femur. Therefore, it is necessary to fluoroscopically visualize the neck in the lateral plane to assess its version. This is accomplished during the reduction by carefully positioning the fluoroscopy unit to eliminate overlying images of the table, peroneal post, and contralateral hip. It is mandatory to accomplish this prior to the surgical scrub and draping.

- The guidewire must be placed accurately to prevent stabilizing the fracture in varus. This is facilitated by placing the patient in the lateral decubitus position. To minimize the possibility of fracturing the proximal fragment during nail insertion the femur is overreamed proximally over a guidewire that is parallel to and centered over the medullary canal in both anteroposterior and lateral planes.

medullary canal; the short guidewire was removed and the femur sequentially reamed. The appropriately sized nail was driven down the femur. Fixation was achieved proximally with a spiral blade and two cannulated screws (Fig. 3–2). Distally the nail was locked with one screw.

Postoperative Management

The patient was up in a chair the day after surgery. Two days after surgery he was allowed to ambulate with a walker, toe touch only on the injured side. At 4 weeks callus was evident on radiographs of the hip and weight bearing was advanced as tolerated on the injured side. By 8 weeks the patient was bearing his full weight on the injured extremity using a cane for support. The nail was not dynamized, and the fracture went on to heal uneventfully (Fig 3–3).

Discussion

Reverse obliquity peritrochanteric fractures can be grouped with intertrochanteric or subtrochanteric fractures. They tend to occur in younger patients and are higher energy injuries than the more commonly encountered two, three, and four part intertrochanteric fractures. Because the plane of the fracture line roughly parallels that of the barrel of a conventional compression hip screw, use of a hip screw may not prevent uncontrolled collapse through the fracture. Regardless of the type of fixa-

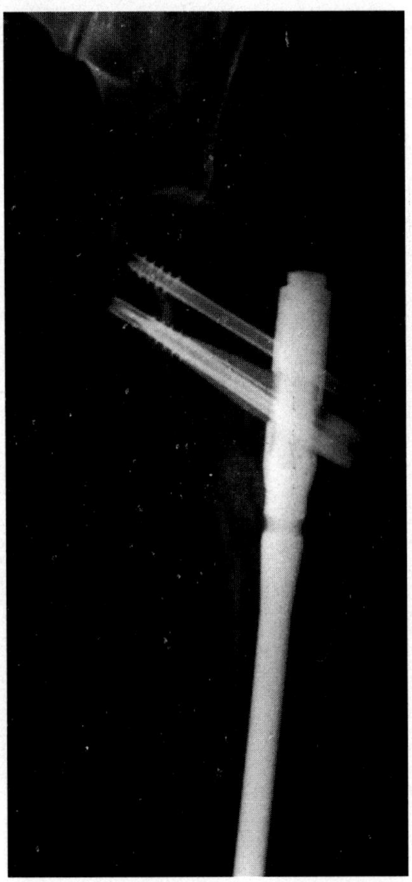

Figure 3–3. Radiograph indicating solid healing of the fracture.

tion, reduction of the medial cortex is an important component of stability of fixation. If accurate reduction is not possible, bone grafting should be considered to minimize the chance of implant failure.

Alternative Methods of Management

Alternatives to a reconstruction type intramedullary nail are conventional compression hip screw, 95 degree blade plate or compression screw, short intramedullary reconstruction type nail, or retrograde nails. Arthroplasty is not an option in most cases because the typical patient with a reverse obliquity peritrochanteric fracture is relatively young and the fracture is relatively distal, requiring a proximal femoral replacement.

Fixation with a conventional compression hip screw has the advantage of being a technique most orthopedic surgeons are very familiar with. However, the device does not reliably prevent uncontrolled collapse when used to stabilize reverse obliquity fractures (Figs. 3–4 through 3–6).

Fixation with a 95 degree blade plate or compression screw will prevent shortening but has a tendency to fail unless there is accurate reduction of the medial cortex or the medial cortex is bone grafted (Fig. 3–7).

Short reconstruction type nails (e.g., Gamma nail) adequately stabilize reverse obliquity fractures but are associated with a high incidence of late fracture of the femur at

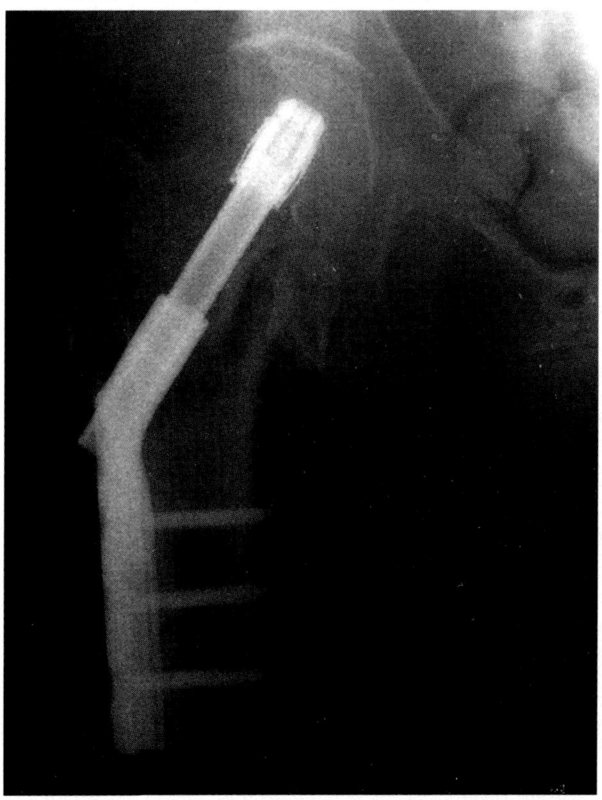

Figure 3–4. Immediate postoperative radiograph of a reverse obliquity intertrochanteric fracture treated with a 135 degree compression screw.

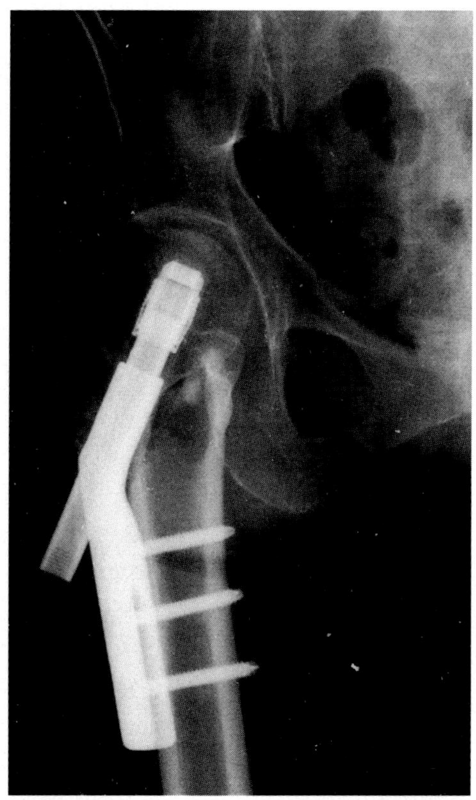

Figure 3–5. The same patient seen in Figure 3–4 following uncontrolled shortening of the fracture.

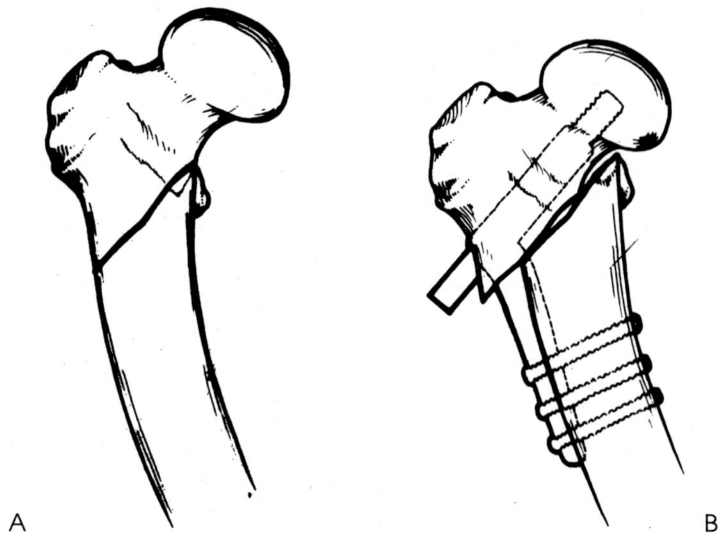

Figure 3–6. (A,B) The mechanism of shortening of a reverse obliquity intertrochanteric fracture stabilized with a 135 degree compression screw and side plate.

their tip. Late fractures result from the combined stress concentration secondary to the very rigid intramedullary nail and the distal locking screw hole (Fig. 3–8).

Long reconstruction type nails stabilize the fracture and should not have the high incidence of associated fractures at their tip. Long reconstruction nails have 2 disadvantages in the management of reverse obliquity fractures. First, the curvature of

Type of Management	Advantages	Disadvantages	Comments
Conventional compression hip screw	Surgeon familiarity	May not prevent uncontrolled collapse at fracture	May not prevent unacceptable shortening; limits use of this device
95 degree blade plate or compression screw	Surgeon familiarity; will prevent shortening	High incidence of implant failure unless nonweight bearing or fracture is bone grafted	High incidence of implant failure limits use of this device
Short antegrade reconstruction nail (e.g., Gamma nail)	Prevents uncontrolled shortening; technically simple; proximally based guide for distal locking screws	Femur fracture at the tip of the implant	Fracture at the end of the implant is a major problem
Long antegrade reconstruction nail (e.g., spiral blade and unreamed nail)	Prevents uncontrolled shortening; eliminates the chance of late femur fracture	Distal locking is freehand	More difficult technique than short antegrade nail, but better because it eliminates midshaft femur fractures
Retrograde nail (e.g., Ender nails)	Intramedullary device that will prevent uncontrolled shortening	Technically difficult procedure; insertion site symptoms	Most surgeons are not familiar with this technique

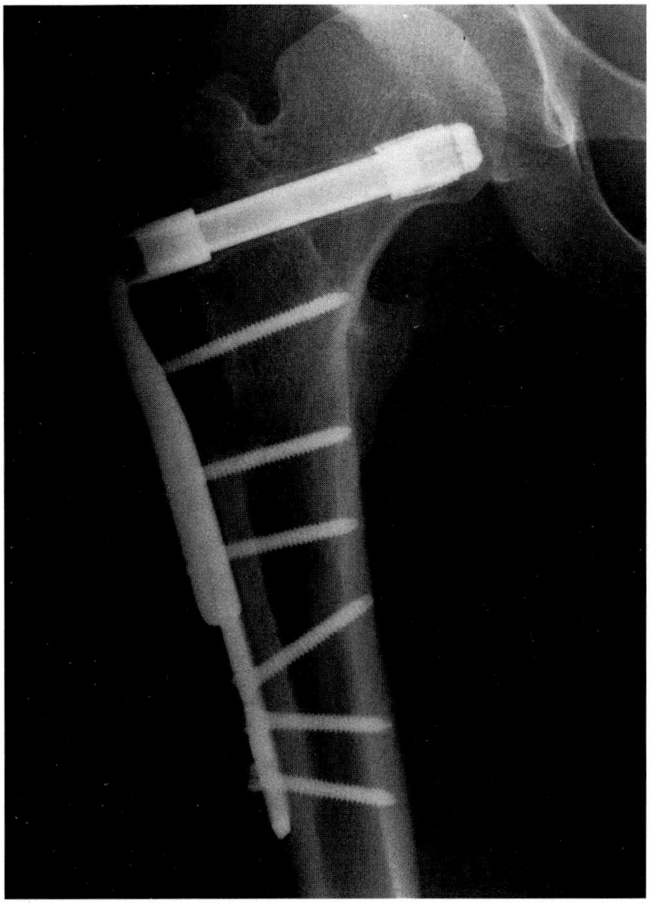

Figure 3–7. Stabilization of a reverse obliquity fracture with a 95 degree compression screw and side plate. This device will not allow collapse, but is susceptible to failure if the medial cortex is comminuted or not bone grafted.

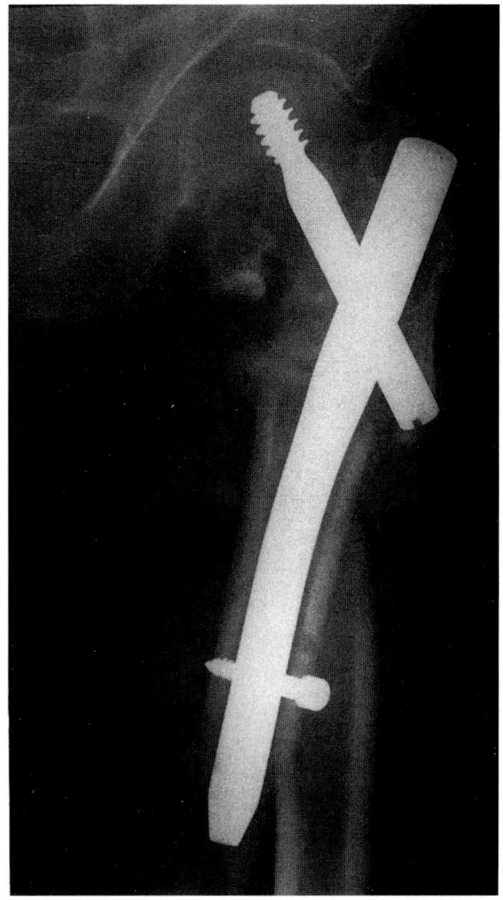

Figure 3–8. A radiograph of a hip following stabilization of a reverse obliquity fracture with a Gamma nail and subsequent fracture at the tip of the nail.

the nail may not mimic that of the patient's femur and therefore there is a risk of the nail breaking through the cortex as it is driven distally. Second, proximal fixation is not as stable as a short reconstruction nail or compression hip screw.

Retrograde nails (e.g., Ender nails) adequately stabilize reverse obliquity fractures but are associated with a high incidence of insertion site problems. Furthermore, retrograde nailing is a technique unfamiliar to most orthopaedic surgeons.

Complications

Complications of reverse obliquity peritrochanteric fracture are uncontrolled collapse through the fracture site, loss of fixation, and fracture below a short antegrade reconstruction nail. Nonunion is extremely rare.

Uncontrolled collapse of the fracture will result in shortening of the extremity. If caught early enough, within 2 to 4 weeks following fixation, the fixation can be revised to a more appropriate device. In cases in which the fracture has healed, management consists of conservative measures such as a shoe lift. In the rare instance when the patient is young and active, an ipsilateral femoral lengthening or contralateral femoral shortening can be performed.

Loss of fixation is most frequently due to uncontrolled collapse at the fracture site, complete telescoping of the implant, followed by cutout. Management consists of hemiarthroplasty if the acetabulum has not been damaged or total arthroplasty if the acetabulum has been damaged. In most cases a calcar replacement prosthesis is necessary.

Fracture below a short antegrade reconstruction nail is managed with revision of fixation to a long antegrade reconstruction nail.

Nonunions are rare. The symptom of an unhealed fracture is pain with weight bearing. If pain persists past 6 months from the time of injury, nonunion should be considered. Methods of management include application of electromagnetic fields or autogenous bone grafting. If the fixation device has failed or cut out, it is removed, replaced, and the fracture is bone grafted. The difficulty is obtaining fixation in the head of the femur. Using a different angle fixation device may increase proximal fixation (e.g., if a 135 degree screw and side plate has failed, it is replaced with a 95 degree screw and side plate). However, this approach results in a large portion of the femoral head being removed during reaming for insertion of the lag screw.

Suggested Readings

Broos PL, Rommens PM, Deleyn PR, Geens VR, Stappaerts KH: Peritrochanteric fractures in the elderly: are there indications for primary prosthetic replacement? J Orthop Trauma 1991; 5(4):446–451.

Evans EM: The treatment of trochanteric fractures of the femur. J Bone Joint Surg 1949; 31B(2):190–203.

Goldhagen PR, O'Connor DR, Schwarze D, Schwartz E: Prospective comparative study of the compression screw and the gamma nail. J Orthop Trauma 1994; 18(5):367–372.

Muller ME, Nazarian S, Koch P: Classification AO des Fractures I, pp 120–121. Springer Verlag, Berlin, 1987.

Perry CR, Brueckmann ER, Pankovich AM, Sanders RW, Waddell JP: Flexible intramedullary nailing of long bone fractures. Instructional Course Lectures 1993; 42:57–65.

Sensheimer F: Subtrochanteric fractures of the femur. J Bone Joint Surg 1978; 60A:300.

Senter B, Kendig R, Savoie FH: Operative stabilization of subtrochanteric fracture of the femur. J Orthop Trauma 1990; 4(4):399–405.

Case 4

History and Physical Examination

An 84-year-old woman slipped and fell in the living room of her house. She experienced the immediate onset of severe pain in the right hip and was unable to walk or crawl. Her daughter found her somnolent and incoherent approximately 12 hours after injury. The patient arrived in the emergency department via ambulance 13 hours after injury.

The patient's right leg was shortened and externally rotated approximately 90 degrees. A large hematoma was evident about the greater trochanter. No other injuries were noted. Specifically, there were no signs of an upper extremity fracture. However, the patient appeared to be extremely fluid restricted with dry mucous membranes, decreased skin turgor, a blood pressure of 90/60, and a pulse rate of 90. The daughter related that the patient had lived by herself and had been a community ambulator. She had a history of mild congestive heart failure that had responded to medication.

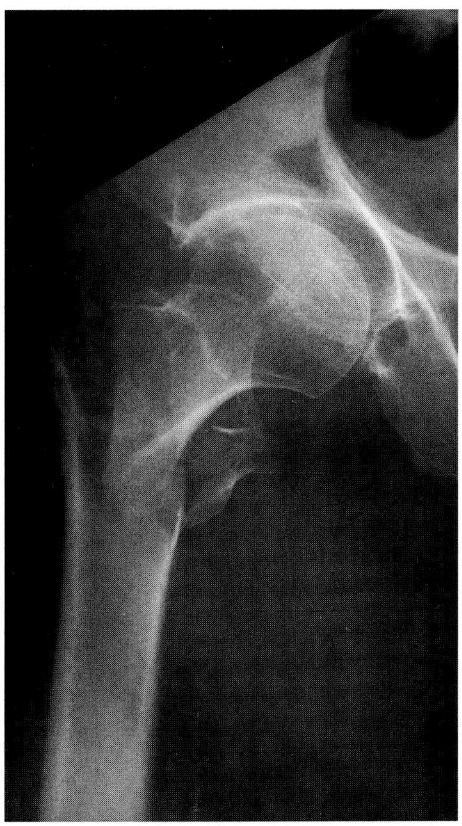

Figure 4–1. Anteroposterior radiograph of the hip.

Radiologic Findings

Radiographs of the hip, femur, and pelvis indicated the presence of an intertrochanteric fracture. The lesser trochanter was fractured. The majority of the greater trochanter and lateral cortex remained attached to the shaft fragment (Fig. 4–1).

Diagnosis

Three part or A-2 intertrochanteric fracture. This is an unstable fracture pattern due to the medial comminution and vertical fracture line. In addition to the fracture the patient was fluid depleted.

Surgical Management

Seven pounds of traction was applied to the extremity via a foam boot applied to the leg and foot. A pillow was placed under the thigh. Intravenous access was obtained. A Foley catheter was inserted and the patient was carefully fluid resuscitated by her internist. She was log rolled from her back to her left side every hour.

The first day postinjury, when the patient had been fluid resuscitated, she was taken to the operating room. A spinal anesthetic was administered and the patient was moved to the fracture table. Surgical management of the intertrochanteric fracture consisted of closed reduction, surgical exposure, a valgus producing osteotomy, and application of a compression hip screw and side plate.

Closed reduction was performed with the aid of fluoroscopy. The extremity was gently externally rotated 45 degrees, "unlocking" the fragments. Traction was then applied and the extremity internally rotated 45 degrees, reducing the fracture. Significant posterior displacement of the distal fragment was evident on the lateral fluoroscopic projection. It became clear that this posterior displacement would have to

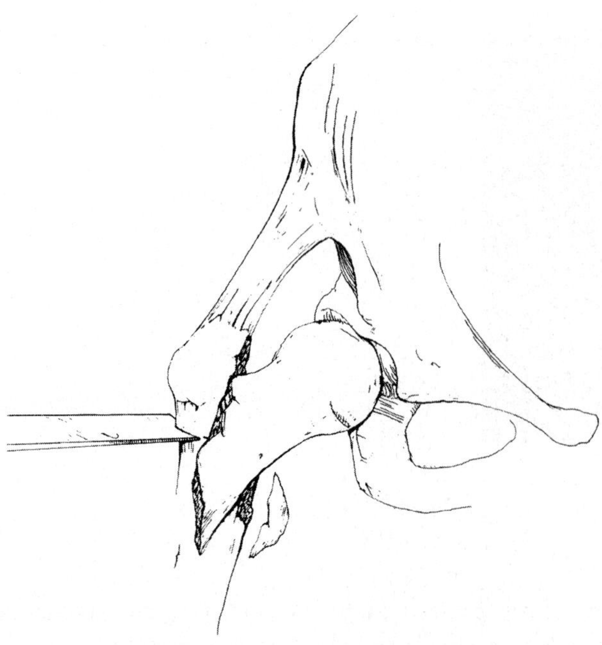

Figure 4–2. The osteotomy is performed at the level at which the barrel of the side plate will be inserted.

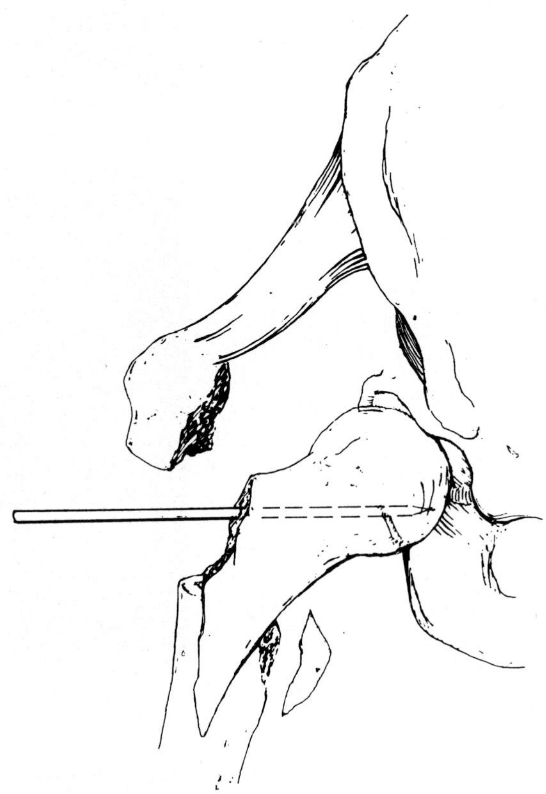

Figure 4–3. Insertion of the guide pin low in the head. Note that the guide pin has been placed at an angle of 90 degrees to the long axis of the femur. Because this angle is less than that of the barrel to the side plate, the fracture will be stabilized in valgus.

PEARL

- There is a temptation to use a higher angle plate with a valgus producing osteotomy. This frequently results in the screw being too superior in the head and can lead to cutout. The key to producing valgus is to position the guide pin at an angle with the long axis of the femur that is less than that of the barrel to the side plate (Fig. 4-3).

be corrected after the fracture had been surgically exposed. Due to the osteopenia and instability of the fracture pattern, the surgeon elected to perform a valgus producing osteotomy prior to reduction and stabilization with a sliding hip screw.

Surgical exposure was via a straight lateral approach. The fascia lata was divided in line with its fibers; the underlying hematoma was evacuated. The vastus lateralis was retracted anteriorly with large blunt rakes. The femur was palpated through the posterior portion of the vastus. The thin posterior portion of the vastus was incised longitudinally, exposing the lateral cortex of the femur.

A *valgus producing osteotomy* was performed with a 1 in. osteotome. The lateral cortex of the femur was osteotomized at the level at which the barrel of the side plate would eventually be located. The location of the osteotomy was determined with the aid of fluoroscopy (Fig. 4–2).

The first step in stabilization of the fracture with a *sliding compression screw* was guide pin placement. The guide pin was inserted freehand, roughly parallel to the axis of the femoral neck, with its tip just inferior to the center of the head. An angle guide was not used, but the pin was positioned at an angle less than 135 degrees with the long axis of the femur, thus ensuring that when the side plate was attached to the femur the neck would be in valgus (Fig. 4–3).

The head and neck fragment were reamed to the appropriate size to within .5 cm of the subchondral bone of the femoral head over the guide pin. The distal fragment was reduced by lifting it anteriorly with a large periosteal elevator. The posterior "sag" at the fracture site was corrected by placing a crutch covered with a Mayo stand cover under the thigh. The compression bolt was inserted into the head over the guidewire. The barrel of the side plate was slid over the compression bolt (Fig. 4–4). The side plate was clamped loosely to the femur. An unscrubbed assistant

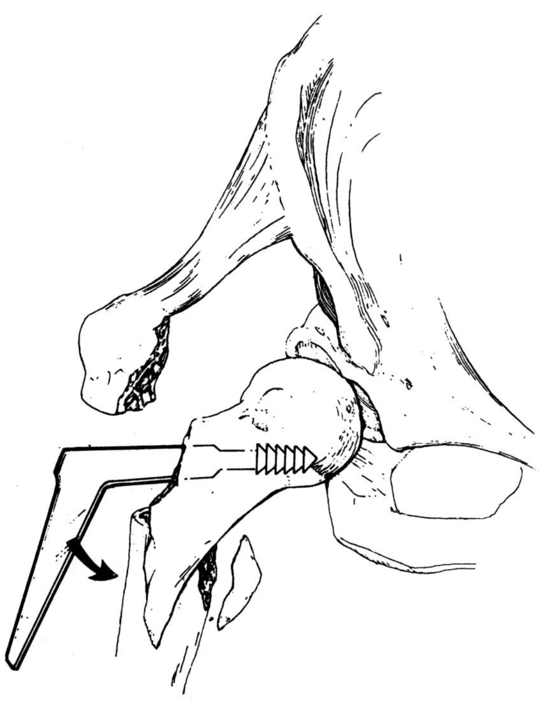

Figure 4–4. The compression screw and side plate are inserted. The side plate should be off the lateral cortex of the femur.

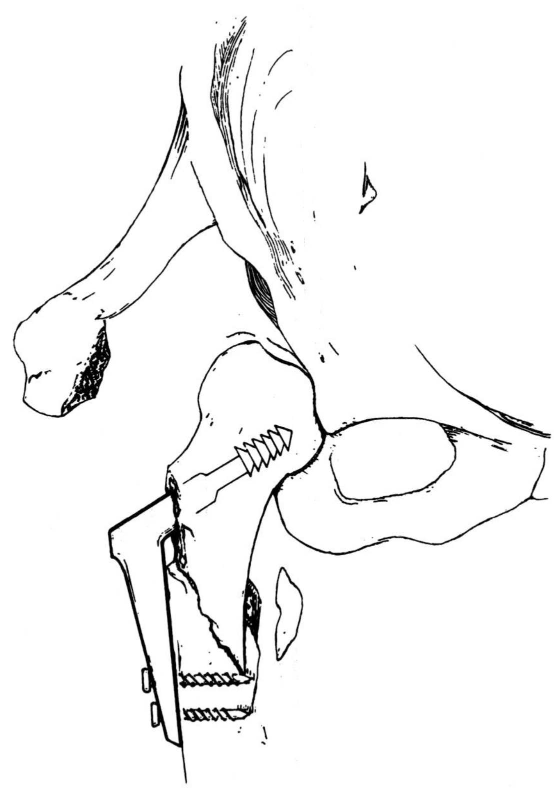

Figure 4–5. As the side plate is approximated to the femur, the head and neck are positioned in valgus.

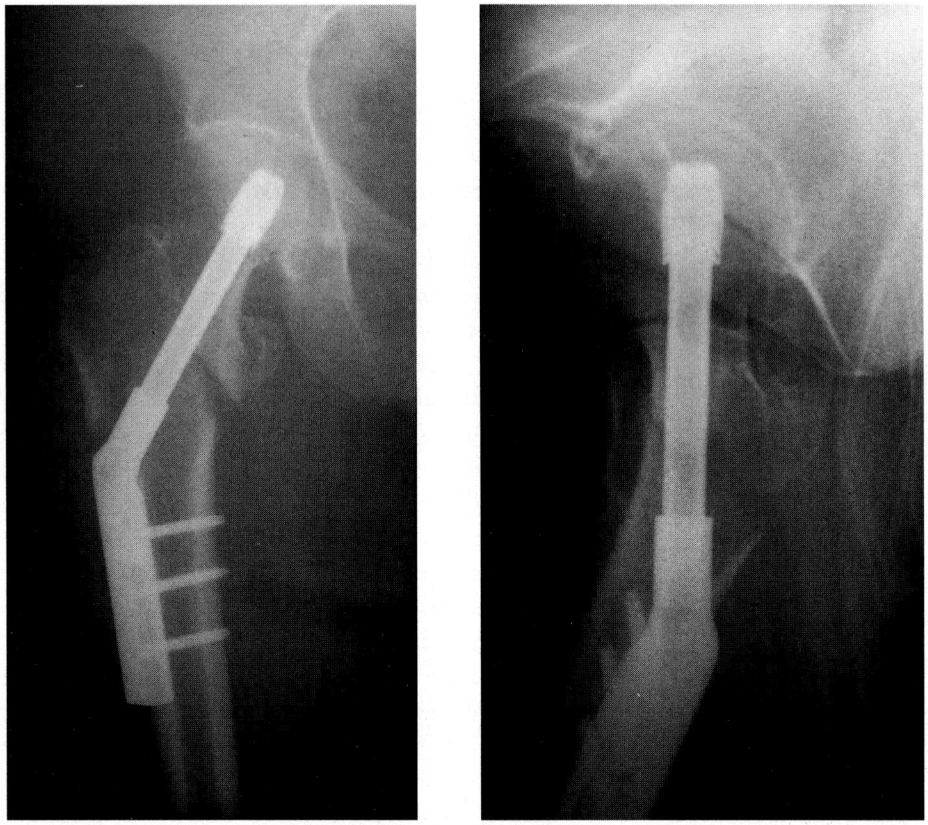

A B

Figure 4–6. Anteroposterior (A) and lateral (B) radiographs obtained postoperatively. The head and neck are in valgus. The screw is centered in the neck on the lateral projection.

then loosened the fracture table and increased hip abduction while the clamp was tightened, thus bringing the head and neck into valgus. The side plate was fixed to the femur with screws (Figs. 4–5 and 4–6). Traction was released, and the wound was closed in layers over a suction drain.

Postoperative Management

The patient was up in a chair on the first postoperative day. On day 2 she was allowed to bear weight as tolerated. The patient was independent with a walker at 3 weeks. Controlled collapse at the fracture site resulted in approximately 2 cm of shortening. At 6 months the fracture was solidly healed (Fig. 4–7).

Discussion

Patients who have sustained low energy intertrochanteric or femoral neck fractures are elderly and frequently debilitated. The physical examination and history should focus on the cardiovascular, pulmonary, and genitourinary systems. The medical status should be optimized as quickly as possible, with the goal being to stabilize the fracture within 24 hours.

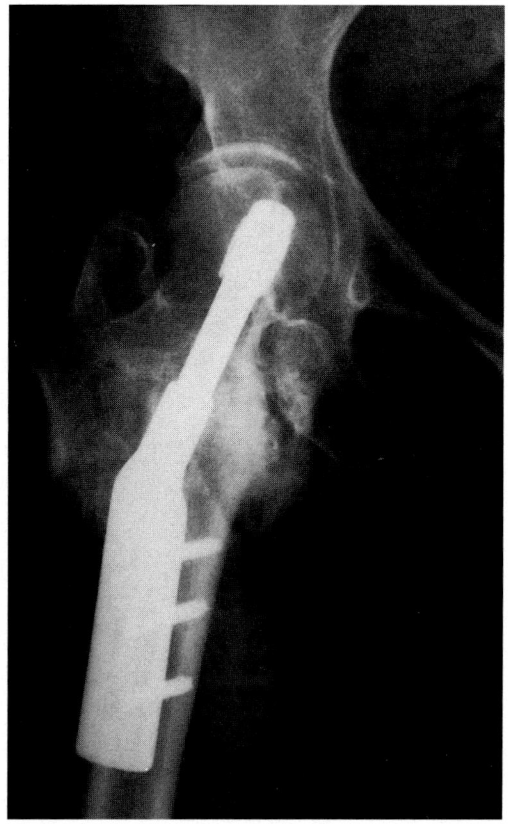

Figure 4–7. Anteroposterior radiograph of the hip after the fracture has healed.

Alternative Methods of Management

Alternatives to the method of management used in this case are anatomic reduction, fixation with an implant other than a sliding compression screw, hemiarthroplasty, augmentation of fixation with polymethylmethacrylate (PMMA), hemiarthroplasty, or nonoperative management with traction.

Anatomic reduction of the fracture increases the stability of fixation without shortening of the extremity. The disadvantage of anatomic reduction is the difficulty in reducing and stabilizing the key posterior medial fragment, which includes the lesser trochanter.

Alternative implants include antegrade reconstruction type intramedullary nails, retrograde intramedullary nails, and compression hip screw with a sliding plate.

Hemiarthroplasty is seldom performed as the primary management of an intertrochanteric fracture. It is performed as a salvage procedure after loss of fixation.

Augmentation of fixation with PMMA increases the surface area of the interface between the implant and the bone of the femoral head, thus decreasing the stress per surface area and the incidence of cutout. The disadvantage of PMMA augmentation is that the PMMA may inhibit healing and eventually fragment. In addition, if not properly placed, it may prevent controlled shortening of the fracture.

Type of Management	Advantages	Disadvantages	Comments
Valgus or medial displacement osteotomy	Technically easy; immediate weight bearing postoperatively	Results in shortening of the extremity	
Anatomic reduction	Maintains extremity length; weight bearing usually delayed	Can be extremely difficult to reestablish medial buttress	
Alternative implants	Biomechanically stronger	Less experience with other devices	
Hemiarthroplasty	Immediate postoperative weight bearing	More extensive procedure than ORIF	
Augmentation with PMMA	Technically easy; weight bearing usually delayed	May retard healing or prevent telescoping of compression screw if cement extrudes into fracture site or along barrel of compression screw	

Alternative Implants	Advantages	Disadvantages	Comments
135 degree angle compression screw	Simple reliable technique that in most cases allows controlled collapse	Controlled collapse may result in unacceptable shortening	Technique with which there is the most experience
Sliding compression screw (e.g., Medoff Plate)	Allows additional collapse along the axis of the femur	Controlled collapse may result in unacceptable shortening	Very little experience with this technique
Reconstruction antegrade nail (e.g., Russell Taylor Nail)	Intramedullary fixation; low incidence of implant failure	Limited proximal fixation; nail may cut out of femur anteriorly during insertion	Limited proximal fixation and possibility of cutout limit the application of this technique
Short antegrade nail (e.g., Gamma nail)	Intramedullary fixation; low incidence of implant failure	2 to 10% incidence of fracture at the tip of the implant	Less blood loss, but when used for 4 part fractures fixation is limited
Retrograde nail (e.g., Ender nails, Harris condylocephalic nail)	Intramedullary fixation; low incidence of implant failure	Difficult technique; high incidence of insertion site symptoms; limited proximal fixation	These devices have been largely abandoned because of their technical demands

Complications

The surgical complications of intertrochanteric fractures are cutout, nonunion, and infection. Cutout of the lag screw from the head occurs when the fracture shortens to the extent that the threads of the lag screw engage the barrel of the side plate preventing further telescoping of the implant. The surgeon should try to prevent cutout by ensuring that there will be controlled collapse with bone to bone contact prior to complete telescoping of the compression hip screw. This may mean that a medial displacement or valgus producing osteotomy is necessary. If cutout becomes evident, but the screw has not yet penetrated the head, weight bearing is discontinued for 1 to 3 months until more healing has occurred. If the lag screw penetrated the head, the fixation is revised to a calcar replacement arthroplasty.

Nonunion (i.e., failure to heal by 1 year) is extremely rare following an intertrochanteric fracture. When delayed union occurs, the fracture may be infected or the patient may be seriously systemically ill. In cases in which fixation is stable, pulsed electromagnetic fields can induce healing. In cases in which fixation has failed, revision to a hemiarthroplasty is necessary.

Infection is a rare complication. When it occurs, fixation is left in place as long as it provides stability. When the fracture has healed, the implants are removed, necrotic and grossly infected tissue eliminated, and systemic antibiotics administered for a minimum of 4 weeks. In cases in which fixation failed, the implants are removed, the wound debrided, and systemic antibiotics administered. The long term prognosis for an infected intertrochanteric fracture with failed fixation is very poor. Fixation usually cannot be revised because of osteopoenia and arthroplasty is not an option because of the risk of reactivating the infection.

Suggested Readings

Baumgaertner MR, Curtin SL, Lindskog DM, Keggi JM: The value of the tip-apex distance in predicting failure of fixation of peritrochanteric fractures of the hip. J Bone Joint Surg 1995; 77A:1058–1064.

Boyd HB, Griffen LL: Classification and treatment of trochanteric fractures. Arch Surg 1949; 58:853–863.

Den Hartog BD, Bartal E, Cooke F: Treatment of the unstable intertrochanteric fracture effect of the placement of the screw, its angle of insertion, and osteotomy. J Bone Joint Surg 1991; 73A(5):726–733.

Dimon JH, Hughston JC: Unstable intertrochanteric fractures of the hip. J Bone Joint Surg 1967; 49A:440.

Elabdien Z, Olerud S, Karlstrom G: Ender nailing of pertrochanteric fractures. Complications related to technical failures and bone quality. Acta Orthop Scand 1985; 56:138–144.

Evans EM: Trochanteric fractures. J Bone Joint Surg 1951; 33B:192.

Harrington KD, Johnston JO: The management of comminuted unstable intertrochanteric fractures. 1973; 55A(7):1367–1376.

Medoff RJ, Maes K: A new device for the fixation of unstable pertrochanteric fractures of the hip. J Bone Joint Surg 1991; 73A:1192–1199.

Singh M, Nagrath AR, Maini PA: Changes in the trabecular pattern of upper end of the femur as an index of osteoporosis. J Bone Joint Surg 1970; 52A:470.

Case 5

History and Physical Examination

A 64-year-old woman was an unrestrained passenger in an automobile accident and sustained an obvious open fracture dislocation of her hip. She was extracted from the wreckage and transported to the emergency department, arriving approximately 45 minutes after the accident. Her blood pressure and pulse rate were stable and she was conscious and alert. She complained of pain only over her right knee and hip. A laceration approximately 10 cm in length, with a spike of bone protruding through the skin edges, was present on her right buttock. Devitalized muscle and tissue were visible in the wound. The right extremity was shortened and externally rotated. A stellate laceration was present over her knee. The patellar tendon was visible in the depths of this wound and appeared to be at least partially lacerated. The neurovascular examination of the right lower extremity was within the limits of normal. Injuries to the chest, abdomen, head, and cervical spine were ruled out.

Medical history was relevant in that the patient smoked heavily, was an insulin dependent diabetic, and had a history of congestive heart failure.

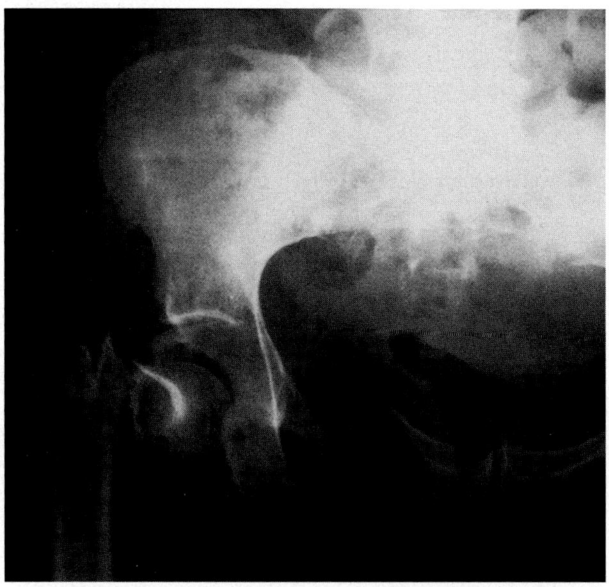

Figure 5–1. Anteroposterior radiograph of the hip and hemipelvis indicating a fracture of the neck and intertrochanteric region of the proximal femur. The femoral head is not concentrically located in the acetabulum. There are fractures of the ischial and pubic rami.

Radiologic Findings

Radiographs of the hip and pelvis indicated a severely displaced comminuted fracture of the proximal femur, involving the neck and intertrochanteric region. Fractures of the posterior lip of the acetabulum and ipsilateral ischial and pubic rami were evident (Fig. 5–1). Radiographs of the knee indicated air within the joint, but there was no evidence of fracture of the patella, proximal tibia, or distal femur.

Diagnosis

Grade III open fracture of the proximal femur; fracture of the posterior lip of the acetabulum; fractures of the ischial and pubic rami, an open injury of the knee joint, and a partial or complete laceration of the patellar tendon. The fracture of the proximal femur was classified as grade III because of the extensive laceration and presence of devitalized muscle. The femoral fracture is not classifiable by the Comprehensive Classification of Fractures because it involves both the extracapsular intertrochanteric region and the intracapsular neck.

Surgical Management

A distal femoral pin was inserted for traction. The hip and knee wounds were cultured, irrigated superficially with a liter of normal saline, and covered with sterile dressings. A second generation cephalosporin and an aminoglycoside were administered intravenously.

Four hours after the accident, injuries to other systems had been ruled out and medical clearance had been obtained. The patient was taken to the operating room. An anesthetic was administered, and she was turned to the lateral decubitus position. The open wound over the buttock was extended proximally toward the posterior superior iliac spine, and distally along the femur. Necrotic tissue and free fragments of bone, including the posterior rim of the acetabulum, were removed. Traction was applied to the leg through the traction pin by an unscrubbed surgeon, and by manipulating the head fragment and proximal femur the fracture was

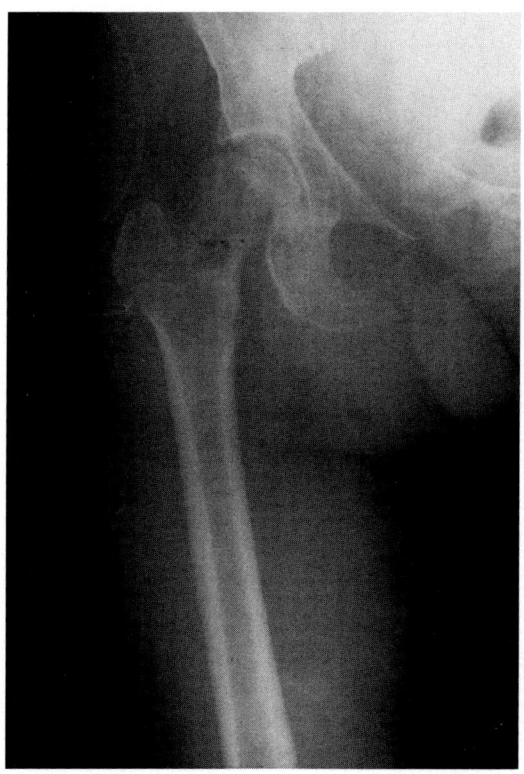

Figure 5–2. Anteroposterior radiograph of the hip following debridement. The extremity is in traction. The femoral head is located in the acetabulum, and the fracture is well aligned. There appears to be an impaction fracture of the dome of the acetabulum.

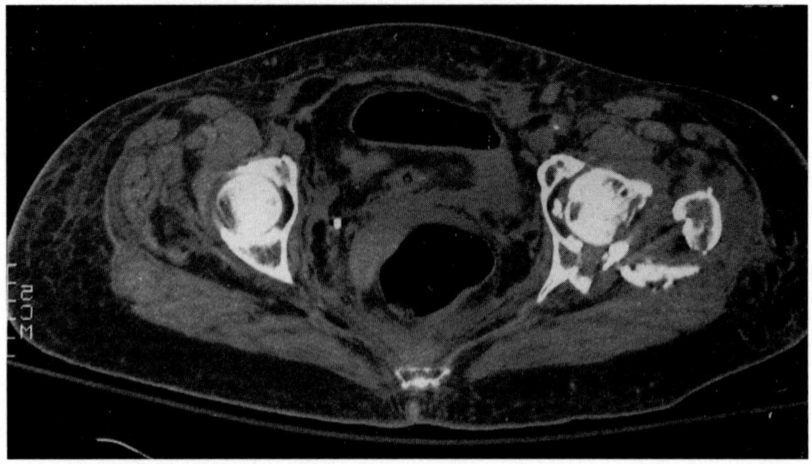

Figure 5–3. Computerized axial tomography of the hip in traction. A fracture of the posterior wall of the acetabulum is present.

aligned. The knee laceration was extended, explored, debrided, and irrigated. The patellar tendon was identified and found to be completely lacerated. The surgical incisions were closed in a single layer with vertical mattress sutures. The lacerations were loosely approximated with simple sutures. Suction drains were left in the wounds. The knee was splinted at 30 degrees with a posterior slab.

The extremity was placed in balanced skeletal traction via the distal femoral pin. Radiographs in traction indicated an adequate reduction, and questionable impaction fractures of the femoral head and of the acetabulum (Fig. 5–2). Computer-

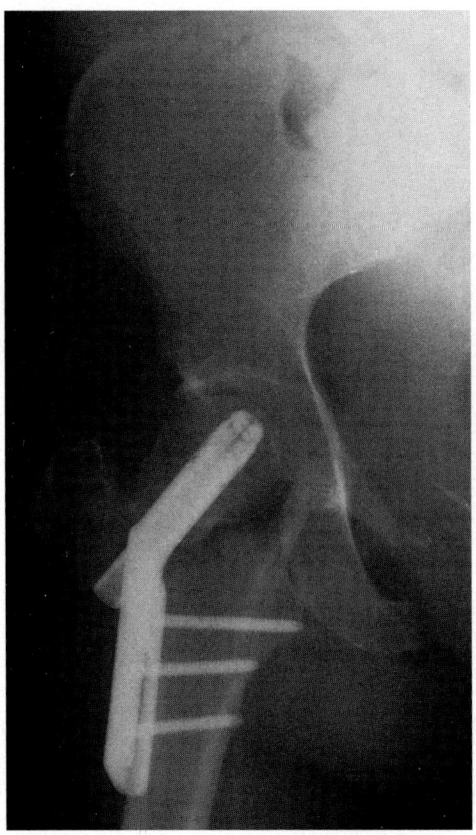

Figure 5–4. Anteroposterior radiograph of the hip following open reduction and fixation. The head appears subluxed very slightly laterally. The compression bolt has shortened maximally.

ized axial tomography confirmed these diagnoses (Fig. 5–3). One week after injury the patient was taken back to surgery where an anesthetic was administered, and the patient moved to the fracture table. The incision over the proximal femur was opened and a 135 degree side plate and compression bolt were used to stabilize the fracture. Traction was released and the fracture was shortened and impacted (Fig. 5–4). The wound was closed over a drain and the traction pin removed from the distal femur. The laceration and incision over the knee were opened and the lacerated ends of the patellar tendon were identified and repaired. The repair was protected with a figure of eight cable that wrapped around the proximal pole of the patella crossed in front of the patellar tendon and went through the tibial tubercle.

Postoperative Management

Postoperatively, five doses of antibiotics were administered. The patient was in a chair on the first postoperative day. She was allowed to be up with a walker "toe touch" weight bearing. Radiographs indicated unchanged alignment of the fracture (Fig. 5–5). The wounds healed. Six weeks after the open reduction and fixation of the hip fracture, radiographs indicated that the head of the femur had dislocated from the acetabulum (Figs. 5–6 and 5–7). The patient noted that her leg seemed

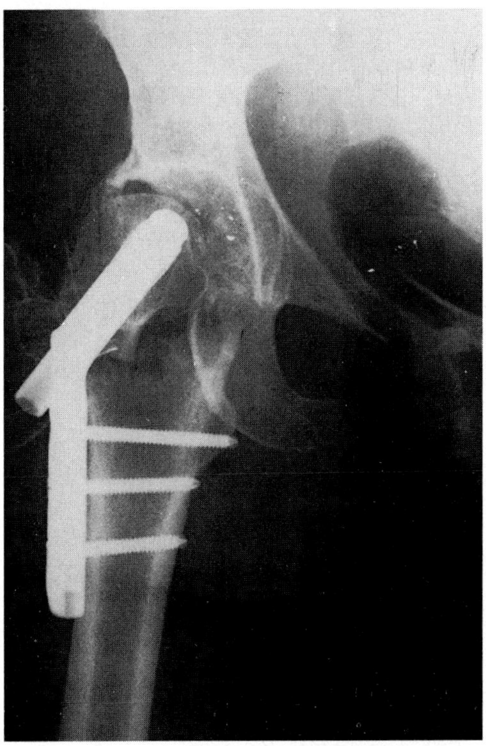

Figure 5–5. Anteroposterior radiograph of the hip 1 week after fixation. There appears to be bone to bone contact between the base of the neck and the lateral cortex of the femur just medial to the plate barrel junction.

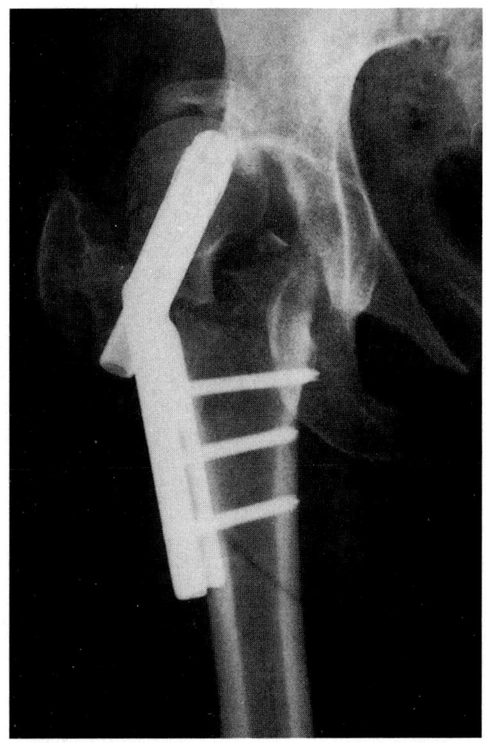

Figure 5–6. Anteroposterior radiograph of the hip 6 weeks following internal fixation. The femoral head is dislocated laterally and superiorly with a fragment of acetabulum. The lesser trochanter appears to be impinging on the medial wall of the acetabulum.

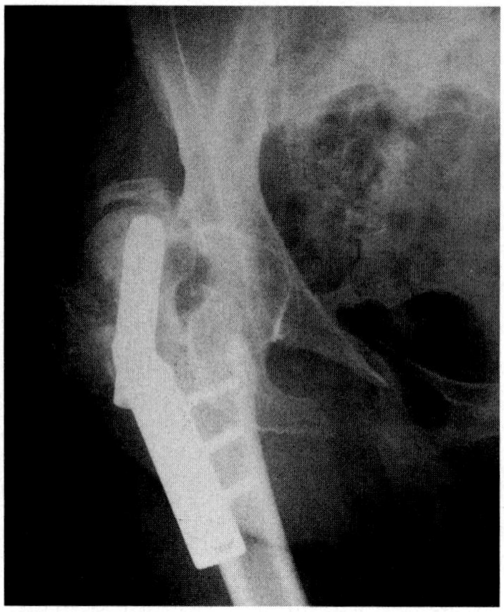

Figure 5–7. Anteroposterior radiograph obtained at 16 weeks following open reduction and internal fixation. Persistent dislocation of the hip is evident. Proximal displacement seems to have increased.

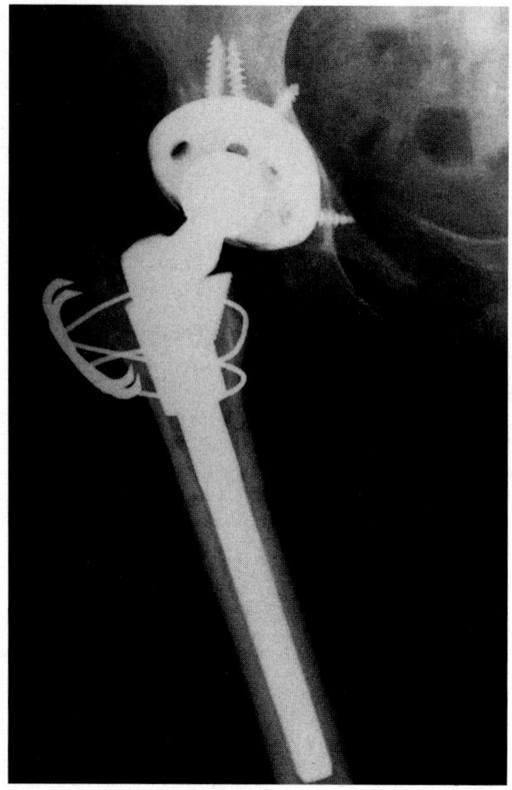

Figure 5–8. Anteroposterior radiograph obtained 20 weeks following hip arthroplasty.

shorter, but she had not experienced an increase in pain or discomfort and in fact felt as though she was improving. Therapy was continued. At 16 weeks the patient had plateaued in therapy and wanted something done to improve her function. Radiographs indicated persistent dislocation of the hip. At 20 weeks a bone ingrowth hip arthroplasty was performed via a posterolateral approach. Postoperatively the patient has done well (Fig. 5–8).

Discussion

There are a number of things that could have been done differently in this case that merit discussion. The decision to delay stabilization of the fracture is controversial. Placing the patient in traction for a week, prior to the definitive fixation, increased the risk of the complications due to prolonged recumbency, including pneumonia, urinary tract infection, and decubitus ulcers. Stabilization of the fractures was not performed on the day of injury because the surgeon wanted to minimize the duration of the procedure.

The decision to debride the posterior wall of the acetabulum contributed to the instability of the hip and the eventual dislocation. However, at the time of the initial debridement it was thought that retaining the devascularized posterior rim of the acetabulum would create an unacceptable risk of infection.

Dislocation of the hip resulted from the combination of an insufficient posterior acetabular wall and the impingement of the lesser trochanter on the ischium. The dislocation was not managed aggressively because it was clinically asymptomatic and the chance of reducing it and maintaining a reduction, without a major surgical procedure, was minimal. Therefore it was elected to perform a hip arthroplasty at a later date if the dislocation became symptomatic.

Alternative Methods of Management

Alternatives to debridement, traction and delayed fixation of the femur are debridement followed by immediate fixation of the acetabulum and femur, and debridement and management of the fracture of the proximal femur in traction.

Debridement followed by immediate internal fixation of the acetabulum and femur has the advantage of allowing early mobilization of the patient. However, it also subjects the patient to an extensive operative procedure. This is particularly worrisome in light of the high energy trauma that this patient had sustained and her medical history of congestive heart failure. Fixation of the acetabulum would have required retention of the avascular posterior rim of the acetabulum, possibly increasing the risk of infection.

Debridement and management of the fracture in traction has the advantage of not placing a foreign body (i.e., plates and screws) in a possibly contaminated wound. In this case, radiographs taken with the patient in traction indicated that the reduction of the femur was acceptable and the femoral head was located in the acetabulum. However, it is unlikely that this fracture would have healed in traction. Factors that mitigate against healing in traction are high energy fractures, open fractures, fractures comminuted with bone loss, and fractures involving the intracapsular portion of the femoral neck. Prolonged traction in this case would have exposed the patient to the risks of prolonged recumbency without a reasonable chance for the fracture to heal.

Type of Management	Advantages	Disadvantages	Comments
Debridement traction and delayed fixation	Spares the patient a major procedure immediately after injury when the extent of injuries is not known	Exposes the patient to the risks of 1 week of bedrest in traction	Because of this patient's age and medical status, it was thought that minimizing the extent of the initial procedure outweighed other considerations
Debridement and immediate fixation	Immediate stabilization of all fractures; allows early mobilization; minimizes complications due to bedrest	Requires an extensive procedure when the patient's medical status is unclear; may increase the risk of infection because of fixation devices in contaminated wound	In this case fixation of the acetabulum may have increased hip stability and prevented dislocation
Debridement and traction	May be necessary if patient is unstable medically	Prolonged bedrest; limited chance for fracture to heal	The least desirable alternative, with the most risk and lowest chance of success

Complications

Complications include infection, nonunion, avascular necrosis of the femoral head, and instability of the hip. The risk factors for infection in this case are the facts that the fracture was open and that the patient was a diabetic and a smoker. If infection had occurred, the management would have been to suppress the infection until healing of the fractures had occurred and then to debride the infected area of implants and necrotic tissue and administer 4 to 6 weeks of intravenous antibiotics. Suppression of the infection ideally would be with dressing changes alone. A short course of intravenous antibiotics followed by an extended course of oral antibiotics would be administered only if necessary. Inability to control the infection would necessitate debridement, possibly a girdlestone procedure, and antibiotic administration prior to healing of the fracture.

The risk factors for nonunion are identical to the risk factors for infection. Nonunion of the proximal femur would be managed initially with nonoperative methods (e.g., pulsed electromagnetic fields). If nonoperative methods failed, the nonunion would be grafted with autogenous bone. The last resort is hip arthroplasty.

The incidence of avascular necrosis of the femoral head following an open proximal femur fracture is high. Disruption of the blood supply to the femoral head results in avascular necrosis. The three groups of vessels that supply the femoral head are the ascending cervical, or retinacular vessel, intramedullary vessels, and the artery of the ligamentum teres. The artery of the ligamentum teres is always disrupted by dislocation of the hip. The intramedullary vessels are always disrupted by a displaced fracture of the femoral neck. This leaves only the retinacular vessels supplying the femoral head; if they are injured, the head will necrose. Management of avascular necrosis in a patient over 65 years of age is hip arthroplasty.

Instability of the hip is managed with hip arthroplasty. It is mandatory to evaluate the acetabulum preoperatively to ensure that the implants necessary to reconstruct it are present. To prevent increasing the hip instability, the surgical approach should be from the direction that the hip dislocates (i.e., in this case the hip dislocates posteriorly, therefore a posterior approach was used to implant the hip).

Suggested Readings

Mariani EM, Rand JA: Nonunion of intertrochanteric fractures of the femur following open reduction and internal fixation. Results of second attempts to gain union. CORR 1987; 218:81–89.

Tabsh I, Waddell JP, Morton J: Total hip arthroplasty for complications of proximal femoral fractures. J Orthop Trauma 1997; 11(3):166–169.

Case 6

History and Physical Examination

A 26-year-old male was an unrestrained passenger in a high speed automobile accident. He arrived in the emergency department 30 minutes after injury. His right lower extremity was shortened and externally rotated. Pulse sensation and motor function of the foot and ankle were intact. He denied loss of consciousness, and the remainder of his physical examination was within the limits of normal.

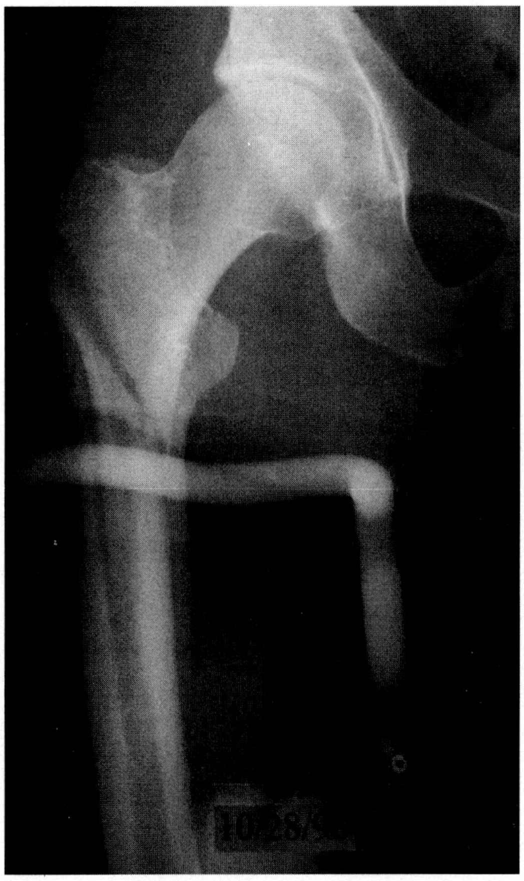

Figure 6–1. Anteroposterior radiograph of proximal femur indicating a subtrochanteric fracture. The fracture extends to 10 cm distal to the lesser trochanter.

Radiologic Findings

Radiographs of the proximal femur indicated a comminuted fracture of the proximal femur, extending from the lesser trochanter distally 10 cm (Fig. 6–1). Radiographs of the contralateral hip, pelvis, and distal femur were within the limits of normal.

Diagnosis

Isolated unstable subtrochanteric fracture. According to the Comprehensive Classification of Long Bones, this is a 31–A2.3 fracture.

Surgical Management

A traction pin was placed in the proximal tibia and the patient put in balanced suspension, with a sling supporting the calf. The patient was most comfortable with the hip slightly abducted and the knee and hip flexed 60 degrees.

The patient was taken to the operating room the first day following injury. An anesthetic was administered and he was moved to the fracture table. Traction was applied through the foot and the tibial pin removed. The circulating nurse was instructed how to internally and externally rotate the extremity, increase and decrease traction, and abduct and adduct the leg.

The area from the ipsilateral lower costal margin to the knee was prepped and draped. A incision was made laterally, parallel with the femur, and extending from the greater trochanter distally midway down the thigh. The vastus lateralis was divided in line with its fibers. Perforating arteries were isolated with their accompanying veins and suture ligated. The anterior two thirds of the vastus lateralis was retracted anteriorly with Bennet retractors exposing the femur. Reduction was accomplished directly by manipulating the fracture fragments and indirectly by manipulating the traction, internal-external rotation, and abduction-adduction on the fracture table. Reduction was held temporarily with tenaculum clamps and interfragmentary lag screws were inserted. A 10 hole 135 degree compression screw was

PEARLS

- The proximal femur tends to abduct and flex following a subtrochanteric fracture due to the unopposed action of the iliopsoas and gluteus medius and minimus. Therefore, when traction is used to maintain alignment, the hip is abducted and the knee and hip are flexed to minimize the patient's pain.
- The two advantages of putting the patient on the fracture table are that indirect techniques can be used and it is easier to obtain the fluoroscopic lateral projection. The disadvantage is that a knowledgeable assistant must be available to adjust the fracture table. An alternative to the fracture table is to position the patient on a radiolucent table with the injured extremity draped free, position the contralateral hip in abduction and flexion (to facilitate obtaining the lateral fluoroscopic projection of the hip), and use the femoral distractor to apply traction across the fracture.
- It is imperative to rule out life threatening visceral injuries associated with high energy injuries such as this. The first step in determining whether an associated injury is present is the physical examination. If there are any signs of visceral injury, a CT scan or diagnostic peritoneal lavage is indicated.

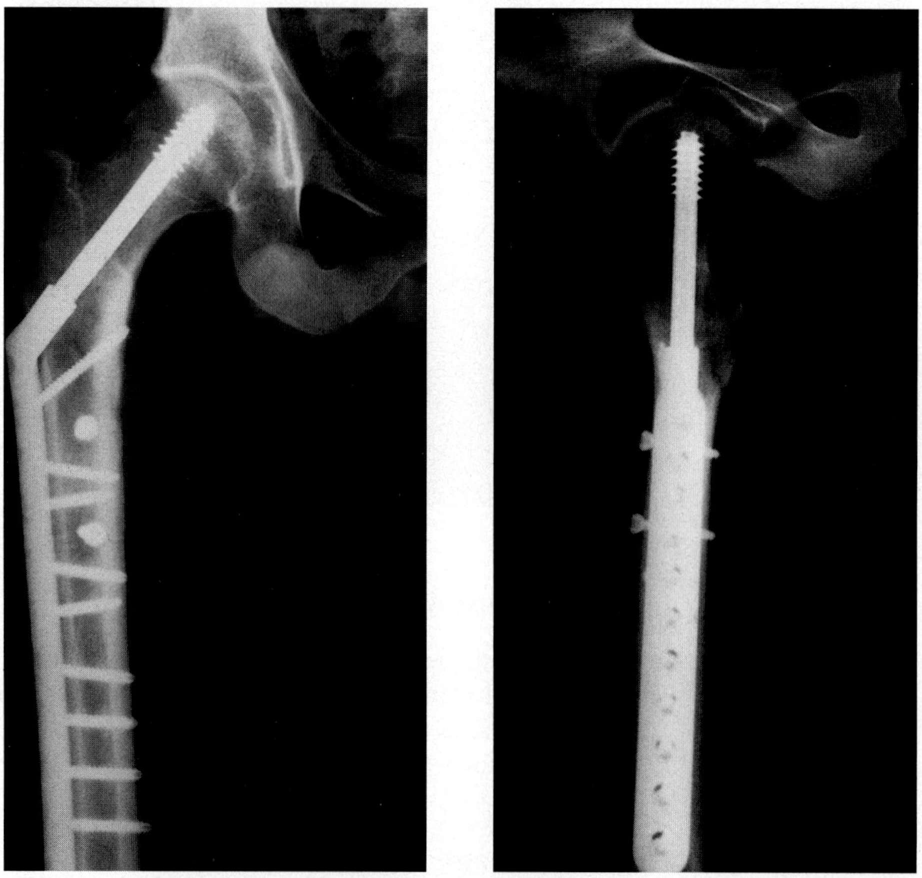

A B

Figure 6–2. Anteroposterior (A) and lateral (B) radiographs obtained 2 months following internal fixation of the fracture with a 135 degree lag screw and 10 hole plate.

applied as a neutralization plate to the lateral cortex of the femur. A keyed lag screw and compression screw were used. The wound was closed over a drain (Fig. 6–2).

Postoperative Management

Postoperatively the patient was kept nonweight bearing until 8 weeks postsurgery when radiographs indicated healing of the fracture. At this point weight bearing was advanced to full over the following 2 weeks.

Discussion

When a patient sustains a high energy subtrochanteric fracture, initially it is important to rule out associated visceral and musculoskeletal skeletal injuries. When these associated injuries have been identified, the optimum treatment plan can be formulated.

Alternative Methods of Management

Management of subtrochanteric fractures is operative stabilization. The two basic methods of stabilization are intramedullary nailing and plating. Subtrochanteric fractures have a high incidence of complications, including failure of fixation and nonunion regardless of the method of management.

Stabilization with nailing is accomplished with either a first generation locked nail or a reconstruction nail. Nailing has the advantage of minimizing the surgical approach and the disadvantage of a difficult closed reduction. Stabilization with plating is accomplished with a 95 degree, 135 degree, or conventional plate.

Type of Management	Advantages	Disadvantages	Comments
First generation locked nail	Technically simple	Limited fixation proximally	The limited proximal fixation outweighs the advantages of this technique
Reconstruction nail	Stable fixation proximally	Difficult to position screws in neck and head	Probably most commonly used procedure for subtrochanteric fractures
Plate and screws	Technically simple, if medial cortex reduced plate acts as tension band	Open procedure; limited proximal fixation	High incidence of nonunion
95 degree side plate and screw	Technically simple, if medial cortex reduced plate acts as tension band	Open procedure	Better proximal fixation than a plate and screws; high incidence of nonunion
135 degree side plate and screw	Technically simple, if medial cortex reduced plate acts as tension band	Open procedure	No advantage of a 135 degree angle over 95 degree plate

Plating has the advantage of an open and therefore relatively simple reduction and the disadvantage of an extensive surgical approach. To decrease the incidence of plate failure, serious consideration is given to bone grafting the medial cortex of the femur if it has not been anatomically reduced. There is no place for management of high energy subtrochanteric fractures with a plate that allows controlled shortening. Unlike low energy intertrochanteric-subtrochanteric fractures, there is no stable configuration to which these high energy fractures can shorten. In general, the most stable configuration is anatomic reduction; when this is achieved, fixation is applied to prevent loss of reduction. Regardless of the method of stabilization, the procedure must be carefully planned to maximize fixation of the proximal fragment.

Complications

Complications include failure of fixation, nonunion, and infection. Failure of fixation occurs because of limited fixation in the relatively small proximal fragment and the high stresses that occur in the subtrochanteric area of the femur. Failure following fixation with a plate and screws, 95 degree side plate, or 135 degree side plate is most often due to the bending stresses being applied to the plate instead of tensile stresses. This occurs when the medial cortex has not been reduced. The plate most often breaks through a screw hole. Management is removal of the broken hardware, bone grafting of the medial cortex, and repeat stabilization, usually with the same type of device that failed. When failure of fixation occurs following stabilization with a 95 degree or 135 degree side plate and screw because of cutout, a large defect is left in the proximal neck and head of the femur. This defect increases the difficulty of achieving proximal fixation. Bone grafting the defect, using a plate and screws, or location of the lag screw in a different part of the head are possible solutions to the problem of proximal fixation. Failure of fixation following intramedullary nailing is managed with removal of the failed fixation device, bone grafting, and repeat stabilization with a reconstruction nail.

Nonunion is signaled clinically by increasing pain with activity and radiographically by fixation that has failed or loosened. In cases in which the fixation has not failed, the nonunion can be managed conservatively with pulsed electromagnetic fields. When the fixation has failed or loosened, management is operative, and consists of removal of the failed or loosened implants, bone grafting, and repeat stabilization.

Infection is more common following open reduction and plating than closed reduction and nailing. Management consists of suppression or control of the infection with dressing changes and oral antibiotics until the fracture has healed. When the fracture has healed, the implants are removed, the infected area is debrided, and systemic antibiotics are administered for 6 weeks.

Suggested Readings

Brien WW, Wiss DA, Becker V, Lehman T: Subtrochanteric fractures: a comparison of the Zickel nail, 95 degree blade plate, and interlocking nail. J Orthop Trauma 1991; 5(4):458–464.

Kinast C, Bolhofner BR, Mast JW, Ganz R: Subtrochanteric fractures of the femur: results of treatment with the 95-degree condylar blade plate. CORR 1989; 238:122–130.

Kraimer WJ, Hearn TC, Powell JN, Mahomed N: Fixation of segmental subtrochanteric fractures. A biomechanical study. CORR 1996; 332:71–79.

Ruff ME, Lubbers LM: Treatment of subtrochanteric fractures with a sliding screw-plate device. J Trauma 1985; 26:75–80.

Case 7

History and Physical Examination

A 46-year-old male fell at home and injured his right thigh. He was unable to put weight on the injured leg but could crawl to the telephone and call for help. He arrived in the emergency department 3 hours after injury. On examination, external rotation and shortening of the leg were present. Attempted motion and palpation of the thigh were extremely painful. Healed scars and several draining sinuses were present laterally on the thigh. The neurovascular examination of the lower extremity was within the limits of normal.

The medical history was relevant because the patient had sustained an open femoral fracture approximately 15 years prior to the present injury. The fracture had been treated with open reduction and internal fixation. The postoperative course was complicated by infection. The fracture healed. Despite aggressive management in the form of multiple debridements, including removal of the implants, and several extended courses of intravenous antibiotics, drainage had persisted. Prior to the most recent injury the patient had been full weight bearing. Cultures of drainage obtained 2 months prior to this injury were positive for methicillin resistant Staphylococcus aureus and Pseudomonas aeruginosa.

Radiologic Findings

Radiographs of the femur indicated a transverse fracture 5 cm distal to the lesser trochanter. The entire proximal femur including most of the femoral head appeared abnormal, with areas of sclerosis and osteolysis. Implants were not present.

Diagnosis

Low energy subtrochanteric fracture through osteomyelitic bone. The osteomyelitis is classified as type IV B according to the classification system described by Cierny and Mader (i.e., an entire segment of femur is diffusely involved) and there is local compromise in the form of dysvascular tissue and scar surrounding the infected bone.

Surgical Management

A traction pin was inserted in the proximal tibia and the extremity placed in balanced suspension with 30 pounds of distally directed traction. The draining sinus was cultured and covered with a dry dressing. Antibiotics were not administered.

The day after injury the patient was taken to the operating room where a general anesthetic was administered. He was moved to an operating table. The hip and thigh were prepped and draped. The lateral femur was approached via the scar from the previous incisions. The lateral muscles were scarred and poorly vascularized. The lateral cortex of the femur was exposed and care was taken not to strip the femur circumferentially of its periosteum. The bone was extremely sclerotic. A high speed burr was used to decorticate the exposed surface of the femur. Pinpoint bleeding from the sclerotic bone was encountered; however, the vessels were widely spaced, indicating that the bone was dysvascular.

PEARLS

- The goal of debridement is to remove necrotic bone and leave living bone behind. Living bone is recognized by bleeding from Haversian systems. Bleeding from the Haversian systems is indicated by pinpoint bleeding from the bone (the "paprika sign" because the bone appears as though it has been sprinkled with paprika). The paprika sign is most clearly seen when an overlying layer of bone has been removed and the bone in question is irrigated with saline. Necrotic bone is removed with osteotomes or a high speed burr. If a high speed burr is used, the field must be constantly irrigated to prevent heat necrosis and cauterization of the Haversian system vessels. Use of an osteotome carries the risk of iatrogenic fracture. In general, osteotomes are used when a large amount of bone is debrided.

- Material for culture that most accurately reflects the pathogenic organisms should be obtained during surgery prior to the administration of antibiotics.

Several pockets of infected granulation tissue were encountered within the bone and were debrided. After tissue was obtained for culture, antibiotics were administered intravenously. The fracture was reduced and two "stacked" plates were applied to the lateral cortex. Antibiotic beads were used to fill the space lateral to the plates, and an antibiotic pump was implanted subcutaneously in the abdomen. The outflow catheters were tunneled subcutaneously and placed in the operative wound. The wound was closed in a single layer with vertical mattress sutures over a large drain (Fig. 7–1).

Postoperative Management

Active range of motion exercises of the knee and hip were initiated 3 days after surgery. The drains were removed 2 weeks after surgery. Antibiotics were administered systemically for 4 weeks and locally via the pump for 12 weeks. The antibiotic beads were removed 3 weeks following stabilization of the fracture and the fracture was grafted with autogenous cancellous bone harvested from the iliac crest.

The drainage gradually decreased and had stopped by the fifth week after stabilization of the fracture. Radiographic signs of consolidation of the fracture were never present. Even though the patient remained nonweight bearing, fixation failed at 6 months (Fig. 7–2). The patient experienced gradually increasing pain and the drainage recurred. The patient underwent another debridement and delayed internal fixation with a 95 degree condylar screw (Figs. 7–3 and 7–4). This fixation also

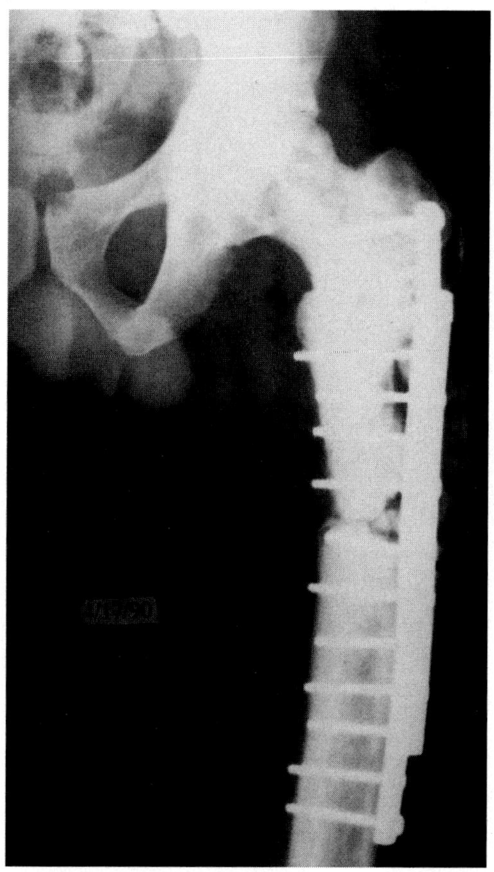

Figure 7–1. Radiograph obtained after stabilization of the fracture with "staked" plates. Beads and the outflow catheters of an antibiotic pump are lateral to the greater trochanter.

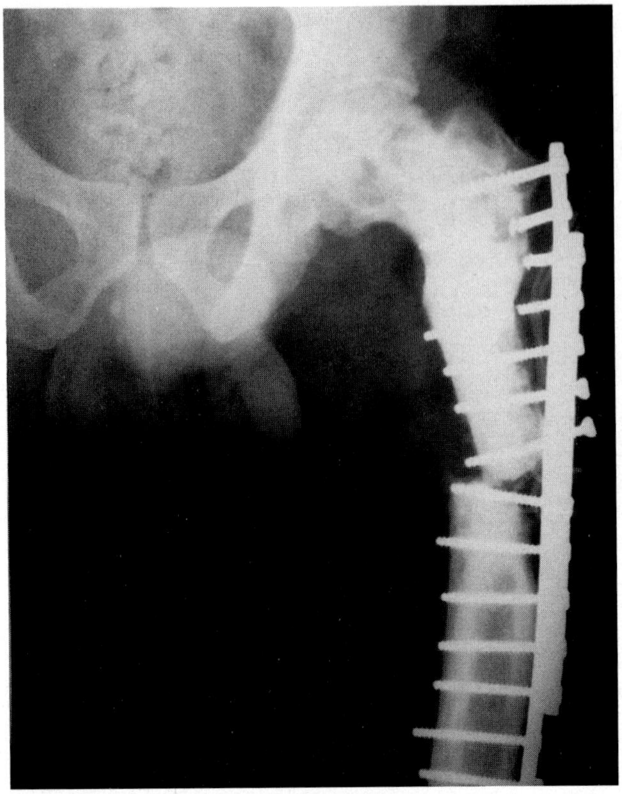

Figure 7–2. *Radiograph obtained following failure of fixation.*

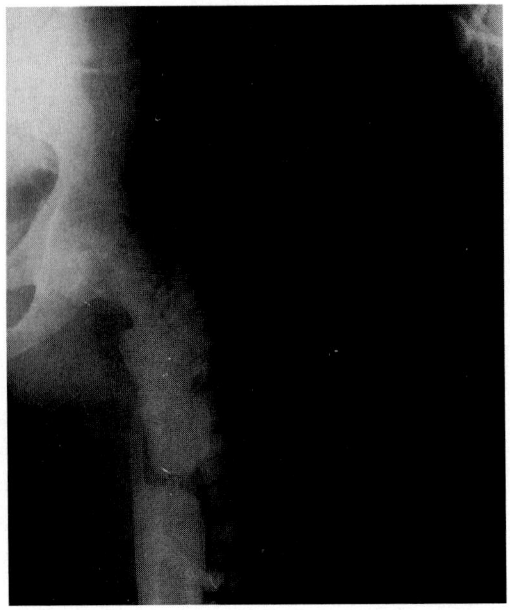

Figure 7–3. Radiograph obtained following debridement and insertion of antibiotic PMMA beads. The fracture is immobilized in traction.

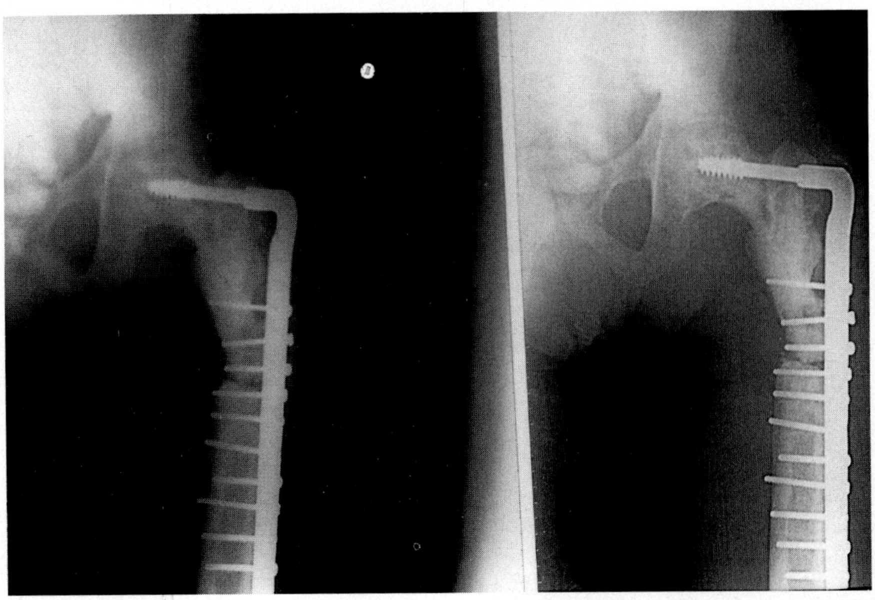

Figure 7–4. Radiograph obtained following stabilization with a 95 degree compression screw and plate.

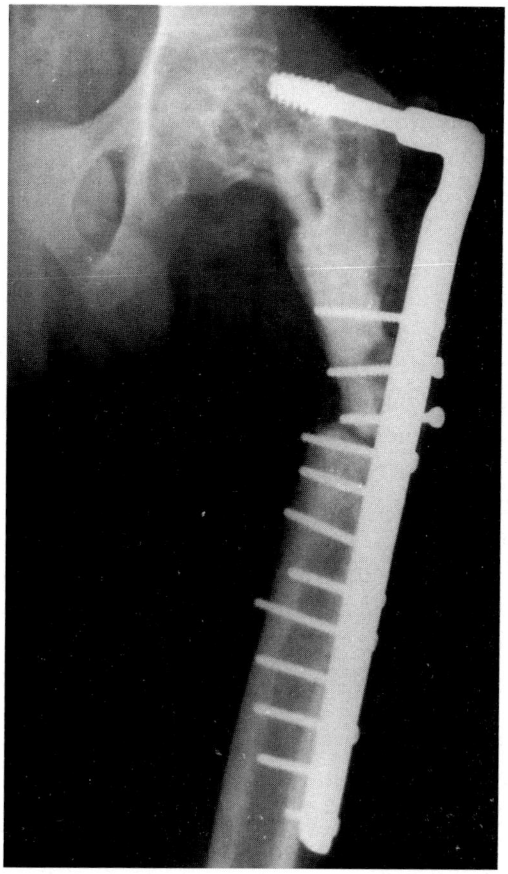

Figure 7–5. Radiograph obtained following failure of fixation.

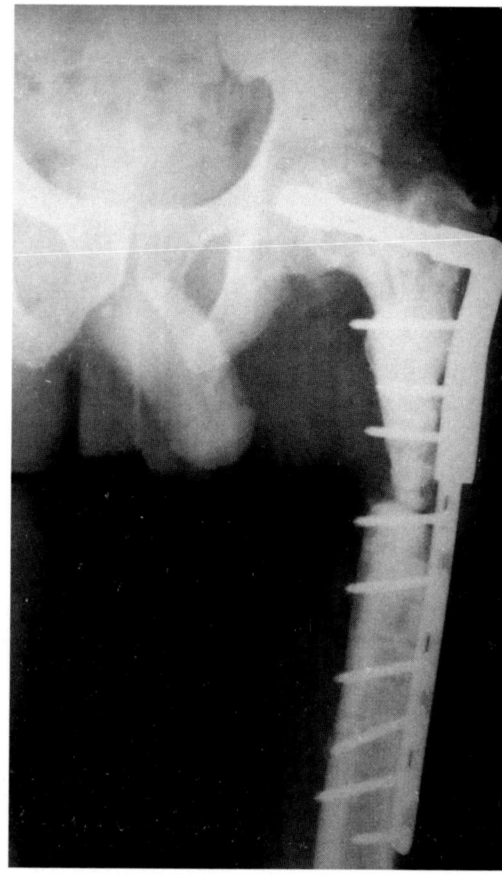

Figure 7–6. Radiograph obtained following revision of fixation with a second 95 degree compression screw and plate.

failed and was revised (Figs. 7–5 and 7–6). Drainage persisted despite systemic and local antibiotic therapy and the fracture did not heal. The patient was left with an infected nonunion of his proximal femur.

Discussion

Fracture through infected bone is an uncommon problem and extremely difficult to manage successfully. The bone fractures because it is weakened by the infectious process. Because the healing potential of the bone seems to be diminished by the infection, there is a significant incidence of delayed union and nonunion. Following fracture, active infections become more symptomatic (e.g., drainage increases) and quiescent osteomyelitis will frequently flare.

Alternative Methods of Management

Two problems have to be managed: the fracture and the infection. In this case the fracture was managed by open reduction and internal fixation. The infection was managed with partial debridement, administration of antibiotics, and delayed bone grafting. Alternative methods of fracture management are closed traction, stabilization with an external fixator, and amputation. The alternative method of management of the infection is resection of the proximal femur with amputation of the leg or reconstruction with intercalary lengthening or sequential bone grafting. In addition, free soft tissue transfer could be performed to convert the patient from a type B host (i.e., locally compromised due to decreased vascularity) to a type A host (i.e., a host without local or systemic compromise).

Management with open reduction, internal fixation, partial debridement, and administration of antibiotics has the advantage of early patient mobilization. It has the disadvantage of not addressing the infection. A partial debridement was performed and antibiotics were administered to suppress the infection during consolidation of the fracture. The best result that this limited approach offers would be a healed fracture and long term suppression of the infection. This approach will not result in cure. Unfortunately in this case the fracture never consolidated and the infectious symptoms continued.

The only advantages of managing the fracture with traction are that the patient is spared a surgical procedure, the infected area is not traumatized further, and no foreign bodies are left in the infected area. The primary disadvantage of traction is the prolonged bedrest. The duration of bedrest is anticipated to be longer than with a fracture through normal bone due to the decreased healing potential of infected bone and because a spica cast cannot be applied at the usual 8 weeks due to the drainage. An additional disadvantage of management with traction is the very low probability that the fracture will heal.

Stabilization of the fracture with an external fixator allows the patient to be mobilized and has the potential advantage of not requiring foreign bodies in the infected area. In this case the entire proximal femur was infected; therefore the advantage of not placing a foreign body in the infected area would not be realized. Pins placed in infected bone are anticipated to loosen quickly, with loss of stability.

Resection of the proximal femur with amputation (i.e., a hip disarticulation) will obviate fracture management and result in resolution of the infection; however, the cosmetic and functional outcomes are poor. Most patients are unwilling to undergo a hip disarticulation unless the infection becomes life threatening or the extremity has no useful function (e.g., the patient is paraplegic).

Resection of the proximal femur with reconstruction by intercalary lengthening in this case is not possible because the femoral head and neck are infected. If they are not resected, the infection will persist. If the neck and head are resected, it will be very difficult to arthrodese the femur to the pelvis, and a painful unstable pseudoarthrosis will almost certainly result. This procedure is possible when only the diaphysis is resected; however, there are many associated complications, including pin tract infections, pain from the lengthening, the prolonged time the patient is required to be in the external fixator, nonunion at the "docking site", ankylosis of surrounding joints, and loss of alignment. In general, segmental defects of the femur are more difficult to manage with intercalary lengthening than segmental defects of the tibia (Fig. 7–7).

Resection of the proximal femur with reconstruction with bone grafting is not possible in this case because the head and neck of the femur are infected. If the head and neck are not resected, the infection will persist. If the head and neck are resected, it is not possible to stabilize the distal femur to the pelvis and a painful pseudoarthrosis will result. In cases in which only the diaphysis is resected, sequential bone grafts are an excellent method of management of segmental femoral defects. Usually the femur is stabilized with an intramedullary rod while the defect consolidates. Free vascularized fibula transfer along with autogenous bone grafting has been utilized to treat segmental femoral defects, but cannot be used in this case because of involvement of the head and neck of the femur.

Resection of the dysvascular tissue and free soft tissue transfer will resolve the local compromise of the patient's ability to fight infection. Soft tissue transfer is an extensive procedure that should be performed with segmental resection of the infected femur. This approach would give the best chance of long term suppression or cure of the infection. In this case the patient did not choose to undergo this therapeutic approach.

Type of Management	Advantages	Disadvantages	Comments
Fracture Management			
ORIF	Allows early mobilization	Leaves foreign body in wound; does not address the segmental infection of the femur	Probably has the best chance for restoring function at the cost of relatively limited surgical procedure
Traction	Does not require a surgical procedure, no foreign bodies left in wound	Prolonged bedrest; minimal chance of fracture consolidation	Minimal chance of fracture consolidation makes this alternative less desirable
External fixation	Stabilizes the fracture	Pins must be placed in infected bone, therefore rapid loosening and loss of stability is anticipated	If pins could be placed out of the infected area this would be the method of choice
Amputation	Early mobilization; will resolve infection	Extreme loss of function; cosmetically unacceptable	Not an acceptable alternative to most patients, unless the infection is life threatening
Infection Management			
Resection, reconstruction with intercalary lengthening	Does not require a second or third operative site for donor bone	Prolonged period in external fixator can injure surrounding joints; extensive procedure	Not indicated in this case because of head and neck involvement
Resection, reconstruction with bone grafting	Does not put surrounding joints at risk	Requires several donor sites; extensive procedure	Not indicated in this case because of head and neck involvement
Free soft tissue transfer	Converts patient from a B host (i.e., with local compromise) to an A host (i.e., no compromise)	Extensive procedure; must be done with resection of proximal femur and reconstruction	Not indicated in this case because of head and neck involvement

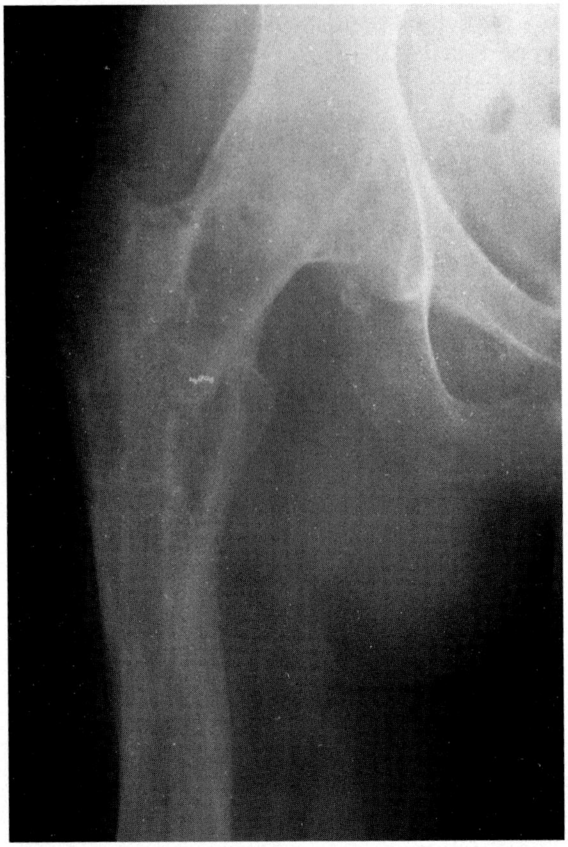

Figure 7–7. Radiograph of a hip that has ankylosed in response to an intercalary lengthening of the femur.

Complications

Complications include loss of fixation, failure of the fracture to heal, and persistence of the infectious symptoms. The patient in this case report, unfortunately, experienced all these complications. Although aware that hip disarticulation would resolve these complications, the patient was unwilling to undergo this procedure. Loss of fixation is managed with revision fixation. Failure of the fracture to heal is managed with autogenous bone grafting and pulsed electromagnetic fields. If bone grafting is performed, antibiotics are mixed into the graft. Persistence of infectious symptoms is managed with dressing changes. If the drainage becomes intolerable and the fracture has healed, the implants are removed and a limited debridement is performed. If the fracture has not healed, the implants should not be removed unless they have failed or the infection is not controllable (i.e., the patient is developing recurrent abscesses or is septic).

Suggested Readings

Cierny G, Mader JT: Adult chronic ostomyelitis. Orthop 1984; 7:1557–1564.

Cierny G, Mader JT, Penninck JJ: A clinical staging system for adult osteomyelitis. Contemp Orthop 1985; 10(5):17–37.

Jupiter JB, Bour CJ, May JW: The reconstruction of defects in the femoral shaft with vascularized transfers of fibular bone. J Bone Joint Surg 1987; 69A:365–374.

Perry CR: Bone and Joint Infections. Martin Dunitz, London, 1996.

Perry CR, Pearson RL, Miller GA: Accuracy of cultures of material from swabbing of the superficial wound and needle biopsy in the preoperative assessment of osteomyelitis. J Bone Joint Surg 1991; 73A:745–749.

Perry CR, Ritterbusch JK, Rice SH, et al: Antibiotics delivered by an implantable drug pump: a new application for treating osteomyelitis. Am J Med 1986; 80:222.

Case 8

History and Physical Examination

A 31-year-old male was admitted to the emergency department after falling asleep behind the wheel of his car and colliding with a truck. On admission he was in shock, with a blood pressure of 70/50 and a tachycardia of 110/minute. Examination showed that he had multiple musculoskeletal injuries of the upper body, including stable fractures of the second and third lumbar vertebrae, a closed right humeral diaphyseal fracture, and closed fractures of the left radius and ulna, as well as numerous injuries to the lower limbs including a closed tibial fracture. After resuscitation with crystalloids and packed red blood cells his condition stabilized and he was transferred to the operating room for treatment of his injuries.

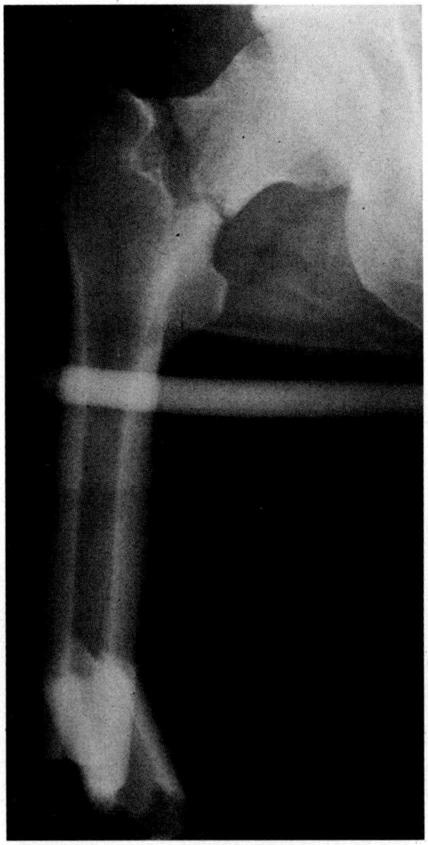

Figure 8–1. An anteroposterior radiograph of the ipsilateral femoral fractures. Note the short femoral segment.

Radiologic Findings

An anteroposterior radiograph of the right femur showed a segmental diaphyseal fracture associated with a minimally displaced basicervical fracture (Fig. 8–1). The lateral radiograph was of poor quality. A separate femoral segment was noted. This was short but appeared intact.

PEARL

- It is particularly important to have adequate radiographs of the hip in any patient who has a femoral diaphyseal fracture. A proximal femoral fracture may follow the accident or intramedullary nailing of the diaphyseal fracture. It may be important to distinguish between the two for medico-legal reasons.

Diagnosis

Ipsilateral fractures of the right femoral diaphysis and neck. AO classification of the basicervical fractures is a 31–B2.1 fracture and the diaphyseal fracture is a 32–C2.1 fracture.

Surgical Management

The patient was taken to the operating room from the emergency department for surgery. By the time the patient arrived in the operating room it was clear that he had developed a compartment syndrome in his right lower leg associated with his tibial fracture. Monitoring of the anterior compartment showed an intracompartmental pressure of 55 mm Hg compared to the diastolic pressure of 70 mm Hg. A four compartment fasciotomy was performed and the tibia stabilized with a unilateral external fixator. It was considered unwise to nail the tibia in view of the high risk of displacement of the femoral neck fracture by placing the patient on a nailing table.

Following stabilization of the tibia the patient was placed on a femoral nailing table and skeletal traction was applied with a distal femoral pin. The segmental fracture could not be reduced closed and an open reduction was undertaken through a midlateral incision. Prior to nailing, the C arm was used to check that the femoral neck fracture remained undisplaced. In view of the presence of the femoral neck fracture care was taken in selecting the entry point for the intramedullary nail. The base of the piriformis fossa was palpated and a narrow bone awl used to make the initial defect in the proximal femur. The exact entry point was determined using fluoroscopic guidance (Fig. 8–2).

The femoral entry point was progressively widened to allow passage of a guidewire followed by the reamers. After the passage of the first reamer the C arm was again used to check for femoral neck displacement. The short femoral segment was held with bone forceps during the reaming process to prevent spinning and consequent devascularization. After the intramedullary nail had been carefully inserted and the locking screws placed appropriately, attention was turned to the femoral neck fracture. This was fixed by passing three cancellous screws into the

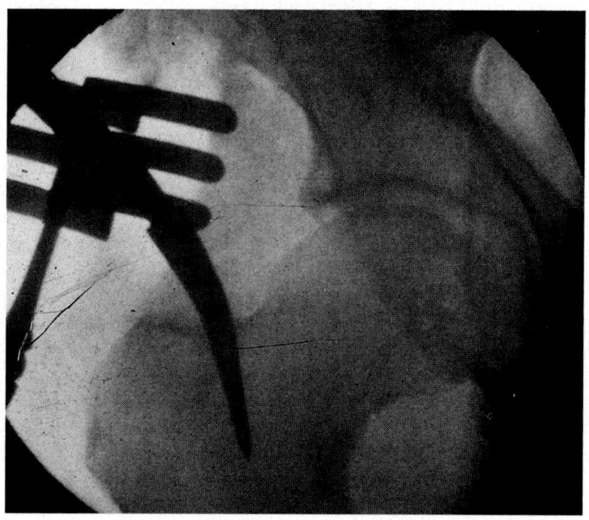

Figure 8–2. The proximal insertion point is very important. A pointer or bone awl should be used to define the optimal point of insertion, which should be above the intramedullary canal.

PEARLS

- Surgeons debate whether femoral nails should be inserted through the greater trochanter or in the piriformis fossa medial to the trochanter. The key to success is to insert the nail in line with the intramedullary canal and the easiest method to check whether this has been achieved is fluoroscopy. The exact location of the entry point does not matter, provided it is not too medial and the nail is not going to have to bend as it passes down the intramedullary canal.

- Surgeons are understandably concerned about spinning a loose diaphyseal segment. In fact this rarely happens because the segment usually has good soft tissue attachments. However, the short length of this segment suggested that spinning was possible.

femoral neck. The screws were placed anterior to the intramedullary nail. Excellent fracture fixation was achieved (Fig. 8–3).

Postoperative Management

The patient was returned to the operating room after 2 days and the tibial external fixator was removed. The tibial fracture was treated by the introduction of a reamed intramedullary nail. The medial fasciotomy wound was closed and split skin grafting used to close the lateral fasciotomy wound. The humeral diaphyseal fracture was treated by the application of a bone plate as were the closed fractures of the left radius and ulna.

In view of the severity of the femoral fracture and the presence of other injuries the patient remained nonweight bearing for 6 weeks. Following this period weight bearing was relatively rapid and he made a good recovery. The femoral diaphyseal fractures and the femoral neck fracture united and after 1 year he had a full range of motion in his right hip and knee.

Discussion

Ipsilateral fractures of the proximal femur and the femoral diaphysis virtually always follow high energy injuries. The patients are therefore seriously injured and early fixation of these fractures is mandatory. It is now universally accepted that early stabilization of femoral diaphyseal fractures is beneficial in severely injured patients because it aids early mobilization and reduces the incidence of pulmonary complications, which have been reported to be as high as 25% with this particular fracture

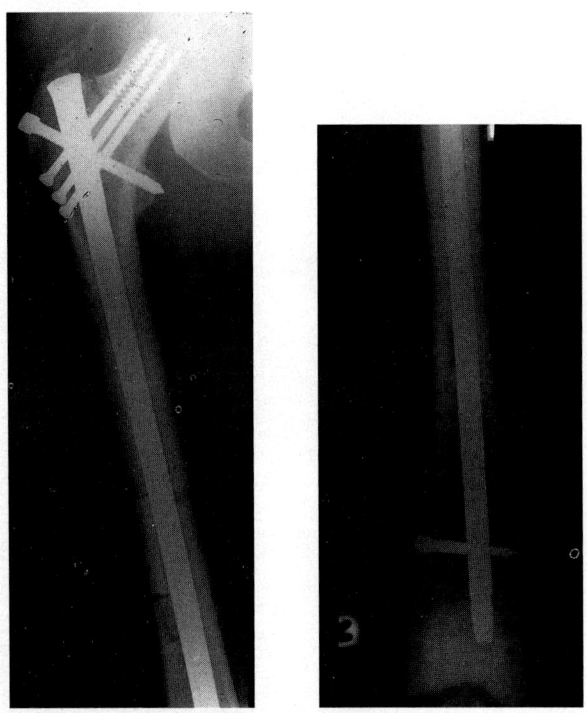

A B

Figure 8–3. Anteroposterior (A) and lateral (B) radiographs after fixation. Excellent reduction and fixation has been achieved.

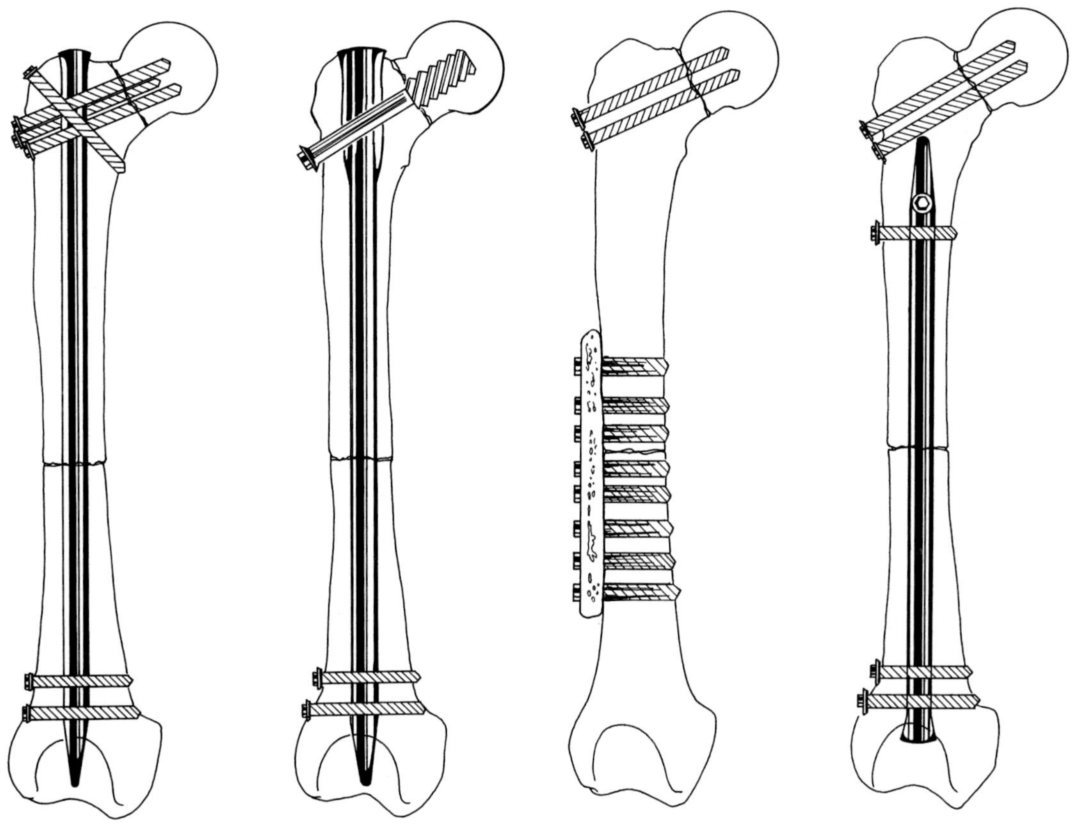

Figure 8–4. Alternative methods of treatment. (A) Conventional nail and proximal screws. (B) Reconstruction or second generation locking nail. (C) Cancellous screws for the proximal fracture and plating for the diaphysis. (D) Cancellous screw and a retrograde nail.

configuration. Another reason for early surgery in this patient is that the femoral neck fracture was undisplaced at the time of admission. If the fracture had displaced before it was fixed, the prognosis would have been much worse, with an increased risk of avascular necrosis and nonunion. Both these complications would probably have necessitated hip arthroplasty and they are best avoided. Early femoral neck fixation is therefore necessary.

There are three main methods of treating ipsilateral fractures of the femoral diaphysis and femoral neck, although the recent introduction of retrograde femoral nailing potentially gives a fourth method (Fig. 8–4). The most common methods involve the use of an intramedullary nail supplemented by the use of cancellous screws to stabilize the femoral neck fracture as illustrated in this case. An obvious alternative is the use of a reconstruction, or second generation, nail in which the proximal lock is gained through the use of a screw passed into the femoral neck and head. The main use of reconstruction nails is in the management of incipient or actual pathological fractures secondary to metastatic deposits in the femur. However, they are also useful in this particular combination of femoral diaphyseal and neck fractures.

If a reconstruction nail is to be used, it is important to be careful about the nail entry point. As with the use of a conventional interlocking intramedullary femoral nail, too medial an entry point may displace the femoral neck fracture. However, if this complication is avoided, the use of reconstruction nails is fairly straightforward.

One other potential complication is that of spinning the femoral head as one drills or inserts the screw. This complication can be avoided by passing a guidewire into the femoral neck about the location of the proximal screw before the track for the screw is drilled. The guidewire should be passed from the anterior femoral cortex over the nail into the posterior femoral neck and head.

The third popular method of dealing with this combination of femoral fractures is to first internally fix the femoral neck fracture using bone screws as if it was an isolated fracture. The diaphyseal fracture can then be plated using AO techniques. Again this is an acceptable method of treating this fracture combination, although considerable soft tissue dissection is required and ideally one of the two intramedullary methods is preferable.

A fourth potential method of managing this fracture combination is to use a retrograde nail to stabilize the femoral diaphyseal fracture and then fix the femoral neck fracture with cancellous screws in the manner already described. The only minor advantage of this technique would be that the tibial fracture could have been nailed fairly easily at the same time as the retrograde femoral nailing was undertaken. However, this has to be balanced against the potential disadvantage of damaging a normal knee in a young adult. There is as yet little literature available on the potential problems of the use of retrograde femoral nailing.

Occasionally a surgeon will encounter the combination of an intertrochanteric fracture and a femoral diaphyseal fracture. Treatment of this combination of fractures is similar to the femoral neck/diaphysis combination, although obviously cancellous screw fixation for the proximal fracture cannot be used. It is suggested that either a reconstruction nail be employed or, if this is not available, the surgeon should use a hip screw and side plate for the intertrochanteric fracture and a plate for the diaphyseal fracture. It should always be borne in mind that if this combination of plates is used, there is a stress riser between the plates where the patient may eventually develop a third fracture. This is a particular problem in elderly patients.

Alternative Methods of Management

Most isolated proximal femoral fractures and femoral diaphyseal fractures should always be treated operatively unless there are unusual circumstances, but the combination of these fractures should never be treated nonoperatively. Traction will probably allow the diaphyseal fracture to unite, but the risk of a proximal femoral nonunion would be considerable. There is also no discernible advantage in using external fixation for these fractures because external fixation of the femoral neck is difficult and external fixation of the femoral diaphysis is accompanied by pintrack sepsis, muscle penetration and joint stiffness.

Complications

The two most serious complications of this combination of fractures are avascular necrosis and nonunion of the femoral head. These are more likely to occur if the femoral head is displaced because the vascularity of the head will consequently be impaired, and the surgeon should be careful that displacement does not occur. If avascular necrosis or femoral neck nonunion does occur, then it is probable that the patient will seek a hip arthroplasty, an operation that has a number of problems when performed in young patients. Nonunion of a femoral neck fracture in a young patient is best treated by bone grafting, but this is not

Type of Management	Advantages	Disadvantages	Comments
Traction	None	Higher incidence of femoral neck and diaphyseal nonunion; malunion; patient immobility	There is no place for nonoperative treatment unless circumstances dictate it
Antegrade nailing and cancellous screws	Technically straightforward; good fixation; early motion	Entry point of the nail critical	Along with reconstruction nails, this is the method of choice for this combination of fractures
Reconstruction nailing	Technically straightforward; good fixation; early motion	Nail entry point is critical	Along with antegrade nailing and cancellous screws, this represents the method of choice
Plate and screw fixation	Fairly simple technique	Soft tissue dissection; higher incidence of nonunion of the femoral diaphysis	A useful technique if intramedullary nailing is unavailable
Retrograde nailing and screw fixation	Potentially an easy technique especially in the multiply injured patients	Unproven technique; knee damage	There is as yet little evidence about the usefulness of this technique

always successful.

The other complications are the same as those encountered in any femoral diaphyseal fracture: infection, diaphyseal nonunion, and malunion. These will be treated in the same way as described in the section on the management of the open femoral fracture.

Suggested Readings

Barquet A, Fernandez A, Leon H: Simultaneous ipsilateral trochanteric and femoral shaft fracture. Acta Orthop Scand 1985; 15:36–39.

Browner BD (ed): The Science and Practice of Intramedullary Nailing, 2nd ed. Williams and Wilkins, Baltimore, 1996.

Casey IJ, Chapman MW: Ipsilateral concomitant fractures of the hip and femoral shaft. J Bone Joint Surg (Am) 1979; 61A:503–509.

Friedl HP, Stocker R, Czermak B, Schmal H, Trentz O: Primary fixation and delayed nailing of long bone fractures in severe trauma. In Court-Brown CM, Christie J (eds): Techniques in Orthpaedics 1996; 11:59–66.

Friedmann RJ, Wyman ET: Ipsilateral hip and femoral shaft fractures. Clin Orthop 1986; 208:188–194.

Swiontkowski MF, Hansen ST, Kellam J: Ipsilateral fractures of the femoral neck and shaft. J Bone Joint Surg (Am) 1984; 66A:260–268.

Case 9

History and Physical Examination

A 21-year-old female was involved in a traffic accident. She was a front seat passenger in a car that had a head on collision with a truck. On presentation to the emergency department she had superficial facial lacerations, a closed fracture of the right radius and ulna, and an open fracture of the right femur associated with a 13 cm wound in the midthigh. She was mildly shocked with a blood pressure of 90/55 and a tachycardia of 95/minute. There was no evidence of neurovascular impairment in the right leg.

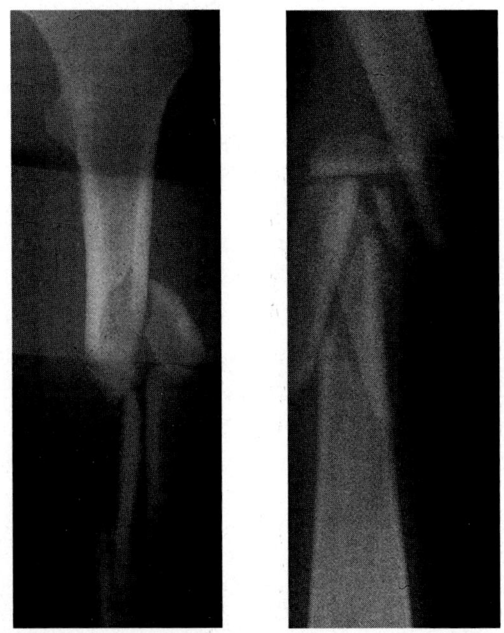

A B

Figure 9–1. Anteroposterior (A) and lateral (B) radiographs of a Gustilo IIIb open femoral fracture.

Radiologic Findings

Anteroposterior and lateral radiographs indicated a comminuted midshaft femoral fracture (Fig. 9–1). Both radiographs showed four loose bone fragments and all four fragments were significantly displaced, suggesting considerable soft tissue damage.

Diagnosis

Gustilo type III open femoral diaphyseal fracture. The extent of the comminution and the associated soft tissue injury strongly suggested that it was a Gustilo type IIIb fracture. AO classification: 32–C3.3 fracture.

Surgical Management

The patient was taken to the operating room and the wound thoroughly cleaned and washed with saline. The patient was placed on a fracture table and the leg was prepped and draped. The wound was explored digitally to check for the presence of degloving as well as confirm the extent of the associated muscle damage. The wound was then extended proximally and distally and the vascularity of the bone fragments examined. The operative findings confirmed the radiological interpretation of soft tissue damage. None of the loose bone fragments had periosteal attachments and the fracture was certainly Gustilo IIIb in severity. Debridement was performed by excision of the skin edges and removal of all contaminated and devitalized soft tissue. All the bone fragments were removed. A standard intramedullary nailing was performed using a statically locked 12 mm diameter reamed intramedullary nail (Fig. 9–2). The wound was left open and a moist dressing was applied to the open wound to cover the exposed muscles. The closed radius and ulna fractures were plated using AO techniques.

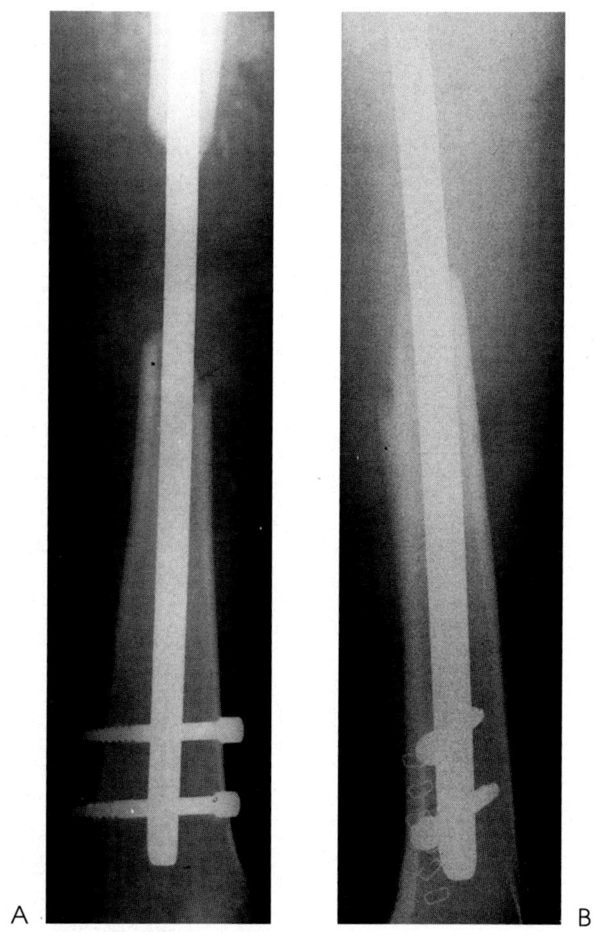

Figure 9–2. Anteroposterior (A) and lateral (B) views of the femur after debridement and removal of the avascular bone fragments. A statically locked reamed nail has been used to stabilize the fracture.

PEARLS

- Most authorities suggest bone grafting open fractures at about 6 weeks. Primary bone grafting can be done, but if there is infection, the graft is lost.
- Union can be surprisingly difficult to determine in some nailed fractures. Surgeons usually rely on the radiological appearance and presence of discomfort to diagnose nonunion. A large nail will prevent discomfort and the X rays may show cortical continuity but that the union is not circumferential. The timing of nail removal under these circumstances may be difficult to determine.

PITFALL

- If the surgeon proposes to perform exchange nailing he or she should be aware of the type of nail to be removed and have the correct extraction equipment. Failure to do this may prove embarrassing.

The patient was returned to the operating room 2 days later and a further wound inspection undertaken. The muscle and bones were carefully reexamined to check for residual contamination and the presence of any myonecrosis. All the soft tissues were found to be healthy and the wound extensions were therefore closed. The original wound could not be closed and a split skin graft was applied.

Postoperative Management

Postoperatively, the patient was mobilized nonweight bearing. The presence of the forearm fracture necessitated the use of gutter crutches for 4 weeks following which she was able to use conventional crutches. The splint skin graft on the lateral thigh healed well and the femur was bone grafted using corticocancellous pelvic autograft 5 weeks after the accident. Nonweight bearing mobilization with crutches was continued and the patient underwent intensive physiotherapy to maintain hip and knee movement. She was pain free until 6 months after the bone grafting procedure when she started to experience some discomfort in the proximal thigh. Radiographs taken at that time (Fig. 9–3) showed that the nail had fractured and that while there was new bone around the fracture site, there was no evidence of cortical continuity.

An exchange nailing was undertaken. This involved removing the broken nail with a long hook, reaming the intramedullary canal to 15 mm, and inserting a statically locked 14 mm nail. At the same time the fracture site was again grafted with

A 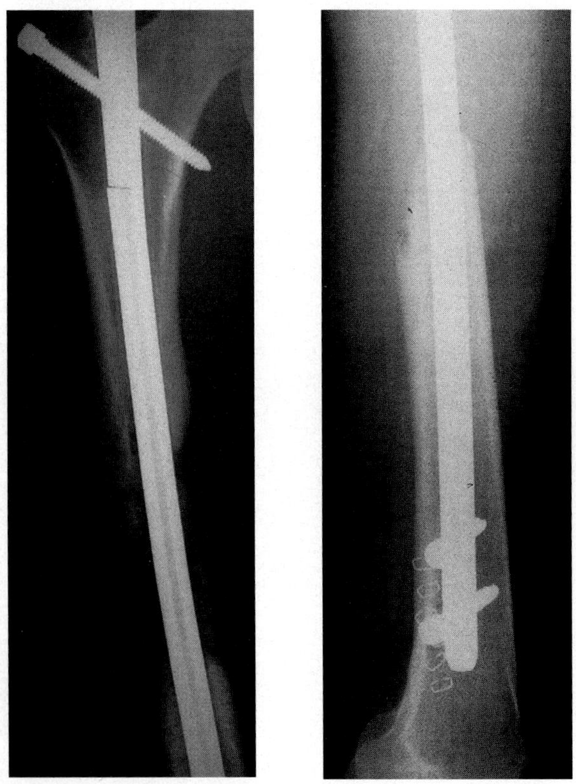 B

Figure 9–3. The nail has broken at the junction of the nonslotted and slotted portions. Some incorporation of the bone graft has occurred. Anteroposterior (A) and lateral (B) views.

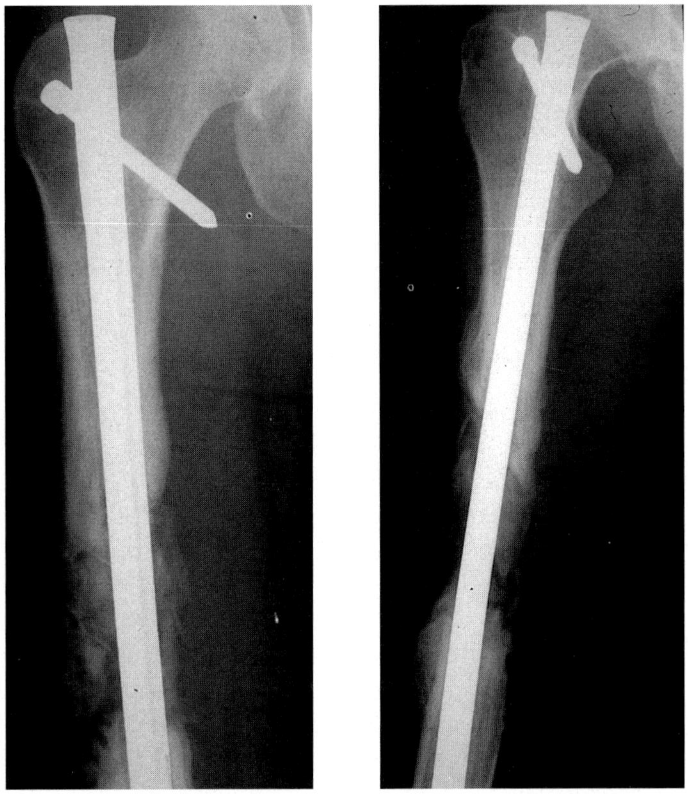

A B

Figure 9–4. A new larger nail has been inserted and the fracture site regrafted. Anteroposterior (A) and lateral (B) views.

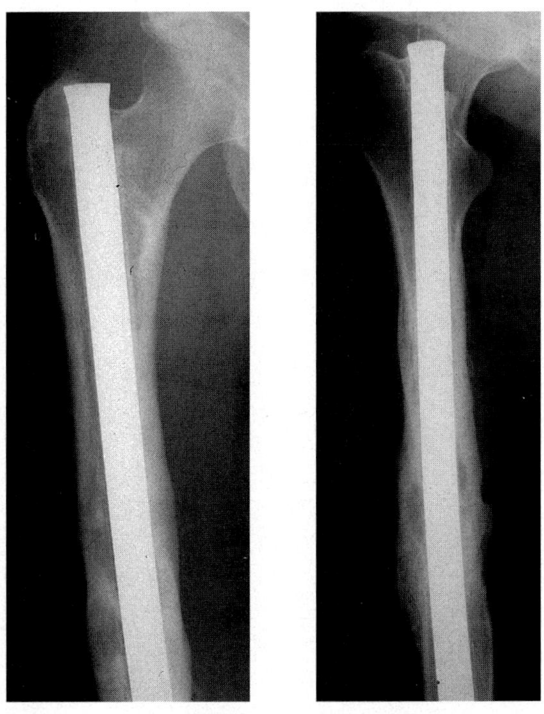

A B

Figure 9–5. Anteroposterior (A) and lateral (B) views showing that the fracture has united well. The patient had excellent function.

pelvic autograft (Fig. 9–4). The patient was allowed to progressively bear more weight on the larger nail and the fracture united after a further 8 months. The proximal cross screw gave rise to some discomfort and was removed 4 months after the second grafting procedure. Radiographs taken 2 years after the fracture showed that the cortices appeared to have remodeled (Fig. 9–5) and the nail was removed. At that time clinical examination showed that the patient had full hip and knee movement and the femora were the same length. Her main complaint was that of occasional discomfort in her contralateral iliac crest where bone was harvested.

Discussion

Open femoral fractures have a reputation for being difficult to treat. In fact the comparatively recent introduction of interlocking intramedullary nails has greatly improved their prognosis. The reason for their poor reputation is straightforward. Open femoral fractures are relatively uncommon and unless surgeons work in a trauma center they are unlikely to encounter many during their career. The incidence of open femoral diaphyseal fractures is about 1.5 per 100,000 per year, which is about 25% of the incidence of open tibial diaphyseal fractures. In addition, most open femoral fractures follow traffic accidents and the patients frequently have multiple injuries. A recent survey of open femoral fractures presenting to the orthopaedic trauma unit in Edinburgh, Scotland, showed that 86.4% of these fractures followed traffic accidents and that 62.7% of the fractures were Gustilo type III in severity. The patients had an average injury severity score of 17 and an average of 2.9 severe musculoskeletal injuries each. Thus the management of patients with open femoral

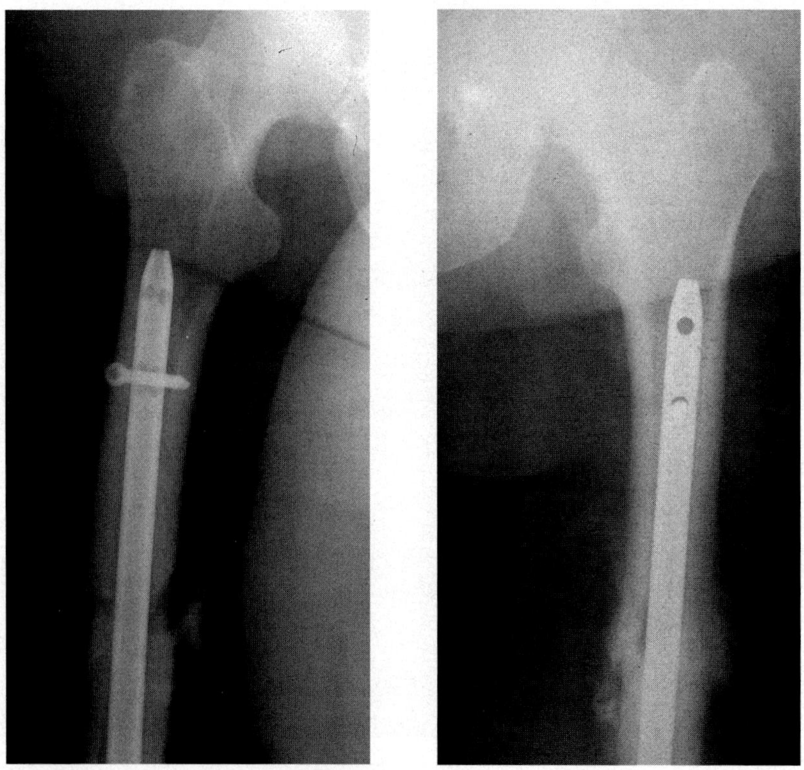

A B

Figure 9–6. Retrograde nailing of a femoral diaphyseal fracture using an unreamed nail. Anteroposterior (A) and lateral (B) views.

PEARL

- Pelvic donor site morbidity can be considerable and may include local pain, infection, and damage to the lateral cutaneous nerve of the thigh. Where possible, small amounts of bone can be removed with a trephine. If a larger quantity of bone graft is needed, it should be taken from the inside of the pelvis. The crest should not be removed unless absolutely necessary.

fractures is often difficult and inappropriate; inadequate patient management frequently leads to poor results.

Regardless of the problems associated with the management of multiply injured patients, the introduction of interlocking intramedullary nails has made the treatment of open femoral diaphyseal fracture fairly straightforward. Virtually all open diaphyseal femoral fractures can be stabilized with a conventional femoral nail as illustrated in this case, and it is strongly recommended that this be passed antegrade if possible. Retrograde femoral nailing (Fig. 9–6) has become popular, but surgeons should consider whether they wish to damage a normal knee in a young person unless circumstances dictate that they must. Many surgeons still consider that retrograde nailing should be reserved for the severely injured patient where operative speed is important.

One of the key differences between the management of open femoral and tibial fractures is that flap cover is rarely required to close the soft tissue defect associated with open femoral fractures. Court-Brown and Quaba (1996) examined 1000 consecutive open fractures presenting to the orthopaedic trauma unit in Edinburgh, Scotland, of which 62 were open femora. Only 29% of these fractures required plastic surgery; the remaining 71% of the wounds were closed secondarily. All the wounds that required plastic surgery were closed using split skin grafting. The need for flap cover in open femoral fractures is extremely rare. This contrasts with the 244 open tibial fractures documented by Court-Brown and Quaba who found that 54.5% of the open tibiae required plastic surgery to close their wounds and 32.4% of all the open tibial fractures required flap cover.

The results of treating open femoral fractures with reamed intramedullary nailing are excellent. A review of the literature indicates that the incidence of infection is between 0 and 5% and the incidence of nonunion between 0 and 7%. Recently, surgeons have been examining the use of unreamed femoral nails but as yet there is little information about their usefulness in the management of open fractures. Krettek et al. (1996) documented the use of an unreamed femoral nail in 15 open fractures. However, only three patients had Gustilo type III open fractures. The overall infection rate for both closed and open fractures was 1.7%, which compares with recent results of the use of reamed nails.

In this case there was extensive bone loss. The management of bone loss has been discussed elsewhere in this book. However, the main methods of treating femoral diaphyseal bone loss are corticocancellous bone grafting, bone transport, and vascularized grafts. Corticocancellous grafting can be effective, but a large defect will usually require more than one graft. The main disadvantages of grafting are donor site morbidity and the fact that the graft takes a considerable time to remodel such that it can bear weight without risk of fracture. However, this latter problem is usually resolved by using a large diameter nail that will allow the patient to bear weight while the bone is remodeling.

Bone transport is becoming more popular now that there are good unilateral frames available. If necessary, a thin intramedullary nail can be used to guide the transported segment. The docking site between the transported segment and the distal femur will usually require cancellous bone graft to facilitate union. The disadvantages of this technique are that femoral fixators are unpleasant to wear and the regenerate bone will require protection until it strengthens sufficiently to permit weight bearing.

In this case the intramedullary nail broke. The strength of intramedullary nails increases with increasing size, and breakage of 12 mm nails is rare. However, it is obvious that the nail fractured because of the presence of the diaphyseal nonunion. Slotted femoral nails usually break at the junction of the nonslotted and slotted portions of the nail, at the fracture site, or at the most proximal of the distal screw holes. They should always be exchanged when the nail fracture is noticed because further damage may occur. Removal is usually straightforward if the nail is cannulated because a long hook can be passed down the nail under radiological control. However, the recent vogue for thin solid nails may provide surgeons with some extraction problems; when these nails break, they must be removed by exposing and taking down the fracture site or windowing the femoral diaphysis.

Alternative Methods of Management

There may be discussion about the relative merits of antegrade or retrograde nailing or the requirement for reaming but virtually all orthopaedic trauma surgeons use intramedullary nailing for the management of open femoral fractures in patients who are not severely injured and therefore at possible risk of acute respiratory distress syndrome. Plating can be used for femoral diaphyseal fractures and has the merit of being a relatively quick procedure. However, as with all plating techniques, femoral plating is associated with significant soft tissue stripping; if the fracture is comminuted, a long plate will be required. A few authors have advocated external fixation, but because femoral fractures may well take between 6 and 9 months to unite external fixation is not a treatment tolerated by many patients. Pin tract sepsis and muscle tethering with consequent joint stiffness are almost inevitable problems.

The traditional approach to open femoral fractures was traction, and the later application of a functional brace. This method still has its advocates, but it means that the patient has a prolonged hospital stay and there is a high incidence of malunion, nonunion, and joint stiffness. It should only be used if there is no access to other forms of management.

Type of Management	Advantages	Disadvantages	Comments
Traction and cast	Readily available	Patient immobility; prolonged hospitalization; nonunion; malunion; joint stiffness	Used only if no other method of management is available
Antegrade nailing	Usually straightforward; early mobilization; early joint mobility; good success rate	None, unless the patient is multiply injured	Method of choice
Retrograde nailing	Straightforward technique; early patient mobilization	Damages knee joint; unnecessary in most fractures	Should only be used in the management of the severely injured patient where speed is required
Plating	None	Soft tissue stripping; knee stiffness; presence of comminution	Useful technique, but only if intramedullary nailing is available
External fixation	Quick; minimal interference with the intramedullary canal	Pin tract sepsis; joint stiffness; muscle tethering	Sometimes useful as temporary fixation in the multiply injured patient

Complications

The most common complications following the intramedullary nailing of open femoral diaphyseal fractures are infection, rotational malalignment, and nonunion. Infection is treated in the same way as other posttraumatic osteomyelitis. Some surgeons believe that posttraumatic osteomyelitis following intramedullary nailing tends to be associated with a panosseous osteomyelitis and is difficult to eradicate. Neither of these beliefs is true, although osteomyelitis can be difficult to eradicate if treatment is delayed. Infection should be treated by incision and drainage of any pyogenic collection, high dose antibiotics, and resection of dead bone followed by later bone grafting. It is recommended that an exchange nailing be performed with reaming of the intramedullary canal to remove any pyogenic membrane that may have formed.

Rotational malalignment usually takes the form of an external rotation deformity that may be troublesome for the patient. Where this is more than 10 degrees, it is suggested that the nailing procedure be redone with appropriate alteration of the axis of rotation. If the femoral fracture has united, a femoral osteotomy and renailing will be required. Nonunion is treated by exchange nailing if it is oligotrophic or hypertrophic. Where the nonunion is atrophic, exchange nailing may be successful; frequently corticocancellous bone grafting is required.

Suggested Readings

Brumback RJ, Stribling EP, Poka A, Lakatos R, Bathon GH, Burgess AR: Intramedullary nailing of open fractures of the femoral shaft. J Bone Joint Surg (Am) 1989; 71A:1324–1330.

Court-Brown CM, Browner BD: Locked nailing of femoral fractures. In Browner BD (ed): The science and practice of intramedullary nailing, pp 161–182. 2nd ed. WIlliams and Wilkins, Baltimore, 1996.

Court-Brown CM, McQueen MM, Quaba AA: Management of Open Fractures. Martin Dunitz, London, 1996.

Grosse A, Christie J, Taglang G, Court-Brown C, McQueen MM: Open adult femoral shaft fractures treated by early intramedullary nailing. J Bone Joint Surg (Br) 1993; 75B:562–565.

Krettek C, Rudolf J, Schandelmaier P, Guy P, Könemann B, Tscherne H: Reamed intramedullary nailing of femoral shaft fractures: operative technique and early clinical experience with the standard locking option. Injury 1996; 27:233–254.

O'Brien PJ, Meek RN, Powell JN, Blachut PA: Primary intramedullary nailing of open femoral shaft fractures. J Trauma 1991; 31:113–116.

Case 10

History and Physical Examination

A 68-year-old man fell in his home and presented to the emergency department with a painful right hip. He had been unable to bear weight on his right leg since the accident. Examination showed the patient to be obese and deaf. His right proximal femur was deformed and very painful, but there was no evidence of neurovascular deficit in the leg. The patient was known to have Paget's disease and was under active treatment at the time of the fall.

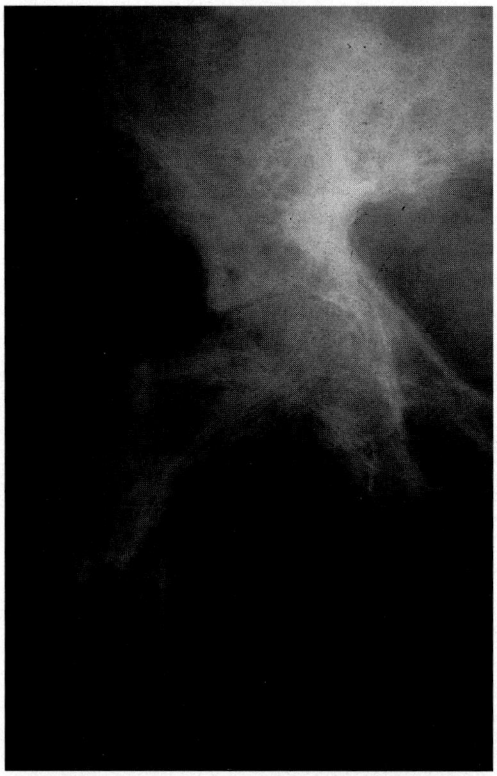

Figure 10–1. An anteroposterior radiograph of a Pagetic proximal femur and hemipelvis. There is a transverse fracture with varus malalignment of the proximal femur.

Radiologic Findings

An anteroposterior radiograph showed a subtrochanteric femoral fracture in a Pagetic femur (Fig. 10–1). An adequate lateral radiograph could not be obtained because of discomfort. Radiographs also showed evidence of Paget's disease in the pelvis and the contralateral femur and there was obvious osteoarthritic change in the ipsilateral hip joint. The proximal femur was in varus and the diaphysis was noted to be wider than normal with a widened intramedullary canal. Examination of the subtrochanteric fracture showed it to be transverse, suggesting that it might well have originated in a pseudofracture occurring in the lateral femoral cortex.

PITFALL

- Intramedullary nailing of Pagetic femora can be very difficult. The bone may alternate between areas of very hard and soft bone and may be difficult to penetrate. Then hypervascularity associated with Paget's disease means that bleeding may also be troublesome and the surgeon should ensure that sufficient blood is available before surgery is undertaken.

Diagnosis

A subtrochanteric fracture in a Pagetic femur. AO classification: 32–A3.1 fracture.

Surgical Management

Initially the patient was treated by the application of skin traction, which eased the discomfort in the right leg. On the following day the patient was taken to the operating room and placed on a conventional flat operating table in the lateral position. A 15 mm proximally locked reamed intramedullary nail was used to treat the fracture (Fig. 10–2). The preoperative radiograph had indicated that the femur had a very wide intramedullary canal and the 15 mm nail had minimal contact with the endosteal surface of the cortex. Following surgery dressings were applied to the wound and the patient was returned to the ward.

Postoperative Management

Postoperatively the patient was mobilized the day following surgery. Full weight bearing was permitted as soon as it could be tolerated by the patient. The patient was pain free 5 months after surgery when an anteroposterior X ray showed abundant medial callus and virtual abolition of the medial fracture line. The lateral fracture line is still open and a degree of varus persists in the proximal femoral fracture (Fig. 10–3).

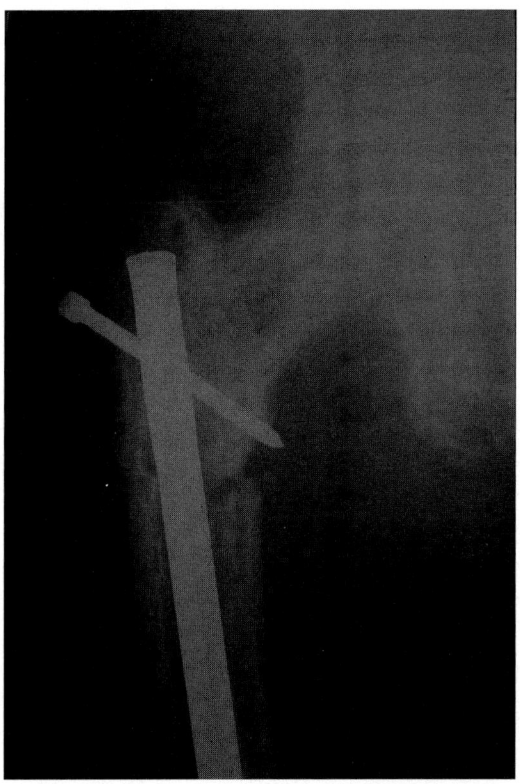

Figure 10–2. After nailing the fracture is stable. A slight varus malalignment persists.

PEARL

- In Pagetic femora it is common to have osteoarthritis in the ipsilateral hip joint. The hip is consequently stiff and there may be a fixed flexion deformity. Under these circumstances the proximal femur cannot be brought down and the femur must be nailed in flexion. This is most easily done with the patient in the lateral position. An alternative but more awkward technique is to use a conventional nailing table with the patient supine and nail the femur from underneath the patient. The former technique is advocated!

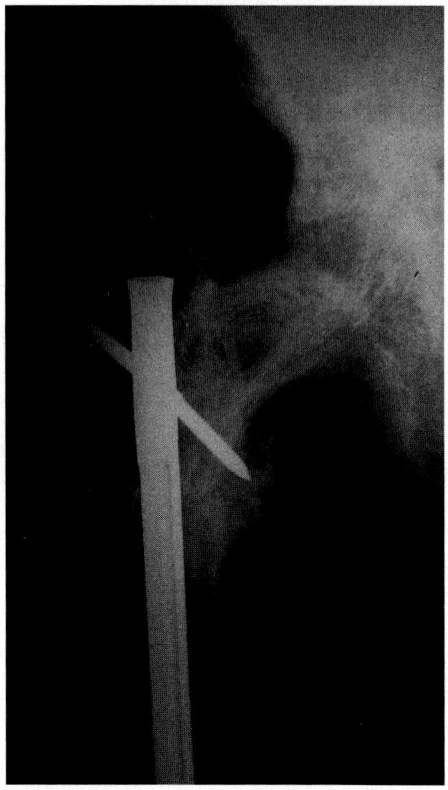

Figure 10–3. Clinical union has been achieved. There is good bone medially, but the lateral fracture line persists. It is likely that this is the site of the original pseudofracture.

Discussion

The most common metabolic bone disease encountered by orthopedic trauma surgeons is Paget's disease. Only metastatic deposits in long bones are a more frequent cause of pathological fractures. Osteomalacia is declining in incidence with better nutrition and therapy but remains relatively common in some institutionalized patients as well as in patients with nutritional and hepatic disorders. Other metabolic bone diseases are relatively rare in adults and are infrequently encountered by trauma surgeons.

The altered bone consistency present in Paget's disease means that intramedullary nailing is the best method of treating diaphyseal fractures of the femur and other long bones. Usually the large diameter of the intramedullary canal means that a large nail is required and the distinction between reamed and unreamed nails is somewhat academic under these circumstances. The surgeon should insert an appropriately sized nail that is probably going to be a reamed nail. Reaming may well induce bone healing, but in this case a 15 mm nail could have been inserted without reaming. There would be little point in inserting a larger nail because the patient will be able to bear weight on a 15 mm diameter nail without any difficulty and the fracture was stable after nailing. The fact that this was a low velocity injury and that the fracture was transverse and not comminuted means that proximal locking is sufficient.

Surgery is frequently difficult in Pagetic bone. The increased bone metabolism associated with Paget's disease often results in perioperative bleeding that may be severe. Thus an appropriate amount of blood should be available for the surgery. The other major problem in the fixation of fractures in Pagetic bone is that the pathological process results in areas of soft and hard bone. Thus the fixation of bone screws or external fixator pins may be difficult and, when possible, intramedullary techniques are advocated.

Pathological fractures are the most prevalent orthopedic complication of Paget's disease. They are relatively infrequent and few surgeons will encounter many during their careers. Fractures such as the one illustrated in Figure 10–1 usually follow the appearance of a pseudofracture on the lateral cortex of the bone. These fractures usually occur during the destructive or osteolytic phase of the disease and may be the initial presentation of Paget's disease. Interestingly, women seem to be more prone to pathological fractures in Paget's disease even though the disease is most commonly seen in elderly males. This may well be due to their smaller bone mass. Pathological fractures associated with Paget's disease are particularly likely to occur in the femur, tibia, humerus, spine, and pelvis, and multiple fractures are not uncommon.

The subtrochanteric area is the most common site for pathological fractures, with about 30% of Pagetic femoral fractures occurring there. Approximately 20% occur in the proximal third of the diaphysis, 20% in the middle third, and 10% in the distal third of the diaphysis. Almost all the remaining fractures are seen in the femoral neck, with only about 3% occurring in the trochanteric area. Patients commonly present with their first Pagetic femoral fracture between 70 and 79 years of age.

Nonunion rates of up to 40% have been reported for Pagetic femoral fractures and, even if the fracture appears to unite, the surgeon should be aware that the callus itself may be involved in the pathological process and can therefore be weak. The hypervascularity of the bone ensures a good callus response that may be impressive on the radiographs but actually provides poor support for the fracture. This is another good reason for choosing an intramedullary technique in the management of Pagetic femoral fractures.

This case is relatively straightforward. After fracture reduction the femur is straight and easy to nail. This, however, is not always possible, and the surgeon should be aware of the problems that accompany a bowed femur. Figure 10–4 shows anteroposterior and lateral radiographs of a patient with mild Paget's disease affecting his left femur. The characteristic transverse femoral fracture is seen, but there is a varus deformity in the lower femur that prevents the passage of a nail down to the distal femur. In this case a short Kuntscher nail was used and the postoperative radiographs (Fig. 10–5) show that there is slight opening in the medial side of the fracture, suggesting that the femur has been straightened by nailing. The nail could only be passed to the distal femoral deformity but good three point fixation was achieved and the fracture united.

It is more common for the femoral deformity to be uniform throughout the length of the diaphysis and for the whole femur to be bowed. Sometimes the proximal half of the diaphysis is more bowed than the distal half. Such a case is shown in Figure 10–6. This shows the anteroposterior and lateral radiographs of a Pagetic femur in a 93-year-old woman who fell out of bed and sustained an oblique fracture of the middiaphysis of the femur. The fracture passed through the proximal screw of one of two plates inserted 22 years earlier as treatment for a previous femoral fracture.

The patient was dependent and demented and a number of treatment options were considered including amputation. However, it was decided to remove the plate and nail the femur at the same operation using the fracture site to correct the femoral bow. This was successfully achieved using an unlocked intramedullary nail

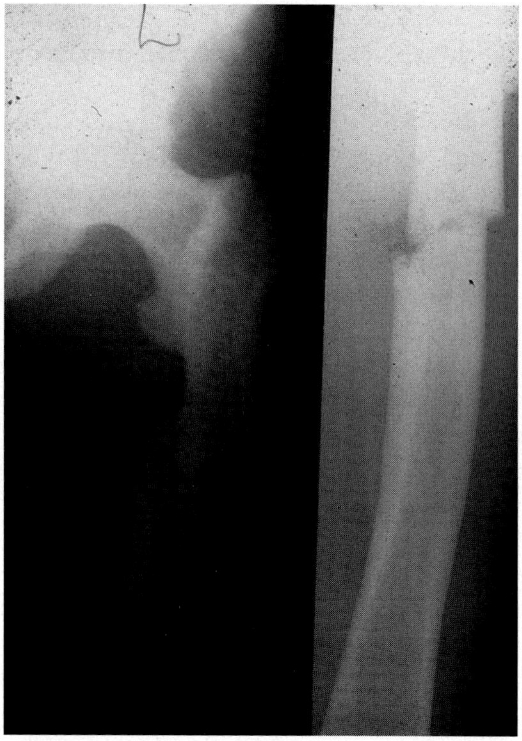

A B

Figure 10–4. Anteroposterior (A) and lateral (B) radiographs of a pagetic femur with a subtrochanteric fracture. The femur is bowed distally.

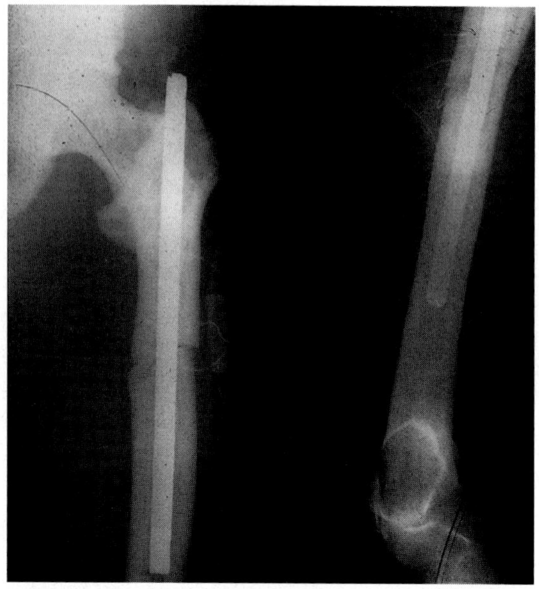

A B

Figure 10–5. Anteroposterior (A) and lateral (B) postoperative radiographs showing that a short Kuntscher nail has been used to stabilize the fracture.

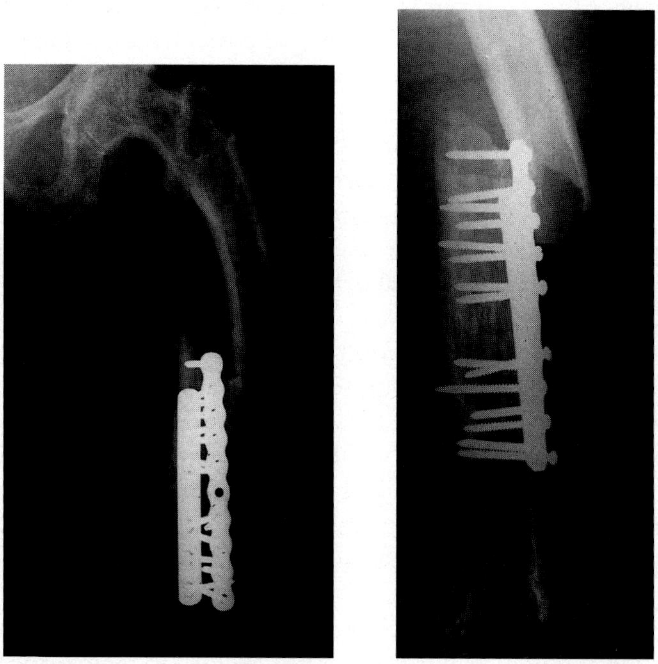

A B

Figure 10–6. Anteroposterior (A) and lateral (B) radiographs showing a diaphyseal fracture in a bowed pagetic femur. The two plates are from a previous fracture.

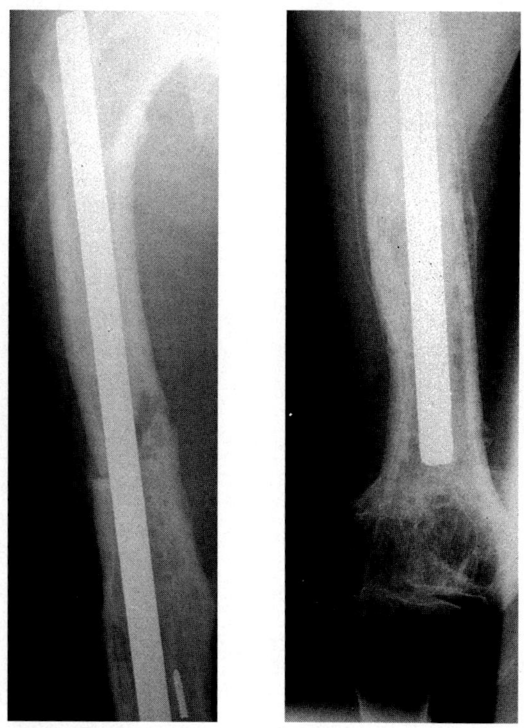

A B

Figure 10–7. The femur has been successfully nailed and straightened. Anteroposterior (A) view; lateral (B) view.

(Fig. 10–7). The patient made a good recovery from the operation. The fracture united but the patient died 1 year later.

The fracture shown in Figures 10–6 and 10–7 allowed the surgeon to correct the femoral bow. However, this does not always happen. The fracture may occur at a point proximal or distal to the apex of the femoral bow, although this is unusual. More commonly the fracture occurs at the apex of the curve because it is the area subject to the greatest stress, but the femur is too deformed to allow the passage of a nail. Under these circumstances it is suggested that a second osteotomy be performed to allow the femur to be nailed. An example is shown in Figures 10–8 through 10–10. A 17-year-old girl presented with severe pain in her right thigh without any antecedent trauma. A radiograph indicated that she had a transverse fracture of the right proximal femoral diaphysis (Fig. 10–8). She had been diagnosed as having juvenile osteoporosis at the age of 14 years and this represented her second pathological longbone fracture. The femur was uniformly bowed throughout its length and it was considered impossible to pass a conventional rigid intramedullary nail. In addition, the deformity of the proximal femur gave rise to concern about the damage that might follow an inappropriate nail insertion point. Accordingly, three Ender nails were passed proximally from the medial femoral condyle and the patient was allowed to mobilize (Fig. 10–9). She continued to complain of thigh pain and a radiograph taken 5 months later clearly indicates that there was an oligotrophic nonunion, presumably as a result of failure to correct the longitudinal axis of the femur. It was decided to remove the Ender nails and then refracture the proximal femur and osteotomize the distal diaphysis under fluoroscopic control. An antegrade intramedullary nail was passed and the proximal fracture and distal osteotomy united within 4 months (Fig. 10–10).

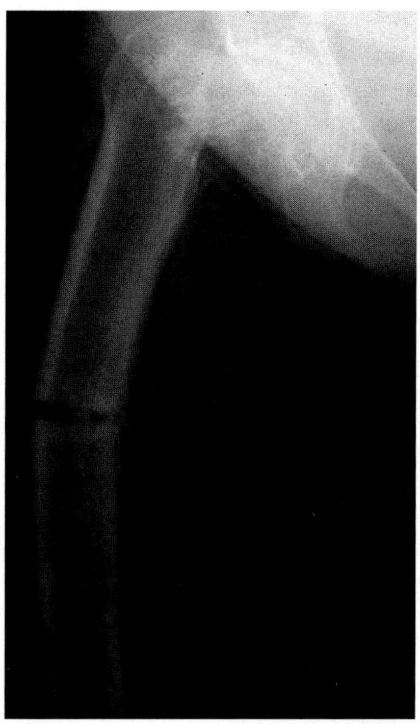

Figure 10–8. A femoral fracture in a girl with juvenile osteoporosis.

PEARL

- Usually only two osteotomies are required to straighten a bowed femur. When planning the osteotomies, the surgeon should allow for the longest diaphyseal length through which he or she can pass the nail. There should be minimal soft tissue stripping and the use of fluoroscopy and minimally invasive osteotomy techniques are recommended.

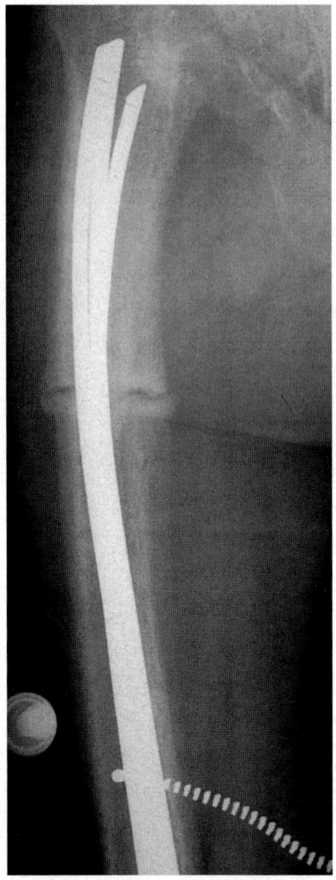

Figure 10–9. Ender nails were used to stabilize the fracture. A nonunion persists because of a failure to straighten the femur.

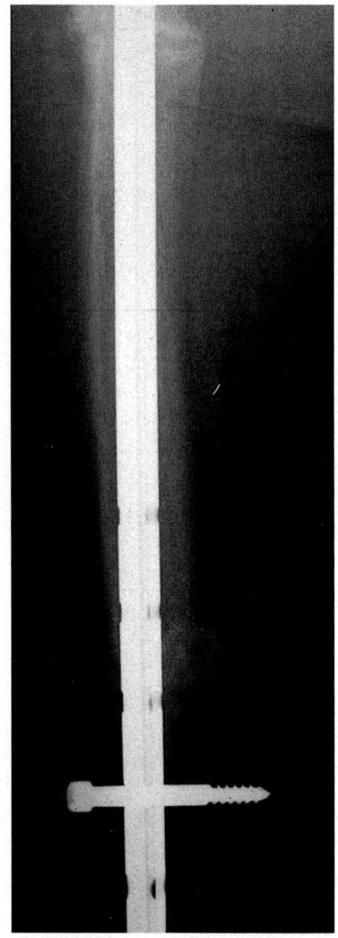

Figure 10–10. After proximal and distal osteotomies and the use of an interlocking intramedullary nail the fracture united.

Alternative Methods of Management

There are no good alternative treatment methods to the use of intramedullary nailing in Pagetic femoral diaphyseal fractures. Traction is sometimes employed, but is associated with the same complications as in non-Pagetic patients. Screws and external fixator pins usually have a poor hold in Pagetic bone and fixation failure is common. Usually the problem with Pagetic femora is not deciding on the type of treatment but determining whether the bone can be nailed at all because of diaphyseal deformity. Some surgeons have suggested the use of appropriately curved nails for these difficult femora. However, it is difficult to predictably curve the nails and, as the last case demonstrates, it is better biomechanically to straighten the femur.

Type of Management	Advantages	Disadvantages	Comments
Traction and casting	Useful as a last resort if surgery is considered impossible because of bone deformity	Patient immobility; malunion; nonunion	Most pathological fractures occur in the elderly and traction is particularly unsuitable for these patients
Intramedullary nailing	Optimal load sharing in osteoporotic bone; good patient function; good joint mobility	May be technically difficult; osteotomies may be required	This is the treatment of choice for pathological femoral fractures
Plating	None	Poor fixation; open surgery; joint stiffness	Technique rarely used in pathological diaphyseal fractures; particularly inappropriate in Pagetic femora
External fixation	None	Poor patient function; pin tract sepsis; joint stiffness	This technique is rarely indicated in pathological fractures

Complications

Many of the complications of operating on Pagetic femora are the same as those seen in normal bone. However, some complications are specific to Paget's disease. The most well known of these is perioperative hemorrhage secondary to the increased bone vascularity. If possible, the surgeon should treat the patient preoperatively with an appropriate drug to decrease bone vascularity. However, this may not be possible and in an emergency situation an adequate amount of replacement blood should be available. Surgeons should also be aware that a fracture may occur at the site of a Pagetic sarcoma but even if this is not the case there may be an area of rarefaction around the fracture that may be mistaken for sarcomatous change.

Other complications of operating on femora affected by a metabolic bone disease are essentially the same as the complications of operating on normal femora except for those induced because the bone is soft. If plating or external fixation is used, there is a high incidence of fixation failure and secondary intramedullary nailing will usually be required.

Suggested Readings

Grundy M: Fractures of femur in Paget's disease of bone. J Bone Joint Surg (Br) 1970; 52B:252–263.

Hamdy RC: Paget's Disease of Bone. Praeger, Eastbourne, 1981.

Kanis JA, Gray RES: Long term follow-up observations on treatment in Paget's disease of bone. Clin Orthop 1987; 217:99–125.

Nicolas JA, Killoran P: Fracture of the femur in patients with Paget's disease. J Bone Joint Surg (Am) 1965; 47A:450–461.

Case 11

History and Physical Examination

A 25-year-old male was admitted to the emergency department following a motor vehicle accident. He had been the driver of a car involved in a high speed collision with another car. He had not been wearing a seat belt at the time of the accident and his car was not fitted with air bags. Examination showed that he had a number of serious injuries. He had been unconscious for a short period but he had a Glasgow Coma Score of 13 on admission to the emergency department. He had significant superficial injuries to his anterior chest wall with evidence of tattooing from the steering wheel (Fig. 11–1). He also had several obvious fractures. On admission the patient was in shock, with a blood pressure of 80/50 and a tachycardia of 100/minute. He was resuscitated with crystalloid solution and red cell concentrate and his clinical state stabilized quickly. CAT scans of his head, abdomen and pelvis showed no significant injuries.

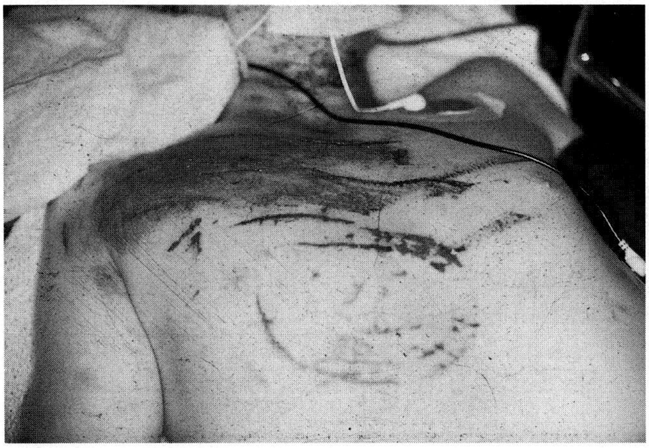

Figure 11–1. Tattooing of the anterior chest wall. This sign is suggestive of underlying pulmonary damage.

A

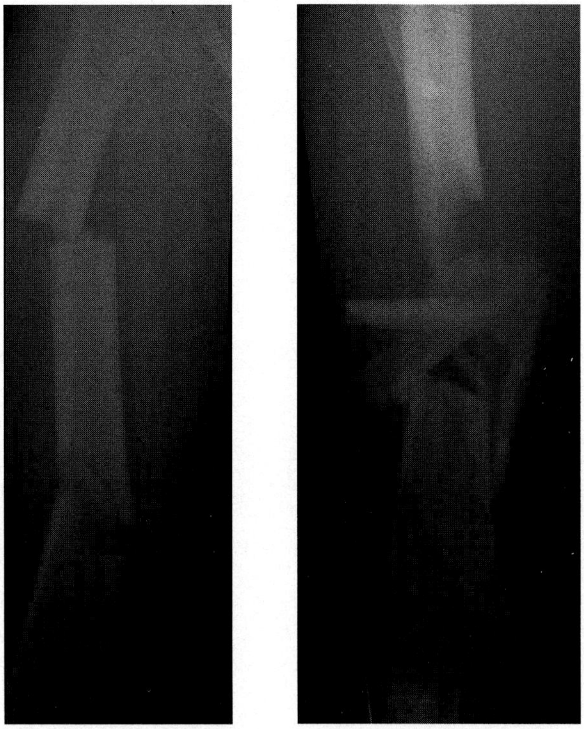

B

Figure 11–2. (A,B) Anteroposterior radiographs of the bilateral femoral diaphyseal fractures.

Radiologic Findings

Radiographs of both femora indicated severe femoral diaphyseal fractures (Fig. 11–2). An anteroposterior chest X-ray showed bilateral opacification in both lungs, suggesting parenchymal lung damage (Fig. 11–3).

PEARL

- Any patient with bilateral femoral fractures, whether open or closed, will be significantly hypovolaemic. Fluid resuscitation is essential, and if an adequate blood pressure cannot be maintained the surgeon should consider the possibility of coexisting pelvic, retro-peritoneal or intra-abdominal injury.

PITFALL

- In severely injured patients it is surprisingly easy to miss both fractures and soft tissue injuries. These injuries are often peripheral and late diagnosis does not significantly affect the patient's prognosis. However, care must be taken not to miss serious injuries and the patient and the radiographs must be examined on several occasions to minimize the risk of this happening.

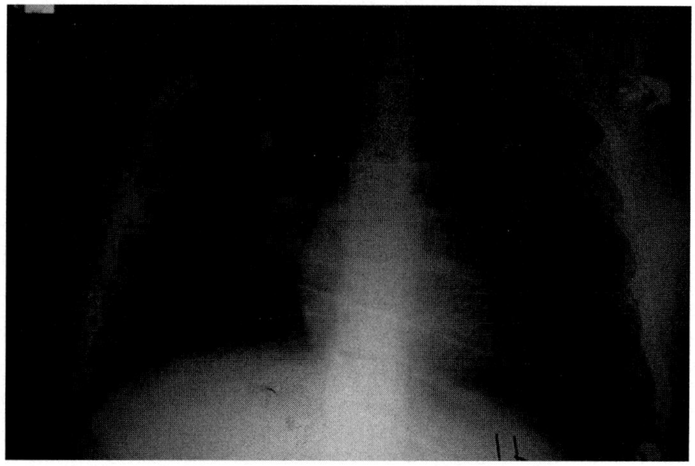

Figure 11–3. A chest X ray showing pulmonary opacification suggestive of parenchymal lung disease.

Diagnosis

Extensive musculoskeletal damage with bilateral closed femoral fractures, a closed left humeral diaphyseal fracture, and a closed left perilunate fracture dislocation. The left femur fracture was classified by the AO classification as a 32—C3.1 fracture and the right as a 32–C2.1 fracture. There was also evidence of early acute respiratory distress syndrome (ARDS).

Surgical Management

After resuscitation in the emergency department the patient was taken immediately to the operating room where it was decided to treat the bilateral femoral fractures first. Accordingly, a splint was placed on the right leg to impart a degree of temporary stability during nailing of the left femur. The patient was placed on a traction table and the surgeon inserted a 12 mm statically locked reamed intramedullary nail using an antegrade technique. The intramedullary canal was reamed to 13 mm in 0.5 mm increments. During the nailing procedure transesophageal echocardiography was used to monitor the passage of any emboli through the heart. During the nailing of the left femur only minor embolic showers were seen in the right ventricle and the anesthetist reported no drop in the patient's oxygen saturation during the procedure. It was therefore decided to stabilize the right femur with a locked intramedullary nail.

The patient was re-prepped and draped and an antegrade nailing procedure was undertaken again. The medullary canal was reamed to 12 mm without any effect on the patient's oxygen saturation or significant emboli noted on the echocardiogram. However, while the 12.5 mm reamer was being passed down the intramedullary canal the oxygen saturation dropped markedly and a shower of large emboli were noted in the right ventricle (Fig. 11–4). The surgeon decided to continue with the nailing procedure and the femur was reamed to 13 mm. A 12 mm nail was inserted and statically locked. The wounds were closed. By this time the anesthetist was having trouble maintaining the oxygen saturation and the humeral fracture was treated by the application of a brace. The perilunate fracture dislocation was quickly manipulated into a better position and a dorsal slab applied.

PEARL

- If the surgeon decides to externally fix the femur because of concern about the pulmonary status of the patient, care must be taken about inserting the external fixator pins. Despite the need for speed under these circumstances it is important that the pins be inserted properly to minimize the risk of pin track infection. If this occurs it may well delay or prevent secondary intramedullary nailing.

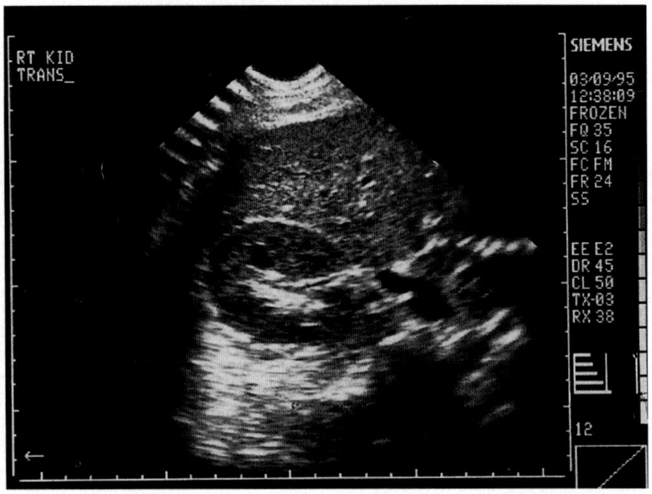

Figure 11–4. Trans-esophageal echocardiogram showing emboli passing through the right side of the heart.

PITFALL

- It is surprisingly easy to nail femora in external rotation in patients with bilateral femoral fractures. This is a serious problem which may require corrective surgery and should be avoided.

Postoperative Management

The patient was transferred to the intensive care unit where he stayed for 3 weeks while his pulmonary condition slowly improved. He was subsequently transferred back to the orthopedic service where he spent a further 12 days and was then discharged. His femoral fractures both united (Fig. 11–5) and he was functioning well within 6 months of the injury. His humeral fracture was eventually plated and the perilunate fracture dislocation was treated by open reduction and Kirschner wiring.

Discussion

This case raises a number of questions. It was known that the patient had significant pulmonary damage prior to the choice of intramedullary nailing as the treatment method. Should the surgeon have elected to use primary intramedullary nailing in a patient who had bilateral femoral fractures, or should another method, such as external fixation, have been selected? If nailing was selected as the optimal treatment method, should a reamed or unreamed nail have been used and is there a level of injury above which nailing is dangerous because of the release of emboli into the pulmonary circulation?

It is currently accepted by most surgeons that intramedullary nailing is the treatment of choice for most femoral diaphyseal fractures, but there is evidence that reaming causes fat and marrow embolization that may impair pulmonary function. This phenomenon is only likely to happen in the presence of preexisting pulmonary injury. Under normal circumstances the pulmonary reserve is enormous. It has been estimated that the surface area of the alveoli is 120 m^2 and that the pulmonary capillary system contains about 25% of all the body's capillaries. Thus under normal circumstances the pulmonary circulation would be able to cope with a considerable amount of particulate matter passing into the lungs without any clinical manifestation; if there is coexisting parenchymal damage, the lungs may be unable to absorb the fat and marrow emboli and pulmonary symptoms may ensue. In addition, the presence of a patent foramen ovale or the opening of subplural and bronchopulmonary shunts may allow particulate matter into the systemic circulation.

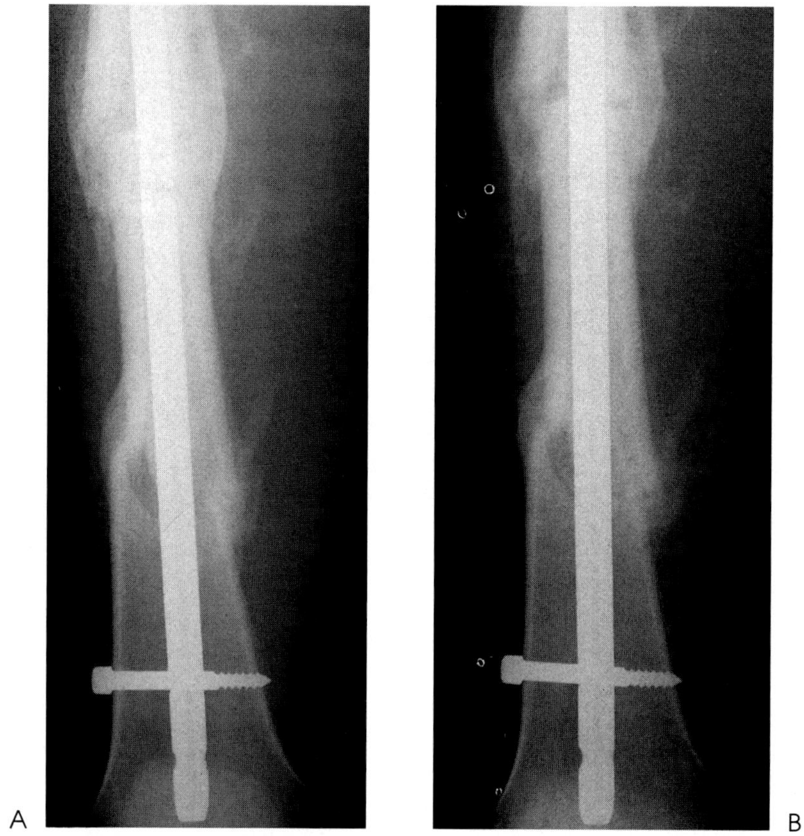

Figure 11–5. Both fractures healed well without further surgery.

There is debate about the exact mechanism of the fat embolus syndrome. It has been shown that reaming enhances the coagulation response. However, the injury itself can cause a consumptive coagulopathy and even traction has been associated with increased activation of fibrinogen degradation products, elastase and protease inhibitor complexes that return to normal after internal fixation. It is likely that the fat embolus syndrome is very complex and the clinical syndrome with which surgeons are familiar is probably a final common pathway stimulated by a number of different pathological events. However, there seems no doubt that fat and marrow debris play a role.

Christie (Court-Brown and Christie, 1996) has used transesophageal echocardiography to observe the passage of particulate debris through the heart during different operative procedures on the femur. He observed marrow embolization in three groups of patients: those who required reaming for traumatic long bone fractures, those patients with metastatic deposits who subsequently underwent intramedullary nailing, whether or not there was a pathological fracture, and those patients who had cemented or uncemented hip arthroplasties. He found that 92% of his patients demonstrated fat and marrow embolization during these intramedullary procedures. However, not all embolic phenomenon were symptomatic. He noted three different types of embolic events. Group 1 consisted of severe prolonged embolic events with substantial and dense embolic showers accompanied by an obvious coagulopathy. In Group 1, patients' clots of up to 8 cm in length passed into the right ventricle and then into the pulmonary circulation. Group 2 consisted of patients who had moderate embolic showers that were also associated with coagulopathy but were less severe and prolonged. The Group 3 patients demonstrated only mild showers that were not accompanied by coagulopathy. The remaining 8% of patients had no embolic response at all. Most of the severe embolic events occurred in patients with metastatic tumor deposits or in patients undergoing cemented arthroplasties. Christie did not encounter any fatality in the hip arthroplasty group or in those patients in whom reamed nailing was used to treat a femoral diaphyseal fracture.

In vitro comparisons of reamed and unreamed nailing suggest that reamed nailing is associated with an increased embolic response, a high degree of platelet activation, and decreased pulmonary function when compared with unreamed nailing. It seems intuitively likely that the passage of an unreamed nail has the same effect as the passage of a reamer of equivalent diameter and it is probably the accumulative effect of passing a number of reamers that accounts for the difference between the two methods.

The problems arise when the clinical literature is reviewed. Despite a reasonable uniformity of opinion that the experimental use of reaming is associated with impaired pulmonary function, this is not confirmed by all the clinical studies. A number of surgeons have examined whether the use of femoral nailing in the management of femoral diaphyseal fractures in the multiply injured patient has been associated with increased pulmonary problems, and the results are conflicting. There is a degree of confusion in the literature because there is no doubt that early long bone stabilization in patients with thoracic trauma leads to a lower incidence of pulmonary complications when compared with delayed fixation. However, this is not the principle argument—whether a primary reamed intramedullary nail is detrimental to pulmonary function in those patients who have coexisting severe pulmonary trauma compared with early diaphyseal stabilization using other methods. Virtually all the articles dealing with this question believe that it is not, but they are all retrospective studies and open to question.

The work of Trentz and his group is, however, of interest (Friedl et al., 1996). This group compared 32 patients who received intramedullary nails within four days of trauma with 23 patients who were nailed between 5 and 14 days after injury and primarily managed with an external fixator. The first group had a significantly lower average injury severity score, but a 25% incidence of ARDS and a 12.5% mortality rate. The second group had no deaths and no pulmonary complications. Thus Trentz and his associates advocate primary external fixation and secondary intramedullary nailing for multiply injured patients with severe pulmonary trauma.

Overall it is difficult to be certain about the role of intramedullary nailing in femoral diaphyseal fractures in multiply injured patients. On balance it is suggested that reamed nailing is the preferred method of treatment in multiply injured patients with no evidence of pulmonary damage. If multiple nailing is required, the anesthetist should monitor the oxygen saturation carefully and if a problem occurs, primary nailing should be abandoned in place of primary external fixation. If there is thoracic trauma, nailing is probably safe in patients with an injury severity score of below 25 but unsafe if the score is above 40 (Friedl et al., 1996). Multiple nailing in the severely injured patient probably produces a cumulative embolic problem and should be avoided in favor of primary external fixation and secondary nailing. However, it must be emphasized that this represents a very small number of patients in the average orthopaedic trauma unit.

Alternative Methods of Management

In view of the uncertainty surrounding the question of intramedullary nailing in femoral fractures in multiply injured patients, it is difficult to make exact recommendations about other treatment methods.

External Fixation

As has already been suggested, it seems reasonable to use temporary external skeletal fixation in multiply injured patients who have thoracic trauma or an injury severity score of more than 40 (Friedl et al., 1996). However, long term femoral external fixation is not advocated by many surgeons, and ideally secondary intramedullary nailing should be undertaken between 5 and 14 days after the initial operation. The surgeon must be aware, however, that the pulmonary complications following trauma may take several weeks to resolve, although only in a few patients will the lung damage prevent secondary nailing for this length of time. It is suggested that if temporary external fixation is used, a simple unilateral frame utilizing a rigid bar and large fixator pins is adequate. Temporary external fixation will often be per-

Type of Management	Advantages	Disadvantages	Comments
Traction casting	None	High morbidity; mortality; patient immobility	There is no place for nonoperative management of femoral diaphyseal fractures in the multiply injured
Reamed intramedullary nailing	Good results in the treatment of isolated femoral fractures	Probably inappropriate in the severely injured patient (ISS >40) or in patients with severe thoracic trauma	Usually the preferred treatment option except for a very small number of patients who have significant thoracic trauma or are very seriously injured
Unreamed intramedullary nailing	Quicker procedure; fewer embolic problems	Nails mechanically weaker than the larger reamed nails	Probably better than reamed nails in very severely injured patients
External fixation	Good temporary fixation	Poor definitive management for femoral fracture; pin tract sepsis; malunion	Best used as temporary fixation with later intramedullary nailing
Plating	None	Time consuming; inappropriate for many femoral fractures	Rarely used

formed in a hurry, but attention should nevertheless be paid to pin insertion technique to minimize the risk of later infection.

Plating

Femoral plating in the multiply injured patient is not normally recommended. Plating is a time consuming procedure that is not suited to the comminuted fractures often seen in the multiply injured patient. It is also likely, though unproven, that the tissue handling inherent in long-bone plating will increase the likelihood of emboli and coagulopathy.

Traction and Casting

There is no place for the nonoperative management of femoral diaphyseal fractures in multiply injured patients. All authorities in the last 20 years have emphasized the need for early surgical stabilization of the femur in the multiply injured patient.

Complications

In view of the association between reaming and intramedullary nailing and pulmonary dysfunction it is important for the surgeon to be aware of potential problems that may arise during and after intramedullary nailing of a femoral diaphyseal fracture in the severely injured patient. If the patient's oxygen saturation is being measured intraoperatively, it is usually relatively easy to detect any problem. However, postoperatively surgeons may have to rely on the clinical signs of fat embolus, with petechial hemorrhage and confusion commonly seen. If a fat embolus occurs, the patient should be transferred to a high dependency or intensive care unit and ventilation commenced when indicated.

Other complications the surgeons may have to treat are posttraumatic osteomyelitis, nonunion, and malunion. These are dealt with in the same way as in a patient with an isolated femoral fracture.

Suggested Readings

Alastair PH, Hughes D, Keating J, et al: Brief report: fulminating fat embolism syndrome caused by paradoxical embolism through a patent foramen ovale. N Engl J Med 1993; 329:926–929.

Browner BD (ed): The Science and Practice of Intramedullary Nailing. Williams and Wilkins, Baltimore, 1996.

Christie J, Robinson CM, Pell ACH, McBirnie J, Burnett R: Transcardiac echocardiography during invasive intramedullary procedures. J Bone Joint Surg (Br) 1995; 77B:450–455.

Court-Brown CM, Christie J (eds): Intramedullary reaming and its physiological effects. In: Techniques in Orthopaedics. 1996; 11.

Friedl HP, Stocker R, Czermak B, Schmal H, Trentz O: Primary fixation and delayed nailing of long bone fractures in severe trauma. Techniques in Orthopaedics 1996; 11:59–66.

Pape HC, Auf'm'Kolk M, Paffrath T, et al: Primary intramedullary femur fixation in multiple trauma patients with associated lung contusion: a cause of post traumatic ARDS. J Trauma 1993; 34:540–548.

Wolinsky PR, Sciadini MF, Parker RE, Plitman JD, Snapper JR, Rutherford EJ, Schulman M, Johnson KD: Effects on pulmonary physiology of reamed femoral intramedullary nailing in an open-chest sheep model. J Orthop Trauma 1996; 10:75–80.

Case 12

History and Physical Examination

A 54-year-old man was in a motor vehicle accident. He was the unrestrained passenger when his vehicle left the road at approximately 50 mph and rolled over. He was extracted from the vehicle without difficulty by paramedics, who noted pain and deformity of both lower extremities. He arrived in the emergency department approximately 1 hour after injury on a board with traction on both lower extremities. He was noted to be awake and alert with complaints only of knee and leg pain. There was obvious instability and external rotation deformity of both lower extremities at the knees with instability and pain to palpation. The left fracture was open. A 6 cm long laceration was present directly anterior. Gross contamination was not present. Distal pulses were present and the neurological examination was intact. The patient's medical history was relevant in that he had a history of systemic lupus erythematosus treated with corticosteroids. He also had undergone bilateral total hip replacements 3 years prior to this injury. The right hip had dislocated 3 weeks after it had been implanted. The dislocation was managed successfully with closed reduction and an abduction brace. Both hips had been painless and functioning well prior to this injury.

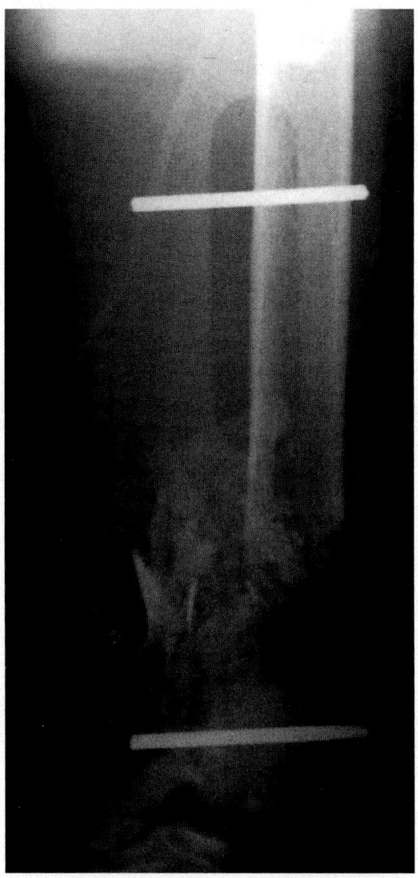

Figure 12–1. Anteroposterior radiograph of the left open supracondylar fracture with undisplaced intraarticular extension.

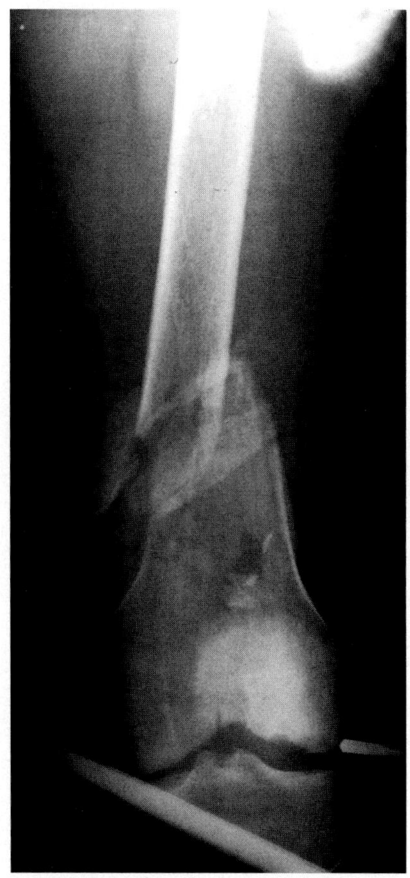

Figure 12–2. Anteroposterior radiograph of the right supracondylar fracture.

Radiologic Findings

Radiographs of the pelvis, hips, femurs, knees, and tibias were obtained. On the left side a very comminuted supracondylar fracture with an undisplaced fracture involving the articular surface was present (Fig. 12–1). The radiographs of the right femur and knee indicated a comminuted fracture of the distal femur. The articular surface was fractured but minimally displaced (Fig. 12–2). Radiographs of both hips indicated bilateral uncemented hip arthroplasties in good alignment. The bone prosthesis interface appeared well preserved. Periprosthetic radiolucencies, signs of osteolysis, and loosening of the prosthesis were not present. The radiographs of the pelvis and tibia were otherwise within the limits of normal.

Diagnosis

Bilateral comminuted supracondylar fractures with undisplaced intraarticular extension (C-2) below a well fixed prosthesis. The left fracture was open grade 3A. It was classified as grade 3 because of the associated comminution. It was further classified as A because the laceration was not grossly contaminated and closure would not require a soft tissue transfer. AO classification: (left fracture) 33–C2.3; (right fracture) 33–C2.2.

Surgical Management

When associated head, neck, and visceral injuries had been ruled out, the patient was taken to the operating room and anesthetized. He was moved to a radiolucent operating table. Both lower extremities were prepped and draped simultaneously. The open left fracture was managed first. The wound was extended proximally and distally. Proximally, the quadriceps was split; distally a lateral parapatellar capsular incision was used to expose the articular surface. All nonviable tissue and avascular bone fragments were removed. The intraarticular fracture was reduced and stabilized with a Kirschner wire. The articular segment was then reduced to the metaphysis and stabilized with a lateral plate. A T plate was applied to the medial side of the femur because of comminution of the medial cortex. Antibiotic beads were used to fill the defect resulting from the debridement, and the wound was closed (Fig. 12–3). The surgical extensions of the injury were closed in layers, taking care to repair the lateral capsule. The laceration was closed in a single layer over a large drain.

On the right side, a straight anterior incision was made centered over the patella. The incision was carried down to the fascia, and a medial flap was elevated. A medial para-patellar capsular incision was performed, and the patella was retracted laterally. Cannulated screws were used to hold the intraarticular fracture reduced, taking care to position the screws anteriorly so that they would not interfere with insertion of a retrograde nail. The leg was placed over a bolster and with the aid of fluoroscopy; the fracture was reduced with manual traction. An entrance portal was made by drilling the distal articular surface just anterior to the origin of the anterior cruciate ligament. A guidewire was passed across the fracture site. The femur was sequentially reamed to 11 mm. An 11 mm nail was driven across the fracture site and locked proximally and distally. Proximal locking was accomplished with one screw only, to decrease the chance of a stress fracture between the tip of the nail and the femoral prosthesis (Fig. 12–4).

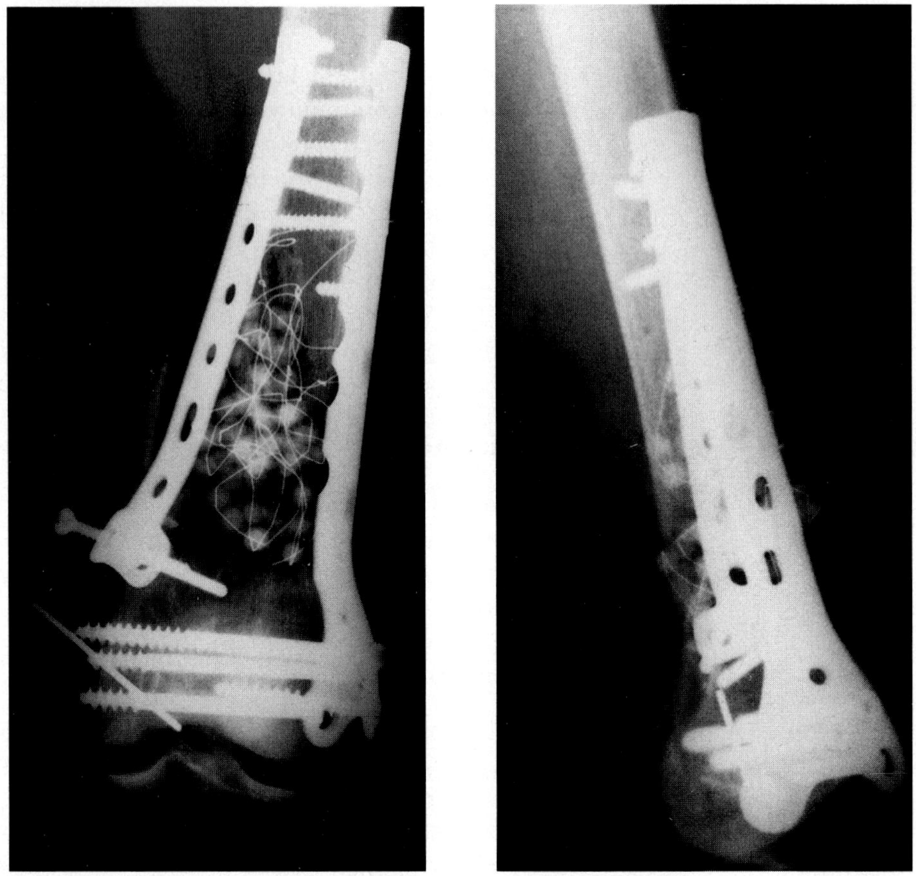

A B

Figure 12–3. Anteroposterior (A) and lateral (B) radiographs of the fracture 4 weeks after fixation just prior to grafting with autogenous bone. The beads are between the plates.

Postoperative Management

Postoperatively gentle passive and active range of motion of both knees was initiated 3 days postinjury. At 3 weeks postinjury the antibiotic beads were removed from the left knee and the defect grafted with autogenous bone obtained from the iliac crest. Nonweight bearing was maintained for 8 weeks on the right (the fracture treated with the retrograde nail) and then advanced to full weight bearing over the next 4 weeks. Nonweight bearing was maintained for 12 weeks on the left side and then advanced to full weight bearing over the following month. Six months after his supracondylar fractures, the patient sustained a bicondylar tibial plateau fracture that was reduced and stabilized with medial and lateral plates. The final range of motion was 0 to 120 degrees on the right and 0 to 90 degrees on the left (Figs. 12–5 and 12–6).

Discussion

This patient sustained bilateral high energy supracondylar fractures below total hip prostheses that were functioning well prior to injury. The goal of treatment was restoration of knee function.

A 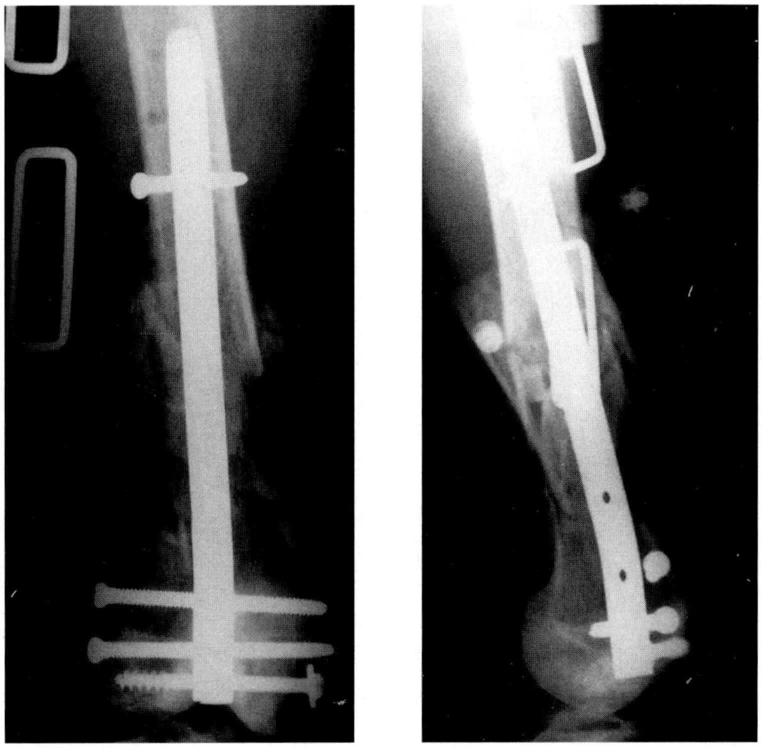 B

Figure 12–4. Anteroposterior (A) and lateral (B) radiographs 4 weeks after stabilization with a retrograde nail.

A 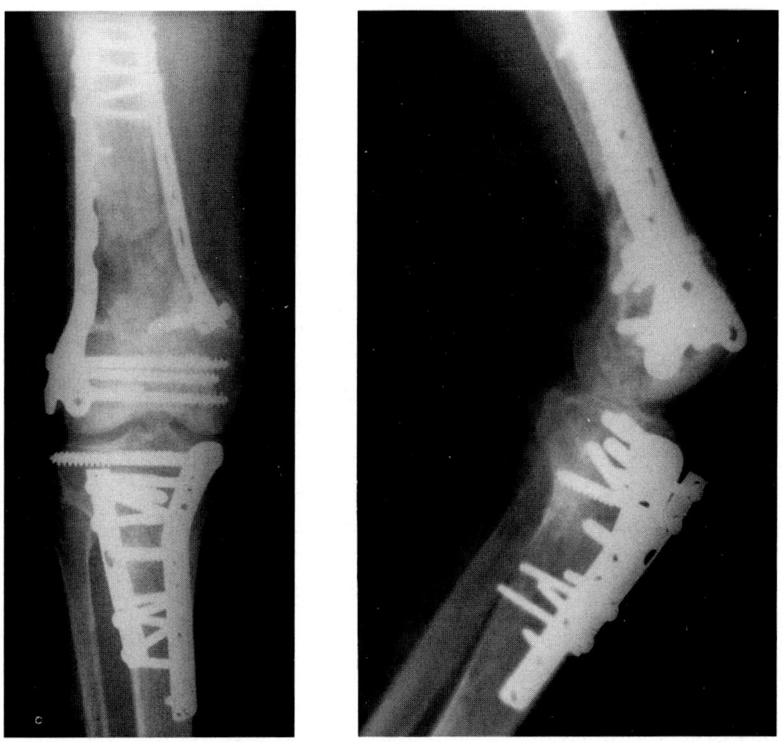 B

Figure 12–5. Anteroposterior (A) and lateral (B) radiographs of the left femur after it had healed. The patient had sustained a bicondylar fracture of the tibial plateau that had been stabilized with medial lateral plates.

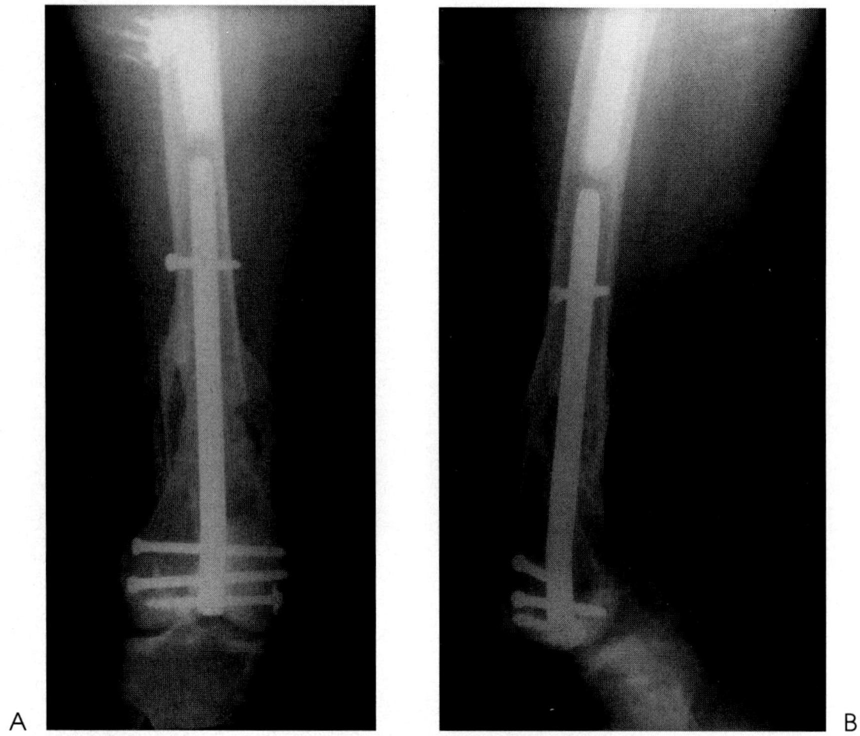

Figure 12–6. Anteroposterior (A) and lateral (B) radiographs of the right femur after it had healed.

Alternative Methods of Management

This patient could potentially have been managed by closed management with traction followed by casting, closed management with an external fixator, a retrograde intramedullary nail, or open management with reduction and fixation with plates and screws. Management with traction has the advantage of being noninvasive with no surgical trauma or morbidity, although its disadvantages include prolonged recumbency, complications, and a low incidence of fracture consolidation.

The disadvantages of management with external fixation include painful postoperative physical therapy due to transfixion of the quadriceps muscle by the fixator pins and proximity of the pin tracts to the zone of injury and femoral component. The proximity of the pin tracts to the fracture and femoral component increases the potential for infection. On the other hand, management with external fixation is minimally invasive with limited operative morbidity. The most effective method of achieving restoration of knee function is reduction and stabilization of the fracture. The two methods of stabilization are retrograde nailing and plating.

Management with a retrograde intramedullary nail requires a limited surgical exposure, and thus minimal operative trauma and a relatively small risk of infection. Retrograde nailing has two major disadvantages. First, it does not rigidly stabilize the fracture. When the fracture is stressed under fluoroscopy following retrograde intramedullary nailing, a surprising amount of motion is found. The fact that fixation is not rigid may add to the patient's discomfort during range of motion exercises in the first month following surgery. Second is the presence of increased stresses on the femur at the tip of the nail and around the proximal locking screw.

This is an area of the femur that is already at increased risk of fracture because of stress concentration around the distal end of the prosthetic femoral stem.

Open management with plates and screws results in anatomic reduction and rigid fixation. The rigidity of fixation decreases the pain associated with physical therapy; however, the extensive surgical exposure necessitated by this technique is associated with an increased risk of infection and nonunion.

Type of Management	Advantages	Disadvantages	Comments
Traction and casting	Minimal operative trauma	Necessity of prolonged bedrest casting; low incidence of fracture healing	Seldom done because disadvantages outweigh advantages
External fixation	Minimal operative trauma	Painful physical therapy; pin tract infection may lead to infection of fracture or arthroplasty	Good alternative when patient cannot undergo open procedure
Retrograde nail	Minimal operative trauma; minimal risk of infection	Not rigid fixation; not applicable to all cases (e.g., comminution of articular surface is contraindication)	Excellent method of management in appropriate cases
Plates and screws	Rigid, stable fixation	Significant operative trauma; increased risk of infection and nonunion	The best method of management when intraarticular comminution and displacement are present

Complications

The complications of fixation of supracondylar fractures below a hip arthroplasty are delayed union with loss of fixation, stress fracture between the prosthesis and fixation device, decreased motion, and infection. Delayed union without loss of fixation is managed conservatively with pulsed electromagnetic fields or iliac crest bone grafting. If the fixation has failed, it is revised and the fracture is bone grafted. The range of motion of the knee is an important prognostic factor. In cases in which knee motion is limited, the chance of successful management of a delayed union is not high. Stress fracture between the prosthesis and fixation device is managed with open reduction, rigid fixation, and bone grafting. Fixation with a plate can be augmented with cables and allograft struts (Figs. 12–7 and 12–8). Decreased range of motion is managed conservatively with physical therapy. Usually the risks of operative intervention outweigh the benefits of increased motion. Infection may involve the fracture alone or the fracture and the prosthesis. If only the fracture is infected, aggressive management with debridement, systemic antibiotics, and early autogenous bone grafting is warranted. If the prosthesis is involved, suppressive therapy with long term oral antibiotics is attempted. In cases in which the infection cannot be controlled, the prosthesis is removed, the fracture fixation is left in place until the fracture has healed. When the fracture heals, the fixation is removed and the infected area debrided. The prosthesis can be reimplanted after a prolonged infection-free interval.

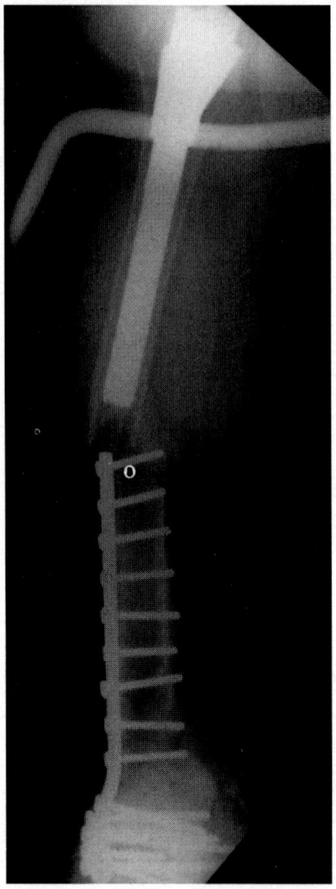

Figure 12–7. Radiograph of a femur that has fractured between a distal plate and prosthetic stem.

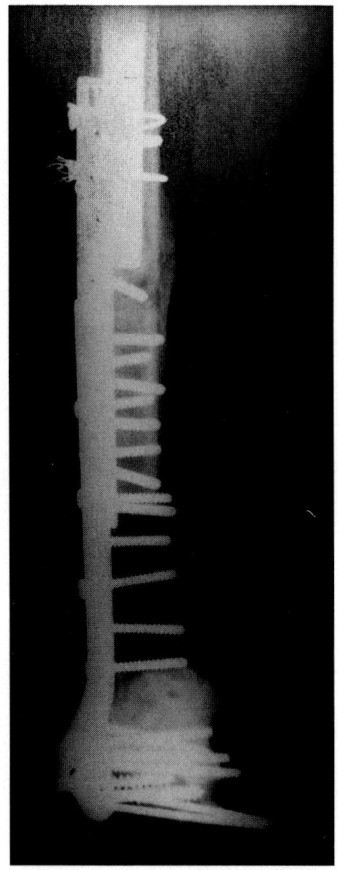

Figure 12–8. Radiograph of a femur that has healed after being stabilized with an anterolateral plate and medial allograft strut.

Suggested Readings

Adolphson P, Jonsson U, Kalen R: Fracture of the ipsilateral femur after total hip arthroplasty. Arch Orthop Surg 19xx; 106:353–357.

Bethea JS, DeAndrade JR, Fleming LL, Lindenbaum, SD, Welsh RB: Proximal femoral fractures following total hip arthroplasty. CORR 1982; 170:95–106.

Serocki JH, Chandler RW, Dorr LD: Treatment of fractures about hip prosthesis with compression plating. J Arthroplast 1992; 7:129–135.

Case 13

History and Physical Examination

An 82-year-old woman tripped and fell in her daughter's home. She experienced the immediate onset of severe thigh pain. The patient arrived via ambulance in the emergency department 1 hour after injury. Her right leg was shortened and externally rotated. Movement of the leg was extremely painful. A well healed scar that was compatible with a posterior lateral approach to the hip was present. The neurovascular examination of the extremity was within the limits of normal. There were no injuries other than that of the lower extremity.

The patient's medical history was significant in that she had undergone a hip arthroplasty 12 years prior to this injury, followed by a revision for loosening 6 years later. She had experienced slowly increasing hip and thigh pain over the last 6 months. The pain was similar to that preceding her revision surgery. It was made worse by weight bearing and had become so severe that the patient had begun to use a walker.

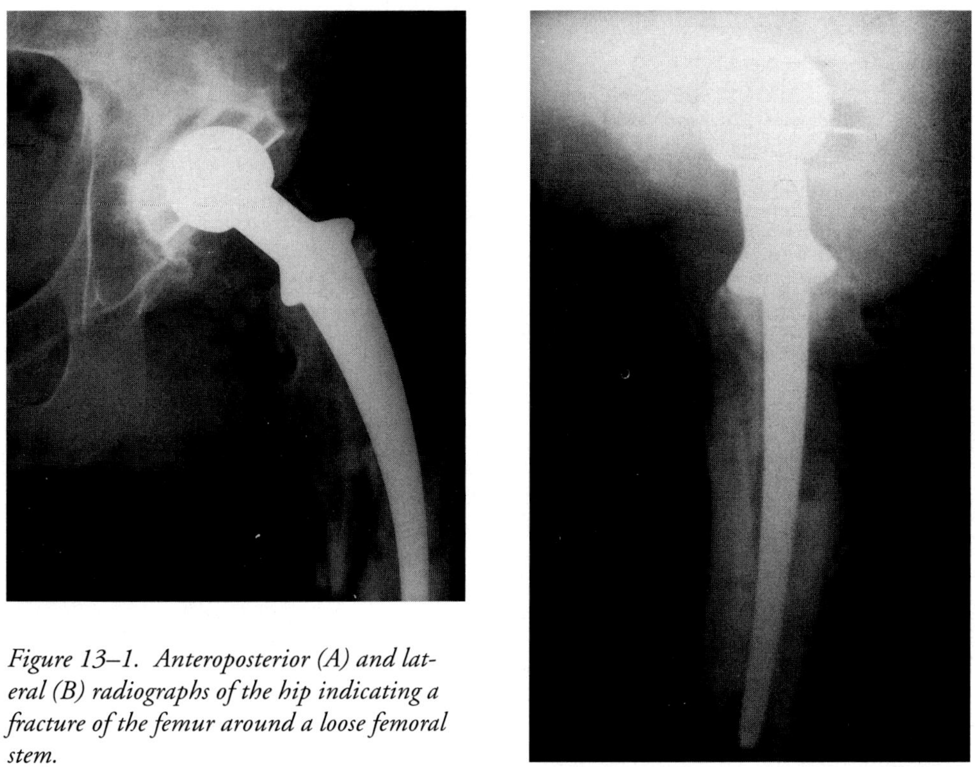

A

B

Figure 13–1. Anteroposterior (A) and lateral (B) radiographs of the hip indicating a fracture of the femur around a loose femoral stem.

Radiologic Findings

Radiographs of the hip and femur indicated an oblique fracture of the femur starting at the tip of the prosthesis and extending proximally. The prosthesis was cemented. The cement mantle had fractured and there was osteolysis and ex-

PEARL

- It is important to determine how the prosthesis was functioning prior to fracture. In this case, the presence of signs and symptoms of loosening necessitated a revision arthroplasty. The fact that the fracture occurred at the tip of the femoral stem, and not proximally around the stem or distal to the stem, necessitated operative management. This is because of the low incidence of healing with closed management.

PITFALL

- The mistake to avoid is attempting to remove the femoral component and salvage the proximal femur (i.e., dislocating the hip and using osteotomes and high speed cutting burrs to cut around the cement mantle). Salvage of the proximal femur increases the duration of the procedure and is not warranted because of the osteolysis.

pansion of the femoral cortex. The acetabular component, which was all polyethylene and cemented, showed signs of wear but did not appear loose (Fig. 13–1).

Diagnosis

Fracture of the femur distal to a total hip with clinical and radiographic evidence of prefracture loosening of the prosthesis. The fracture extended from the tip of the prosthesis proximally.

Surgical Management

The patient was put in bed. A pillow was placed behind the knee and 5 pounds of traction applied through a foam boot to the injured extremity. She was log rolled every 4 hours, a Foley catheter was inserted, knee-high sequential compression stockings were placed on both lower extremities, and she was encouraged to use an incentive spirometer.

The day after injury, the patient was placed on a conventional operating table, anesthetized, and turned on her side. The leg and hip were prepped and draped with the leg free. The incision was made incorporating the existing scar, extending from the lateral condyle of the femur, proximally along the lateral aspect of the femur to the greater trochanter, where it curved posteriorly. The femur was exposed by incising the fascia lata, splitting the gluteus maximus and fascia lata in line with their fibers, and retracting the vastus lateralis anteriorly. The fracture site was identified. The lateral cortex of the femur proximal to the fracture was cut with an oscillating saw parallel to the long axis of the femur. The osteotomy included the greater trochanter. Using two broad osteotomes, surgeons wedged open the proximal femur laterally, fracturing the medial cortex longitudinally and exposing the femoral component and cement. The femoral component and cement were removed, exposing the acetabular component. Osteotomizing the proximal femur longitudinally and "booking" it open is a relatively quick and atraumatic way of removing the femoral component and exposing the acetabulum.

The acetabular component was examined and found to be firmly fixed to the pelvis. The cortex of the proximal femur was extremely thin. Staining of the surrounding tissue, compatible with metallosis, was present. Although there were no signs of infection other than the loosening of the prosthesis, tissue samples were sent for culture. A proximal femoral allograft was then cut to the length appropriate to replace the patient's proximal femur. The allograft was reamed, broached, and a long stem prosthesis was cemented into it with approximately 10 cm of the stem extending beyond the allograft. The distal femur of the patient was then reamed. The stem of the prosthesis was cemented into the distal femur, taking care that the allograft bone was in contact with the host bone. The patient's proximal femur, which had previously been osteotomized longitudinally, was curetted and shaped to fit over the allograft and held in place with cerclage wires, thus reattaching the abductors to the femur. For additional stability, a plate was applied laterally with cables around the proximal femur and screws in the distal femur. The hip was located and the wound closed over drains.

Postoperative Management

Postoperatively the patient was fit with a brace designed to hold the hip slightly abducted and prevent greater than 45 degrees of flexion. The brace was discontinued at 6 weeks. Nonweight bearing was maintained for 2 months. At 2 months weight bearing as tolerated was initiated. Although all cultures were negative, intravenous antibiotics were continued while the patient was hospitalized. Oral antibiotics were continued a total of 6 months following surgery. Weight bearing was initiated at 12 weeks. At 1 year the patient was walking with a cane (Fig. 13–2).

Discussion

The patient sustained a low energy fracture below a hip arthroplasty. The arthroplasty had become painful due to osteolysis at the bone cement interface. Closed management was not an option because of the patient's age, the negligible chance that the fracture would heal, and the loose and painful condition of the prosthesis. Because of osteolysis it was clear, prior to surgery, that the proximal femur was inadequate to support the femoral component.

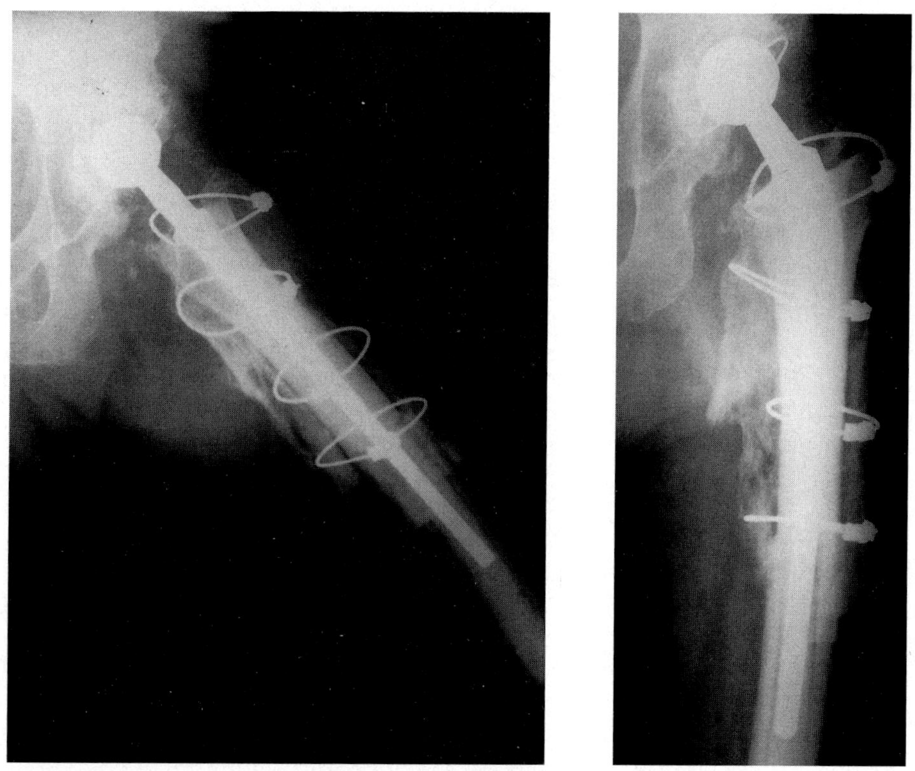

A B

Figure 13–2. Anteroposterior (A) and lateral (B) radiographs 1 year after injury. The allograft appears to be incorporating and the prosthesis is in good position.

Alternative Methods of Management

The two choices of prosthesis are a prosthetic proximal femur, used primarily for reconstruction following tumor resection, and a long stem conventional prosthesis and allograft. The advantage of the proximal femoral prosthesis is that the procedure is relatively simple; reduction and stabilization of fractures and allografts are not required. The primary disadvantage of the proximal femoral prosthesis is that it can be difficult to achieve durable, stable fixation of the prosthesis to the femur, especially in an elderly osteopoenic patient with a large medullary canal. Use of the prosthesis and allograft was elected because this was the familiar technique. Use of an allograft and long stem prosthesis restores bone that has been lost; however, it is questionable how useful or how important this bone is in an 82-year-old patient. Use of an allograft and long stem prosthesis is a more difficult technique than use of a proximal femoral prosthesis. The allograft must be accurately fit to the host femur. We added a lateral cable plate to the construct to increase the stability of fixation and closed the remnants of the patient's proximal femur around the allograft to increase the host bone growth into the allograft.

Type of Management	Advantages	Disadvantages	Comments
Allograft and long stem prosthesis	Bone growth into allograft	More complex procedure; requires exact cuts of allograft and host bone; may require additional fixation for stability	Seems more physiologic because it restores bone stock
Prosthetic proximal femur	Technically simpler procedure	Bone prosthesis interface is likely to fail	Indicated for patients with low demands

Complications

The complications of reconstruction with an allograft and long stem prosthesis are infection and dislocation. Infection is due to inoculation of the wound at the time of surgery or hematogenous seeding postoperatively. One other possibility is that the osteolysis present in this case was due to low grade sepsis. This possibility was ruled out by the negative intraoperative cultures obtained prior to administration of antibiotics. We routinely administer prophylactic antibiotics for 6 months to patients who have undergone implantation of an allograft to minimize the incidence of hematogenous seeding of the allograft with bacteria. When infection does occur, it is disastrous for the patient. To eradicate the infection, surgeons remove the prosthesis and allograft and cement and administer long term antibiotics. The result is a useless lower extremity that usually cannot be reconstructed because of the massive tissue loss. Failure to eradicate the infection or a fulminate course may necessitate a hip disarticulation.

The extensive surgical exposure complicates postoperative rehabilitation and increases the risk of dislocation; therefore a brace that holds the hip abducted and prevents flexion is prescribed. If the hip does dislocate, immediate closed reduction is performed and the hip is examined under fluoroscopy to assess the position of the components and where the dislocation occurs. If there is malposition of the components, a revision arthroplasty is performed.

Suggested Readings

Bethea JS, DeAndrade JR, Fleming LL, Lindenbaum SD, Welch RB: Proximal femoral fractures following total hip arthroplasty. CORR 1982; 170:95–106.

Kolstad K: Revision total hip replacement after periprosthetic femoral fractures. An analysis of 23 cases. Acta Orthop Scand 1994; 65:505–508.

Martin WR, Sutherland CJ: Complications of proximal femoral allografts in revision total hip arthroplasty. CORR 1993; 295:161–167.

Case 14

History and Physical Examination

An 81-year-old female presented to the emergency department, having slipped in the bathroom of her home 2 days earlier. She had been unable to bear weight and complained of severe left knee pain. Her medical history included mild cardiac failure and an intertrochanteric fracture of her left hip about 18 months earlier. This had been successfully treated with a hip screw and side plate. Otherwise her general health was good and she lived on her own with some social support. Examination showed a painful swollen left knee and lower leg. She had normal neurovascular function in the leg.

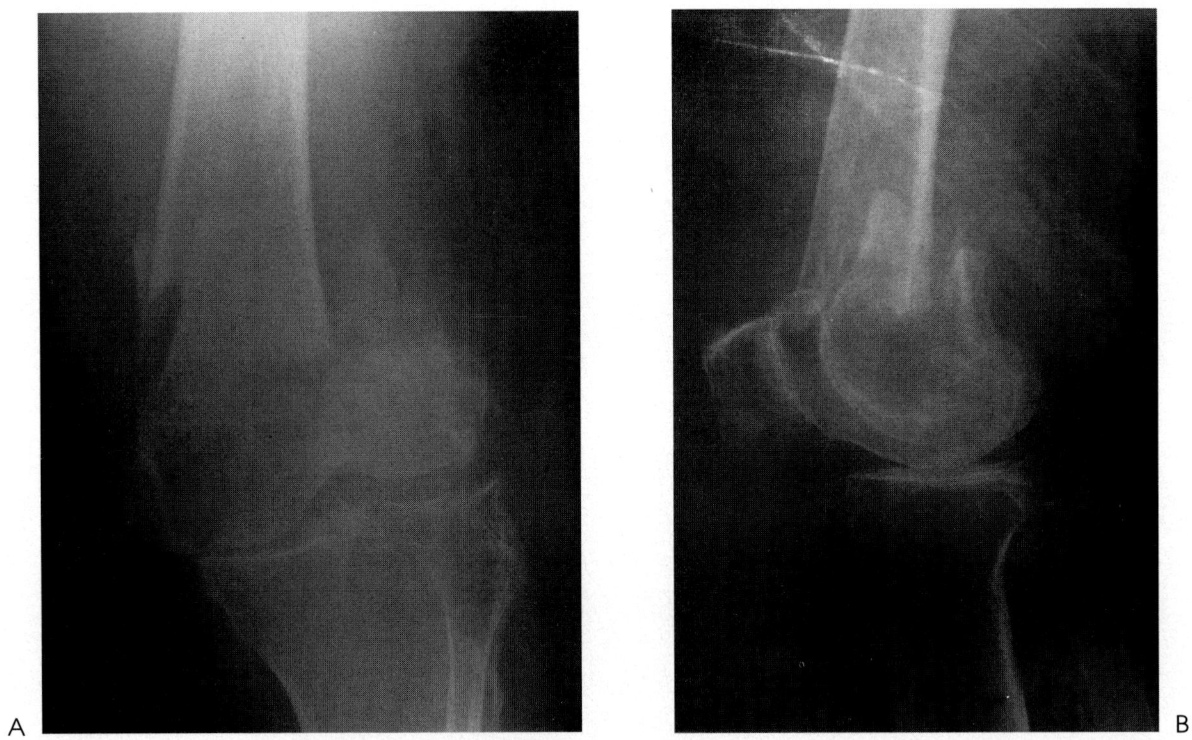

Figure 14–1. Anteroposterior (A) and lateral (B) radiographs of an osteoporotic supracondylar femoral fracture.

Radiologic Findings

Anteroposterior and lateral radiographs showed a supracondylar femoral fracture with some metaphyseal comminution (Fig. 14–1). The bone was obviously very osteoporotic. The anteroposterior radiograph demonstrated some osteoarthritic change in the knee that particularly affected the medial compartment. The lateral radiograph indicated that the diaphysis was displaced anteriorly in relation to the metaphysis and that there was patellofemoral osteoarthritis.

PEARLS

- In a busy trauma unit it can often be difficult to assess the degree of social dependence of the elderly fit patient. A useful simple question concerns their ability to do their own shopping. If they can it should be assumed that they are fit and they should be treated appropriately.
- Supracondylar fractures in the elderly may often have an occult intercondylar component. If retrograde nailing is proposed the surgeon should be aware of this possibility and obtain appropriate preoperative radiographs or scans.
- To ensure that the locking screws are through the nail, the nail is scanned flouroscopically at the conclusion of the procedure. In the lateral projection, when the leg is rotated so that only the profile of the nail is seen on flouroscopy (i.e., the head or leading end of the screw is not visualized), then the surgeon has confirmed that the screw is through the nail.

PITFALL

- Careful inspection of the postoperative anteroposterior radiograph shows that the lowest interlocking screw has not been placed through the nail. At first sight the screw looked satisfactory on both anteroposterior and lateral views but on the anteroposterior view it can be seen that the screw is in fact lying below the waist in the nail that represents the location of the screw hole. On the lateral view the screw is lying diagonally and does look to be through the nail.

Diagnosis

Displaced supracondylar femoral fracture with some minor metaphyseal comminution. AO classification: 33–A1.2 fracture.

Surgical Management

This is a very difficult fracture to treat. In this case a decision was made to use a supracondylar femoral nail to stabilize the fracture. The knee was prepped and draped and flexed to 90 degrees. A small midline incision was made just below the inferior pole of the patella. Digital examination indicated the position of the intercondylar notch and a bone awl was used to make the appropriate entry point. A guide wire was inserted after closed reduction of the fracture, the femur was reamed, and subsequently a supracondylar nail was inserted and locked proximally and distally using two screws proximally and distally. Postoperative radiographs (Fig. 14–2) showed that a good position had been achieved on the anteroposterior radiograph, but that the femoral shaft was still anterior to the

A

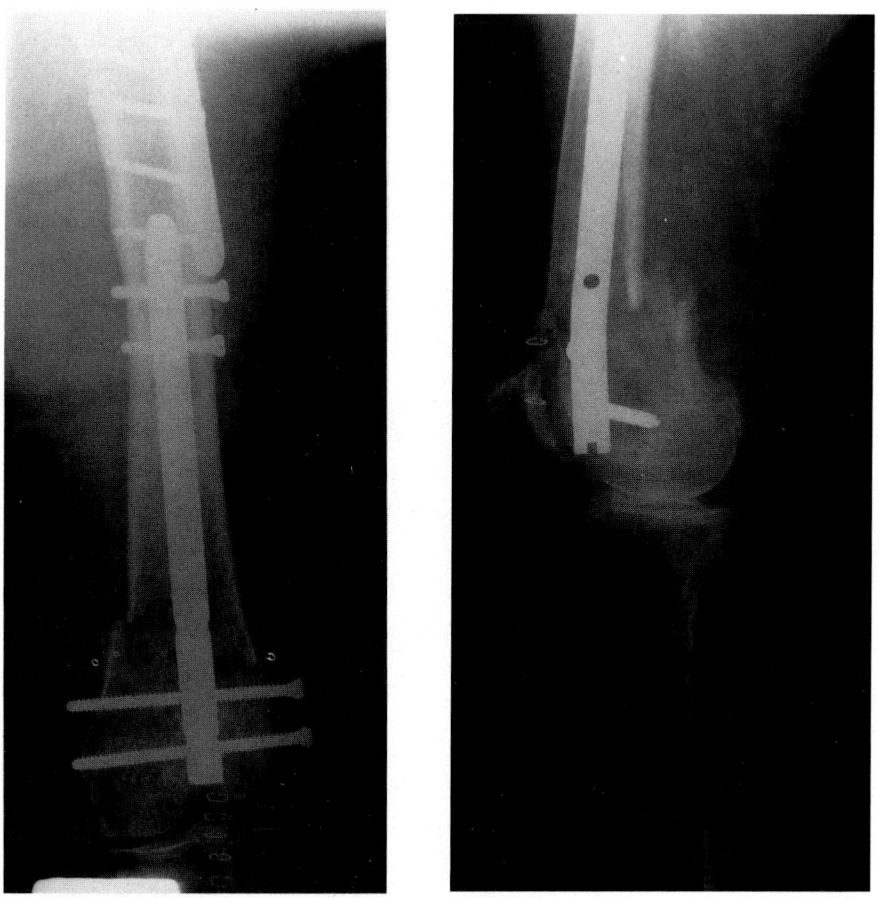

B

Figure 14–2. Fixation is with a supracondylar nail; anteroposterior (A) and lateral (B) views. The fracture is not adequately reduced and the lowest cross screw has missed the nail.

PITFALL

- It can be surprisingly difficult to decide whether a supracondylar femoral fracture in an elderly patient has an intercondylar component. In the elderly many of these fractures are low energy injuries and there is little, if any, displacement of the condylar fragments. Failure to diagnose an intercondylar component may lead to difficulties with retrograde nailing.

condylar fragment on the lateral radiograph. Because of the residual anterior displacement the nail had been placed into the anterior part of the condylar fragment. The surgeon recognized that the fixation was poor and protected the fixation in a knee brace. The patient was also mobilized nonweight bearing to lessen the forces acting on the fracture.

Postoperative Management

Unfortunately, despite the use of a knee brace and the nonweight bearing status of the patient, radiographs taken 2 weeks after the initial surgery indicated that the fracture fixation had failed (Fig. 14–3). The nail had cut out through the anterior cortex of the condylar fragment and even the correctly placed distal interlocking screw had cut through the bone. The fracture had also shortened.

The patient was returned to the operating room and the supracondylar nail and cross screws were removed. A condylar screw and side plate were applied with autogenous bone graft being used to fill the small medial defect. The side plate had to be cut to prevent overlap with the previously inserted hip plate. The postoperative radiograph showed an iatrogenic fracture of the distal femoral diaphysis that was stabilized by the plate and screws (Fig. 14–4).

Postoperatively the knee was braced for several weeks and the patient remained nonweight bearing. The fracture healed in good alignment (Fig. 14–5) and the patient required 60 degrees of knee flexion after 3 months and 90 degrees of flexion after 1 year.

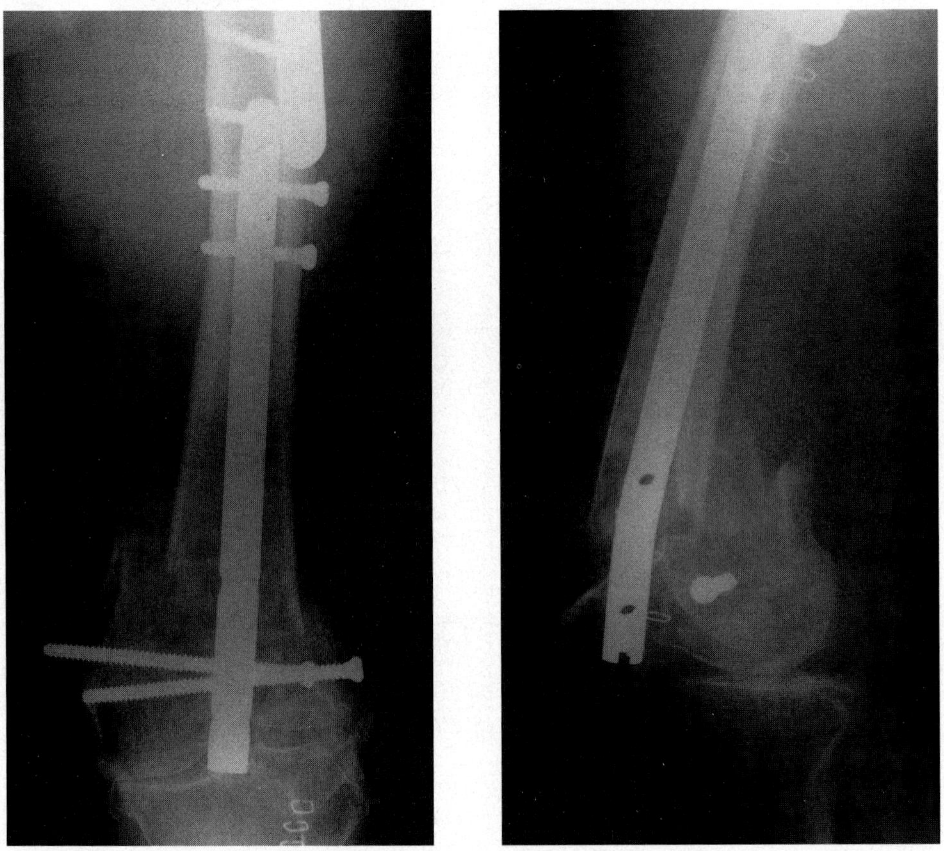

A B

Figure 14–3. The nail and screws have cut out of the bone. Anteroposterior (A) and lateral (B) views.

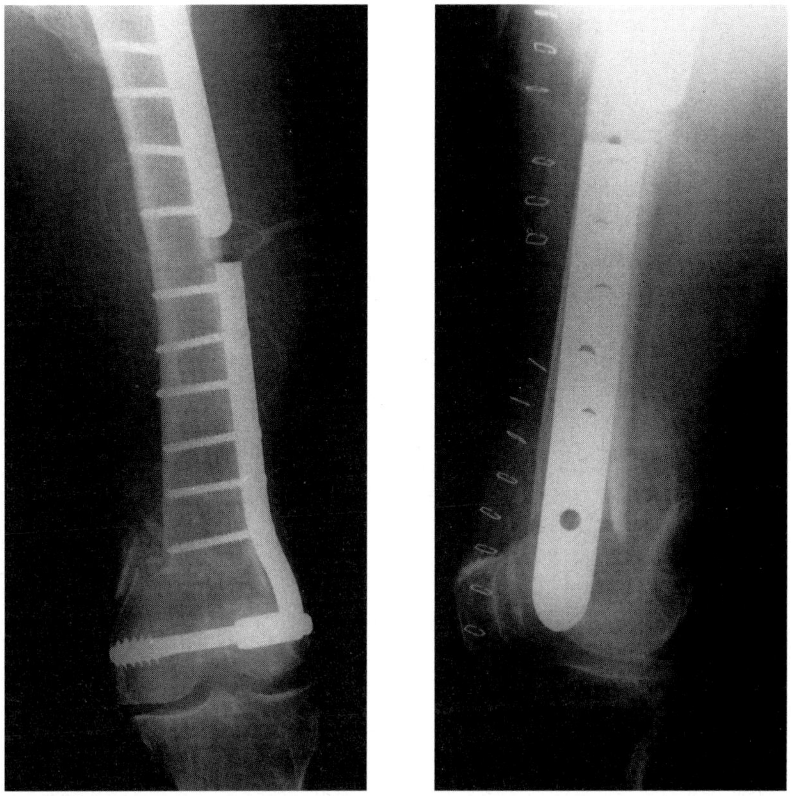

A B

Figure 14–4. A supracondylar screw and side plate have been used to stabilize the fracture. Anteroposterior (A) and lateral (B) views.

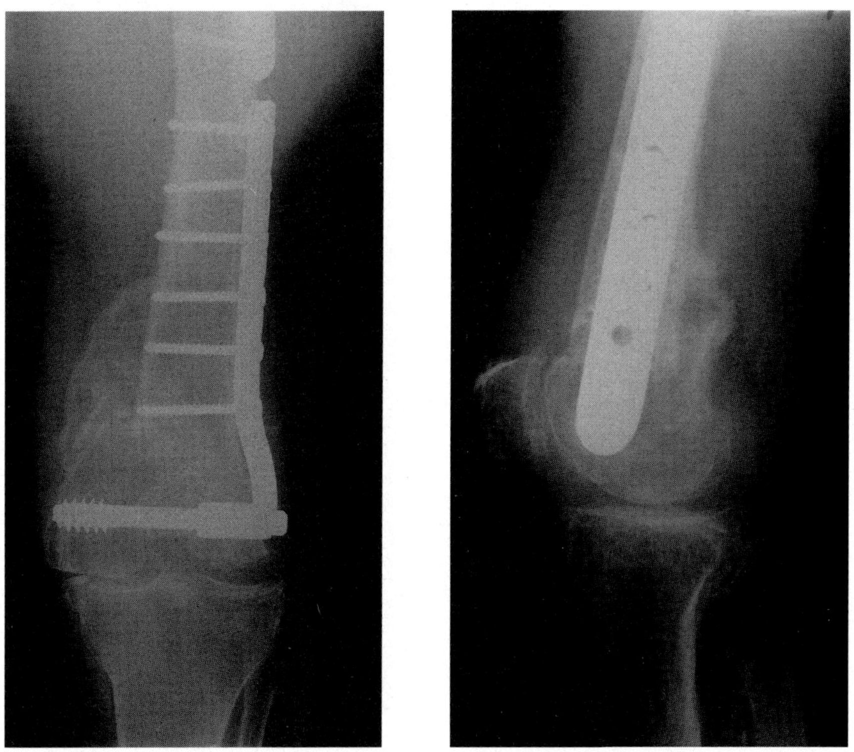

A B

Figure 14–5. Successful union was achieved, anteroposterior (A) and lateral (B) views.

Discussion

Fractures in the elderly are assuming considerable clinical and economic importance. Elderly patients tend to be medically fitter than in previous years and demand good surgical treatment so that they can regain optimal function. However, the bone in very elderly patients is extremely osteoporotic and fixation failure is common. For this reason a case of failed fracture fixation has been selected to illustrate the management of this difficult fracture. Supracondylar femoral fractures are relatively common. Like other fractures they follow a typical bimodal distribution. They occur either in young people as a result of high energy trauma or in the elderly population usually following low energy trauma. A relatively high proportion occur in elderly people and a review of the Edinburgh database indicates that 50% of all supracondylar fractures in the population are over the age of 70 years and 36% are over the age of 80 years.

Unfortunately there is no one method of treating these fractures that will guarantee success. The use of traction in the very elderly is to be avoided because it leads to the consequences of immobility. Surgeons often refer to the physical consequences of immobility including bed sores, pneumonia, urinary infection, renal calculi, and increased osteoporotic change. In reality, however, it is the psychological consequences of prolonged immobilization that not infrequently prove detri-

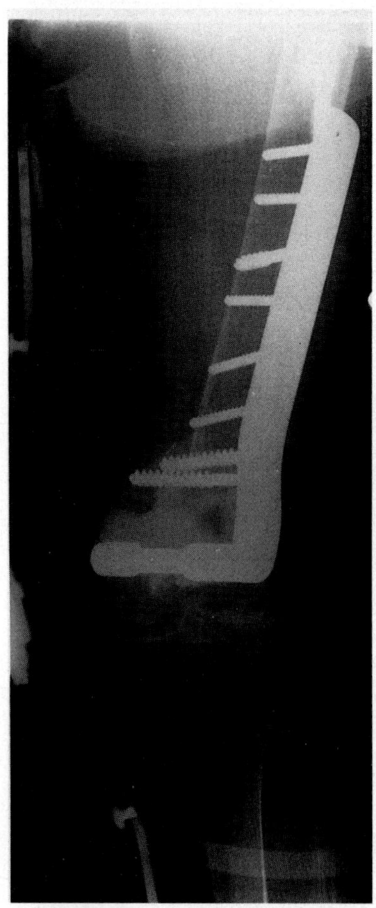

Figure 14–6. The use of bone cement to enhance bone fixation.

mental, or even fatal, to the patient. Once an elderly patient is confined to a hospital for a prolonged period they often lose their independence and become dependent on the hospital system. Most surgeons have now abandoned nonoperative management for these fractures. Unfortunately most of the literature dealing with the surgical management of supracondylar fractures considers patients who are usually less than 60 years of age and whose bone is therefore of much better quality.

In uncomplicated supracondylar fractures in younger patients most surgeons would either use a 95 degrees blade plate or a condylar screw and side plate like those eventually used in this patient. These implants are associated with good results in the younger patient. In recent years surgeons have adopted intramedullary nailing for the management of diaphyseal femoral fractures in older patients and both antegrade and retrograde nailing techniques can be used to treat supracondylar fractures. In this case the use of an antegrade nail would have been difficult because of the presence of the proximal hip screw and side plate and the distal location of the fracture. Thus retrograde nailing was selected. Both antegrade and retrograde nailing are technically difficult procedures when used in the management of supracondylar femoral fractures. The fixation gained by both antegrade and retrograde nailing is purely dependent on the adequacy of the fixation of the distal blocking bolts in the osteoporotic metaphyseal bone and therefore it is inevitable that some fixation will fail.

If closed nailing techniques are to be used, it is important to reduce the fracture to prevent the complication illustrated in this case. However, even good reduction might not prevent the nail from cutting out of the osteoporotic bone. Supracondylar nailing is a relatively new technique and the instrumentation is still being refined. Thus failure of the interlocking screws to penetrate the nail does occur from time to time and the surgeon should be aware of this.

Plating of fractures in the elderly is also associated with several problems. Screw cutout is fairly common and surgeons not infrequently use bone cement to improve the fixation of the condylar screw in the condyles. An example of this is shown in Figure 14–6. An 84-year-old woman had a supracondylar fracture below a hip prosthesis. A condylar screw and side plate was used and good stability achieved. The fracture healed without displacement. If bone cement is to be used, every attempt must be made to place a reasonable amount of cement in the condyles. A thin film of cement is of little value. Cement can also be used to enhance the diaphyseal screws if required.

Alternative Methods of Management

External Fixation

External fixation can be used to treat supracondylar femoral fractures and examples of two cases where its use was indicated are presented in this book. In general, however, external fixation has the same problem as internal fixation, namely, pin failure. The osteoporotic bone does not hold external fixation pins well and pin sepsis and loosening are not uncommon. If external fixation is to be used for fractures in osteoporotic bone, it is advisable to use a rigid triangular frame utilizing half pins or a small wire frame. However, both techniques are likely to result in knee stiffness. External skeletal fixation is rarely indicated in the management of elderly osteoporotic supracondylar femoral fractures.

Arthroplasty

It is perhaps surprising that more use has not been made of knee arthroplasty to treat supracondylar and intercondylar fractures in the elderly population. The fact that 36% of supracondylar fractures occur in patients of over 80 years of age who often have limited goals and a limited life expectancy suggests that this method of management may be useful. Bell et al. (1992) published the results of a series of 14 arthroplasties used to treat supracondylar and intercondylar femoral fractures in a group of female patients whose average age was 84 years. All but one patient had significant medical problems and 78% of the patients had significant coexisting rheumatoid arthritis or osteoarthritis. Eleven of the 13 patients reviewed returned to their original level of independence in the community within 12 weeks of the operation. All the patients regained full extension and mean knee flexion at 6 months was 80 degrees. Only one patient returned with a significant complication, which was a fracture around the femoral stem of the hinged arthroplasty 5 years after it was inserted. It was successfully treated by the insertion of another hinged arthroplasty.

Clearly, more work is required to evaluate the usefulness of primary arthroplasty in the management of these difficult fractures, but it is likely that as our patient population gets older arthroplasty will be adopted as a useful treatment method. An example of the use of a hinged arthroplasty is shown in Figure 14–7. It illustrates an intercondylar fracture in an 86-year-old woman treated by primary hinge arthroplasty. Postoperative weight bearing was allowed on the third postoperative day and the patient had returned to her nursing home 8 days after surgery. She mobilized well and resumed her normal activities. She died of unrelated causes two years after the surgery.

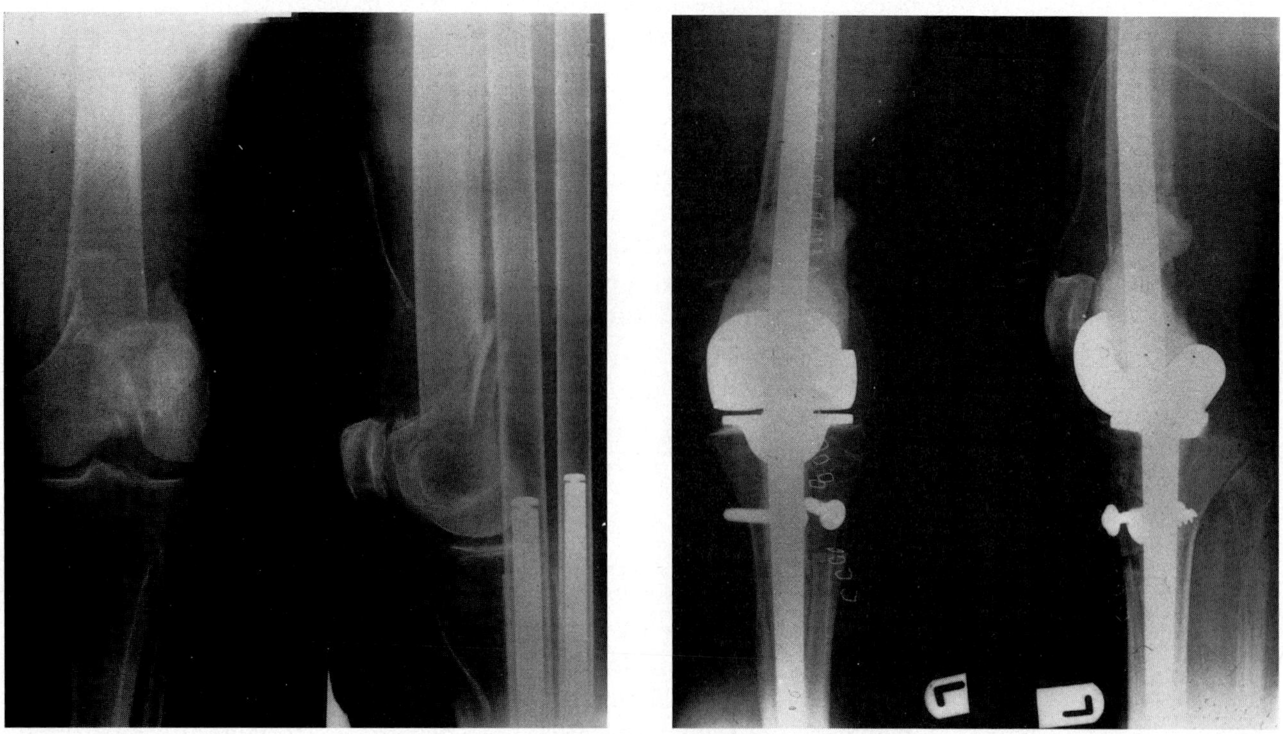

A B

Figure 14–7. An intercondylar fracture in an elderly patient (A). A successful result after hinged arthroplasty (B).

Type of Management	Advantages	Disadvantages	Comments
Casting and traction	None	Prolonged immobility; malunion; nonunion; joint stiffness; psychological dependence	This is not a suitable technique for elderly patients unless operative fixation is impossible
Plating	May permit early joint motion if the bone is of reasonable quality	A difficult technique in osteoporotic bone; patient may require supplementary bone cement to secure fixation	Despite potential disadvantages, probably the best method available. The surgeon should be aware of the requirement for bone cement and also that knee movement and patient mobility may be restricted for some considerable period after surgery
Intramedullary nailing	Small skin incision; less soft tissue damage; in good bone may allow early joint motion	Technically difficult; antegrade nailing may be impossible because of proximal implants; pin tract sepsis	Retrograde supracondylar nailing is a technique gaining in popularity. Surgeons should not forget that the essential problem is the quality of the bone, not the implant itself
External fixation	Technically straightforward	If an appropriately rigid frame is used, joint stiffness is inevitable; difficult to wear; pin tract sepsis	External skeletal fixation is not easily tolerated in the elderly and the pins are likely to cut out of the osteoporotic bone.
Arthroplasty	Potentially a very useful technique in elderly patients; early mobility; good results	Salvage surgery very difficult; potential for infection	Probably will become a more important technique in the future. A hinged prosthesis is required as the collateral ligaments are removed

Complications

The most important complication of treating supracondylar or intercondylar femoral fractures in the elderly is failure of the implant to hold the bone fragments. The osteoporotic nature of the bone means that all implants are liable to fail. To prevent this, the surgeon may brace the knee postoperatively and keep the patient nonweight bearing, but the incidence of fixation failure remains high. If the primary implant fails to hold the fracture, further surgery using a different technique is advocated. If this fails, or secondary surgery is impossible, nonoperative management may be the only alternative. However, the physical and psychological consequences of this are considerable.

The surgeon should always bear in mind that a proximal femoral implant may have already been inserted. This is usually either a hip screw and side plate inserted for proximal femoral fracture or an arthroplasty inserted for osteoarthritis or rheumatoid arthritis. Under these conditions the use of a distal implant, whether an intramedullary nail or a condylar screw and side plate, will cause a stress riser in the short bone length between the implants. This is of particular importance in elderly bone and it is not uncommon for the surgeon to have to treat a third fracture between the two implants, which can be extremely difficult. There is often little that can be done about the presence of a stress riser, but the surgeon should always bear in mind that a third fracture in the femur is a possibility.

The other problems associated with the supracondylar or intercondylar fracture in the elderly are usually malunion, because of the difficulty in securing bone fixation, nonunion, and infection. Osteoarthritis may occur, but many of the patients who will be treated already have arthritic knee joints and the fact that these patients are very elderly and have limited functional goals means that arthroplasty is only infrequently required.

Malunion should be avoided by careful surgery, adequate radiological examination, and reoperation as necessary. However, if malunion does occur, it is usually wise to accept the malunion unless it is particularly severe. In this group of patients osteotomy is difficult and a slight malunion is unlikely to lead to significant secondary problems.

Infection is a particular problem in the very elderly patient and if a severe infection occurs, it may well lead to amputation. Thus any infection should be treated aggressively with debridement and antibiotics, but if a septic arthritis or significant osteomyelitis occurs, consideration should always be given to amputation.

Suggested Readings

Bell K, Johnston A, Court CM, Hughes SPF: Primary knee arthroplasty for distal femoral fractures in elderly patients. J Bone Joint Surg (Br) 1992; 74B:400–402.

Benum P: The use of bone cement as an adjunct to internal fixation of supracondylar fractures of osteoporotic femurs. Acta Orthop Scand 1977; 48:52–56.

Firoozbakhsh K, DeCoster TA, Moneim MS, Naraghi FF: Mechanics of retrograde nail versus plate fixation for supracondylar femur fractures. J Orthop Trauma 1995; 9:152–157.

Healy WL, Siliski JM, Incavo SJ: Operative treatment of distal femoral fractures proximal to knee replacements. J Bone Joint Surg (Am) 1993; 75A:27–34.

Mize RD: Surgical management of complex fractures of the distal end of the femur. Clin Orthop 1989; 240:77–86.

Seligson D, Malkani AL (eds): Supracondylar femur fractures. Techniques in Orthopaedics. 1994; 9.

Case 15

History and Physical Examination

A 19-year-old male was the driver of a motorcycle involved in a collision with an automobile. Following the accident he was unable to walk and was taken to the emergency department. Examination showed that he had a swollen painful right knee with a skin graze overlying the lateral side of the joint. The graze did not communicate with the joint. There was no other injury and examination of the right leg showed normal neurovascular function.

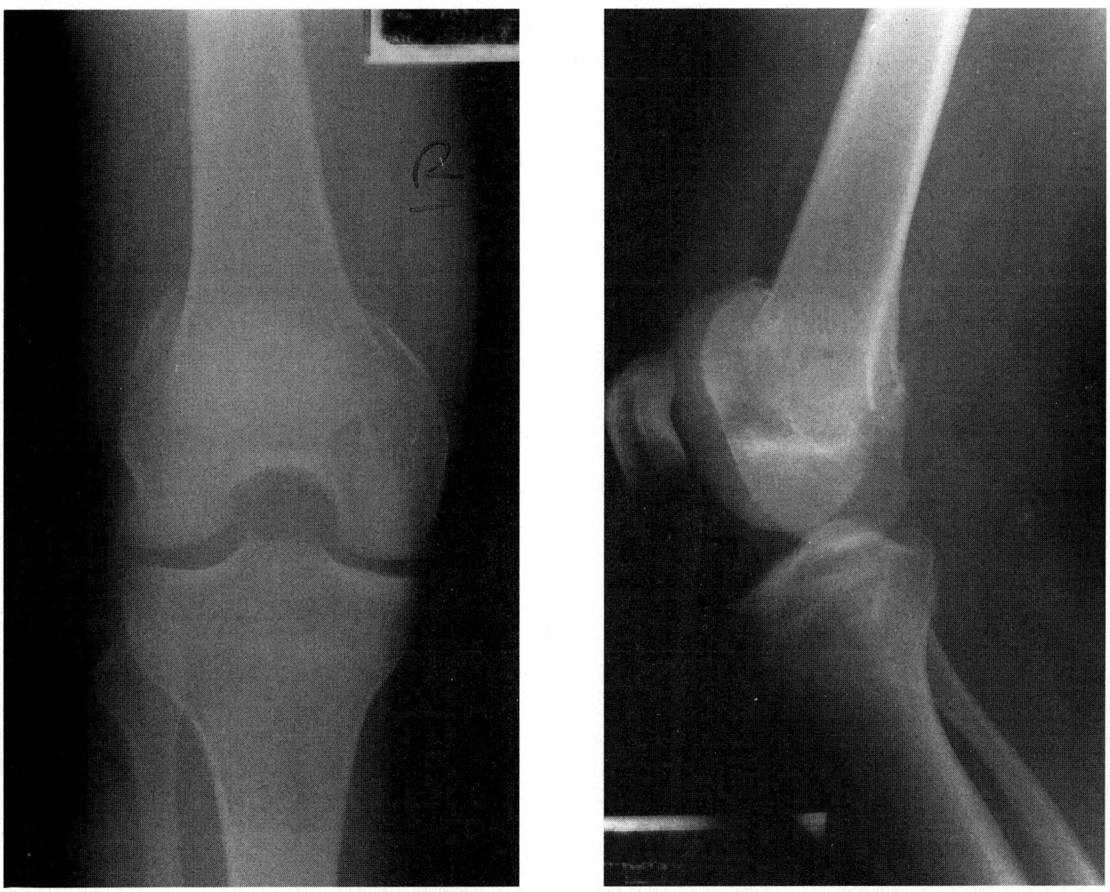

A B

Figure 15–1. Anteroposterior radiograph of the distal femur (A). The overall alignment is apparently good but this appearance of the distal femur is normally seen with the knee in flexion. The lateral and medial bone fragments are also abnormal. The lateral radiograph shows a rotational malalignment of the distal femur (B). Both condyles are split in the coronal plane.

Radiologic Findings

Anteroposterior and lateral radiographs showed an intercondylar fracture of the right distal femur (Fig. 15–1). A cursory examination of the anteroposterior radiograph (Fig. 15–1A) suggests that the distal femur looks relatively normal but closer

PITFALL

- This case illustrates the importance of reading the initial X rays correctly. A superficial examination of the anteroposterior radiograph might have suggested nonoperative management. Close inspection indicates that this would be a poor method of managing this fracture.

PEARL

- The goal of this type of internal fixation is rigid fracture fixation to allow early joint movement. A single plate would have reduced the fracture but not allowed early movement.

inspection shows that the intercondylar notch is deeper than normal and resembles the appearance of the notch on a radiograph taken with the knee in flexion. Bone is also seen on each side of the femoral condyle. The reasons for these appearance are obvious when the lateral radiograph is inspected (Fig. 15–1B). This radiograph shows that the condyles are facing forward and that the posterior part of the femoral condyles is articulating with the tibial plateau. Both femoral condyles are split in the coronal plane.

Diagnosis

A closed intercondylar femoral fracture with significant displacement of the articular surfaces. This fracture is not easily classified with the AO system. Impaction is not recognized in conventional classifications but equating impaction with comminution suggests that this is a 33–C2.3 fracture.

Surgical Management

The initial management was splintage to reduce movement of the fracture site, thereby relieving pain and minimizing further soft tissue and bone damage. On the

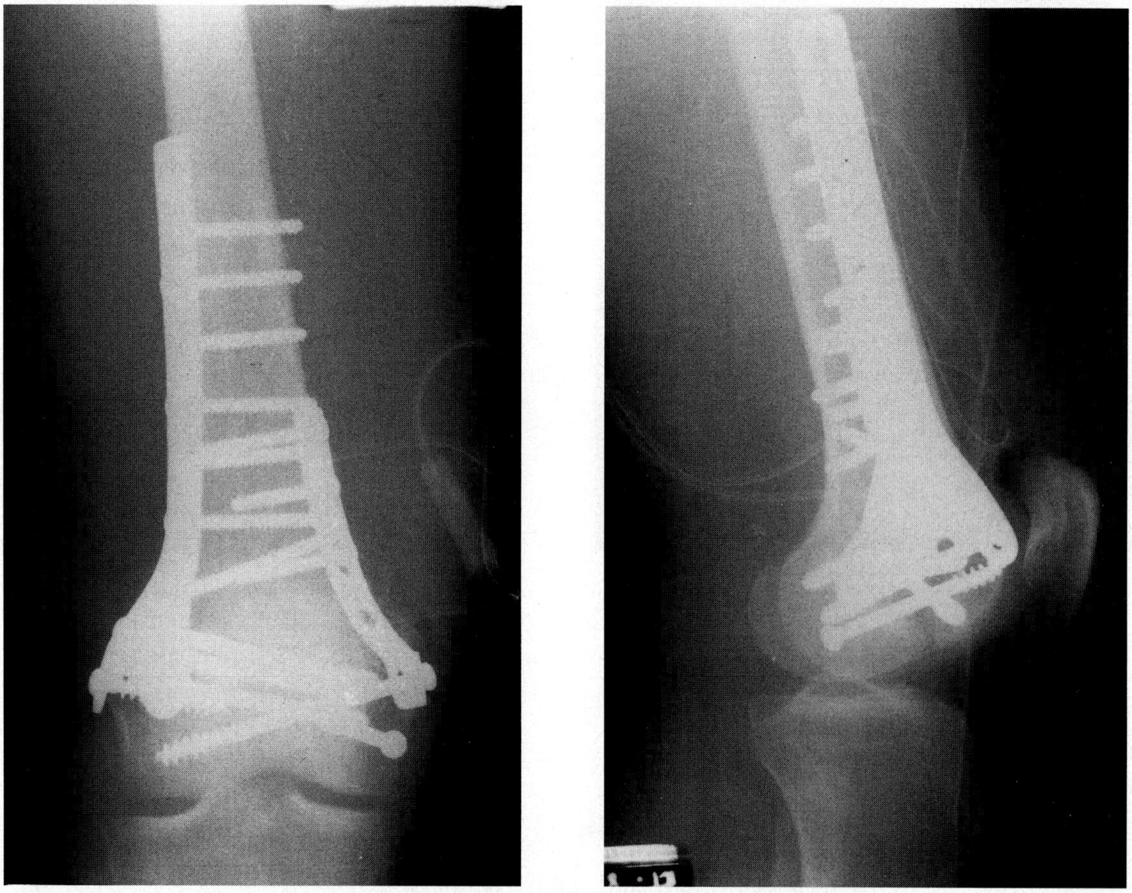

A B

Figure 15–2. Anteroposterior (A) and lateral (B) postoperative radiographs show that excellent alignment has been achieved. The lateral view confirms that the joint surface has been reconstructed.

PITFALL

- In retrospect, the lateral radiograph (Fig. 15–1B) does suggest the possibility of some metaphyseal impaction because there is a bone defect noted in the area of the coronal condylar fracture. It would have been sensible to prepare the iliac crest preoperatively rather than perioperatively and, where possible, the surgeon should always do this. It is of course possible to prepare the iliac crest perioperatively, but that constitutes a break in surgical technique and, if undertaken, prophylactic antibiotics should be given.

day after the accident the patient was taken to the operating room and after prepping and draping the fracture was exposed through a long anterior midline incision. The patella was dislocated laterally to allow exposure of the condyles and once the knee was flexed a good view of the medial and lateral condyles was obtained. The findings of the preoperative X-rays were confirmed. The condyles had rotated almost 90 degrees and there was a coronal fracture of both the medial and lateral condyles. The two halves of the medial condyle were significantly displaced, but the articular surface over the lateral condyles was virtually intact; the lateral condyle had hinged, with the intact articular cartilage acting as the fulcrum. It was also noted that the metaphyseal bone in the condyles had been compressed by the force of the injury and that after reduction of the fracture there was a large defect in the metaphysis.

The coronal fracture in the medial condyle was reduced and stabilized with a cancellous bone screw. This resulted in reduction of the coronal fracture in the lateral condyle. The condyles were then repositioned by rotating them posteriorly and the impaction defect in the metaphysis was filled with a tricortical bone block and supplementary cancellous bone chips taken from the ipsilateral iliac crest. Because the requirement for bone grafting had not been determined preoperatively the iliac crest had to be prepped and draped peri-operatively.

After the tricortical bone block was inserted and the condyles reduced on the metaphysis, a lateral condylar buttress plate was applied and the distal screws were placed anteromedially and posteromedially into the two halves of the medial

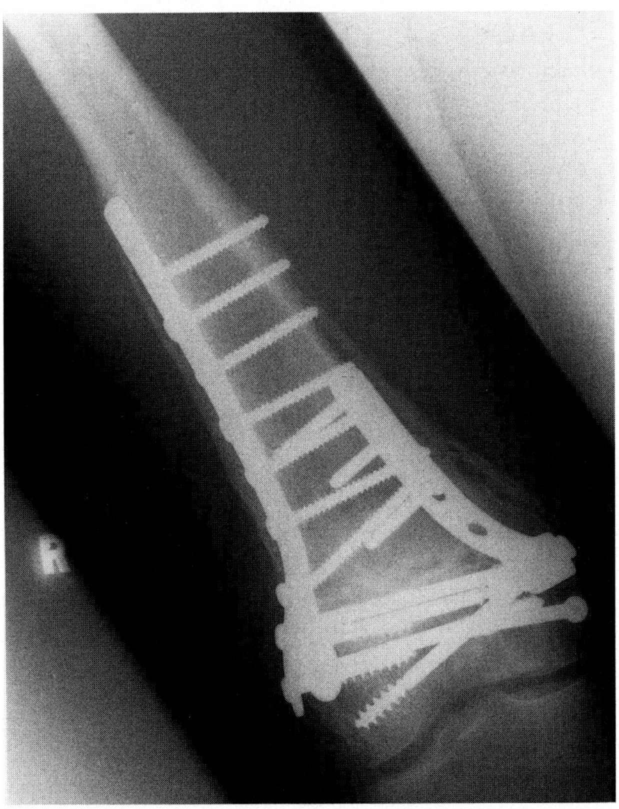

A

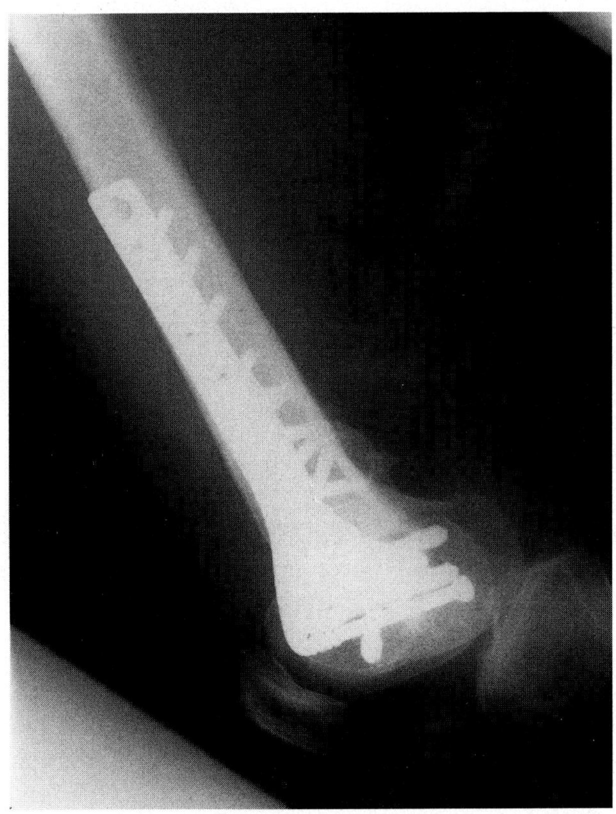

B

Figure 15–3. Anteroposterior (A) and lateral (B) views of the knee 9 months post-injury show good union. The patient had excellent function. The plates were not removed.

condyle. This resulted in improved stabilization of the two medial condylar fragments. After the condylar buttress plate had been applied it was noted that there was some residual movement at the fracture site and a supplementary medial buttress plate was therefore applied to ensure rigid fixation. The lowest screw in this plate was placed into the posterior part of the lateral condyle. Good fracture stability was achieved and postoperative radiographs were satisfactory (Fig. 15–2).

Postoperative Management

Postoperatively the right leg was placed on a knee mobilizer to facilitate knee flexion. The patient's rehabilitation was complicated by a deep venous thrombosis that was successfully treated by anticoagulants; a physiotherapy regime was instituted after a few days. The patient had an extensor lag of 20 degrees after 3 months but by 9 months he had full extension and 130 degrees of flexion with no pain and virtually normal function. Radiographs at that time showed good union (Fig. 15–3).

Alternative Methods of Management

There is no place for nonoperative management of this fracture. It would be impossible to reduce the coronal condylar fracture and maintain alignment of the condyles on the metaphysis without internal fixation. Failure to reduce and fix this fracture would virtually guarantee posttraumatic osteoarthritis, malunion, and joint stiffness. Intramedullary nailing would be impossible in this case. The two alternative options are to use another form of plating or external skeletal fixation. The preoperative radiographs highlight the difficulty of using a 95 degree blade plate because the central metaphyseal bone where the blade would be placed is deficient. A single lateral condylar buttress plate was used initially in this case, but did not provide adequate function.

External skeletal fixation would be extremely difficult in view of the small size of the condyles. The main fracture is a very low supracondylar fracture and unlike

Type of Management	Advantages	Disadvantages	Comments
Casting and traction	None	Joint stiffness; malunion; osteoarthritis	There is no place for nonoperative management of this fracture
Intramedullary nailing	None	Impossible	This technique cannot be used in this fracture
Plating	Rigid fixation; early joint motion; good fracture reduction; reduced incidence of osteoarthritis	A higher rate of infection; technically difficult	This is the treatment of choice for this fracture; two plates are required because of the position of the supracondylar fracture
External fixation	None	Technically difficult; a small wire fixator would be required; joint stiffness; pin tract sepsis; risk of septic arthritis	Technically possible if a small wire external fixator is used but would represent a triumph of technique over reason

other cases in this book in which external fixation was used it would be difficult to achieve any bone stability unless a small wire fixator was employed. It would be difficult to place multiple small wires in this small supracondylar fragment without transgressing the articular surface; in addition, if adequate stability was to be achieved using an external fixator, wires or pins would have to be placed through the thigh musculature, resulting in joint stiffness.

Complications

In any operation that requires a large amount of soft tissue dissection there is a risk of sepsis. This is avoided by meticulous adherence to surgical technique, but, if it occurs, it should be treated by debridement and the use of high dose antibiotics. Every attempt should be made to maintain the plate fixation unless loosening of the plate occurs, in which case external fixation would probably be employed. Given the low location of the supracondylar fracture, infection might well lead to septic arthritis and the prognosis would be poor.

The other obvious complication of this type of fracture is posttraumatic osteoarthritis. Fortunately, the intraarticular component was relatively straightforward. There was only minor articular damage and osteoarthritis did not ensue. The patient was reviewed at 5 years after the injury and it was noted that there was no osteoarthritic changes in the knee joint. If osteoarthritis had occurred in a young male, it would be treated by nonsteroidal antiinflammatories, occasional intraarticular steroid injections, and arthroscopic washouts. Knee arthroplasty or arthrodesis should be avoided as long as possible.

Given adequate primary management, the incidence of malunion and nonunion could reasonably be expected to be low in this fracture. If a malunion occurred, it would have to be treated by osteotomy and plating; if a nonunion occurred, it would be treated by corticocancellous bone grafting.

Suggested Readings

Gellman RE, Paiement GD, Green HD, Coughlin RR: Treatment of supracondylar femoral fractures with a retrograde intramedullary nail. Clin Orthop 1996; 332:90–97.

Giles JB, DeLee J, Heckman J, Keever JE: Intracondylar fractures of the femur treated with a supracondylar plate and lag screw. J Bone Joint Surg (Am) 1982; 64A:864–870.

Helfet DL: Fractures of the distal femur. In Browner BD, Jupiter JB, Levine AM, Trafton PG (eds): Skeletal Trauma, pp 1643–1683. Vol 2. WB Saunders, Philadelphia, 1992.

Sanders R, Swiontkowski MF, Rosen H, Helfet DL: Double plating of comminuted unstable fractures of the distal part of the femur. J Bone Joint Surg (Am) 1991; 73A:341–346.

Schatzker J, Lambert DC: Supracondylar fractures of the femur. Clin Orthop 1979; 138:77–83.

Seligson D, Malkani AL (eds): Supracondylar fractures. Techniques in Orthopaedic. 1194; 9(3).

Case 16

History and Physical Examination

A 53-year-old man was driving a car that was involved in a traffic accident. His injuries were an undisplaced fracture of his left scaphoid and a right supracondylar femoral fracture with an undisplaced intraarticular extension. He was a known hemophiliac with a Factor VIII inhibitor. He was HIV negative but hepatitis C positive. Adequate examination of the right knee was impossible, but the patient stated that he normally had a block to full extension of 20 degrees with a flexion arc of 20 to 50 degrees only. The neurovascular status of the leg was normal.

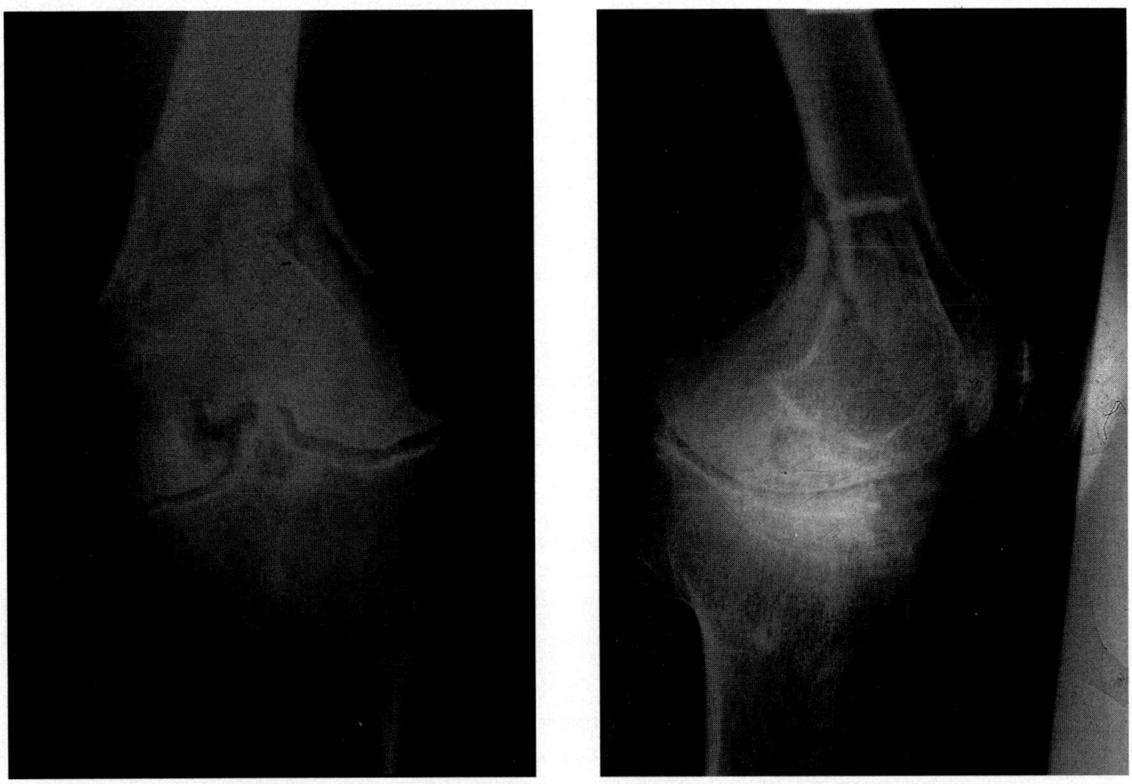

A B

Figure 16–1. Anteroposterior (A) and lateral (B) radiographs of a supracondylar femoral fracture with an undisplaced intercondylar extension. There is marked hemophilic arthropathy.

Radiologic Findings

Anteroposterior and lateral radiographs (Fig. 16–1) confirmed the presence of a comminuted supracondylar femoral fracture with an undisplaced intraarticular extension. There were obvious signs of a severe hemophilic arthropathy secondary to recurrent hemarthroses.

PEARL

- Surgeons often become preoccupied about the minutiae of different implants and lose sight of the established principles of fracture treatment. This is certainly true of external fixation and the literature is full of papers extolling the virtues of particular fixators, often on flimsy evidence. In this case the type of external fixator used by the surgeon does not matter as much as the requirement to avoid muscle penetration and bleeding and to preserve knee motion.

PITFALL

- Care must be taken in the insertion of external fixator pins close to joints. Ideally not only must they miss the local nerves and blood vessels but they should also be placed so as to minimize the penetration of the gliding tissues around the joint to maximize joint movement.

Diagnosis

A comminuted supracondylar fracture with an intercondylar extension in a severe hemophiliac. AO classification: 33–C2.3 fracture.

Surgical Management

Because the patient was known to have an inhibitor to Factor VIII, he was treated with Feiba preoperatively. Several therapeutic options were considered. It was clearly desirable to avoid open surgery and the obvious alternative was nonoperative management in a long-leg cast. This alternative was seriously considered in the belief that because he already limited knee flexion the loss of a few more degrees of movement might not prove troublesome. It was thought that a secondary arthroplasty could be performed if necessary. However, the patient pointed out that his knee was painless and he did not wish to have an arthroplasty that, given his hematological status, might be a very difficult operation. He also stated that the 20 to 50 degrees of flexion allowed him to drive and if he lost this movement, his mobility would be seriously impaired.

It was therefore decided to externally fix the fracture and surgeons considered which external fixator configuration would be optimal. Conventional unilateral configuration utilizing half pins in the condyles and the femoral diaphysis would lead to muscle penetration that would increase the likelihood of troublesome bleeding and virtually ensure knee stiffness. The same argument applied to the use of small wire external fixation and it was therefore decided to use a half ring and half pin configuration around the condyles, with the proximal pins being placed in the greater trochanter. This configuration minimized the amount of muscle dissection and therefore decreased the risk of bleeding and increased the potential for knee movement. The external fixator is shown in Figure 16–2. Before the fixator was ap-

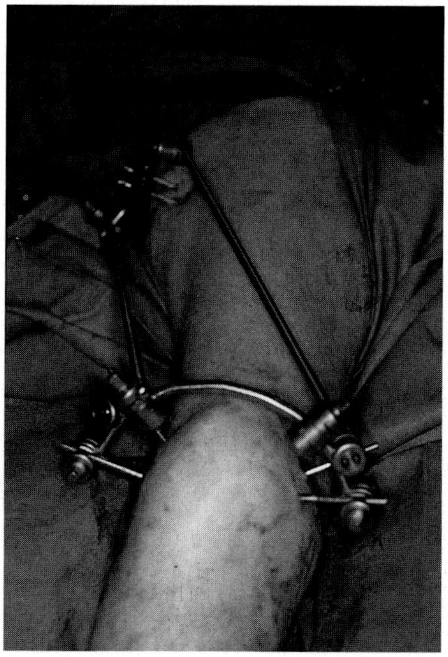

Figure 16–2. The external fixator used to stabilize this fracture. The distal pins are in the distal femoral fragment; the proximal pins are in the greater trochanter.

PITFALL

- This case illustrates the importance of taking an adequate history and acting appropriately. The easiest method of management would be the application of a long-leg cast but loss of only 30 degrees of knee movement would have rendered the patient virtually housebound. Consultation between the orthopedic surgeon and the hematologist permitted the use of external fixation and allowed the maintenance of knee movement.

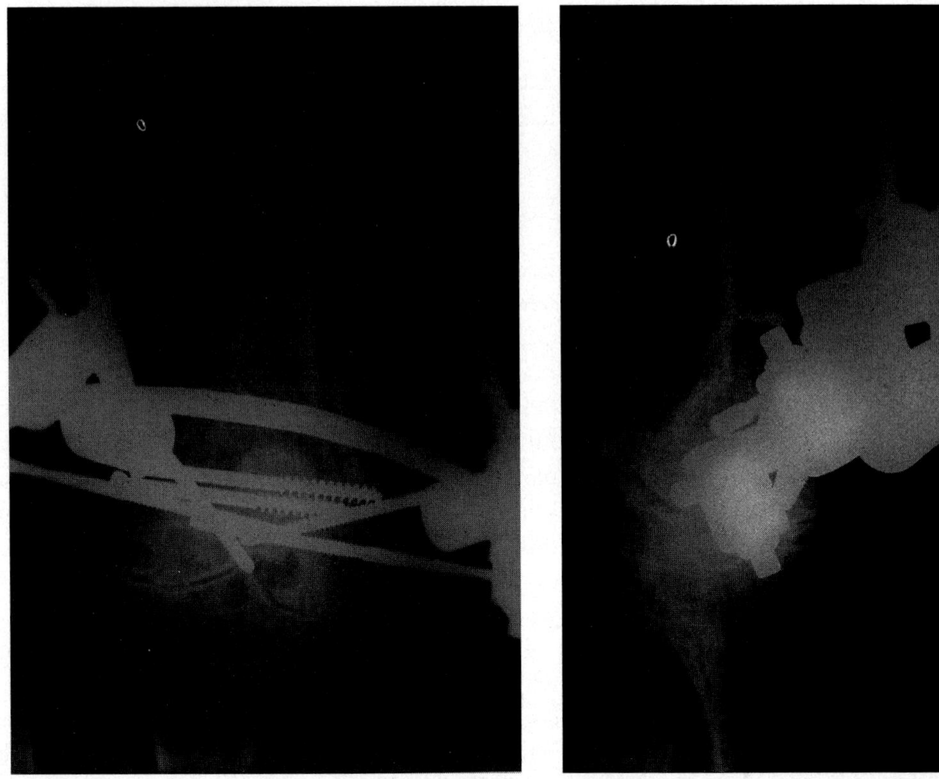

A B

Figure 16–3. Anteroposterior (A) and lateral (B) postoperative radiographs show that a good position was achieved.

plied, two interfragmentary screws were used to fix the femoral condyles. These were inserted under fluoroscopy. Postoperative radiographs showed a good reduction (Fig. 16–3).

Postoperative Management

The external fixation device was maintained for 12 weeks until fracture union occurred (Fig. 16–4). Physiotherapy was employed throughout the period of external fixation and in the postoperative period. One year after union the patient had flexion from 20 to 40 degrees and had lost about 10 degrees of flexion. He was, however, able to drive and had no other functional impairment. Radiographs showed the fracture to have united in a good position.

Discussion

This case represents a very unusual problem with a high energy injury occurring in a hemophiliac who has an inhibitor to Factor VIII. Hemophiliacs rarely present with fractures, but there are other more common coagulopathies that orthopaedic surgeons may encounter. Today many patients take Warfarin, usually because of cardiovascular problems, or nonsteroidal antiinflammatory drugs that cause a mild coagulopathy. Thus although it is often possible to reverse the coagulopathy preoperatively, surgeons will be faced from time to time with an untreated or poorly treated coagu-

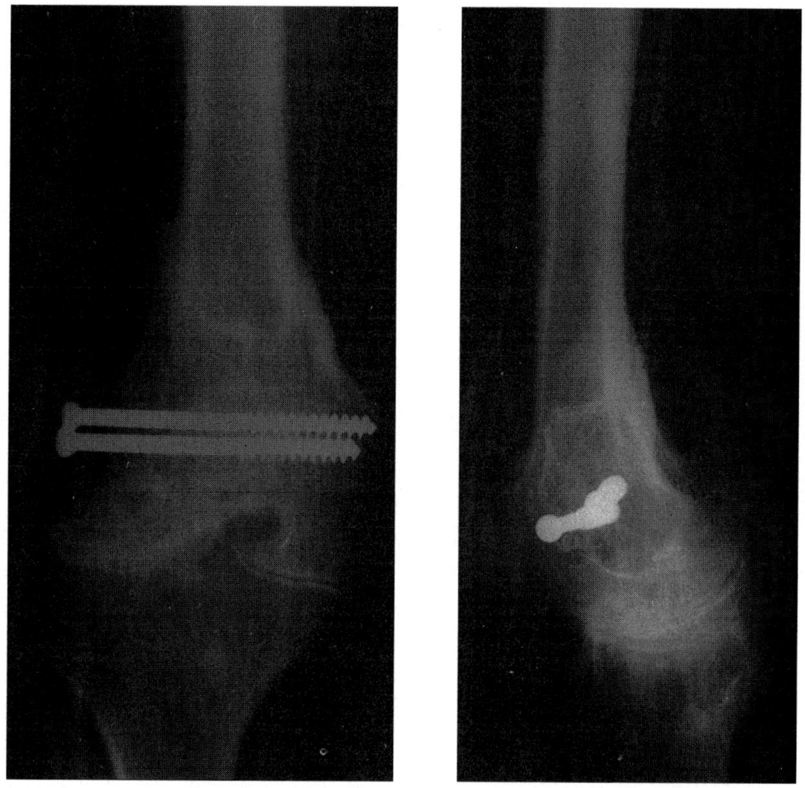

Figure 16–4. Final anteroposterior (A) and lateral (B) radiographs showed that the fracture had united in a good position.

lopathy. Under these circumstances the surgeon must consider nonoperative management or external skeletal fixation. If the latter treatment method is chosen, care must be exercised in placing the fixator pins because muscle transfixion will cause bleeding.

The particular external fixation configuration chosen was less rigid than more conventional frames such as a unilateral frame or a small wire fixator. However, the use of four pins placed in an arc around the condyle permitted good fracture fixation and the postreduction fracture position was maintained despite early knee movement.

Alternative Methods of Management

As already discussed, the use of a long-leg cast is superficially attractive when a knee joint is already stiff as the method involves no surgery. Plaster wedging could be used to achieve alignment. One of the problems with the use of cast management is joint stiffness, although knee stiffness is not all that common following a relatively short time in plaster. However, in this particular patient it was considered that knee stiffness would be inevitable, virtually untreatable, and would lead to significant impairment of function. Traction could have been employed to regain alignment and hold the fracture out to length until union. However, in addition to the usual problems of immobility the knee joint would have inevitably been stiff and the skeletal pin used for the traction would probably have given rise to bleeding problems.

Plating is obviously to be discouraged in this type of patient. The dissection required makes bleeding inevitable and knee stiffness very likely. Antegrade intramedullary femoral nailing involves considerable muscle dissection around the proximal end of the femur, which again would lead to bleeding. Retrograde femoral nailing using either a conventional long retrograde femoral nail or a shorter supracondylar nail would further damage an already compromised knee joint.

Type of Management	Advantages	Disadvantages	Comments
Traction and casting	No surgery required and therefore little risk of bleeding	Immobility; knee stiffness; malunion	Of little practical use in this particular case
Plating	Good fixation; early knee movement	Considerable potential for bleeding; probable knee stiffness secondary to soft tissue mobilization	This method of management should be avoided principally because of the potential for severe bleeding
Intramedullary nailing	Good fracture fixation; early knee movement	Bleeding	As with plating, this method is not indicated because of the potential bleeding problems
External fixation	Technically straightforward; less potential for bleeding than with plating or intramedullary nailing	Rigid frames require muscle penetration, thus less rigid frames must be employed	Overall the best method of management of this difficult case

Complications

In cases such as this it is important for the surgeon to attempt to predict complications and thereby avoid them. The obvious complication associated with this fracture is prolonged bleeding, whose treatment is outside the scope of this book. However, malunion, increased degenerative change in the knee, joint stiffness, and pin track sepsis are all practical problems the surgeon may face.

It is particularly important to attempt to avoid a significant malunion because an osteotomy would be a hazardous procedure. If malunion occurs, it would probably be prudent to accept it rather than undertake an osteotomy and plating.

Increased degenerative change in the knee would obviously be treated by arthroplasty. In a hemophiliac with an inhibited Factor VIII this might well be a risky operation and again it would be wise to delay arthroplasty for as long as possible.

If significant joint stiffness had occurred, then this patient might have lost the ability to drive and therefore would become relatively immobile. However, treatment of knee stiffness would be extremely difficult. There would be little point in undertaking the potentially dangerous operation of quadricepsplasty without first carrying out a knee arthroplasty, and the combination of these two operations might well be hazardous to this patient. Thus it is better to attempt to avoid the complication of joint stiffness. Inevitably with this type of problem and treatment some joint stiffness will occur, but in this case it did not significantly interfere with the patient's mobility.

Pin tract sepsis would be treated in the usual way by local cleaning, the use of antibiotics, and occasional pin replacement if clinically indicated.

Suggested Readings

Heim M, Horoszowski H (eds): Musculoskeletal problems in haemophilia. Clin Orthop 1996; 328.

Helfet D: Fractures of the distal femur. In Browner BD, Jupiter JB, Levine AM, Trafton PG: Skeletal Trauma, pp 1643–1683. WB Saunders, Philadelphia, 1992.

Seligson D, Malkani AL (eds): Supracondylar femoral fractures. Techniques in Orthopaedics 1994; 9.

Case 17

History and Physical Examination

A 14-year-old male was injured in a traffic accident. He was a rear seat passenger in a motor vehicle that was involved in a high speed head on collision and was not wearing a seat belt. On admission to the emergency department it was obvious that he had a severe open fracture of the right distal femur with an 8 cm laceration on the anteromedial aspect of the right lower thigh. The only other injuries were a Salter-Harris II fracture of the left distal radius and a soft tissue injury to the left foot. Examination of the right leg showed no evidence of neurovascular compromise or compartment syndrome. CAT scans of the abdomen and pelvis showed no significant injury.

A B

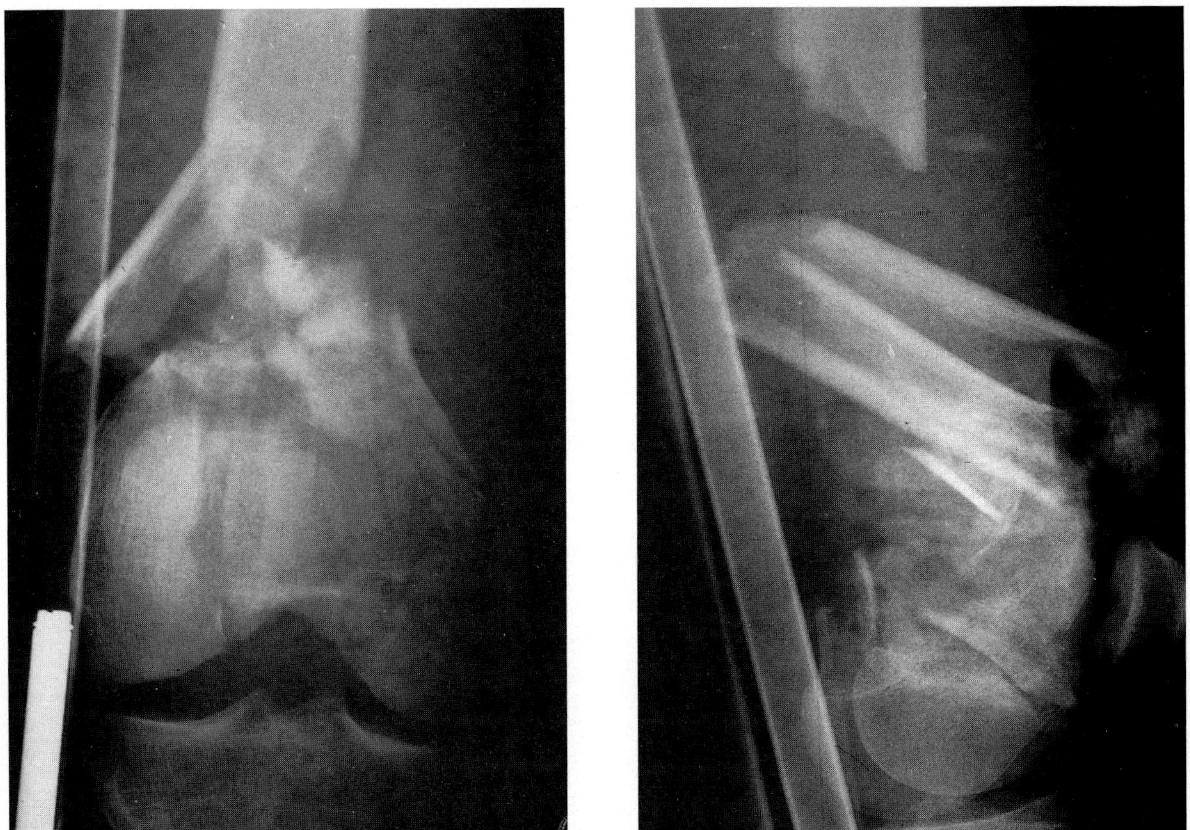

Figure 17–1. Anteroposterior (A) and lateral (B) radiographs of a Gustilo IIIb open distal femoral fracture.

Radiologic Findings

Anteroposterior and lateral radiographs showed a comminuted intraarticular distal femoral fracture with supracondylar metaphyseal comminution (Fig. 17–1). The severity of the metaphyseal comminution suggested extensive periosteal stripping and that this was a Gustilo type IIIb open fracture. The anteroposterior radiograph showed at least two intercondylar fractures that appeared to be only minimally displaced. It was considered unlikely that a two or three dimensional CAT scan would help the surgeon prior to the initial debridement and fracture fixation.

Diagnosis

Gustilo type IIIb open distal femoral fracture with supracondylar comminution and intraarticular extensions. AO classification: 33–C3.3 fracture.

Surgical Management

The patient was taken to the operating room immediately after admission. Under general anesthesia the leg was cleaned and the wound lavaged. The leg was then prepped and draped. A tourniquet was applied around the proximal thigh in case major vascular damage was encountered during surgery, but the tourniquet was not inflated for the initial debridement. The anteromedial wound was extended proximally and distally and a quantity of road dirt and devitalized muscle removed. The wound was then lavaged again with saline. Virtually all the supracondylar fragments were completely stripped of soft tissue and removed. The femoral condyles were in four pieces, with the lateral condyle being split into two by a fracture in the sagittal

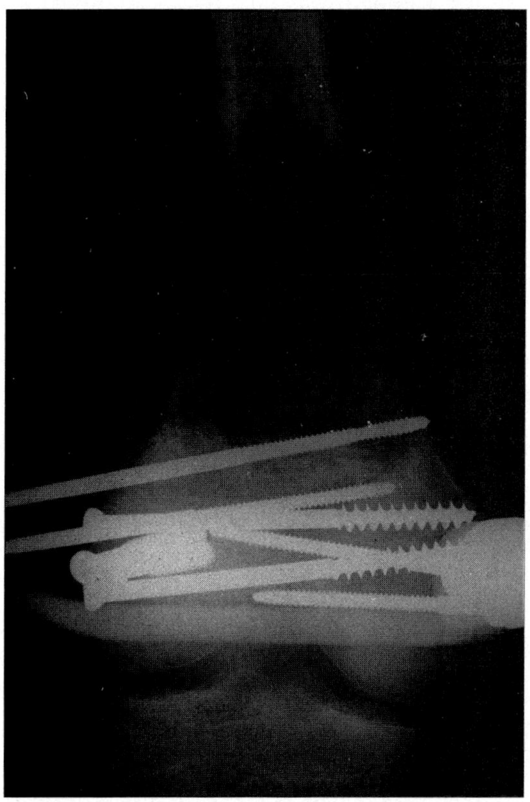

Figure 17–2. An anteroposterior radiograph of the distal femur showing the reconstructed condyles and the external fixator pins.

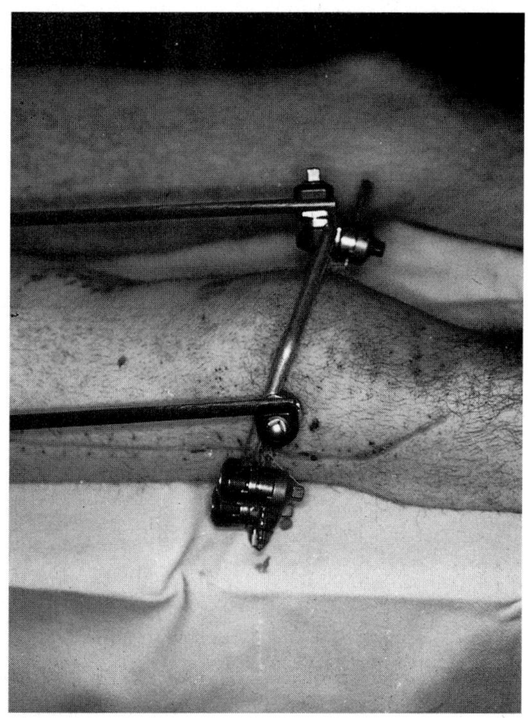

Figure 17–3. The semicircular external fixator used to stabilize the reconstructed condyles.

plane. Because of the contamination it was decided not to undertake definitive management and the fracture was therefore stabilized with a temporary transarticular external fixator applied on the lateral side of the leg; pins were placed in the midfemoral diaphysis and the proximal tibial diaphysis. The wound was packed and the patient returned to the ward.

Two days after the initial debridement the patient was returned to the operating room and further wound inspection performed. At this time it was seen that the wound was clean and healthy; there was no residual contamination or devitalized tissue present. Accordingly, it was decided to proceed with definitive fracture management. A number of alternatives had been considered preoperatively, but surgeons decided to use interfragmentary screws to fix the condyles and a condylar screw and side plate to attach the condyles to the diaphysis.

The four condylar fragments were reduced and fixed with cancellous screws. Four screws were required to secure fixation; the bone quality was excellent and good fixation was achieved. An attempt was made to insert the condylar screw, but the number and position of the cancellous screws prevented its passage. The surgeon was faced with the option of replacing the interfragmentary screws or choosing another method of stabilizing the metaphyseal fragment. It was thought that screw replacement would be difficult and an external fixator was therefore applied to maintain length and alignment. A distal half ring was employed and four distal half pins were used to secure fixation. This is illustrated in Figures 17–2 and 17–3.

Because of the problems associated with muscle transfixion, the external fixator was fixed proximally to the greater trochanter. More rigid external fixation would have been gained by inserting pins into the diaphysis, but it was thought that this would significantly interfere with already compromised knee function. The soft tissues were sutured. Postoperatively the leg was placed in a resting splint with gentle physiotherapy employed to restore some knee motion.

The fixator was maintained for 6 weeks to allow the condylar fragments to unite and was then removed. The four condylar screws were also removed and the condyles were noted to have united. A condylar screw and side plate were then used to fix the femoral fracture and good stability was achieved. The defect was filled with a mixture of femoral head allograft and corticocancellous pelvic autograft.

PITFALLS

- Surgeons should be aware that primary definitive fracture management is not mandatory under all circumstances; indeed, when there is significant contamination or evidence of significant soft tissue damage in a juxta- or intraarticular fracture, temporary fixation can be used. In some circumstances a delay in definitive management may be worthwhile to allow time for the surgeon to assess the problem in depth and choose an appropriate method of treatment. This course of action should not be confused with nontreatment and whatever temporary fixation is chosen should provide pain relief, adequate rigidity, and protection for the soft tissues. These conditions are not provided by traction or the application of a cast.
- This case illustrates the importance of the surgeon being familiar with all methods of fracture fixation. In the majority of fractures it will be possible to determine the optimal method of fracture fixation preoperatively, but inevitably the surgeon will occasionally encounter unforeseen problems perioperatively and have to select a different fixation technique. It is therefore not only important that orthopedic trauma surgeons be skilled in all techniques of surgery, but that the treatment of this type of difficult case is undertaken in a center where surgical expertise and appropriate equipment are available.

Postoperative Management

Because good stability had been achieved, the leg was only immobilized in a plaster back shell for a few days postoperatively. Subsequently a functional brace was applied, with the hinges carefully placed at the knee joint line. Passive motion was encouraged followed by active motion after 2 weeks. The brace hinges were initially set at 40 degrees of flexion but gradually the flexion was increased. Serial X-rays showed good bone incorporation, but 3 months after the initial grafting procedure it was thought that the grafted area was deficient and a further autogenous bone graft was undertaken. Six months after the accident the patient was pain-free and had 90 degrees of flexion. Weight bearing was instituted at that time. Eighteen months after the injury that patient had 110 degrees of flexion and no pain. Examination showed a 1 in. leg length discrepancy. He had not returned to sporting activities, but otherwise functioned well. Radiographs showed satisfactory union (Fig. 17–4).

PEARL

- Do not undertake definitive osseous reconstruction in a contaminated wound until the wound is completely free of contaminated or devitalized tissue. Successive debridements over several days may be required.

PITFALL

- When using a condylar screw and side plate system in a fracture associated with metaphyseal bone loss, the surgeon must be careful to avoid a varus or valgus malunion. The small size of the condylar fragment and the relatively large area of bone loss make it difficult to align the leg. The condylar screw must be inserted parallel to the knee joint and this may be facilitated by placing a thin Steinmann pin or guidewire across the knee joint. If, however, there is any doubt about the alignment of the leg, a temporary external fixator can be used to align the condylar fragment prior to applying the condylar screw and side plate.

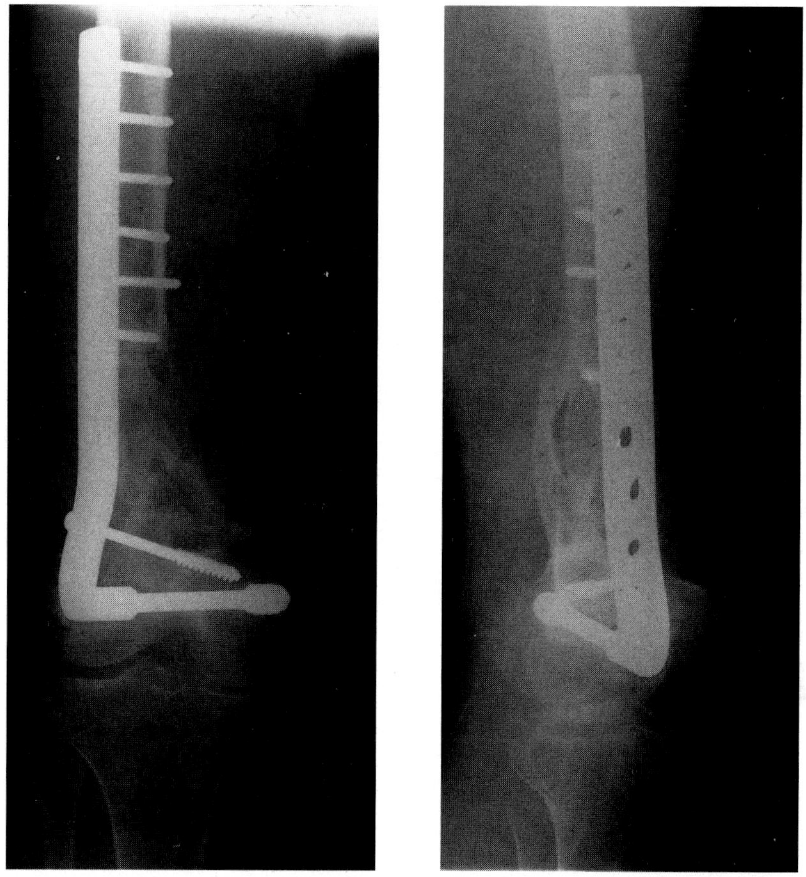

A B

Figure 17–4. Anteroposterior (A) and lateral (B) radiographs of the femur 18 months after the injury.

Discussion

This case illustrates the complexities of dealing with a complex juxta- or intraarticular fracture associated with metaphyseal bone loss. Even though this was a Gustilo IIIb open fracture, the soft tissue defect was straightforward to treat. Unlike the tibia, most soft tissue defects associated with open femoral fractures require only secondary closure or split skin grafting to close the wound and very few open femoral fractures need flap cover. However, the combination of bone loss and significant intercondylar comminution does provide the surgeon with some problems. Obviously, the key is to reconstruct the condyles; if this is difficult, it may alter the management of the metaphyseal or diaphyseal component of the fracture. There is no practical alternative to the use of interfragmentary screws to reconstruct the distal femur, but once this has been done a number of alternatives can be used to stabilize the condylar fragment and the proximal femoral shaft. However, all are associated with potential problems.

Two different types of external skeletal fixation were used in this case. Transarticular external fixation was initially employed to provide temporary fixation between the first and second wound debridements. Subsequently periarticular external fixation was used while the condylar fragments united. Theoretically, there is no reason why the periarticular external fixator could not have been maintained until fracture union. However, the particular external fixator configuration that was used could not have been maintained for long in view of the relative instability inherent in spanning the distance between the condyles and the greater trochanter. If definitive external fixation was used, it would require pins in the midfemoral diaphysis. Distally, the condylar fragment could be held with a half ring configuration as shown in Figure 3 or with lateral half pins attached to a unilateral frame. However, the use of these fixators would necessitate muscle penetration, leading to stiffness in an already compromised knee. The other problems of maintaining an external fixator for a prolonged period are pin track sepsis and malunion, and the chances of these complications developing in this fracture would be high. A small wire circular external fixator could also be used, either as a full circular frame or a hybrid frame utilizing proximal half pins. This would provide a more stable construct than other external fixator configurations, but the muscle penetration of multiple small wires would unquestionably lead to knee stiffness. Patient mobilization is also difficult with a full circular frame on the thigh.

Alternative Methods of Management

Plating

A condylar screw and side plate were used in this case. However, other lateral plates could have been used. The most common alternatives would be the lateral condylar buttress plate (Fig. 17–5A), or the 95 degree angled blade plate (Fig. 17–5B). One advantage of the lateral condylar buttress plate is that theoretically it could be used to fix the condylar fragments as well as reattach the reconstructed condyles to the femur. If this technique was used, the condyles could be reconstructed with temporary Kirschner wires and a plate and screws then applied. Superficially, this is an attractive concept, but there are hazards in attempting to make the plate perform two different functions and the chances of a malunion and knee dysfunction are high. The 95 degree angled blade plate is a fixed angle plate, but is otherwise similar to the condylar screw and plate used in this case. The same potential problems with the initial placement of the interfragmentary screws might occur if the 95 degree angled blade plate was used primarily, but it could have been used as a secondary device in the same way the condylar screw and plate were used here.

Another alternative is the use of two plates on the lateral and medial sides of the femur (Fig. 17–5C). This provides maximum rigidity of fracture fixation and bone graft could have been placed between the plates. The main advantage of this technique is that the knee could be mobilized very early; the disadvantage is that considerable soft tissue dissection is required on both sides of the femur. This degree of soft tissue dissection may well negate the benefits of early joint movement. In general, double plating is not a popular technique, although its use is highlighted elsewhere in this book.

Bone Shortening and Subsequent Lengthening

In theory, the condyles could be reconstructed with interfragmentary screws and the reconstructed condylar fragment placed on the end of the femoral diaphysis and held either with an external fixator or a lateral plate. This would result in an immediate shortening of about 3 in. With the condylar fragment securely fixed, it would be possible to lengthen the femur by undertaking a corticotomy in the subtrochanteric area and, using a unilateral femoral lengthening fixator, length could be restored. This

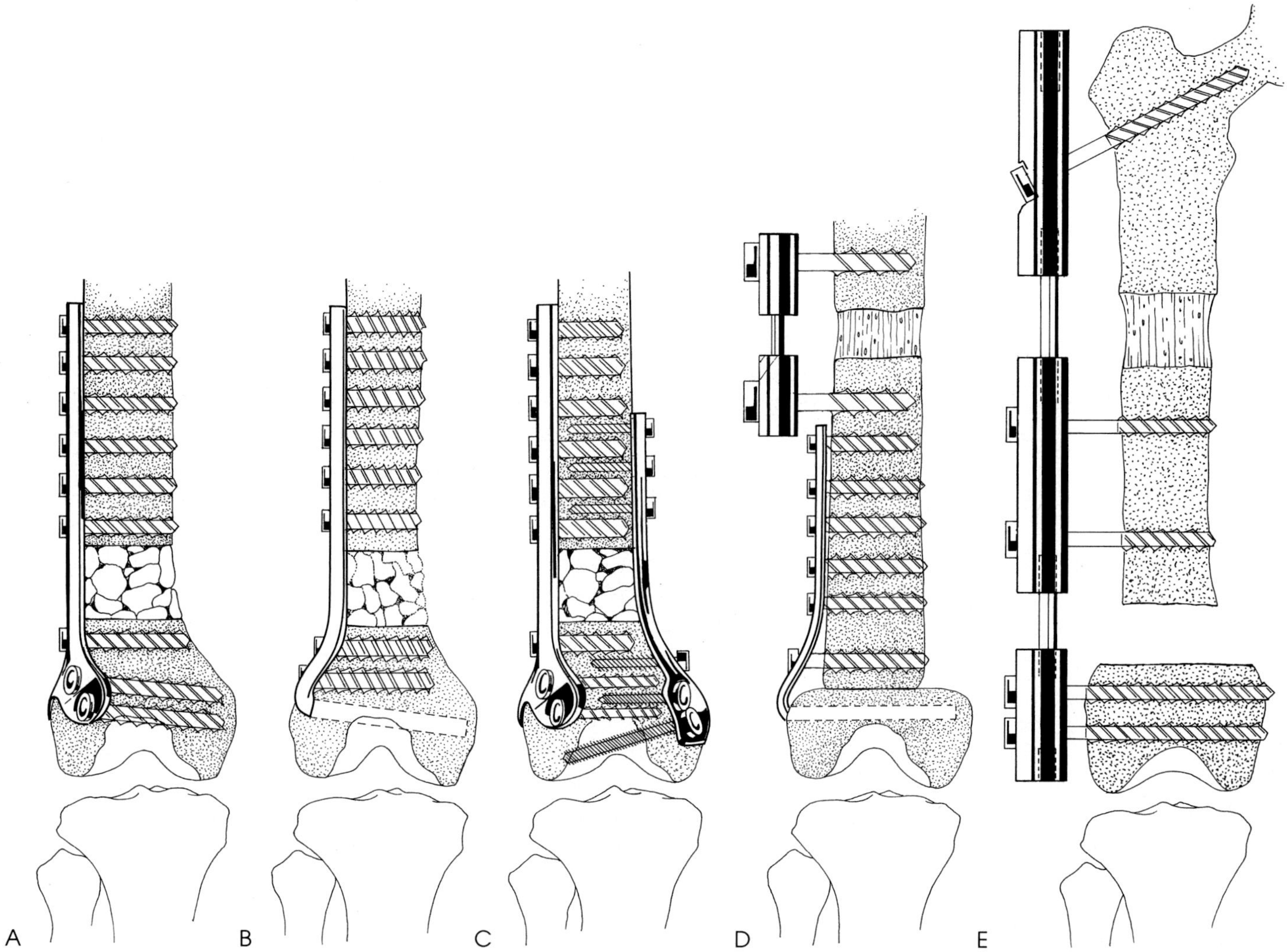

Figure 17–5. A lateral condylar plate (A). A 95 degree angled blade plate (B). Medial and lateral distal femoral plates (C). A diagrammatic representation of primary fracture shortening and proximal femoral lengthening (D). Note that the external fixator should have more than one pin in each bone segment. A diagrammatic representation of bone transport using a unilateral frame (E).

technique is illustrated diagramatically in Figure 17–5D. It is probable that the interface between the condyles and the diaphysis would require bone grafting.

Unfortunately, very little information exists about the use of bone shortening and subsequent lengthening for primary fractures associated with bone loss. It is possible that the immediate shortening of the quadriceps and hamstrings followed by relatively slow lengthening would result in abnormal muscle tension and knee dysfunction, but more clinical results are required to determine this. The other problems the surgeon might encounter are distal malunion and difficulty in maintaining alignment of the regenerate bone.

Bone Transport

Once the condyles have been reconstructed with interfragmentary screws, the metaphyseal defect could be filled by transporting a femoral segment downward after making a corticotomy in the subtrochanteric area. This could be achieved by using a unilateral fixator with the proximal pins placed in the femoral neck and the distal pins in the condylar fragment (Fig. 17–5E). Central pins would be inserted into the diaphysis to facilitate diaphyseal movement. Bone transport is now used extensively by surgeons to regain bone length. As yet its inevitable disadvantages have not been adequately documented, but malunion and the need to bone graft the docking site are relatively common. This is a complicated technique and should only be undertaken by surgeons experienced in its use.

Bone Grafting Techniques

One of the problems in using corticocancellous bone graft to span large bone defects is that, even if successful, it takes a considerable time before the graft is mature enough to permit weight bearing. The bone that is laid down following grafting is disorganized and will not stand up to the same loads as normal bone. Thus the fixation device will need to be retained for a considerable period. However, Figure 17–4, taken 1½ years after the injury, clearly shows a lucent line around the condylar screws, suggesting that it is loose and that the bone is taking much of the load.

A number of options are available for grafting this femoral defect. A combination of autograft and allograft was used in this case. This combines the improved results of autografting with the availability of allograft and in this case it was certainly successful. Autograft by itself would be preferable, but the surgeon might need to harvest a considerable quantity of pelvic bone to fill the femoral defect. Allograft by itself has less potential for incorporation than a mixture of allograft and autograft. If corticocancellous graft is to be used, the surgeon and patient must be aware that more than one grafting procedure might be required.

Other alternative grafting procedures can be used. A shaped block of cadaveric allograft supplemented by autograft proximally and distally is a relatively straightforward way of filling this type of bone defect. In this case the graft would best be held by a plate. Disadvantages of this method include difficulty in getting the allograft block to unite to the normal femoral bone. Vascularization of the allograft is slow, if it occurs at all, and allograft fracture can easily occur. A further grafting method is to use vascularized fibular grafts. In the distal femur two fibular grafts would probably by required. This method depends on having intact local vessels in which to anastomose the afferent and efferent fibular vessels. In experienced hands this is a relatively straightforward technique that is associated with good results. The major disadvantage is that fibular hypertrophy is slow and it is likely that the patient would be nonweight bearing for a considerable period.

Complications

This fracture is almost certain to be complicated by two major problems, limb shortening and knee stiffness. Limb shortening will occur because of the destruction of the distal femoral physis and the knee stiffness will occur because of the local soft tissue damage, damage to the articular cartilage, and the need for prolonged treatment. Other possible complications are knee osteoarthritis, graft or bone transport problems, infection, and malunion.

The distal femoral physis was destroyed by the fracture and 1½ years after the injury the patient had a discrepancy of 1 in. between his femora. This was treated by the use of a shoe raise, but the patient may wish a lengthening procedure in the future.

Type of Management	Advantages	Disadvantages	Comments
Traction and casting	None	Higher infection rate; fracture instability; patient immobility; difficulty of grafting	There is no place for nonoperative management in a severe open fracture complicated by bone loss
Open reduction and internal fixation	Accurate reduction of condylar fragment; good fracture stability; permits movement of local joints; high patient acceptability given that the treatment method will be prolonged	Potential infection risk; varus or valgus malunion; technically difficult	Certainly the treatment of choice for rebuilding the condylar fragment; probably the treatment of choice for stabilizing the distal femur
Temporary external fixation	Useful for stabilizing the condyles while the condylar fragments unite	Pin tract sepsis	The method will not provide adequate long term rigid stabilization of the fracture unless proximal pins are placed in the diaphysis, thus restricting knee function. If the proximal pins are placed in the greater trochanter, this construct can probably only be used for a few weeks
Definitive external fixation	Better control over varus or valgus malunion; permits leg lengthening or bone transport	Muscle penetration and resulting knee stiffness; pin tract sepsis; patient acceptability if external fixation retained for a prolonged period	This type of severe fracture is often associated with a prolonged union time, making external fixation difficult to use
Intramedullary nailing	None	A virtually impossible technique for this fracture	The use of intramedullary nailing in this fracture is purely theoretical. In practical terms there is no place for this method
Bone transport	Avoids extensive bone graft	Inadequate results reported for the use of bone transport in primary fracture management	This is probably a useful technique, but only in experienced hands; more information is required
Bone shortening and lengthening	Avoids extensive bone grafting	The literature contains adequate results for the use of this technique in primary management; technically difficult	This technique may well have a place in fractures associated with bone loss, but only in experienced hands
Bone grafting	Straightforward; good results in literature	Unpleasant morbidity associated with harvesting bone graft; prolonged time to graft maturity	Probably the method of choice at the moment, but may well be superseded by bone transport techniques over the next few years

Knee stiffness after a Gustilo IIIb femoral intraarticular fracture is virtually inevitable and interference with normal social and sporting activities is likely. This patient regained 110 degrees of flexion and was able to return to his studies without any problems, but 1½ years after the injury he had not restarted any form of athletic activity.

Knee osteoarthritis would be treated initially using nonsteroidal antiinflammatory drugs and local intraarticular steroid injections. Arthroscopic debridement might help, but if the condition worsened the patient, would have to be offered an arthroplasty or arthrodesis. The decision between these two options is difficult, but few patients today opt for an arthrodesis!

Other likely complications concern the bone grafting or bone transport technique. More than one grafting operation was required in this case and if any infection of the bone graft had occurred, this could have been catastrophic. Bone lengthening is often straightforward, but one needs to be careful to dock the regenerate segment properly and bone grafting is frequently required at the interface between the regenerate segment and the condylar fragment.

Suggested Readings

Chao EYS, Cooney WP (eds): Newest knowledge of external fixation devices. Clin Orthop 1993; 293.

Green S (ed): Ilizarov method. Clin Orthop 1992; 280.

Helfet DL: Fractures of the distal femur. In Browner BD, Jupiter JB, Levine AM, Trafton PG (eds): Skeletal Trauma, pp 1643–1683. Vol 2. WB Saunders, Philadelphia, 1992.

Leung P-C: Current Trends in Bone Grafting. Springer Verlag, Berlin, 1989.

Sanders R, Regazzoni P, Rüedi TP: Treatment of supracondylar-intercondylar fractures of the femur using the dynamic compression screw. J Orthop Trauma 1989; 3:214–222.

Seligson D, Malkani AL: Supracondylar femur fractures. Techniques in Orthopaedics 1994; 9(3).

Case 18

History and Physical Examination

A 16-year-old male was admitted to the emergency department after being tackled while playing soccer. He had been struck on the right knee by an opponent's shoe. Clinical examination showed a right knee with an obvious valgus deformity. Neurovascular examination indicated no evidence of either vascular or neurological damage. No other injury was noted.

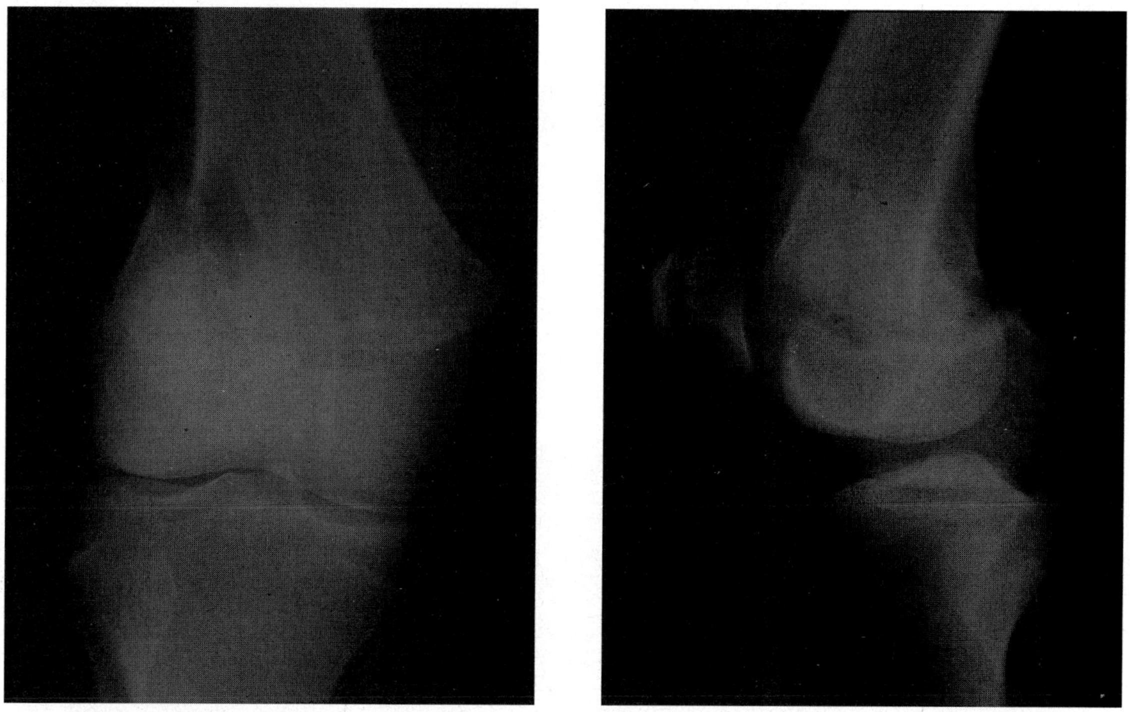

A B

Figure 18–1. Anteroposterior (A) and lateral (B) radiographs of a Salter-Harris II physeal fracture of the distal femur.

Radiologic Findings

Anteroposterior and lateral radiographs of the distal femur showed a Salter-Harris II fracture through the distal femoral physis with the metaphyseal spike attached to the lateral femoral condyle (Fig. 18–1).

Diagnosis

Salter-Harris II distal femoral physeal fracture.

PITFALL

- Oblique radiographs may be required to determine minor fracture displacement. Stress views or MRI scans may also be used if radiographs are negative but the clinical picture suggests a fracture separation.

Surgical Management

The right leg was placed in a supporting plaster back shell to relieve discomfort and the patient was admitted to the orthopaedic ward. He was prepared for open surgery in case the closed manipulation was impossible, but it proved easy to reduce the fracture that was held with two crossed percutaneously inserted Kirschner wires (Fig. 18–2). Check radiographs were satisfactory.

Postoperative Management

Postoperatively the patient's leg was splinted in a long-leg cylinder for 3 weeks to allow the pain to settle and facilitate mobilization. Following cast removal the wires were retained for a further 2 weeks and then removed. Two weeks are wire removal he had full extension and 100 degrees of knee flexion. This increase to 130 degrees of flexion 4 weeks later and knee motion was full after a further 4 weeks, 15 weeks after the injury. Check radiographs showed good fracture union (Fig. 18–3).

Discussion

Separation of the distal femoral epiphysis has received much attention in the literature, but there has been little interest in this condition in recent years. Between 1

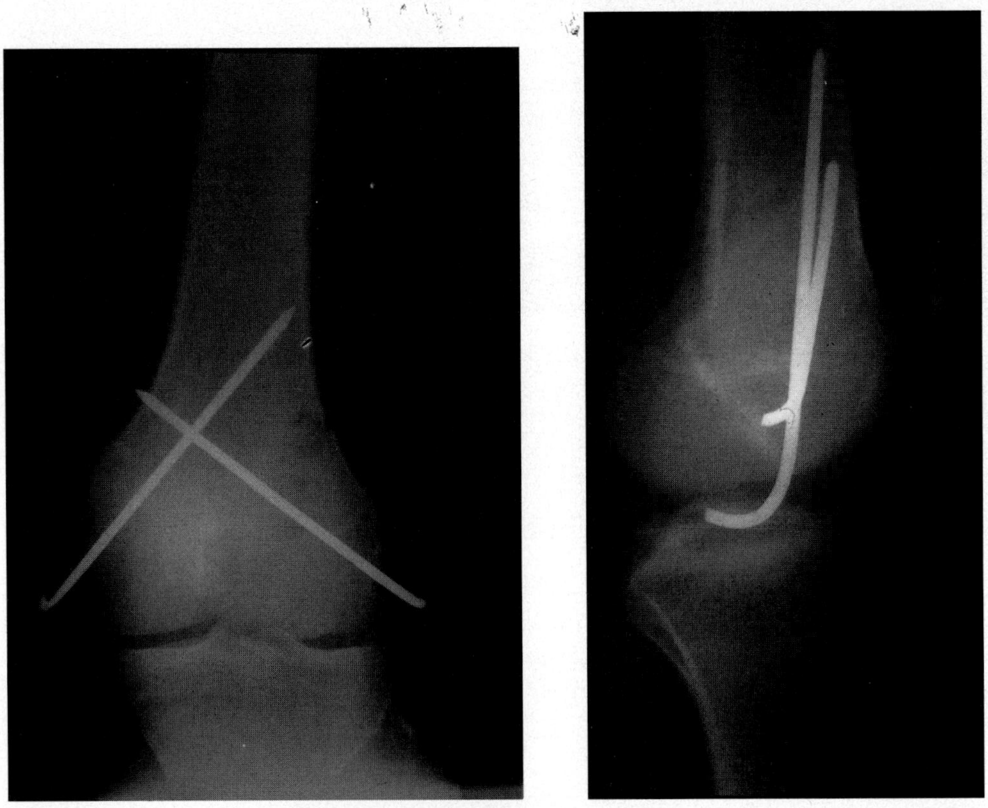

A B

Figure 18–2. A closed manipulation was performed. Postoperative anteroposterior (A) and lateral (B) radiographs show that a good reduction has been achieved.

A 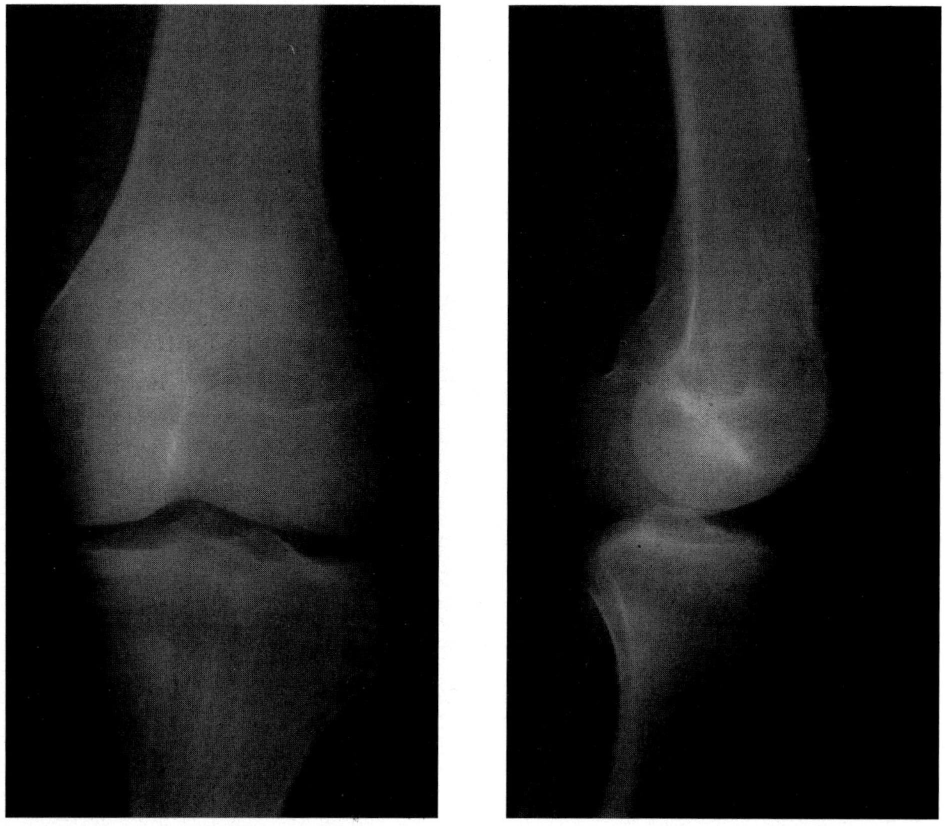 B

Figure 18–3. Good union was achieved and the patient regained full knee function. Anteroposterior (A) and lateral (B) views.

and 6% of all epiphyseal fractures occur in the distal femur and it is likely that distal femoral physeal fractures account for about 1% of fractures of the growing skeleton.

This case illustrates a fairly classical presentation of the problem. One of the main causes of distal femoral physeal fracture is a bending force applied to a leg that is fixed to the ground by a cleated shoe. Usually the force is produced by an opponent's foot. The epiphysis pulls apart on the tension side and there is an oblique metaphyseal fracture on the compression side. This produces the characteristic Salter-Harris II fracture.

Sports related distal femoral physeal fractures tend to occur between 10 and 19 years of age, with younger patients often sustaining the injury in traffic accidents. Lombardo and Harvey (1977) showed that 60% of a group of 35 patients presenting with distal femoral physeal fractures were at least 12 years of age.

All types of physeal fractures can occur in the distal femur, although the Salter-Harris II fracture is by far the most common. In Lombardo and Harvey's series these accounted for 68.6% of all distal femoral physeal fractures. The Salter-Harris I fracture separation is seen in newborns or adolescents when it presents as an undisplaced separation. In these cases the diagnosis may only be made retrospectively when new bone formation is apparent. Lombardo and Harvey documented a 2.8% incidence of Salter-Harris I fractures in their series. The Salter-Harris III fracture is more common, accounting for 14.3% of Lombardo and Harvey's series, while the Salter-Harris IV fracture was seen in 8.6% and the Salter-Harris V fracture in 2.8% of the patients.

PEARL

- Bright (1984) lists trauma as the most common cause of partial growth arrest. He also states that the distal femoral epiphysis is the most frequent site of partial growth arrest. This is followed by the distal tibia, proximal tibia, and distal radius.

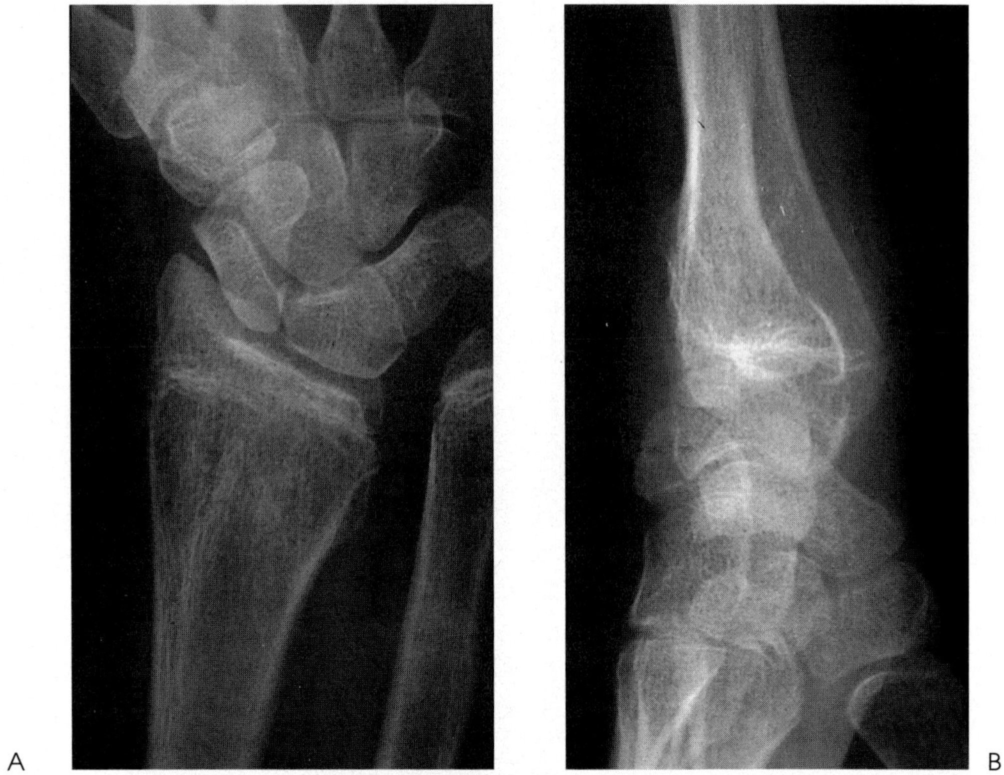

Figure 18–4. Anteroposterior (A) and lateral (B) radiographs showing partial growth arrest in a distal radial fracture.

Salter-Harris II fractures are commonly assumed to be benign provided the surgeon can achieve a good reduction. Salter and Harris (1963) suggested that only 10% would have growth limitation. Growth arrest is often assumed to be an unusual problem because the fractures tend to occur in the zone of hypertrophy of the physis. However, it is dangerous to assume that all Salter-Harris II fractures are similar and a useful rule of thumb is that the larger the bone the more force is required to disrupt the physis and the more force that is required the higher the incidence of damage to the germinal layer of the physis. Thus growth arrest following Salter-Harris II fractures is not infrequently seen. Surgeons should always follow up these patients until growth has ceased. This is not required for the common simple Salter-Harris II phalangeal fracture where growth arrest is very unlikely. An example of growth arrest in the distal radius following a physeal fracture is shown in Figure 18–4.

The other misconception regarding Salter-Harris II fractures is that they can all be treated nonoperatively. This misconception has arisen because of the relative ease with which Salter-Harris II fractures of small joints such as the phalanges can be reduced and held. However, the greater energy involved in physeal fracture separation of larger bones means that the soft tissue damage is greater and the potential for fracture instability therefore higher. Thus surgeons should consider internal fixation in Salter-Harris II fractures affecting larger epiphyses if there is any suggestion of fracture instability. In Salter-Harris II fractures of the distal femoral epiphysis it is accepted that fixation is essential if redisplacement is to be prevented. Many authorities advocate cross wire fixation as used in this case, although screws can also be used.

PEARL

- Open reduction should be undertaken through a longitudinal incision centered over the palpable end of the metaphysis. There may well be an interposed flap of periosteum between the epiphysis and the metaphysis.

It is important that the surgeon is sure that an accurate reduction has been achieved because failure to achieve an accurate reduction in younger patients will lead to malunion. If a closed reduction cannot be achieved because of interposed soft tissue, an open reduction must be undertaken.

Alternative Methods of Management

The only commonly used method of management of physeal fractures, other than internal fixation, is nonoperative management. This can be used if a perfect reduction can be obtained and maintained. A well molded long-leg cast from toes to groin is used. It can be removed after 5 or 6 weeks following which a physiotherapy program is instituted. If this method of management is chosen, the surgeon must be fastidious in taking weekly postoperative radiographs to check for fracture malalignment.

In theory, external skeletal fixation could be used, but this has not been commented on in the orthopedic literature. Clearly intramedullary fixation is not an option for this particular fracture.

Type of Management	Advantages	Disadvantages	Comments
Nonoperative management	Closed treatment	Malunion; joint stiffness	Can be used but the incidence of malreduction and malunion is high in the distal femur
Internal fixation	Straightforward operation; good alignment; good knee function	Minor risk of infection	This is the method of choice for Salter-Harris II fractures of the distal femoral physis. Crossed wires are normally used but screws can be employed

Complications

Because Salter-Harris II distal femoral fractures will tend to damage the germinal layer of the physis, leg length discrepancy may follow. If, as in this case, the patient is within 2 years of skeletal maturity, the shortening will probably be insignificant, but if there is more than 2 years of growth left the leg length discrepancy may progress at a rate of 1 cm per year. Lombardo and Harvey (1977) stated that the development of leg length discrepancy is related to the amount of displacement and the quality of reduction rather than to the type of fracture. They documented leg length discrepancy in 75% of their Salter-Harris II distal femoral fractures with the range being between 0.3 and 7 cm. They also found a 33% incidence of varus or valgus malunion and a high incidence of knee stiffness. However, it must be remembered that a number of these patients were nonoperatively treated.

Other complications associated with Salter-Harris II distal femoral fractures are popliteal artery thrombosis and peroneal nerve injuries. A review of the literature suggests that popliteal artery thrombosis is now rare. Peroneal nerve injury is somewhat more common and is thought to occur in about 3% of cases. The only other complication to occur with any frequency is partial growth arrest that can be treated by excision of the bone bridge.

Suggested Readings

Bright RW: Physeal injuries. In Rockwood CA, Wilkins KE, King RE (eds): Fractures in Children, pp 87–172. JP Lippincott, Philadelphia, 1984.

Lombardo SJ, Harvey JP: Fractures of the distal femoral epiphysis. J Bone Joint Surg [Am] 1977; 59A:742–751.

Roberts JM: Fractures and dislocations of the knee. In Rockwood CA, Wilkins KE, King RE (eds): Fractures in Children, pp 891–982. JP Lippincott, Philadelphia, 1984.

Salter RB, Harris WR: Injuries involving the epiphyseal plate. J Bone Joint Surg [Am] 1963; 45A:587–662.

Case 19

History and Physical Examination

A 75-year-old woman caught her foot on a carpet and fell, injuring her right knee. She experienced immediate onset of pain and was unable to rise, but crawled to the telephone and called for help. She arrived at the emergency department approximately 90 minutes after injury. Physical examination revealed deformity, instability, swelling, and pain just proximal to the right knee. The neurovascular examination of the right leg was intact. The patient's medical history was notable in that she had undergone a right total knee arthroplasty for osteoarthritis 4 years prior to injury. The right knee had been painless and functioning well since her surgery.

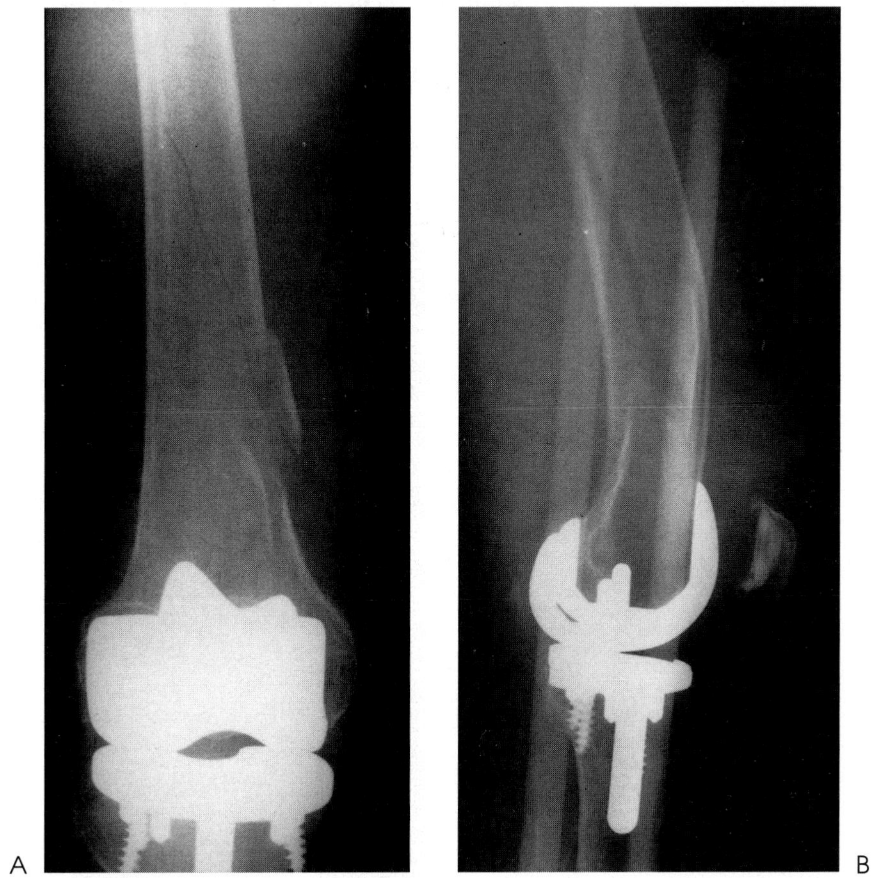

Figure 19–1. Anteroposterior (A) and lateral (B) radiographs of the distal femur indicating a fracture of the femur proximal to a total knee prosthesis. The prosthesis appears to be in good alignment with no sign of loosening. The bone appears osteopenic.

Radiologic Findings

Anteroposterior and lateral radiographs of the entire right lower extremity revealed a long oblique supracondylar fracture of the femur proximal to a total knee prosthesis (Fig. 19–1). The bone appeared extremely osteopenic. Comminution of the medial cortex was evident. The prosthesis was properly aligned, the femoral and tibial components were uncemented. The patella had been resurfaced. There was no sign of loosening at the prosthesis bone interface.

PEARL

- A splint will not immobilize a supracondylar fracture of the femur. Even though the patient was very thin, a splint would have extended just proximal to the fracture and actually would have increased stresses and motion at the fracture site, thus increasing pain. Gentle longitudinal traction with the knee flexed approximately 20 degrees will relieve most of the patient's pain.

Diagnosis

Low energy supracondylar femoral fracture above a stable well aligned prosthesis. In addition, the patient's bone was osteopenic.

Surgical Management

The patient was put in bed with a pillow behind the knee. Five pounds of traction was applied to the injured extremity via a foam boot. The patient was log rolled every 4 hours and encouraged to use an incentive spirometer. A Foley catheter was placed.

In the operating room the patient was anesthetized and placed supine on the operating table. The injured extremity and ipsilateral hip were prepped and draped. A straight anterior approach was used to expose the fracture. Distally, the scar through which the arthroplasty had been inserted was incorporated in

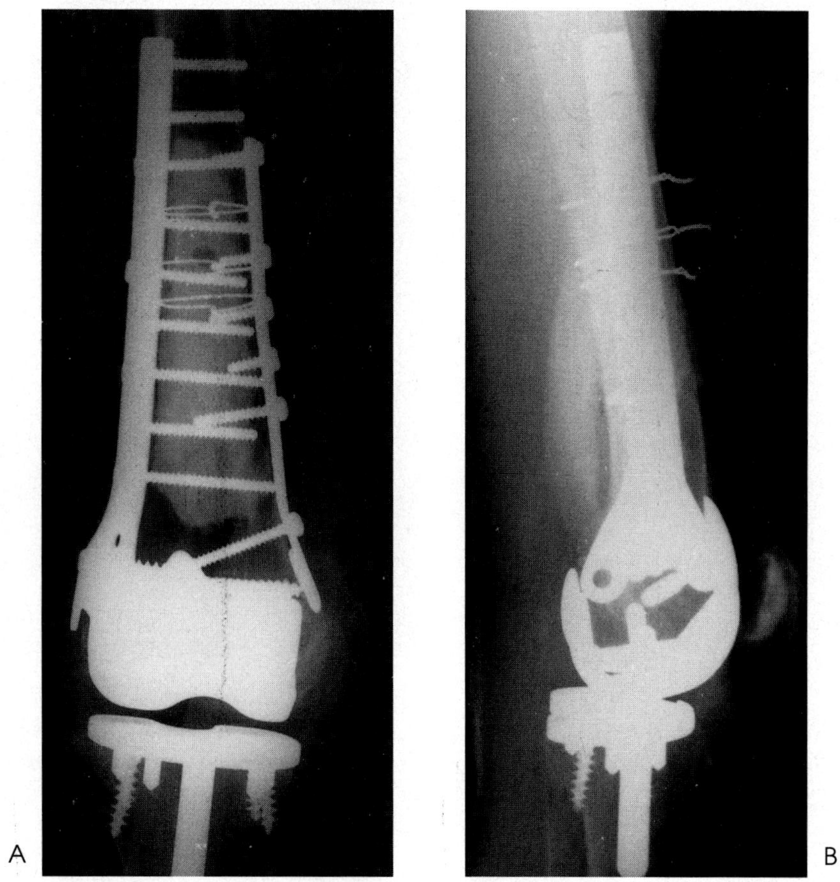

Figure 19–2. Anteroposterior (A) and lateral (B) radiographs obtained intraoperatively. The fracture has been reduced: the medullary canal has been packed with methylmethacrylate and stabilized with medial and lateral plates. The cerclage wires were used to temporarily hold the reduction while the methylmethacrylate was hardening.

PEARLS

- The technique of using PMMA as an adjunct to fracture fixation is as follows. To create space for the PMMA, the cancellous bone of the distal fragment is lightly compacted and the medullary contents of the proximal fragment (mostly fat) are removed with a curette. The PMMA is mixed. When it reaches a doughy state, it is finger packed into the medullary canal via a window through the anterior cortex of the femur. It is very important to have an accurate reduction and use doughy PMMA to minimize extravasation of PMMA through the fracture. After packing the medullary canal, the femur is continuously irrigated while the PMMA hardens to minimize thermal necrosis of bone and soft tissue. When the PMMA has hardened, it can be drilled and tapped for screw placement. When drilling, the PMMA may melt and adhere to the drill bit; if the bit is not cleaned frequently, it will bind and break. When tapping, more resistance is encountered with PMMA than with bone. The tap is advanced slowly to minimize torque and therefore decrease the incidence of tap breakage.

- The surgical approach used splits the quadriceps muscle. To prevent the quadriceps from scarring to the femur it is necessary to obtain a significant arc of flexion at the knee relatively early postoperatively. This is most easily accomplished with continuous passive motion.

the incision. A lateral parapatellar incision was used to open the capsule. The incision was carried proximally, medially splitting the quadriceps tendon and the quadriceps muscle directly over the femur. The fracture was curetted of hematoma and reduced anatomically. The cortex of the femur was extremely thin, and the fracture was stabilized with polymethylmethacrylate (PMMA).

Medial and lateral plates were applied to the femur. The medial plate functioned as a buttress to resist varus stresses. Therefore it was not necessary to utilize all the screw holes. The distal screw of the medial plate was inserted percutaneously through a stab incision to avoid injuring the overlying skin and subcutaneous tissue with excessive retraction. The fracture site was grafted anteromedially and laterally with autogenous bone harvested from ipsilateral iliac crest. The wound was closed over a drain (Fig. 19–2).

Postoperative Management

Postoperatively the patient was placed in a bulky dressing. The dressing was changed on postoperative day two, and continuous passive motion was initiated. The range of passive motion was increased as tolerated to 60 degrees.

Active motion was initiated at 1 week when incisional pain had become bearable. Nonweight bearing was maintained until 10 weeks postsurgery when radiographs indicated consolidation of the fracture. The fracture healed uneventfully (Fig. 19–3).

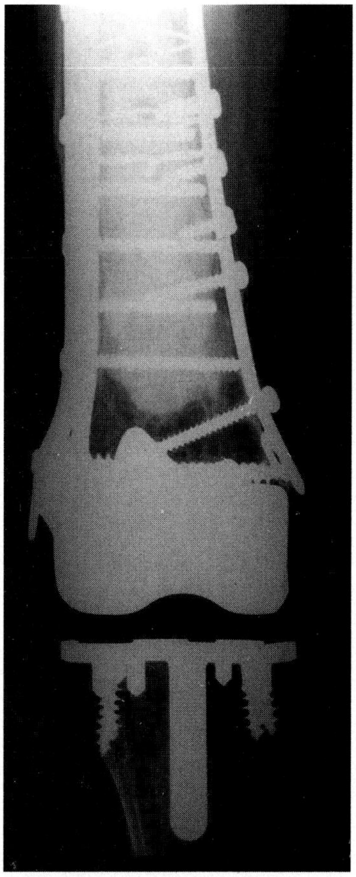

Figure 19–3. Sixteen months later the fracture is solidly healed.

Discussion

Fracture of the femur proximal to a total knee is clearly associated with two risk factors: notching of the anterior cortex and neurological disorders (e.g., Parkinson's disease). The goals of management are to return the patient to his or her prefracture status and minimize the complications of loss of motion, failure of fixation, and infection.

Alternative Methods of Management

Methods of management are divided in two groups: open or semi-open methods and closed methods. In addition, when open methods are used, fixation can be augmented with PMMA or allograft. The open and semi-open methods are closed reduction and retrograde nailing, open reduction and plating, and revision with a custom prosthesis. These methods stabilize the fracture and allow early rehabilitation and potentially a more complete recovery of function. However, they also expose the patient to the risks of loss of fixation and infection.

Closed methods are external fixation and traction. Both methods usually include prolonged cast immobilization after an initial period of external fixation or traction, resulting in loss of motion. In addition, alignment of the fracture is not as easily controlled with these methods, and the incidence of malunion is greater than with open or semi-open methods. External fixation offers the disadvantages of open and closed methods. The fracture is not immobilized adequately to allow early motion. The pins prevent quadriceps excursion, compounding the problem of early mobilization. Pin tract irritation can result in osteomyelitis and infection of the fracture and prosthetic joint.

When open reduction and internal fixation with a plate is used to manage the fracture, fixation can be augmented with PMMA or allograft struts. Augmentation with PMMA yields the most stable construct, but may decrease the healing potential of the fracture; therefore it should always be used with autogenous bone grafting. Allograft struts can be applied medially to reconstitute the medial cortex. They

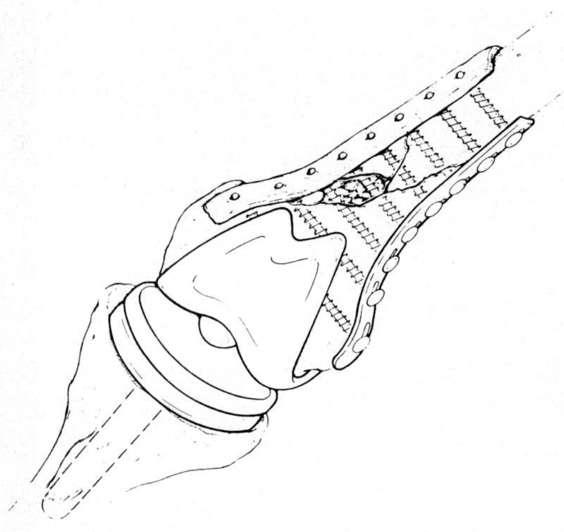

Figure 19–4. An alternative method of management would have been to use an allograft strut medially and insert screws into the allograft to increase the strength of fixation.

are used in conjunction with a lateral plate. The patient's bone is sandwiched between the lateral plate and medial allograft. While the allograft does not provide as much stability as PMMA, it does not decrease the healing potential of the fracture and eventually is partially incorporated (Fig 19–4).

Type of Management	Advantages	Disadvantages	Comments
Closed reduction and retrograde nail (Fig. 19–5)	Closed procedure, therefore decreased risk of infection and blood loss	Stability is limited, therefore postoperative motion is painful; not possible with all types of prosthesis	The advantages of minimizing the surgical approach frequently outweigh the disadvantage of limited stability
Open reduction and stabilization with plates and screws	Most stable type of fixation, allows early motion; total joint surgeon may feel more comfortable with this method	Major surgical exposure, therefore increased risk of infection and blood loss	Stable anatomic reduction may maximize rehabilitation potential
Revision with custom prosthesis	Allows early motion	Surgery is delayed until prosthesis is manufactured; extensive surgical procedure	Seldom done because of the extent of surgical procedure
External fixation	Minimizes exposure and surgical trauma	Pin tracts communicate with fracture, therefore increased risk of infection; limited stability; soft tissue tethering prevents early active motion	Disadvantage of pin tract infections outweighs advantages
Traction	Minimizes risk of infection	Prolonged enforced bedrest and its complications of decubiti, emboli, urinary tract infections, and pulmonary infections	The disadvantages of enforced bed rest outweigh advantages; used only when patient is moribund
Augmentation with PMMA	PMMA acts as spacer, can be drilled and tapped	Heat of polymerization can cause heat necrosis; must be used in conjunction with autogenous bone graft	Excellent method to augment fixation, but must be bone grafted
Augmentation with allograft struts	Reconstitutes the medial cortex	Makes medial plate unnecessary; may not be as strong as PMMA	Excellent method to augment medial cortex

Complications

Complications of a fracture proximal to a total knee arthroplasty are loss of fixation, loss of motion, fracture above the fixation, and infection. Loss of fixation occurs because of instability due to osteopenia, decreased healing potential due to the patient's age and prior surgery, and increased stresses across the fracture due to the prosthesis acting as a stress riser in concert with decreased range of motion at the knee. When loss of fixation occurs, revision is necessary, usually with augmentation

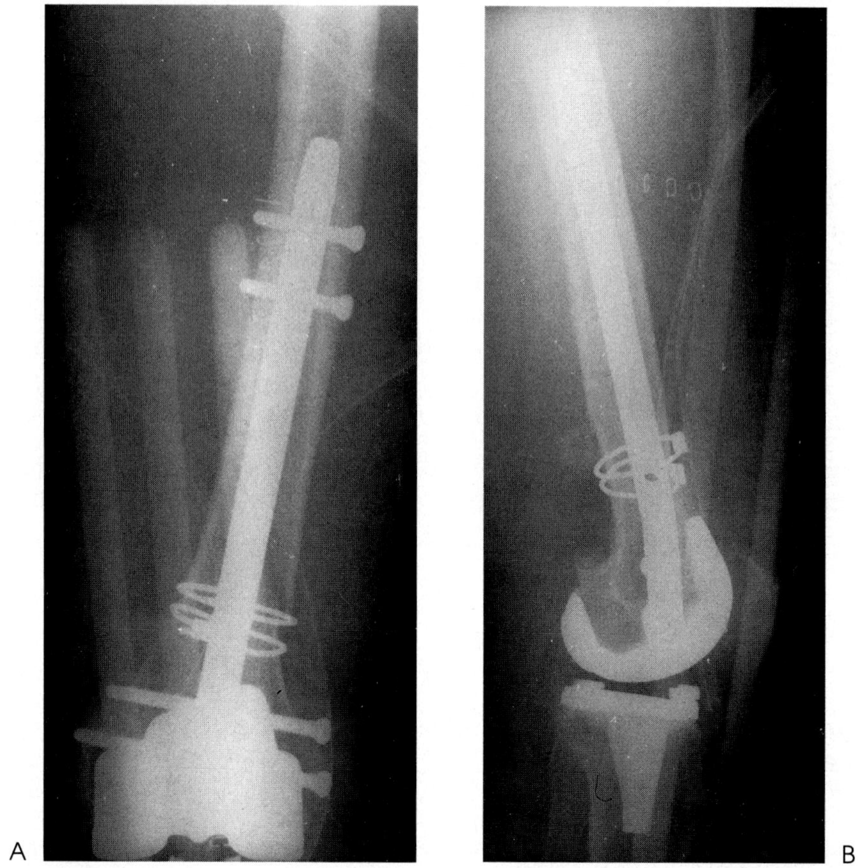

Figure 19–5. Anteroposterior (A) and lateral (B) radiographs showing that an alternative method of fixation is utilizing a retrograde femoral nail. This method of fixation is not as stable as plates and screws.

using either PMMA or cortical allograft. Revision surgery increases the incidence of infection and loss of motion of the knee. Loss of fixation may be a relative indication for revision with a custom prosthesis.

Some degree of loss of motion is inevitable following a periprosthetic fracture. Stable fixation and early postoperative motion will minimize loss of motion. When loss of motion occurs, it is best managed conservatively with range of motion exercises and educating the patient regarding the risk factors of aggressive management. Closed manipulation and surgical release carry the risk of refracture and postoperative infection.

Fracture above the fixation occurs because the bone is osteopenic, decreased knee motion results in increased stress in this area, and the fracture fixation implants act as a stress riser. The incidence of fracture is minimized by selection of implants, proper placement of the implants, and achieving early postoperative motion. When fracture occurs, the fixation must be revised or augmented (Figs. 19–6 and 19–7).

Infection usually involves not just the fixation, but also the prosthesis. Debridement results in such extensive bone loss that salvage of the knee is frequently not possible. Usually, the only partial solution is to achieve suppression of symptoms by surgical drainage of abscesses and long term administration of systemic antibiotics. In cases in which the infection cannot be controlled, massive debridement and temporary stabilization of the knee with an external fixator followed by arthrodesis are necessary.

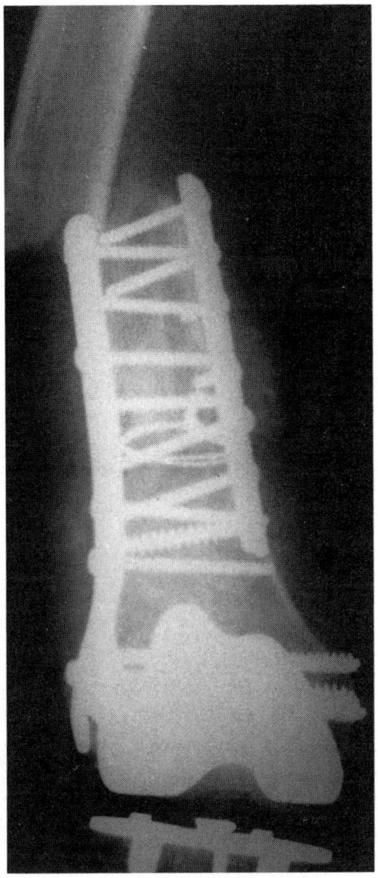

Figure 19–6. Following fixation of a femoral fracture proximal to a total knee arthroplasty, the femur fractured again at the proximal end of the plates. Fracture was partially due to the increased stresses caused by the medial and lateral plates both ending at the same level.

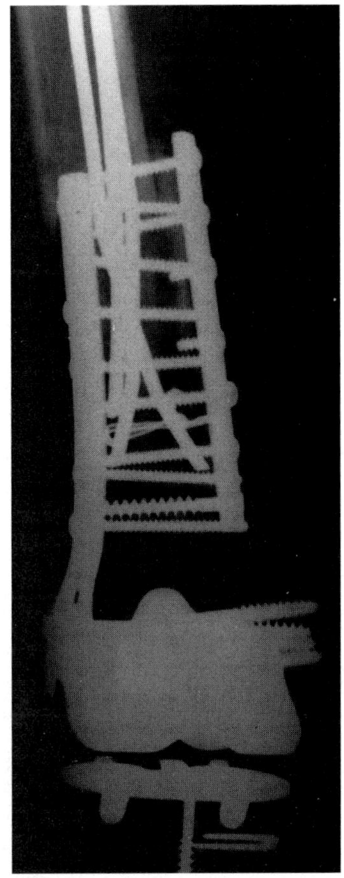

Figure 19–7. The fracture was aligned with two antegrade Ender nails.

Suggested Readings

Cull RW, Schmidt RG, Hanks G, Mak A, Esterhai JL, Heppenstall B: Supracondylar fracture of the femur following prosthetic arthroplasty. CORR 1987; 22:212–222.

Figgie MP, Goldberg VM, Figgie HE, Sobel M: The results of treatment of ipsilateral supracondylar femoral fracture above total knee arthroplasty. J Arthroplast 1990; 5:267–276.

Healy WL, Siliski JM, Incavo SJ: Operative treatment of distal femoral fractures proximal to total knee replacements. J Bone Joint Surg 1993; 75A:27–34.

Madsen F, Kjaersgaard-Andersen P, Juhl M, Sneppen O: A custom-made prosthesis for the treatment of supracondylar femoral fractures after total knee arthroplasty: report of 4 cases. J Orthop Trauma 1989; 3(4):333–337.

Merkel KD, Johnson EW: Supracondylar fracture of the femur after total knee arthroplasty. J Bone Joint Surg 1986; 68A:29–43.

Ritter MA, Faris PM, Keating EM: Anterior femoral notching and ipsilateral supracondylar fracture in total knee arthroplasty. J Arthroplast 1988; 3:185–187.

Case 20

History and Physical Examination

A 69-year-old male was the unrestrained passenger in a one-car accident. On impact his right knee struck the dashboard. He arrived in the emergency department 30 minutes after injury. His only complaints were of right knee pain. A stellate laceration was present over the anterior aspect of the patella. The laceration was 3 cm in length and bleeding freely. It was not possible to determine if the patient was able to actively extend his knee because of pain. Ligamentous stability was not assessed because of pain. There was no pain to palpation or with motion of either hip. The neurovascular examination of the injured extremity was within the limits of normal.

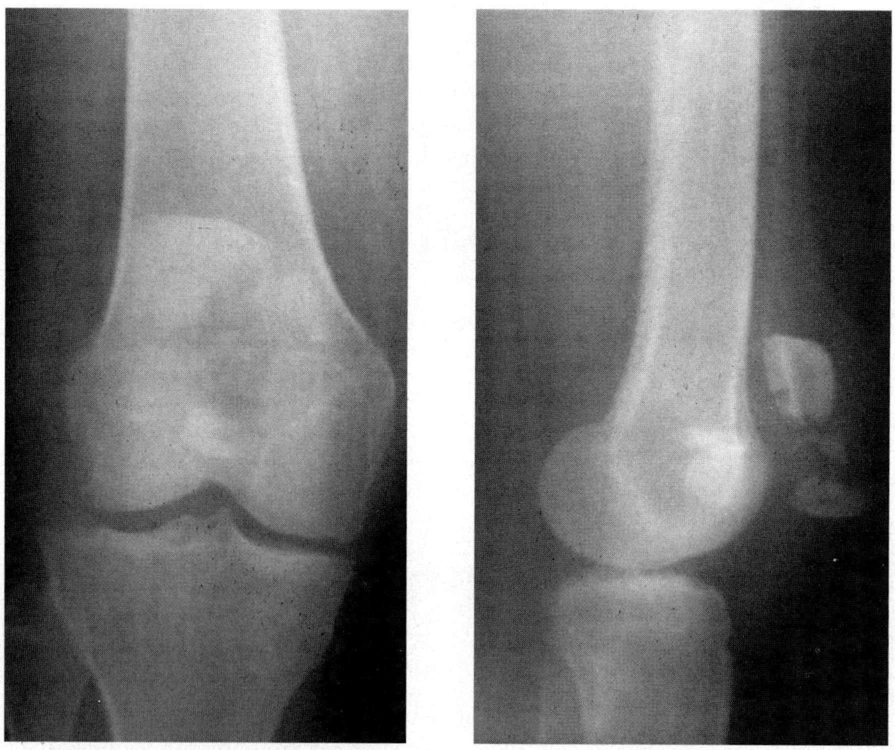

A B

Figure 20–1. Anteroposterior (A) and lateral (B) radiographs of the knee.

Radiologic Findings

Radiographs of the right knee, tibia, femur, hip, and pelvis were obtained. Radiographs of the knee indicated a comminuted fracture of the patella with a "step off" of the articular surface and a gap of over 1 cm between fragments (Fig. 20–1). No other fractures were present.

PEARL

- Injury to the anterior aspect of the knee in a patient who was an unrestrained passenger in a motor vehicle accident is often part of the "dashboard injury." This injury occurs when sudden deceleration results in the anterior aspect of the knee striking the dashboard. The energy of impact is often transmitted proximally along the femur, resulting in a fracture or dislocation of the hip. An injury to the anterior aspect of the knee should direct attention to the proximal femur and hip.

Diagnosis

Grade III open fracture of the patella. The fracture involved the distal pole and was extremely comminuted. Displacement and a significant intraarticular step off were present. Although not able to be accurately assessed due to pain, the extensor mechanism was probably disrupted based on the displacement of the fragments.

Surgical Management

The patient was taken to the operating room where an anesthetic was administered. Examination of the knee revealed that the ligaments were intact; specifically, there was no sign of posterior cruciate instability. The leg was prepped and draped free. A straight anterior incision was made extending from 5 cm proximal to the patella to 2 cm distal to the tibial tubercle. Loose fragments of bone were removed, severely damaged soft tissue was excised, intraarticular hematoma was sent for culture, and the knee was irrigated. The medial and lateral retinacula were found to be torn. Almost all of the distal pole of the patella was removed in the debridement. A locking whipstitch was used to secure the patellar ligament. Two holes were drilled through the proximal patella from distal to proximal. The sutures were brought through these holes and tied over the proximal pole of the patella. The retinacula were repaired with figure of 8 sutures. A "neutralization cable" was implanted to protect

A

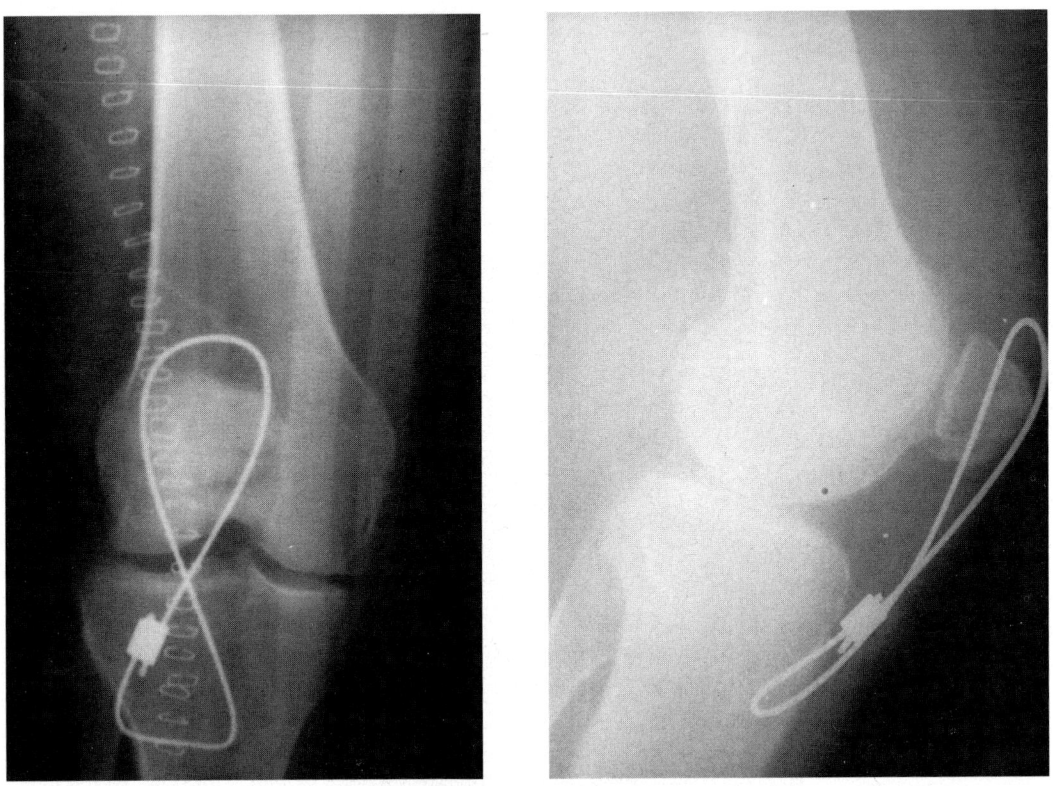

B

Figure 20–2. Anteroposterior (A) and lateral (B) radiographs of the knee following excision of the distal pole, attachment of the patellar tendon to the patella, and protection of the repair with a figure of eight neutralization cable.

PEARL

- It is important to rule out associated ligament damage prior to repairing the patellar tendon. This injury was caused by a blow to the anterior aspect of the knee; the posterior cruciate is therefore the most likely ligament injured. The locking whipstitch is utilized because it is the strongest method of anchoring suture to tendon. The patellar ligament is reattached to the patella in such a way that the patella is not "tilted" during contraction of the quadriceps. Tilting of the patella will result in the rapid onset of osteoarthritis and is usually due to anterior placement of the holes by which the ligament is attached to the patella. The neutralization cable is designed to neutralize stresses across the repair during flexion of the knee. This allows early rehabilitation of the knee. The keys to implanting the cable are to place it as close as possible to cortex of the proximal pole of the patella to minimize its "pulling through" the quadriceps tendon and thus loosening, and to cross the cable over the anterior aspect of the tendon to prevent the cable from displacing posteriorly during flexion.

the repair (Fig. 20–2). The surgical extensions of the wound were closed. A drain was left in the joint, and the stellate skin laceration was left open.

Postoperative Management

The cultures from the emergency department and operating room were negative. Antibiotics were continued for 3 days. Active range of motion and weight bearing as tolerated were started on day 3. By day 4 the patient was able to extend the knee to 5 degrees and flex to 30 degrees with some discomfort. The stellate laceration, which had been left open, was skin grafted at 4 days. The knee was immobilized in extension for 2 days following skin grafting, after which physical therapy was resumed. All wounds healed. At 6 months, when the neutralization cable was removed, the range of motion was from 0 to 105 degrees. The final range of motion at 1 year was 0 to 130 degrees (Fig. 20–3).

Discussion

This fracture presents two problems: an open injury to the knee joint and disruption of the extensor mechanism. The intraarticular step off is not a major consideration because it involves the distal pole of the patella. This part of the patella does not articulate with the femoral condyles, and therefore a step off will not result in osteoarthritis. Management of the *open injury to the knee* is the first priority. Devi-

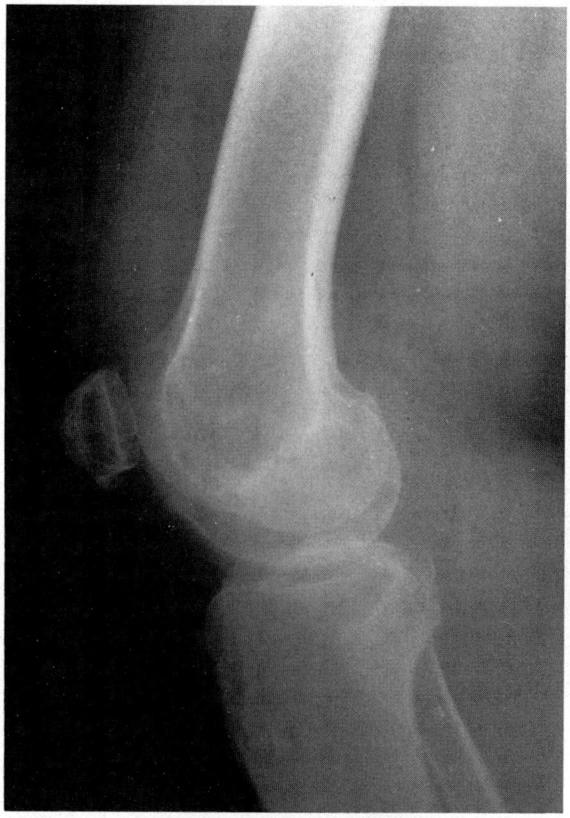

Figure 20–3. Lateral radiograph at 1 year following injury. The neutralization cable has been removed and the patella is healed.

talized tissue and hematoma are debrided and the wound is cultured. After a clean wound has been achieved, reconstruction of the *disrupted extensor mechanism* can proceed. Regardless of the method used to reattach the patellar ligament to the patella, reapproximation of the medial and lateral retinacula increase the strength of the repair. Closure of the stellate laceration was not attempted because the surrounding skin was traumatized and tension on the edges of the laceration might have caused necrosis.

Alternative Methods of Management

Alternative methods of management of the extensor mechanism disruption were delayed repair, immediate repair without a cable, or immediate repair with a cable, as in this case. Delayed repair may decrease the chance of infection, but in most cases the difficulties of late reconstruction of the extensor mechanism outweigh the advantages. The quadriceps tendon and patellar ligament will both retract and shorten, making reconstruction extremely difficult. Only in cases in which an extensive wound is severely contaminated should delayed repair be considered. Immediate repair without a neutralization cable has two advantages. First, the exposure does not have to be extended distally to the tibial tubercle. Second, the cable does not have to be removed after the ligament has healed. Immediate repair with a neutralization cable has the overwhelming advantage of allowing early aggressive physical therapy. Usually the cable is removed because it prevents the last 10 to 20 degrees of flexion. Cable removal is an outpatient procedure.

Type of Management	Advantages	Disadvantages	Comments
Delayed repair	Decreased chance of infection	Difficulty reconstructing extensor mechanism	Indicated with grossly contaminated, very severe soft tissue injuries
Immediate repair without cable	Less extensive approach	Limited rehabilitation until 4–6 weeks	The disadvantages outweigh the advantages
Immediate repair with cable	Aggressive rehabilitation is possible	Often necessary to remove the cable	Major advantage of allowing early aggressive range of motion

Complications

Complications of an open comminuted patella fracture include infection and loss of fixation. Infection usually involves the knee joint. It is managed with incision and drainage of the knee and closure over drains. The patellar ligament is not debrided unless the infection is uncontrollable. Coverage is obtained with rotation of the medial head of the gastrocnemius or free vascularized tissue transfer. Systemic antibiotics are administered for 4 to 6 weeks. Immobilization of the knee may be necessary, but will result in a permanent loss of motion. Loss of fixation is most frequently due to the sutures pulling out of the patellar ligament. A less common reason for loss of fixation is fracture of the patellar remnant (Figs. 20–4 and 20–5). Fracture is usually through the suture holes. Use of a neutralization cable minimizes

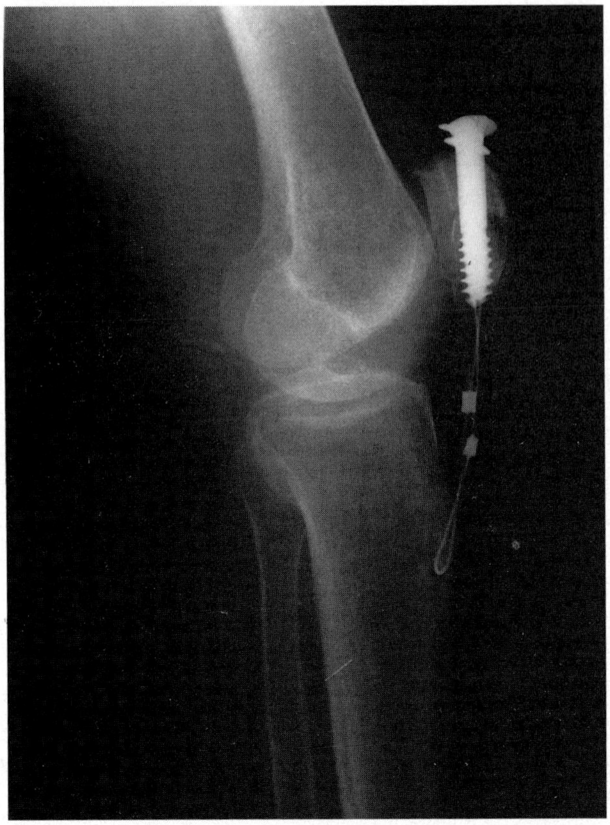

Figure 20–4. Lateral radiograph of a knee following fixation of a transverse patellar fracture with cancellous screws and a neutralization cable.

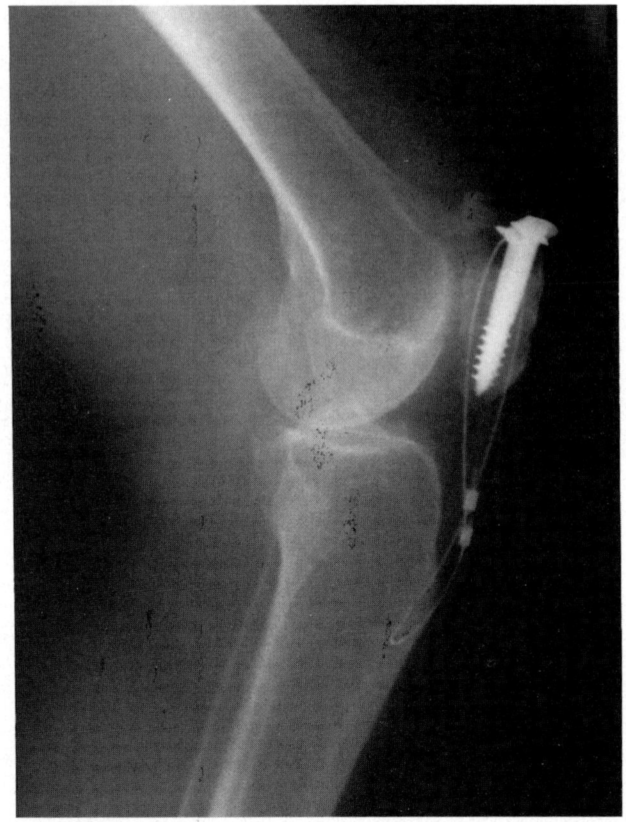

Figure 20–5. Lateral radiograph of the knee. The quadriceps tendon has avulsed the proximal pole of the patella. This is due to weakening of the proximal pole by insertion of the cancellous screws.

the chance of loss of fixation. When fixation is lost, management involves revision and protection with a neutralization cable.

Suggested Readings

Burvant JG, Thomas KA, Alexander R, Harris MB: Evaluation of methods of internal fixation of transverse patella fractures: a biomechanical study. J Orthop Trauma 1994; 8:147–153.

Liang QY, Wu JW: Fracture of the patella treated by open reduction and external skeletal fixation. J Bone Joint Surg 1987; 69:83–89.

Perry CR, McCarthy JA, Kain CC, Pearson RL: Patellar fixation protected with a load-sharing cable: a mechanical and clinical study. J Orthop Trauma 1988; 2:234–240.

Weber MJ, Janecki CJ, McLeod P, Nelson CL, Thompson JA: Efficacy of various forms of fixation of transverse fractures of the patella. J Bone Joint Surg 1980; 62A:212–220.

Case 21

History and Physical Examination

An 89-year-old female was admitted to the emergency department after falling about 4 feet from a small ladder that she had climbed to allow her to clean a window in her home. She was in good health, took no medication, and lived alone without support. On examination in the emergency department she had a very painful right knee with no evidence of distal neurovascular abnormality. There was no other injury. She gave a history of having had slight knee pain before the accident, particularly on ascending and descending stairs or slopes.

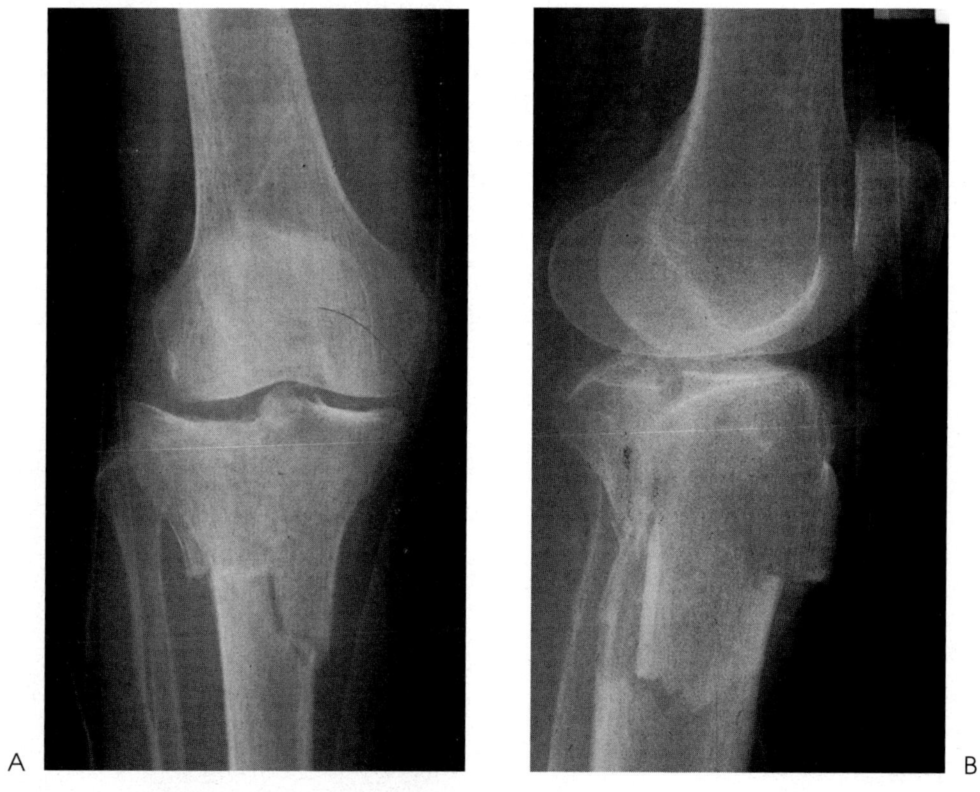

Figure 21–1. Anteroposterior (A) and lateral (B) views of a complex intraarticular tibial plateau fracture in an 89-year-old female with very osteoporotic bone.

Radiologic Findings

Anteroposterior and lateral radiographs (Fig. 21–1) of the right knee indicate a bicondylar tibial plateau fracture. The anteroposterior view shows some depression and subluxation of the lateral tibial condyle. The medial condyle was slightly displaced. The complexity of the fracture is further highlighted in the lateral radio-graph. The medial tibial condyle is split in the coronal plane and the posterior depression of the lateral condyle can be clearly seen. In addition, the tibial tubercle containing the insertion of the patella tendon is fractured and there is evidence of fairly extensive metaphyseal comminution. There is no evidence of a lateral metaphyseal wedge.

Diagnosis

A bicondylar tibial plateau fracture associated with metaphyseal comminution, a coronal fracture of the medial condyle, and depression of the lateral condyle. AO classification: 41–C2.1.

Surgical Management

When deciding on the initial management a number of factors were taken into consideration. The age and degree of dependency of the patient were considered. At 89 years of age the bone is profoundly osteoporotic and it was thought that there was little likelihood of gaining adequate fixation with bone screws. However, because the patient was in excellent health, it was believed that she merited active treatment to allow her to continue her independent existence. After considering the advantages and disadvantages of surgery, it was considered that in view of the complexity of the fracture and the fact that the fragments were well approximated and reasonably aligned, nonoperative management would be undertaken. It was thought that a knee replacement could be undertaken after union if her symptoms suggested that this was a reasonable option. Both the surgeon and patient accepted that she might lose some joint mobility.

A well padded cylinder cast was applied and the patient was mobilized to be nonweight bearing using a zimmer frame. Radiographs were taken 4 days after ad-

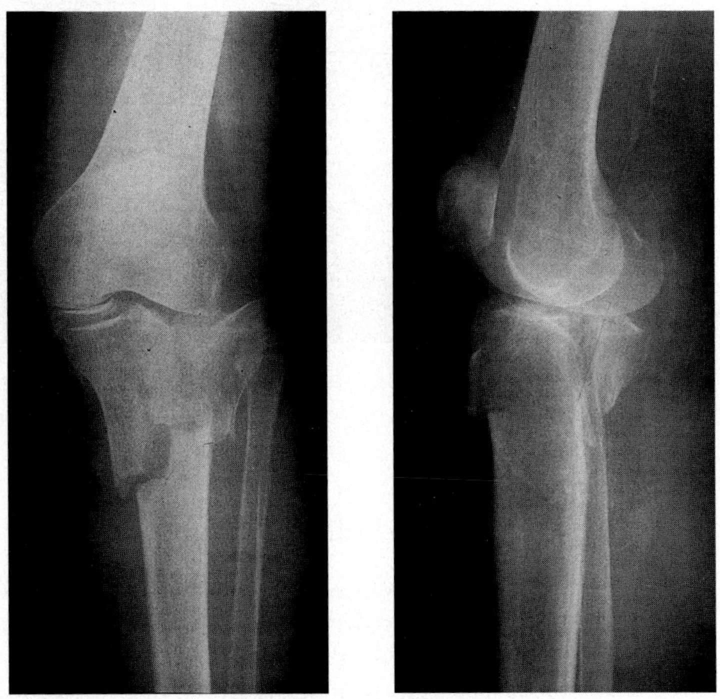

Figure 21–2. After a short period of nonoperative management, it is obvious that the fracture is displacing. (A) Anteroposterior and (B) lateral views.

PEARL

- Nonoperative management should not be confused with nontreatment. There may well be circumstances when the surgeon considers that the patient is too old or frail for the optimal treatment method to be undertaken. However, the surgeon may decide that nonoperative management is the optimal method of treatment. Nonoperative management may be more difficult than operative management because there may be late displacement of the fracture fragments. This must be looked for with serial radiographs. Failure to diagnose fracture displacement early may result in the fracture being inoperable later.

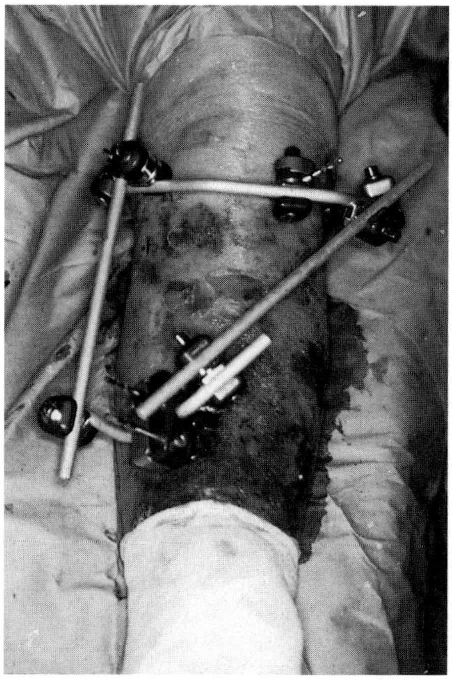

Figure 21–3. The fixator used to stabilize this fracture. Note the poor condition of the soft tissues.

mission to check on the fracture position (Fig. 21–2). The anteroposterior view indicates significant displacement of the tibial condyles with marked lateral subluxation of the lateral condyle. The lateral view suggests that the coronal split in the medial condyle has widened and that the tibial tuberosity may also have moved anteriorly. The overall alignment was seen to be drifting in valgus and if nonoperative management is continued, it is probable that the lateral femoral condyle will descend into the defect in the lateral tibial condyle, creating a significant valgus deformity.

It is obvious from these radiographs that continuing a nonoperative regime is unreasonable in a fit elderly person. It was thought that the osteoporotic nature of the bone precluded the use of two bone plates and it was decided to treat the fracture by percutaneous screw fixation to reduce the condyles and external fixation to maintain the alignment of the tibia. Late arthroplasty was still considered an option, although it was accepted that the risk of infection was higher following the use of external skeletal fixation.

The patient was taken to the operating room and the leg was prepped and draped. Under fluoroscopy the condyles were reapproximated with a percutaneous bone clamp and a 6.5 mm cancellous screw was placed across the condyles to maintain reduction. The osteoporotic nature of the bone was illustrated by the fact that the first external fixator pin touched the cancellous screw and pushed it out. This occurred even though the pin was inserted gently by hand.

A second 6.5 mm cancellous screw was placed into the slightly harder cortical bone in the metaphyseal area to maintain condylar alignment and a half ring external fixator utilizing half pins was applied. Three half pins were placed into the condyles and connected in a triangular configuration to the diaphysis (Fig. 21–3). Radiographs showed a reasonable approximation of the joint (Fig. 21–4).

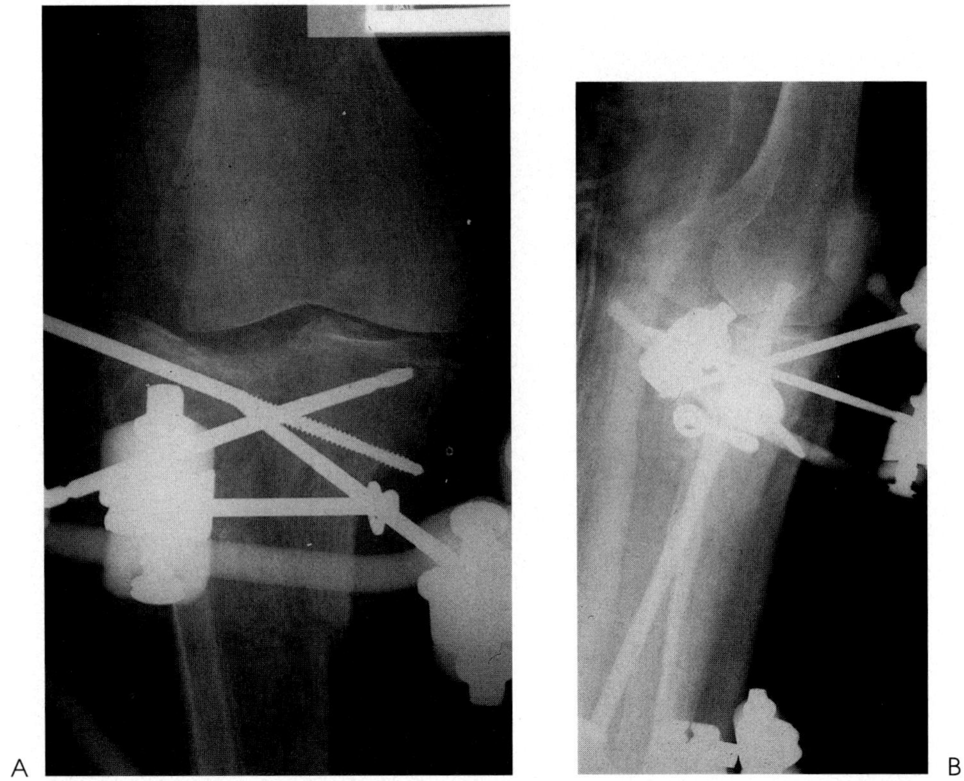

Figure 21–4. Anteroposterior (A) and lateral (B) postoperative radiographs show reasonable alignment. This position was maintained throughout the treatment.

Postoperative Management

Postoperatively dressings were applied and because of the osteoporotic nature of the bone a back slab was also applied to supplement the external fixation. This was maintained for 4 weeks and then used as a resting splint with active and passive physiotherapy exercises instituted. After 5 weeks one of the external fixator pins loosened and required replacement, but reasonable alignment was maintained, although check radiographs showed a persistent lateral subluxation of the tibia.

The patient was allowed to weight bear at 10 weeks and the external fixation device was removed at 15 weeks. Six months after the injury the patient had 80 degrees of knee flexion and could walk with the aid of one crutch. She had more knee pain than she had experienced preoperatively. She was offered an arthroplasty but declined. She returned home but required social support.

Discussion

Tibial plateau fractures are very common in the elderly. A review of 225 tibial plateau fractures admitted to the orthopedic trauma unit in Edinburgh, Scotland, over a 3 year period showed that the most common decade for patients to present with tibial plateau fractures was between 60 and 70 years of age. Overall 48.6% of the patients with tibial plateau fractures were over 60 years of age and 30.9% of the patients were over 70 years of age. About 10% of patients of more than 70 years of

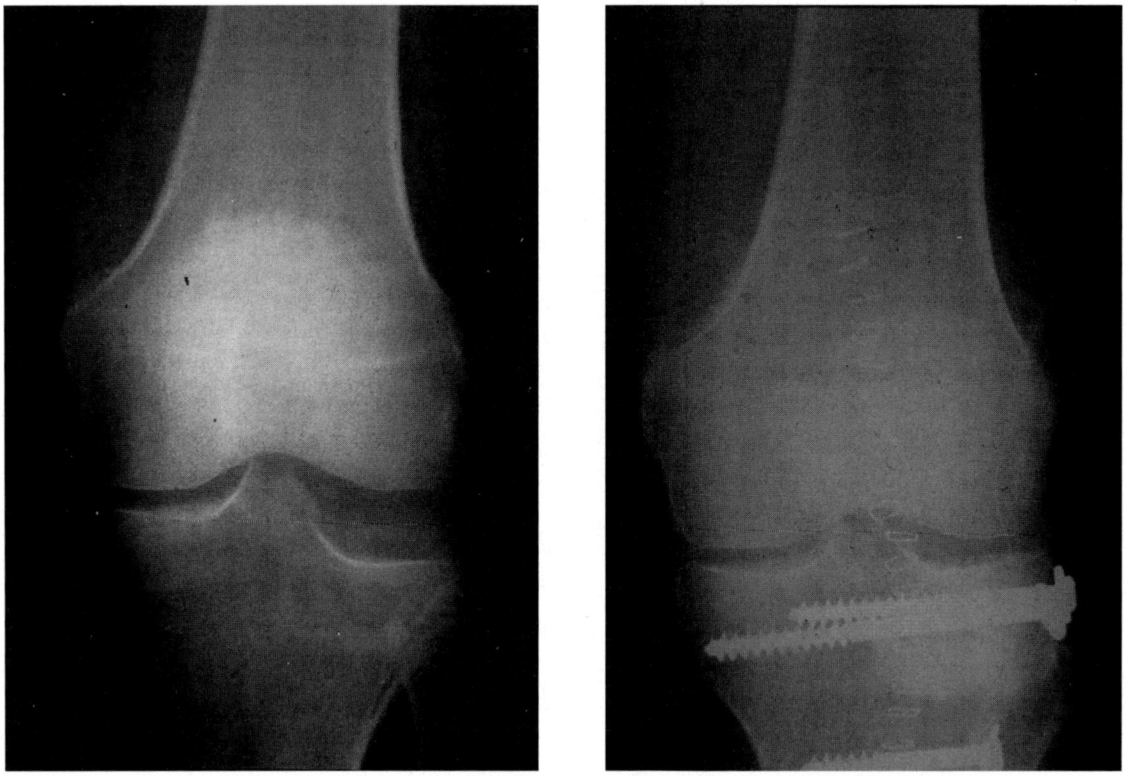

A B

Figure 21–5. Anteroposterior radiographs showing the use of Norian SRS in the management of a depressed lateral condyle fracture. Preoperative (A); postoperative (B).

PITFALL

- Surgeons commonly assume that the more severe fracture configurations occur in younger patients after high energy injuries. This is not the case. In many fractures the average age of the AO-C2 and AO-C3 fractures is more than 50 years. This is true of tibial plateau fractures. The epidemiological data from Edinburgh show that the average age of patients with C2 or C3 fractures is 55 years. The osteoporotic bone makes the fractures more difficult to treat than in younger patients.

age present with AO type C bicondylar fractures. Of the remaining 90% of patients almost 70% were either pure depression partial articular fractures (AO–B2 fractures) or partial articular split depression fractures (AO–B3 fractures). About 53% of all patients over 70 years of age present with pure depression fractures. This highlights the osteoporotic nature of elderly bone and also demonstrates why surgeons are faced with considerable difficulties when treating tibial plateau fractures in the elderly.

There is often debate about the optimal method for elevating the depressed articular cartilage in tibial plateau fractures. However, elevation of the cartilage is usually straightforward. It is maintaining the elevated position that is often impossible. The usual method of supporting the articular surface of a depressed tibial condyle is by using autogenous bone graft from the iliac crest. Unfortunately, the bone graft is also osteoporotic and experience suggests that it rarely maintains the articular cartilage in a reduced position. Surgeons have been seeking alternatives to osteoporotic autogenous cancellous bone graft, but allograft and bone cement have their own inherent problems. Recent interest has centered around the use of bone substitutes such as Norian SRS, an example of which is shown in Figure 21–5. As yet there is little data about the usefulness of these bone substitutes in depressed metaphyseal fractures such as those seen in the calcaneus and proximal tibia, but early results in the distal radius are encouraging.

Obviously, many tibial plateau fractures in elderly patients do not require any surgery. A number of fractures present in patients who are debilitated, demented, or have profoundly limited function. These patients often have limited goals and surgery is frequently inappropriate. However, this case illustrates the dilemma that orthopedic trauma surgeons increasingly face. Modern medical techniques and increasing affluence have meant that patients in many parts of the world are not only living longer but are medically fit enough to pursue a range of fairly strenuous activities well into advanced old age. Thus while a generation ago it might have been considered reasonable to treat this patient by "benign neglect" because of her age this is no longer justifiable. Even very elderly patients are demanding to be returned to their prefracture level of function. This is usually much more difficult than in younger patients and demands expensive and time consuming surgery that society is going to find increasingly difficult to finance. These patients not infrequently require multiple operations and in this case of a very complex bicondylar fracture both surgeon and patient must reconcile themselves to a 6 or 9 month treatment period if even reasonable function is to be regained.

Alternative Methods of Management

Many tibial plateau fractures in the elderly will be treated nonoperatively. This may well be appropriate, but this case highlights one of the complications of the use of a cast in a displaced multifragmented proximal tibial fracture. Traction, using a split bed and early joint motion, was popular at one time, but this technique is very labor intensive and is unlikely to result in the reduction of the intraarticular fragments. In addition, prolonged bed rest is universally acknowledged to be harmful to the elderly.

The conventional management for a bicondylar tibial plateau fracture in a younger patient involves open reduction and the application of medial and lateral bone plates. Autogenous bone graft is used if required. As its name implies, osteoporotic bone is more porous than younger bone and bone screws frequently gain a

Type of Management	Advantages	Disadvantages	Comments
Cast/traction	Straightforward technique; useful in simple fractures	Traction not tolerated by the elderly; malunion; joint stiffness; pain	The treatment of choice for uncomplicated tibial plateau fractures in the elderly
Internal fixation; plates/screws	Useful in the less common split condylar fracture of the elderly	Technically difficult in the elderly; may need a supporting cast; high failure rate	Useful in split condylar fractures, but much less so in depression fractures or bicondylar fractures
External fixation	Useful method in maintaining bone alignment; easy to apply	Unlikely to maintain articular congruity; joint stiffness; pin tract sepsis	Probably most useful as temporary fixation but does play a part in definitive management of tibial condylar fractures in the elderly
Arthroplasty	Good range of motion; loss of pain	Technically difficult; unproven	May well become a much more popular method of managing these fractures in the future

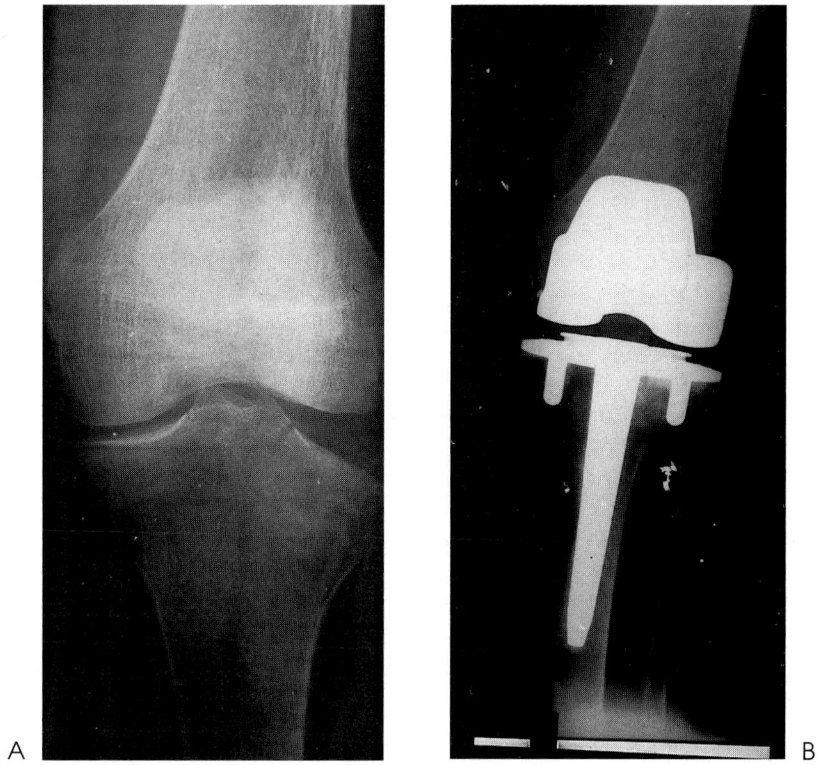

Figure 21–6. Anteroposterior radiographs showing the use of a primary arthroplasty in the management of a depressed lateral condyle fracture in an elderly patient. (A) Preoperative; (B) postoperative.

poor hold. In addition, the soft tissue dissection required to insert two plates is considerable and there is an increased risk of infection.

In recent years surgeons have explored the possibility of using primary arthroplasty to treat these complex fractures. Many elderly patients already have arthritic changes in their knee joints prior to the plateau fracture and thus arthroplasty seems doubly attractive. In this case the detached tibial tuberosity was considered to mitigate against a successful primary arthroplasty. If primary arthroplasty is to be used in bicondylar tibial plateau fractures, surgeons will need to use long stem or hinged prostheses. However, conventional arthroplasty prostheses can be used in the common depressed lateral condylar fracture. An example of this is shown in Figure 21–6.

Complications

The most frequent complication of the management of proximal tibial fractures in the elderly is posttraumatic osteoarthritis. This is very common, but usually the patient will be treated successfully with nonsteroidal antiinflammatory drugs and alteration of their activities. Occasionally, however, arthroplasty is required. The surgeon should always be aware of this possibility when planning the original surgery. If internal fixation is to be used, it is always wise to use a midline incision to make the secondary arthroplasty easier and safer.

Nonunion is unusual because the fracture is in cancellous bone, but malunions are not uncommon following nonoperative management. These must be assessed individually and the advantages and disadvantages of surgery discussed with the patient. The patient, however, may take the view that the morbidity associated with osteotomy and possible bone grafting is not worthwhile at their advanced age. Infection is unusual, but if it occurs, it would be treated as described elsewhere in this book.

Suggested Readings

Delamarter R, Hohl M, Hopp E: Ligament injuries associated with tibial plateau fractures. Clin Orthop 1990; 250:226–233.

Hohl M, Luck J: Fractures of the tibial plateau: a clinical and experimental study. J Bone Joint Surg (Am) 1956; 38:1001–1018.

Honkonen SE: Degenerative arthritis after tibial plateau fractures. J Orthop Trauma 1995; 9:273–277.

Schatzker J: Tibial plateau fractures. In Browner BD, Jupiter JB, Levine AM, Trafton PG: Skeletal Trauma, pp 1745–1769. WB Saunders, Philadelphia, 1992.

Schatzker J, McBroom R: Tibial plateau fractures. The Toronto experience. Clin Orthop 1979; 138:94–104.

Weiner LS, Kelley M, Yang E, et al: The use of combination internal fixation and hybrid external fixation in severe proximal tibia fractures. J Orthop Trauma 1995; 9:244–250.

Case 22

History and Physical Examination

A 34-year-old man sustained an open injury of his right leg involving the knee and proximal tibia. The injury occurred when the patient's leg was crushed between a brick wall and a truck bumper while the truck was moving at approximately 5 miles per hour. The injury occurred 1 hour prior to the patient's arrival in the emergency department.

The initial physical examination revealed no injuries other than those to the knee and proximal tibia. There was obvious deformity and instability of the proximal tibia. The skin overlying the proximal tibia was contused and "tented" by displaced fragments of bone. A 3 cm long laceration was present and actively bleeding. The dorsalis pedis and posterior tibial pulses were palpable. Sensation was decreased in the first web space, but otherwise intact. Gentle passive stretch of the dorsi and plantar flexors of the ankle resulted in severe pain. The patient was unwilling to actively move his toes or ankle due to pain. Compartment pressures measured 55 mm Hg in the lateral compartment, 45 mm Hg and 40 mm Hg in the posterior deep and posterior superficial compartments, respectively, and 60 mm Hg in the anterior compartment.

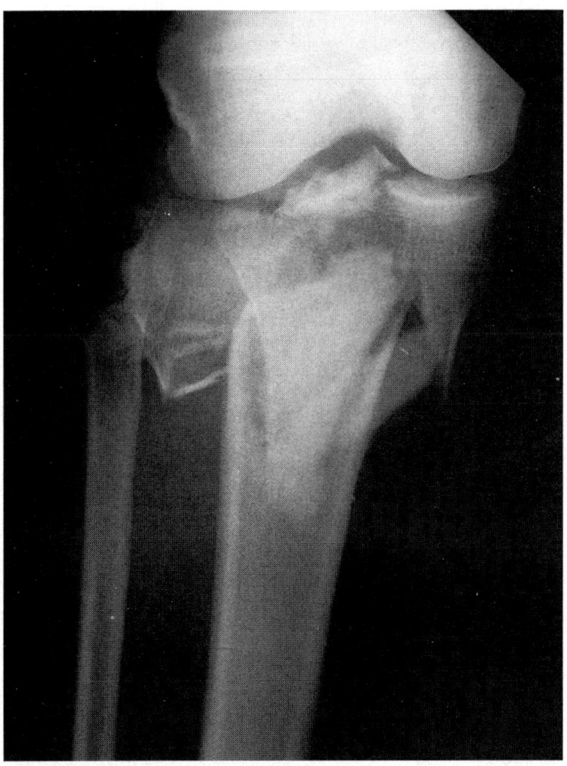
A

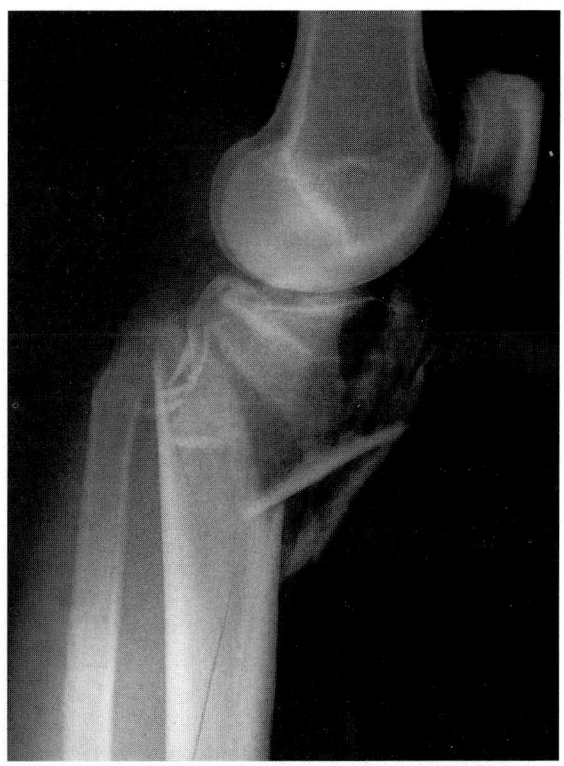
B

Figure 22–1. Anteroposterior (A) and lateral (B) radiographs of the proximal tibia. A comminuted fracture involving the articular surface is present.

PITFALL

- Neurovascular injuries are frequently associated with high energy fractures of the proximal tibia. Therefore it is mandatory to perform a complete examination to determine if a neurological or vascular injury is present. Compartment syndrome and vascular injuries are managed emergently because delay often results in amputation. The presence of a neurological injury does not alter the initial management, but is documented for legal reasons and because a dense global neurological deficit that does not resolve is a *relative* indication for amputation.

Radiologic Findings

Radiographic assessment consists of plane films of the knee, tibia, and ankle in the anteroposterior, lateral, and oblique projections. In this case, radiographs indicated a comminuted displaced fracture of the proximal tibia with involvement of the articular surface (Fig. 22–1). A CT scan obtained the first postinjury day indicated the plane of the fractures and degree of comminution of the articular surface.

Diagnosis

Open proximal intraarticular tibial fracture (Schatzker type VI) with elevated pressures in all four compartments. The open fracture was classified as grade III because of comminution and the associated compartment syndrome. It was not possible to further classify the fracture as grade IIIA or B until surgical exploration.

Surgical Management

The patient was taken to the operating room where a general anesthetic was administered. The leg was held by an assistant while it was scrubbed and then draped. The laceration was extended proximally and distally. Hematoma, devascularized bone, and soft tissue were removed from the fracture site. Fasciotomies of all four com-

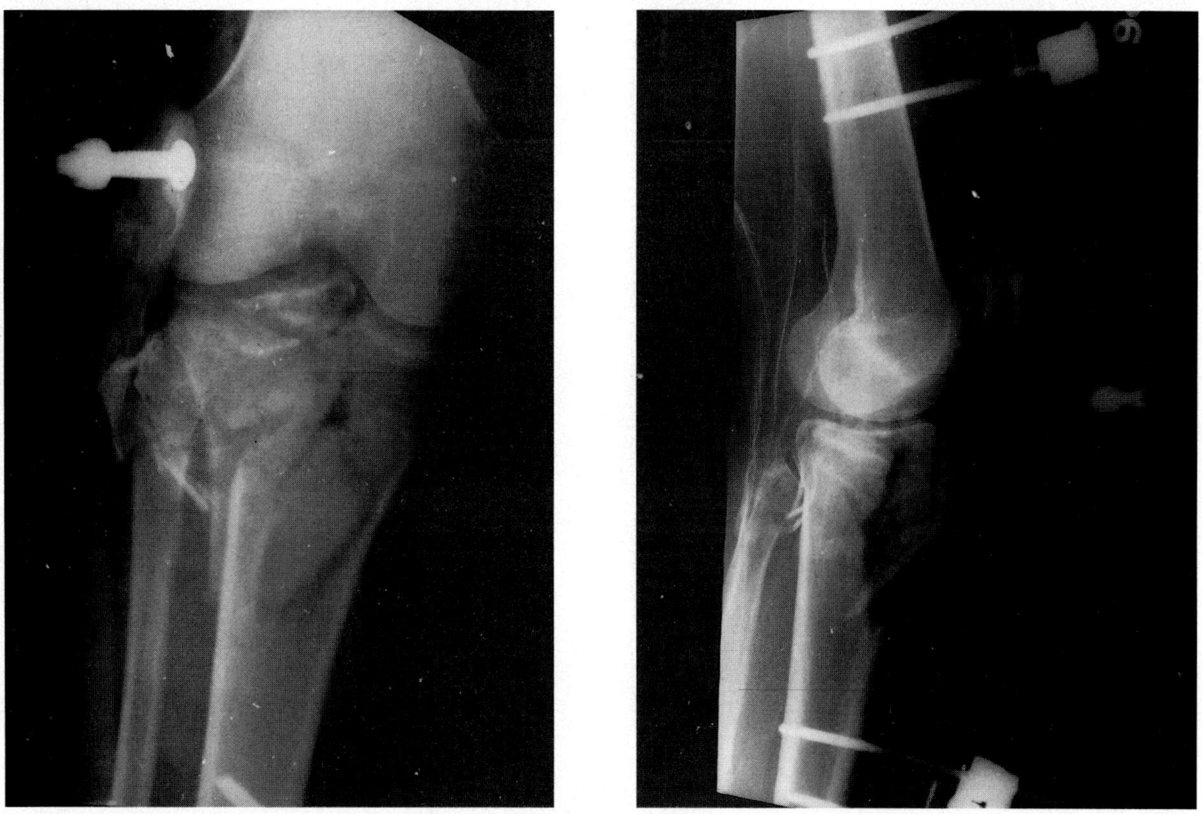

A B

Figure 22–2. Anteroposterior (A) and lateral (B) radiographs following temporary stabilization with a bridging frame. In addition, the compartments of the leg were surgically decompressed.

PEARL

- Computerized axial tomography is invaluable in identifying the plane and direction of fractures involving the articular surface in complex fracture patterns, but is not necessary for relatively simple fracture patterns with *undisplaced intraarticular extension.*

partments were performed through medial and lateral incisions and a bridging external fixator with two pins in the distal femur and two pins in the midtibia was applied. The fracture was aligned with longitudinal traction and the fixator tightened (Fig. 22–2). The fasciotomy incisions were packed open. Reduction and fixation of the intraarticular fractures were planned with the aid of a CT scan obtained the first postinjury day.

The second postinjury day the patient was returned to the operating room for limited open reduction and fixation with screws and the addition of a small wire circular frame to the bridging fixator. Reduction of the joint surface was achieved via the existing incisions. Fluoroscopy was used to confirm reduction and guide the placement of percutaneous screws and wires. Four days after injury a split thickness skin graft was applied to the fasciotomy sites (Fig. 22–3).

The *technique of external fixation with a small wire circular frame and limited internal fixation* is performed with the patient supine on a radiolucent operating table and has two stages. The first stage is reduction and stabilization of the articular surface. The second is fixation of the proximal tibia, including the reconstructed joint surface, to the distal tibia with an external fixator.

Stage 1 (reduction and stabilization of the articular surface). When intraarticular fractures are minimally displaced without a step off, lag screws or olive wires are inserted percutaneously and used to achieve interfragmentary compression. In cases in which there is a step off, the articular surface is exposed through a parapatellar ap-

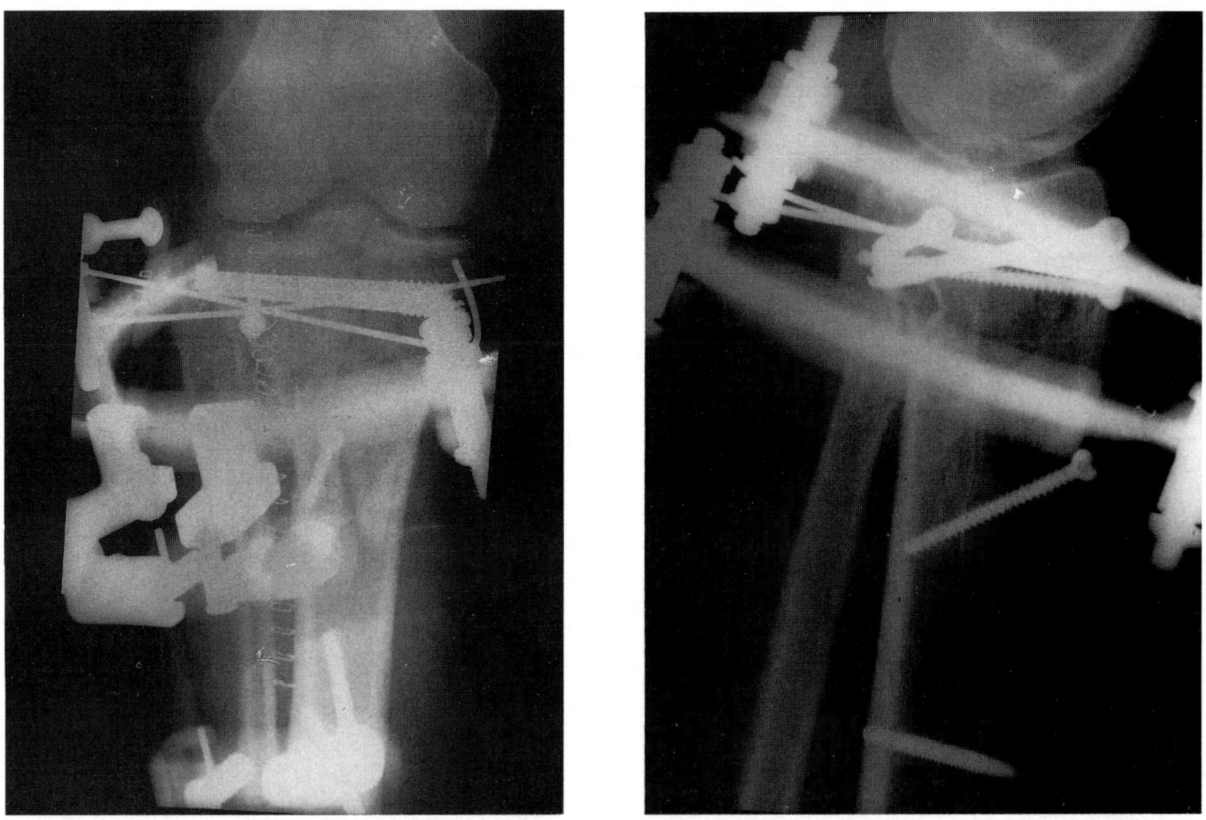

A B

Figure 22–3. Anteroposterior (A) and lateral (B) radiographs following reduction and stabilization with limited internal fixation and a small wire circular frame. A component of the external fixator is bridging the knee joint and holding it is distraction.

PEARL

- To ensure that the wires are not intracapsular, they should be at least 1 cm distal to the articular surface. Placement of the wires within 1 cm of the joint surface may be necessary, but exposes the patient to the risk of septic arthritis.

proach and the fracture is reduced under direct vision. Provisional fixation with Kirschner wires is supplemented with lag screws or olive wires.

Stage 2 consists of fixation of proximal tibia to distal tibia. The goal of the second stage of the procedure is stabilization of the reduced proximal tibia to the distal tibia with an external fixator. It is important to align the articular surface correctly with the tibial shaft and, most important, to avoid varus malalignment. A radiolucent grid is helpful in assessing alignment. There are two types of fixator frames, small wire circular and hybrid. When a small wire circular frame is used, at least one more ring is applied distally and fixed to the proximal ring. When a hybrid frame is used, large cantilever pins are inserted in the distal tibia via its subcutaneous border. These pins are fixed to the proximal ring via the fixator frame.

Postoperative Management

The goal of postoperative management is to prevent loss of reduction and regain a functional range of motion. The bridging component of the fixator was removed 6 weeks after injury and active range of motion exercises were initiated. The wounds healed without evidence of infection. Ten weeks after injury, partial weight bearing was initiated and advanced to full weight bearing over the next 2 weeks. The fixator was removed 14 weeks after injury. At 6 months the knee range of motion was to 90 degrees. Ankle plantarflexion was 60, dorsiflexion was 10 (Fig. 22–4).

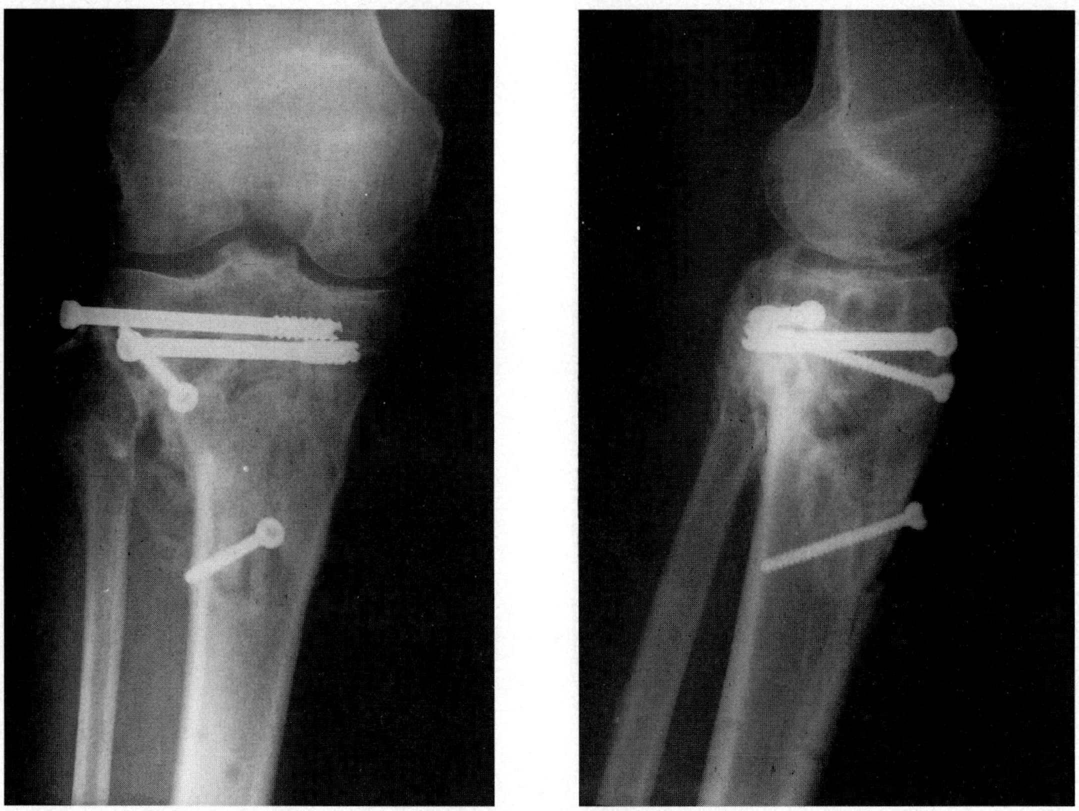

Figure 22–4. Anteroposterior (A) and lateral (B) radiographs at 1 year.

Discussion

This patient sustained a high energy fracture of the proximal tibia due to direct trauma. In the spectrum of proximal tibia fractures, this is the most severe type of injury. Significant soft tissue injuries are invariably associated with this type of fracture, including injury of the popliteal, posterior tibial, peroneal, or anterior tibial arteries; injury of the posterior tibial or peroneal nerves; injury of the overlying skin or muscle that compromises coverage; and elevated intracompartmental pressures.

Alternative Methods of Management

Management of high energy proximal tibial fractures evolved from the noninvasive techniques of traction, casting, and intensive physical therapy, to the invasive techniques of extensive surgical exposure, anatomic reduction, and application of plates and screws to achieve bony stability. The most recent method utilizes the techniques of indirect reduction via ligamentotaxis; limited surgical exposure; interfragmentary fixation with percutaneous screws, antiglide plates, and olive wires; external fixation, and bridging frames. Each of these methods of management has unique advantages, making the method applicable in certain clinical settings.

Traction and casting are used infrequently because of the prolonged hospitalization and residual deformity, even though Apley, Connolly, and others have shown that the presence of residual deformity does not correlate with a poor result.

Open reduction of high energy fractures of the proximal tibia has the advantage of facilitating accurate reduction of the articular surface and stable fixation of the articular segments to the metaphysis. Stable accurate reduction permits early active range of motion. Disadvantages of this method include devascularization of fracture fragments that are exposed subperiosteally and exposing the patient with a closed fracture to the risk of infection.

There are two methods of external fixation with limited internal fixation: small wire circular frames with interfragmental screws or pins and large pin cantilever frames applied medially or laterally with a plate applied to the contralateral cortex. Both these methods of external fixation with limited internal fixation have the advantage of limiting the surgical exposure, theoretically decreasing the chance of wound problems and possibly nonunion. Because the joint surface is often not visualized as completely with limited open reduction and external fixation as it is with open reduction and internal fixation, the incidence of posttraumatic arthritis secondary to incomplete reduction of intraarticular fractures may be higher with limited open reduction and external fixation. Limited open reduction and external fixation have the additional disadvantage of subjecting the patient to the possibility of pin tract infection. Because the pins are in the zone of injury, and often actually traverse the fracture site, pin tract infections can result in an infected fracture. Similarly, infected pin tracts that traverse the joint capsule of the knee can lead to joint sepsis.

Small wire circular frames with interfragmental screws or pins is a flexible method of stabilization that is applicable to all types of bycondylar tibial plateau fractures. When a large pin cantilever frame with a contralateral plate is used, the fixator functions as a plate but without the soft tissue dissection. Large pin cantilever frames are not applicable to fractures with a displaced intra articular component, as in this case.

Bridging external fixators extend from the distal femur across the knee distal to the tibial fracture. Bridging frames are useful in two settings: prior to the definitive reduction and stabilization and following the definitive procedure to prevent late loss of reduction. Bridging frames applied prior to the definitive procedure are used to hold the fracture out to length and stabililize the extremity when the definitive procedure is delayed. Bridging frames applied following the definitive procedure are used when the fracture fixation is tenuous. The frame is applied with the joint slightly distracted. It is designed to isolate the fracture from external forces, in particular, axial loads and to a lesser extent rotational and angular loads. In this setting, early motion is sacrificed to minimize the chance of loss of reduction. In general, because bridging frames are used as a last resort in the most severe cases, it is difficult to compare the final result of cases in which they are used with cases in which they are not used.

Type of Management	Advantages	Disadvantages	Comments
Traction and casting	Low incidence of infection	Higher incidence of malunion; osteoarthritis	More applicable to low energy fractures; frequently residual displacement is seen on X ray; this technique is not used frequently because of displacement
Open reduction and internal fixation	Anatomic reduction of articular surface; stable fixation allows early motion	Slower fracture healing because of devascularization of bone fragments; higher incidence of wound complications and infection	Most acceptable method to patient and can yield the best result, but has the risk of extremely severe complications
External fixation with limited internal fixation, small wire circular frame	Limited devascularization of bone; limited surgical exposure may decrease incidence of infection and nonunion	Frame is bulky and patients do not like them; pins traverse fracture and capsule; if pin infection occurs, it can lead to an infected fracture or septic joint	The articular surface must be reduced, and fixation must be stable or results are poor
External fixation with limited internal fixation, large pin frame and contralateral plate	Limited devascularization of bone; limited surgical exposure may decrease incidence of infection and nonunion	Large pin frames are better tolerated than circular frames, but patients still do not like them	Limited application i.e., the fracture cannot be intraarticular
Bridging frame	Prevents loss of reduction	Prevents early range of motion; patients do not like frame	Prevents loss of reduction when stability is not achievable because of osteopenia or comminution

Complications

Complications of high energy fractures of the proximal tibia are infection, nonunion, malunion, and arthritis. Infection is the result of the severe soft tissue injury associated with these injuries. The soft tissue injury in conjunction with an extensive surgical exposure and additional subperiosteal exposure results in devascularization of large segments of bone and increases the possibility of infection. When infection occurs, loss of motion, nonunion, and postinfectious arthritis are likely to occur. In addition, secondary procedures such as debridement and bone grafting are often necessary. A reasonable protocol is to leave the hardware in place as long as it is stabilizing the fracture and the infection is controllable with local wound care in the form of dressing changes and whirlpool. Orally administered antibiotics are used, but long term intravenous antibiotics are not an option because the limited chance of success does not justify the risks (i.e., induced tolerance, infected intravenous lines, and toxic side effects to the antibiotics). Nonweight bearing is maintained until the fracture is healed. When the fracture has healed, the proximal tibia is debrided, implants are removed, soft tissue coverage is obtained, and systemic antibiotics, based on the sensitivities of the pathogenic organisms, are administered for 6 weeks. In cases in which the infection cannot be controlled or is controllable only with intravenous antibiotics, debridement and stabilization with a bridging external fixator are performed. Delayed soft tissue coverage with a free vascularized flap or rotational flap, autogenous bone grafting, and reconstruction of the joint surface or arthrodesis are performed.

Nonunion of proximal tibial fractures is rare. It is usually diagnosed when there is increasing deformity and pain with weight bearing. When the diagnosis of nonunion is made prior to loss of alignment, management is noninvasive, consisting of pulsed electromagnetic fields and nonweight bearing. If this regimen is not successful, or there has been loss of alignment, management is invasive, consisting of reduction, bone grating, and stabilization with plates and screws.

Malunion is managed with osteotomy and plating.

Arthritis is managed conservatively with nonsteroidal antiinflammatories and local injection of steroid and anesthetic. If this regimen is not successful, older patients are managed with a total knee arthroscopy and younger patients are managed with an arthrodesis. In most cases arthrodesis is not well tolerated by the patient, so it is performed only as a last resort.

Suggested Readings

Apley AG: Fractures of the lateral tibial condyle treated by skeletal traction and early mobilization. J Bone Joint Surg 1956; 38B(3):699–708.

Benirschke SK, Agnew SG, Mayo KA, Santoro VM, Henley MB: Immediate internal fixation of open, complex tibial plateau fractures: treatment by a standard protocol. J Orthop Trauma 1992; 6(1):78–86.

Drennan DB, Locher FG, Maylahn DJ: Fractures of the tibial plateau. Treatment by closed reduction and Spica cast. J Bone Joint Surg 1979; 49A:989.

Duwelius PJ, Connolly JF: Closed reduction of tibial plateau fractures: a comparison of functional and roentgenographic end results. CORR 1988; 230:116–126.

Fernandez DL: Anterior approach to the knee with osteotomy of the tibial tubercle for tibial fractures. J Bone Joint Surg 1988; 70A (2):208–219.

Lansinger O, Bergman B, Korner L, Anderson GB: Tibial condylar fractures: a twenty year follow-up. 1986; 68A(1):13–18.

Mallik AR, Covall DJ, Whitelaw GP: Internal versus external fixation of bicondylar tibial plateau fractures. Orthop Rev 1992; 1:1433–1436.

Rasmussen PS: Tibial condylar fractures: impairment of knee joint stability as an indication for surgical treatment. 1973; 55A(7):1331–1350.

Ries MD, Meinhard BP: Medial external fixation with lateral plate internal fixation in metaphyseal tibia fractures: a report of 8 cases associated with severe soft tissue injury. CORR 1990; 256:215–223.

Schatzker J, McBroom R, Bruce D: The tibial plateau fracture: the Toronto experience 1968–1975. CORR 1979; 138:94–104.

Stamer DT, Schenk R, Staggers B, Aurori K, Aurori B, Behrens FF: Bicondylar tibial plateau fractures treated with a hybrid ring external fixator: a preliminary study. J Orthop Trauma 1994; 8(6):455–461.

Case 23

History and Physical Examination

A 42-year-old man was admitted to the emergency department with a painful left leg after being involved in a motor vehicle accident. He was a pedestrian struck by an automobile. Following the accident he was unable to weight bear and examination showed that he had local swelling, skin discoloration, and deformity around the left knee. There was no evidence of impaired distal neurovascular function.

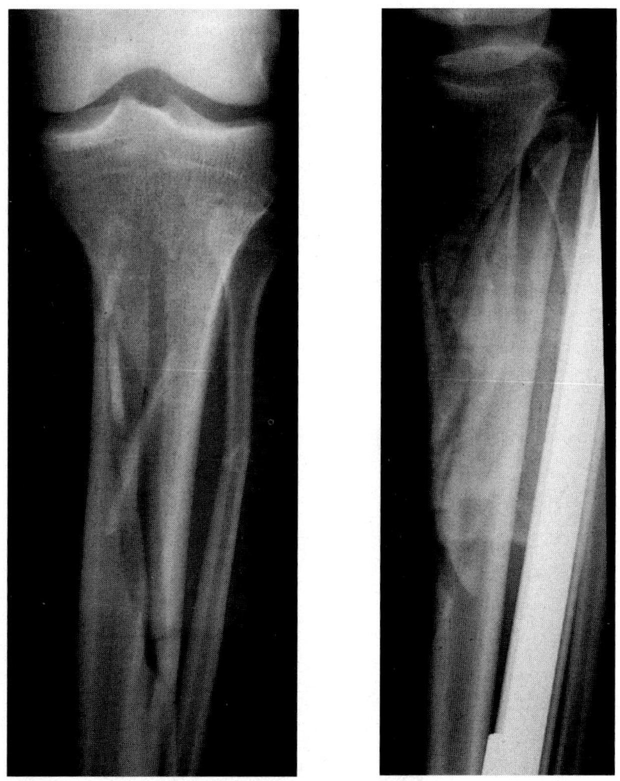

A B

Figure 23–1. Anteroposterior (A) and lateral (B) radiographs showing the extraarticular proximal tibial fracture with the extensive comminution. The proximal fragment is very small.

Radiologic Findings

Anteroposterior and lateral radiographs showed a fracture of the proximal tibial diaphysis with extensive comminution of the proximal third of the tibial diaphysis (Fig. 23–1). There was no evidence of intraarticular involvement.

Diagnosis

A closed extraarticular fracture of the proximal tibia associated with extensive comminution of the upper third of the tibial diaphysis. AO classification: 41–A3.3

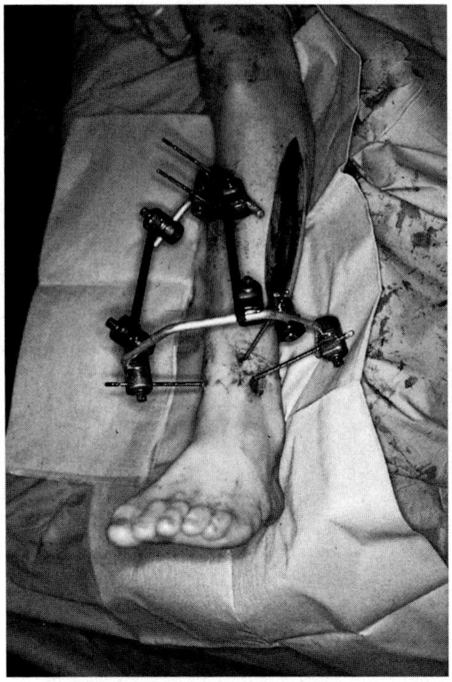

Figure 23–2. The half ring fixator used to treat the fracture.

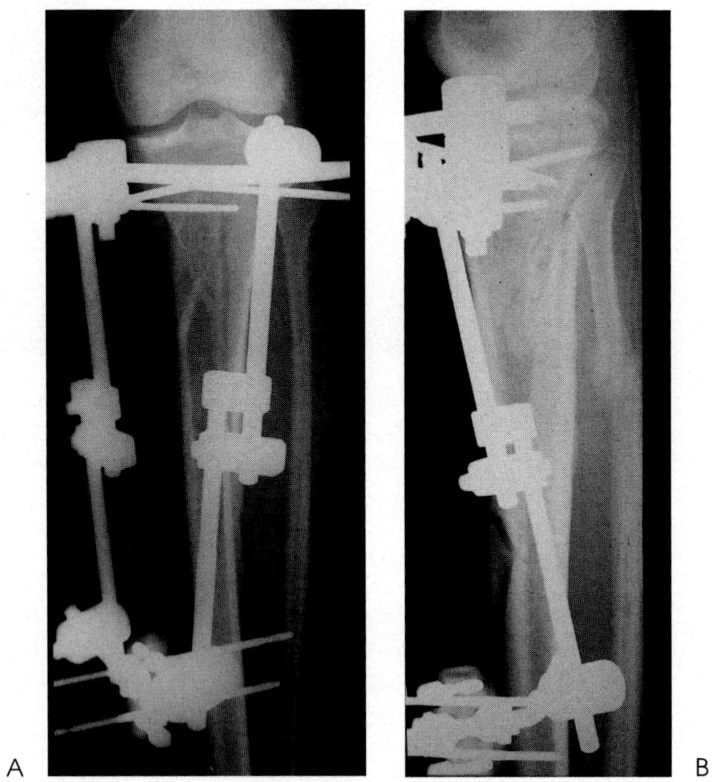

Figure 23–3. Anteroposterior (A) and lateral (B) postoperative radiographs showing that good reduction has been achieved.

PEARLS

- It is important to remember that these are high energy injuries. There may be significant soft tissue damage including vascular injury and compartment syndrome. The patients are often multiply injured.

- This type of external frame is relatively easy to apply. Three pins provide sufficient hold in the proximal fragment. It is important to set the frame up in a triangular configuration with side bars passing down from the lateral and medial sides of the proximal half ring to be secured to the tibial diaphyseal clamp.

PITFALL

- Proximal tibial fractures are associated with a relatively high incidence of neurovascular damage and an adequate preoperative assessment must always be undertaken. This may have both clinical and medicolegal implications.

Surgical Management

Initially the leg was splinted to relieve discomfort and minimize further bone and soft tissue damage. A compartment pressure monitor was inserted into the anterior compartment with the tip of the slit catheter over the comminuted proximal third of the tibia. This recorded a pressure of 8 mm Hg compared with a blood pressure of 130/90 mm Hg. The patient was admitted to the orthopedic trauma unit and the compartment pressure and neurovascular status of his left leg were carefully observed.

On the day after the accident the patient was taken to the operating room and the fracture was stabilized with an external fixator. The frame design consisted of a proximal semicircular bar with four individually placed half pins to hold the proximal fragment. A triangular configuration allowed the proximal fragment to be secured to the tibial diaphysis (Fig. 23–2). Check radiographs (Fig. 23–3) showed that good alignment had been achieved, and clinically the external fixator provided stable fixation.

The half pins were inserted through 1 cm incisions. After the skin incisions were made, dissecting scissors were used to open the tissue down to the bone. External fixator pins were inserted by hand to minimize any heat generation and avoid local soft tissue damage. Care was taken to avoid placing any pins near the common peroneal nerve and to angle all the pins so that they would not emerge posteriorly near the area of the neurovascular bundle.

Postoperative Management

After the external fixator had been applied, the pin sites were dressed. The patient was returned to the ward and early knee mobilization encouraged by the establishment of a physiotherapy program. Full knee movement had been regained by 8 weeks (Fig. 23–4) and the fracture was united after 16 weeks (Fig. 23–5). The patient was kept nonweight bearing until about 10 weeks when it was thought that there was sufficient signs of fracture union to allow progressive increasing weight bearing to be instituted.

Discussion

Surgeons often underestimate the difficulty of treating proximal extraarticular fractures of the tibia. These fractures are relatively uncommon and a recent epidemiological survey of tibial diaphyseal fractures showed that only 6.9% of 523 consecutive tibial diaphyseal fractures presenting to the orthopedic trauma unit in Edinburgh, Scotland, were extraarticular fractures of the proximal third of the tibia. They are almost all high energy injuries and there is often significant comminution. Comparison with tibial fractures in other locations shows that the descriptive indices of extraarticular fractures of the proximal third of the tibia are very different from fractures of the middle or distal third of the tibia and in fact they most resemble the descriptive indices of segmental tibial fractures. The comparative characteristics of tibial diaphyseal fractures according to their location are shown in Table 23–1.

In recent years surgeons have turned to intramedullary nailing to treat tibial diaphyseal fractures. This technique is particularly applicable to fractures of the middle and distal third of the tibial diaphysis, but is less useful in fractures of the proximal

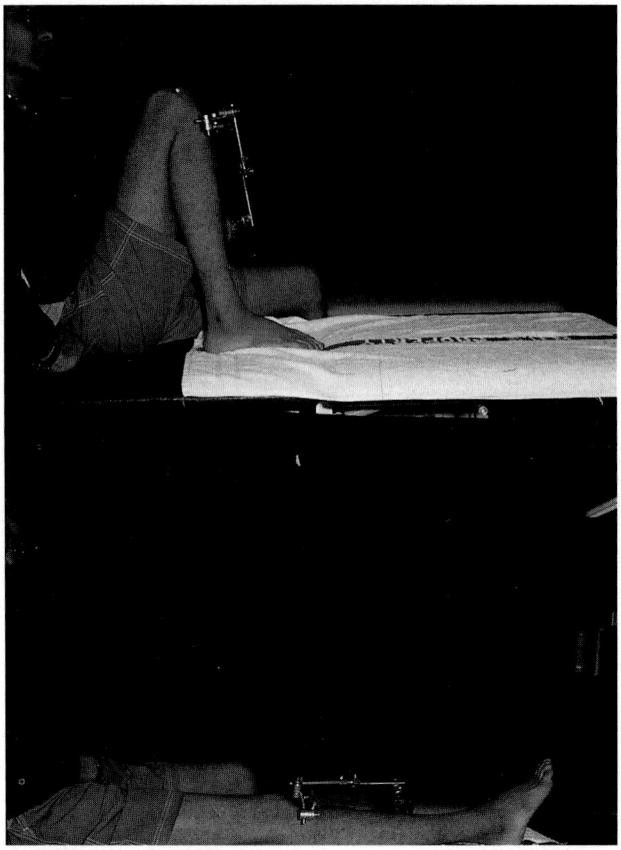

Figure 23–4. After 8 weeks the patient had excellent joint movement.

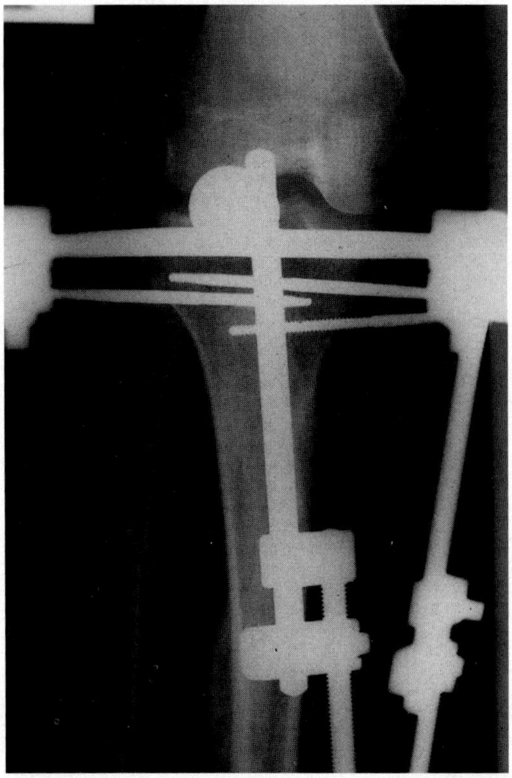

A

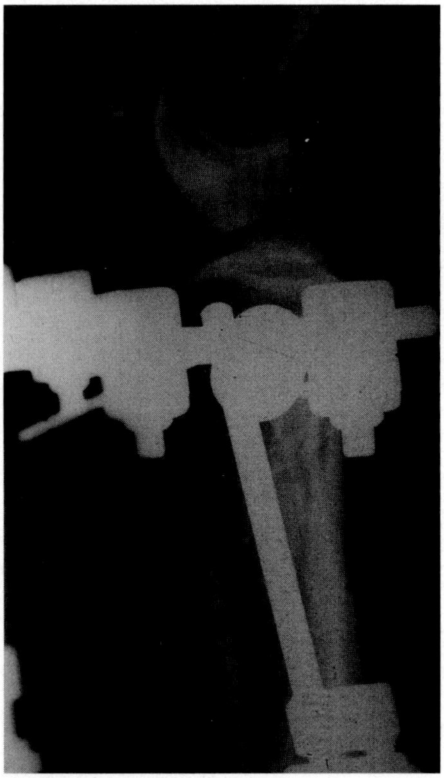

B

Figure 23–5. The fixator was left on for 16 weeks. The good postoperative alignment was retained for this period. Anteroposterior (A) and lateral (B) views.

third of the tibia. In fractures such as the one illustrated here there is a very small intact proximal tibial segment and the chances of gaining adequate stability with an intramedullary nail are slight. If plating was used, the surgeon would have to use two plates to gain sufficient stability to allow early joint movement and in the fracture illustrated here the area of comminution would mean that the length of the plates and therefore the degree of soft tissue dissection would be considerable.

External skeletal fixation provides the best method of stabilizing this very proximal fracture. There are three main fixator configurations that surgeons can employ for this type of fracture. A unilateral frame could be used with the proximal fragment held by two pins placed in the coronal plane (Fig. 23–6A). This type of frame is easy to construct, but does not provide very stable fracture fixation, particularly if there is fracture comminution. The second type of frame frequently advocated by orthopaedic surgeons for this type of fracture is a hybrid frame utilizing small transfixion wires in the proximal fragment and half pins distally (Fig. 23–6B). The transfixion wires are secured to a proximal ring and tensioned. This type of frame provides good fixation; its only disadvantage is that while the surgeon can choose the entry portals for the transfixion wires, these wires can damage nerves and blood vessels as they emerge from the other side of the proximal tibia. Great care must therefore be exercised when using small transfixion wires. The third type of frame is the one used in this case. The principle is essentially the same as the small wire hybrid frame, but half pins are used. The fact that they can be independently placed reduces the chance of soft tissue damage.

The problems of using external skeletal fixation in the diaphysis—namely, malunion, nonunion, and pin tract sepsis—are less evident when external fixation is used to stabilize metaphyseal fractures. The vascularity of the metaphyseal cancellous bone is better than in cortical bone and the time to union and the incidence of nonunion are consequently lower. In high extraarticular proximal tibial fractures the surgeon can usually remove the external fixator after about 8 weeks. In lower extraarticular proximal tibial fractures or in fractures such as this one where there is associated diaphyseal comminution the fixator may have to be maintained for a prolonged period. If this is unacceptable to the surgeon or the patient, it is usually possible to change the fixation method once the metaphyseal fractures have healed.

Table 23–1. Characteristics of Tibial Diaphyseal Fractures

	Proximal	Middle	Distal	Other*
Incidence (%)	6.9	44.0	37.8	11.3
Average age (year)	49.8	31.3	40.4	42.4
AO type A (%)	47.2	63.5	60.5	–
AO type B (%)	36.1	28.9	28.7	7.2
AO type C (%)	16.6	7.4	10.8	92.8
Open fracture (%)	13.9	14.9	12.2	38.1
Tscherne types 2 and 3 (%)	41.6	18.8	24.0	36.4
Winquist-Hansen grades 3 and 4 (%)	41.6	19.3	20.5	50.9
Road traffic accident (%)	80.6	36.4	20.4	70.9
Tibia only (%)	22.2	28.9	20.4	9.1

*Segmental fractures combined with those extending over more than one third of the diaphysis.

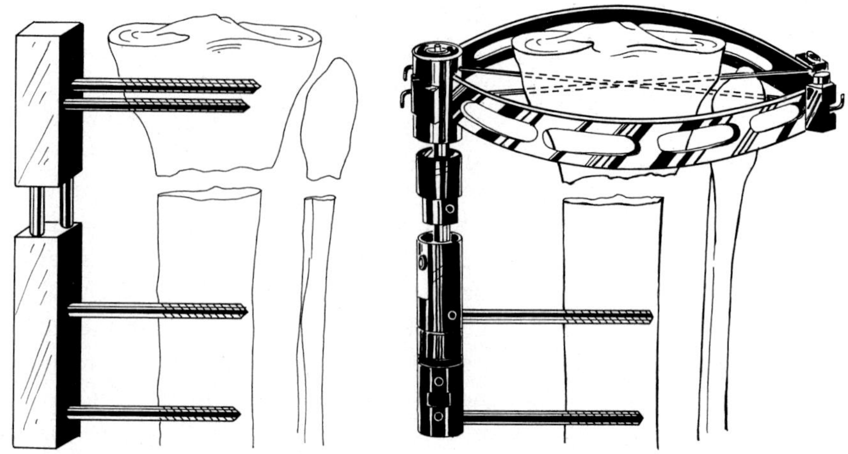

Figure 23–6. Alternative forms of external fixation. (A) A unilateral frame utilizing two pins in each fragment. (B) A hybrid frame utilizing tensioned small wires in the proximal fragment and half pins distally.

Alternative Methods of Management

The obvious alternative treatment method for fractures of the proximal third of the diaphysis is intramedullary nailing. However, as mentioned previously, this can be a very difficult technique and not infrequently the surgeon will be unable to hold the fracture in alignment, resulting in a varus or valgus malalignment. To minimize the chances of this occurring, the surgeon must ensure that the fracture is perfectly reduced before inserting the nail. Unlike fractures of the middle third of the diaphysis, the surgeon cannot rely on the intramedullary nail reducing the fracture as it travels down the intramedullary canal. Even if the fracture is reduced well, the surgeon may still find that the distal fragment is malaligned after passage of the nail and he or she must be particularly careful about the position of the nail insertion point. Surgeons have attempted to compensate for an axial malalignment by using an eccentric entry point. This maneuver is not always successful and the surgeon should take care to get a perfect reduction and central entry point before the operation is undertaken. Sometimes the overall alignment of the tibia is difficult to define using fluoroscopy because the area of the image is too small.

It is also important to use two proximal locking screws when nailing a high tibial fracture. There is a risk that if only one screw is used in the coronal plane, the nail will travel along the screw and thereby cause a malalignment. One technique that is occasionally useful is to use one or two anteroposterior screws to minimize the chance of the proximal end of the nail drifting in the proximal fragment before the locking screws are inserted. The use of a blocking screw is shown in Figure 23–7. These screws are easily inserted and may help prevent fracture malalignment. With care, intramedullary nailing can be used for fractures of the proximal tibial diaphysis, but very high fractures such as the one illustrated here are best treated by external skeletal fixation.

Type of Management	Advantages	Disadvantages	Comments
Cast/traction	None	Malunion; nonunion; joint stiffness	An inappropriate technique for the management of extraarticular proximal tibial fractures
Intramedullary nailing	Early joint movement; good union rate	Technically difficult; malunion	Technically a difficult procedure and impossible in very high extraarticular tibial fractures
External fixation	Straightforward technique; good stability; early joint movement	Pin tract sepsis; may need to be used for prolonged period in high extraarticular tibial fracture	The treatment of choice for high extraarticular tibial fracture
Plating	None	Soft tissue damage; joint stiffness	Limited use in the management of extraarticular proximal tibial fractures

Plating

Some surgeons advocate the use of plates for high tibial diaphyseal fractures and indeed bone plates may be useful for the rare combination of a lateral tibial condylar fracture that needs plate fixation and a high diaphyseal fracture. In general, plating is not the ideal choice for high energy proximal tibial fractures associated with comminution and soft tissue damage.

Casting/Traction

It is difficult to treat high tibial diaphyseal fractures with a cast. Both malunion and nonunion are relatively common and the fact that a long-leg cast may be required for a prolonged period virtually ensures joint stiffness.

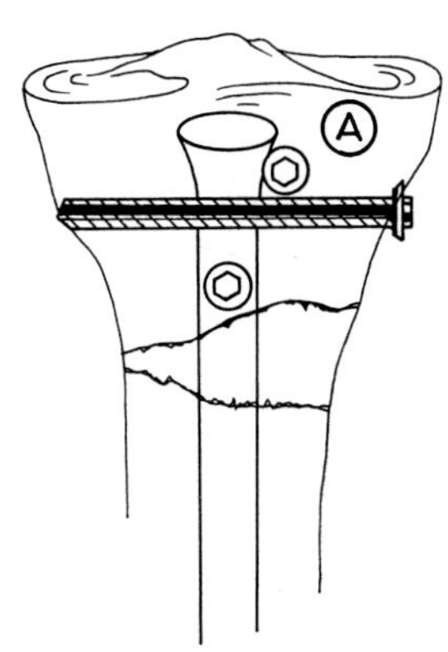

Figure 23–7. The use of a blocking screw (A) to prevent drift of the intramedullary nail. In such a small fragment two locking screws are essential.

Complications

As previously mentioned, the most common problem the surgeon will encounter is malalignment following intramedullary nailing of a proximal tibial diaphyseal fracture. If this occurs, the surgeon should renail the fracture or select a different treatment method, usually external fixation. Renailing is very difficult, particularly for inexperienced surgeons, because there is always a tendency for the nail to pass down the original tract. Unless the surgeon is experienced, it is probably better to use external fixation if intramedullary nailing has failed. The other complications occasionally encountered are nonunion and infection. Nonunion following an externally fixed proximal tibial fracture is best treated by nailing if the bone is aligned and the pin tracts are satisfactory. Nonunion following an initial nailing is best treated by exchange nailing. Bone infection is treated conventionally using high dose antibiotics, drainage of infected foci, reaming to remove the infected endosteal membrane, and bone resection and grafting as indicated.

Suggested Readings

Benirschke SK, Henley MB, Ott JW: Proximal one-third tibial fracture solutions. Orthop Trans 1995; 18:1055–1056.

Browner BD (ed): The Science and Practice of Intramedullary Nailing. Williams and Wilkins, Baltimore, 1996.

Court-Brown CM, McBirnie J: The epidemiology of tibial fractures. J Bone Joint Surg (Br) 1995; 77B:417–421.

Freedman EL, Johnson EE: Analysis of tibial malalignment following intramedullary nailing of the tibia. Clin Orthop 1995; 315:25–33.

Lang GJ, Cohen BE, Bosse MJ, Kellam JF: Proximal third tibial fractures. Should they be nailed? Clin Orthop 1995; 315:64–74.

Puno RM, Vaugh JJ, Stetten ML, Johnson JR: Long-term effects of tibial angular malunion on the knee and ankle joints. J Orthop Trauma 1991; 5:247–254.

Case 24

History and Physical Examination

A 48-year-old woman fell down three steps, injuring her right leg below the knee. The patient was brought to the emergency department 2 hours after injury. A well healed vertical midline scar extended from 4 cm proximal to the patella to 3 cm distal to the tibial tubercle. Pain was elicited at the knee and distal to the knee with palpation and gentle passive flexion and extension. Obvious deformity and a knee effusion were not present. There was an ecchymosis over the pretibial area midway down the calf; otherwise the skin was intact. The neurovascular examination of the leg was within the limits of normal. There were no other injuries.

The patient had a history of rheumatoid arthritis and had undergone multiple joint replacements, including a right total knee arthroplasty 4 years prior to this injury. She had recovered from the arthroplasty with no signs of infection. The arthroplasty had successful relieved the patient's pain, increased her knee motion, and increased her ability to ambulate. At the time of injury the rheumatoid arthritis was being managed medically with corticosteroids and methotrexate.

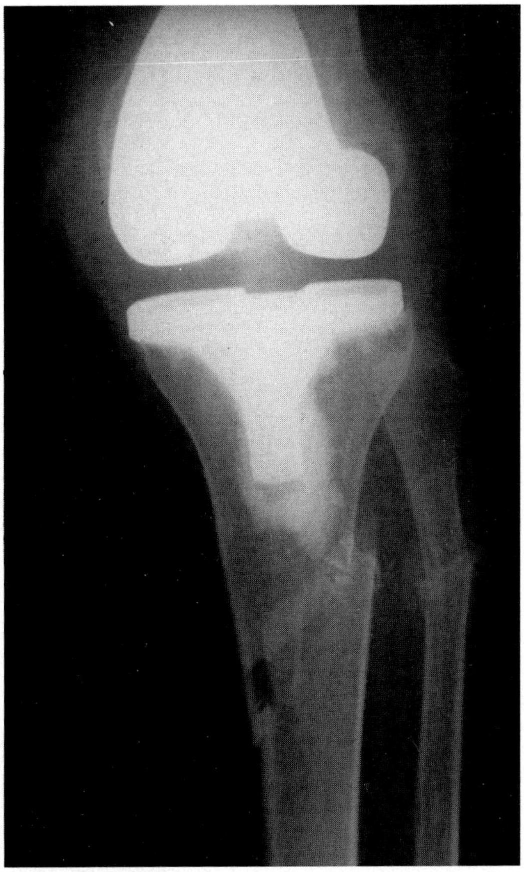

Figure 24–1. Oblique radiograph of the proximal tibia. There is a fracture of the tibia distal to the tibial component.

PEARL

- The fact that the prosthesis was well aligned and had relieved the patient's pain until the fracture of the tibia occurred is important. If the prosthesis were loose or maligned and symptomatic, a revision arthroplasty would be considered. In this case because the prosthesis was functioning well the prosthesis was left in situ.

PITFALL

- The fact that the fracture is minimally displaced and caused by low energy does not decrease the chance of compartment syndrome. In fact, proximal metaphyseal tibial fractures are prone to be complicated by compartment syndrome.

Radiologic Findings

Radiographs of the tibia femur and knee were obtained. A long oblique fracture of the tibia just distal to the tibial component was present. The femoral, tibial, and patellar components were in good position, with no signs of periprosthetic lysis or loosening of the prosthesis (Fig. 24–1).

Diagnosis

Low energy fracture of the tibia distal to the tibial component of a knee prosthesis. The prosthesis was well aligned and firmly fixed to the underlying bone.

Surgical Management

The leg was placed in a padded long leg splint and the patient was admitted for surgery the next day. Overnight the patient was monitored every 2 hours for compart-

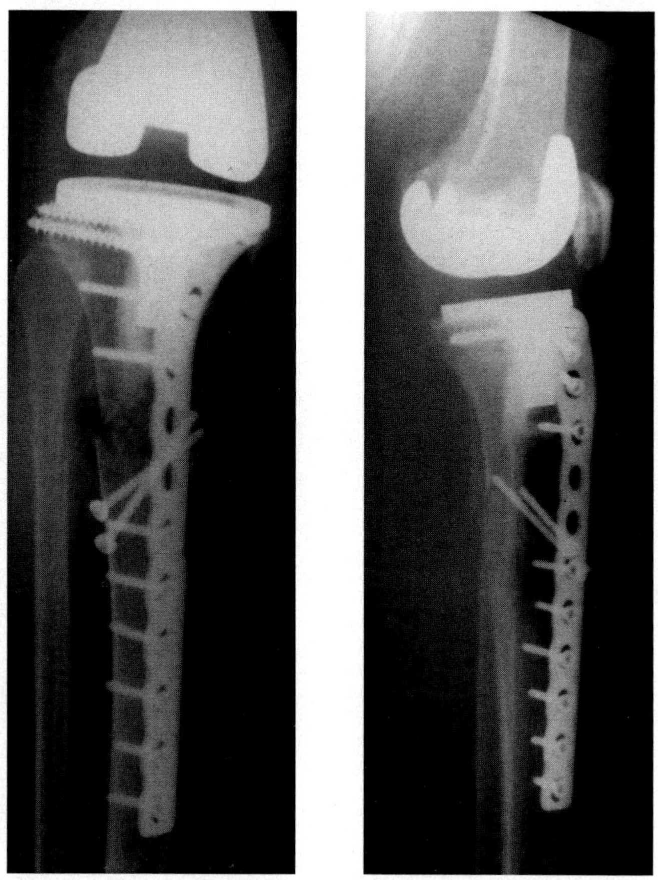

A B

Figure 24–2. Anteroposterior (A) and lateral (B) radiographs intraoperatively during reduction and stabilization with interfragmental screws and a plate.

ment syndrome. She was examined for increasing pain at rest and pain with gentle passive stretch of the anterior and posterior compartment muscles of the calf.

The first day postinjury, the patient was taken to the operating room where a general anesthetic was administered. The injured leg and ipsilateral hip were prepped and draped. An incision was made anteriorly in the midline starting at the patella and continuing distally to the mid tibia. The proximal portion of the incision incorporated the scar through which the total knee had been inserted. The medial side of the tibia was exposed subperiosteally. The lateral side of the tibia was not exposed. The fracture was curetted of hematoma, reduced, and stabilized with two interfragmentary screws and a large fragment compression plate with five screws proximal to the fracture and six distal to the fracture. Iliac crest graft was obtained from the ipsilateral hip and placed laterally at the fracture site (Fig. 24–2). A direct current bone growth stimulator was implanted.

Postoperative Management

The lower extremity was splinted with the knee at 15 degrees and the ankle in neutral. Active knee and ankle motion was initiated on postoperative day 3. Nonweight bearing was maintained until radiographic signs of healing were present; this occurred at 12 weeks. Despite the use of a platform walker, the patient

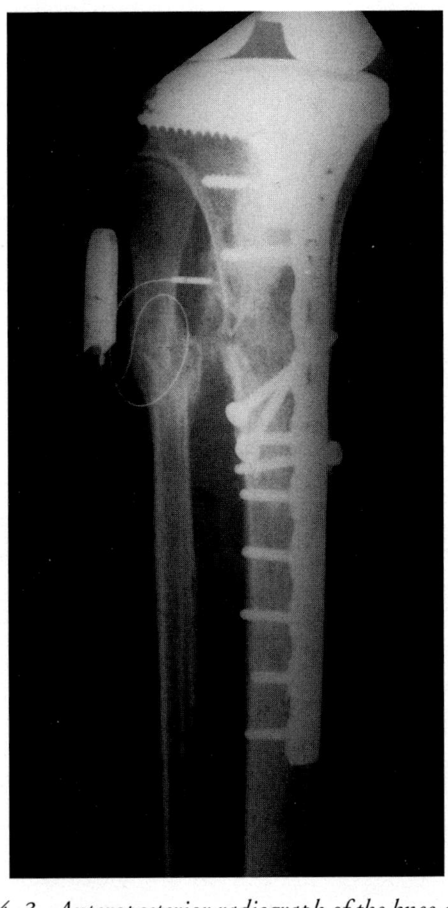

Figure 24–3. Anteroposterior radiograph of the knee at 4 months following injury.

was confined to a wheelchair for most of the 12 weeks because of extensive rheumatoid involvement of the upper extremities. The fracture healed uneventfully (Fig. 24–3).

Discussion

Fractures of the tibia distal to a total knee arthroplasty occur less frequently than other periprosthetic fractures (i.e., femoral fractures below a total hip arthroplasty or above a total knee arthroplasty). Although periprosthetic femoral fractures often have identifiable risk factors such as perforation of the lateral cortex during a total hip arthroplasty or notching of the anterior cortex of the femur during a total knee arthroplasty, this is seldom the case with tibia fractures below a total knee arthroplasty. Like other periprosthetic fractures, the prognosis for healing is poor due to the advanced age of the patient, decreased local vascularity secondary to prior surgery and the presence of the prosthesis, stress concentration at the fracture site secondary to the prosthesis, and decreased range of motion of the knee.

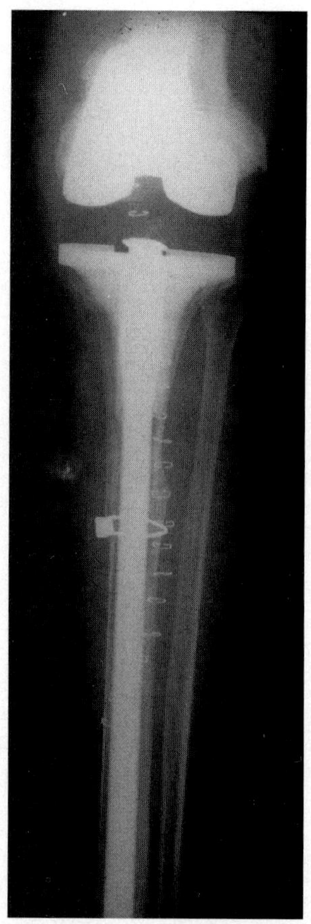

Figure 24–4. Anteroposterior radiograph of a knee following fracture of the tibia and stabilization with a long stem tibial component and a cerclage cable.

Type of Management	Advantages	Disadvantages	Comments
Open reduction, internal fixation with plates and screws	Facilitates accurate reduction; stable fixation allows early mobilization	Prosthesis may limit fixation; exposes patient to risk of infection; delayed weight bearing	If prosthesis is not loose, this is most common method of management
Cast immobilization	Closed procedure; no risk of infection	Stiffness secondary to immobilization; risk of nonunion	Limited application because patient is not able to ambulate with cast
External fixation	Limited procedure; results in some stability; allows postoperative motion	Osteopenia limits stability; pin tracts communicate with prosthesis; increased risk of infection	The limited stability and risk of infection limit the application of external fixation
Revision arthroplasty (Fig. 24–4)	Early mobilization and weight bearing	Extensive procedure	Indicated when the prosthesis is loose

Alternative Methods of Management

Alternatives to open reduction and fixation are casting, external fixation, and revision arthroplasty. The goal of management of periprosthetic fractures is a stable painless lower extremity that has a functional range of motion of the involved joint. To obtain this goal in cases in which the prosthesis was functioning well prior to fracture, it is not necessary to perform a revision arthroplasty. On the other hand, if the prosthesis was not functioning well, because of malalignment, instability, or loosening, revision arthroplasty is considered. Ideally, management should allow motion of the knee. Prolonged immobilization of the knee is likely to result in permanent loss of motion and function. In addition, a stiff knee makes it extremely difficult to successfully manage a nonunion, should one occur. Therefore closed management with casting should be used sparingly. Infection of a periprosthetic fracture seldom has an acceptable outcome; consequently, the method of management should minimize the risk of infection of the prosthesis. Although any surgical procedure entails a risk of infection, it would seem that external fixation of a periprosthetic fracture has an unacceptably high risk because of the proximity of the pins to the prosthesis. One of the major problems with internal fixation with a plate is fixation proximally. There should be a minimum of six cortices on each side of the fracture. This is addressed by careful placement of the plate to maximize screw holes, drilling and tapping cement, and directing screws posterior and anterior to the prosthesis. The major complication of open reduction and internal fixation is loss of fixation and nonunion. Autogenous bone grafting should minimize this complication.

If rigid fixation with a plate is used, weight bearing is delayed until there is radiographic evidence of healing (i.e., trabeculae crossing the fracture site). It is important to realize that clinical signs are not reliable; the patient will feel as though the fracture is healed as soon as the incision pain subsides. However, weight bearing to any degree prior to radiographic healing will result in loss of fixation.

Complications

Complications of management with open reduction and internal fixation with a plate are loss of fixation, postoperative infection, and loosening of the prosthesis. The incidence of loss of fixation is decreased by achieving adequate purchase in the proximal fragment, protecting the vascularity of the fracture (e.g., limiting periosteal elevation), and grafting with autogenous bone. Once loss of fixation has occurred, the options are to revise the fixation and graft with autogenous bone, revise the arthroplasty with a long stem prosthesis, or immobilize the extremity and stimulate healing with pulsed electromagnetic fields.

To decrease the incidence of postoperative infection, postoperative wound problems are managed aggressively. Hematomas are drained, and wound sloughs are debrided and covered with well perfused soft tissue. Once infection has occurred, management includes debridement, stabilization of the fracture, soft tissue coverage, and appropriate antibiotic coverage. Persistent infection often can be successfully suppressed with long term oral antibiotics. Failure of suppression of infection often leads to amputation.

Loosening of the prosthesis is managed with revision arthroplasty. In cases in which loosening first becomes evident or accelerated following fracture fixation, infection should be suspected.

Suggested Readings

Makela EA: Capacitively coupled electrical field in the treatment of a leg fracture after total knee replacement. J Orthop Trauma 1992; 6(2):237–240.

Case 25

History and Physical Examination

A 19-year-old male was admitted to the emergency department having sustained a closed fracture of his right tibia and fibula during a tackle in a soccer match. There was no other injury. On admission it was noted that his right leg was deformed and painful. Examination showed that he had normal sensation in the leg and foot and could dorsiflex and plantarflex his toes without significant increase in his pain. Power was difficult to assess because of discomfort, but clinically there was no objective evidence of significant muscle weakness. Palpation of his dorsalis pedis and posterior tibial pulses showed them to be present. His blood pressure was 120/75.

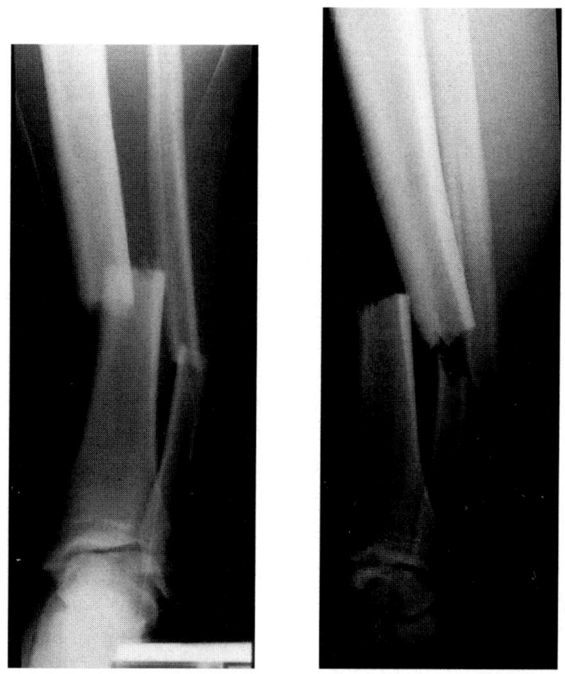

A B

Figure 25–1. Anteroposterior (A) and lateral (B) radiographs showing transverse fractures of the tibia and fibula.

Radiologic Findings

Anteroposterior and lateral radiographs showed transverse fractures of both the tibia and fibula (Fig. 25–1).

Diagnosis

Closed fracture of the right tibia and fibula. The fractures were at approximately the same level indicating that this was an AO classification 42–A3.3 fracture.

PEARLS

- There is debate about whether fracture stabilization or fasciotomy should be performed first and also whether the fasciotomy should be undertaken on the nailing table with the leg under traction. The application of traction will increase the intracompartmental pressure, but provided the nailing is performed expeditiously, it is unlikely that any clinical problem will ensue. However, if the surgeon relies on clinical signs and the compartment syndrome is therefore diagnosed late or the nailing is likely to be prolonged, it is probably safer to undertake the fasciotomy on a conventional flat table and then transfer the patient to a nailing table. It is of course possible to nail the tibia on a flat table using a distractor.
- It is rare to be able to close both fasciotomy wounds. Usually it is possible to close one of the wounds and treat the other with progressive closure using a rubber banding technique or one of the commercially available skin closure machines. Alternatively, split skin grafting can be used, but this technique provides added cosmetic problems and delays hospital discharge.

Surgical Management

Initially the tibia was splinted with a plaster back slab to reduce the discomfort and minimize any further soft tissue damage. The patient was taken to the operating room where a slit catheter was placed into the anterior compartment musculature of the leg under local anaesthetic (Fig. 25–2). The tip of the catheter was placed about 2 to 3 cm from the fracture. The slit catheter was connected to a pressure recorder via a fluid filled tube and a continuous readout of the pressure in the muscles of the anterior compartment pressure was obtained. The initial pressure recorded in the anterior compartment was about 30 mm Hg and the blood pressure was 120/80.

It was decided to stabilize the fracture with a reamed intramedullary nail on the following day. However, the continuous pressure recording showed a steady increase in the intracompartmental pressure. About 8 hours after admission the pressure in the anterior compartment was 75 mm Hg and the patient's blood pressure was recorded at 130/90 mm Hg (Fig. 25–3). Because the pressure rise was consistent and the difference between the diastolic blood pressure and intracompartmental pressure was less than 30 mm Hg a compartment syndrome was diagnosed. Clinical examination at this time showed no evidence of sensory abnormality and the patient was able to move his toes satisfactorily. However, the nurses had noted an increase in his analgesic requirements.

The patient was taken to the operating room and placed on a tibial nailing table using calcaneal traction. Fluoroscopy confirmed fracture reduction and the tibia was reamed and nailed in a conventional manner (Fig. 25–4). An 11 mm nail was inserted after reaming the intramedullary canal to 12 mm. After the insertion of the cross screws a four compartment fasciotomy was undertaken through medial and lateral incisions. Initially, a lateral incision was made and the anterior and lateral compartments were decompressed. Subsequently the superficial and deep posterior compartments were decompressed through the medial incision. Clinically it was considered that the anterior and deep posterior compartments showed the highest intracompartmental pressures. After the fasciotomies had been undertaken, dressings were applied to the fasciotomy wounds and the operative incisions and the patient returned to the ward.

Two days later the fasciotomy wounds were reexamined in the operating room and noted to be healthy. There was no evididence of devitalized muscle. The lateral wound was sutured and the medial wound partially closed using a banding technique. The medial wound was sutured without difficulty 2 days later.

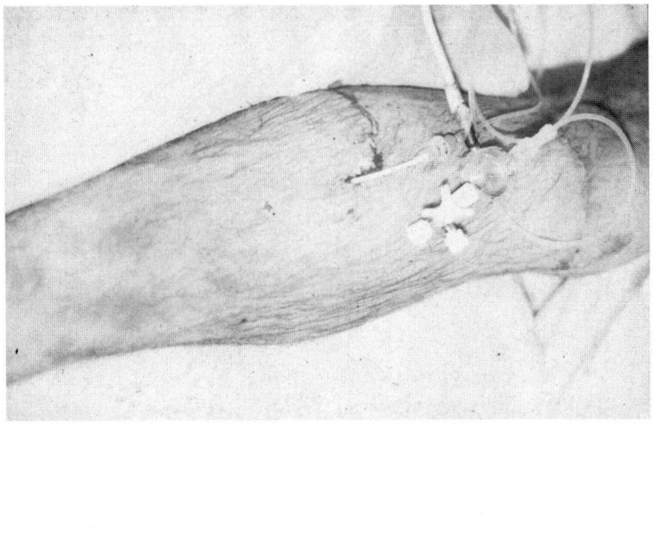

Figure 25–2. A slit catheter has been placed in the anterior compartment.

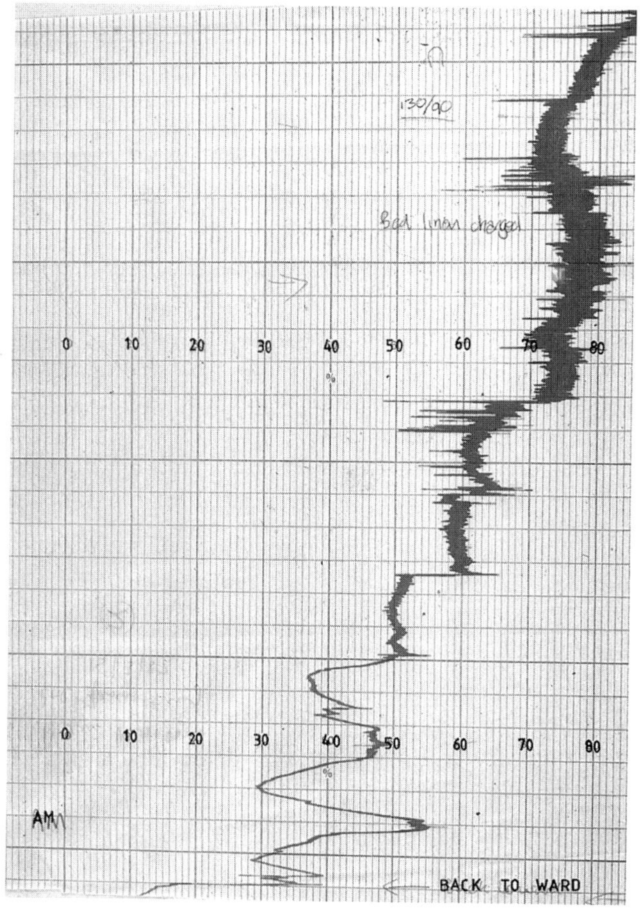

Figure 25–3. A pressure trace showing a gradual rise in the intracompartmental pressure.

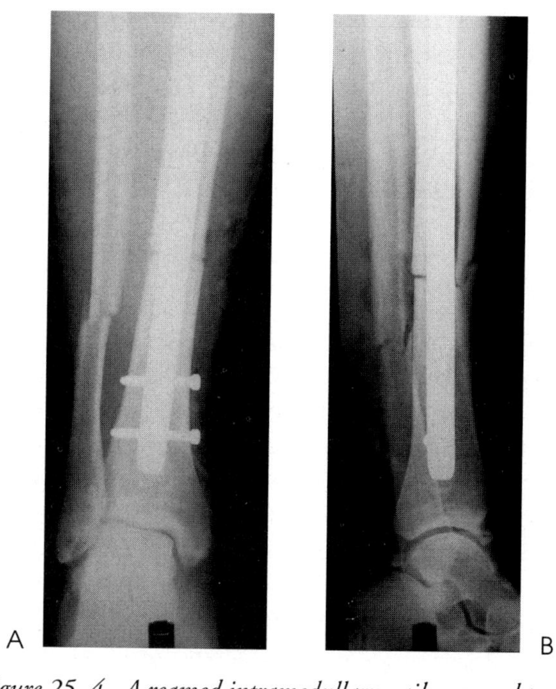

Figure 25–4. A reamed intramedullary nail was used to stabilize the fracture. Anteroposterior (A) and lateral (B) views.

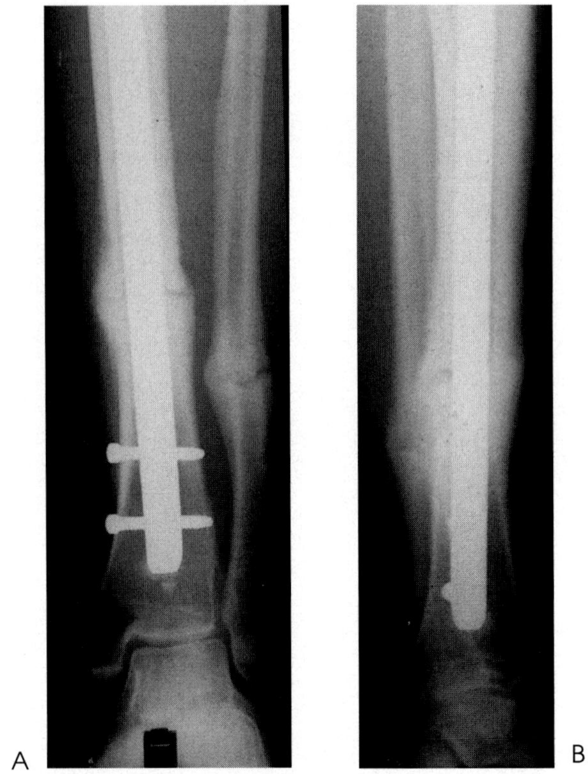

Figure 25–5. The fracture united and the clinical result was excellent. Anteroposterior (A) and lateral (B) views.

Postoperative Management

The patient was allowed to bear weight as tolerated. Because of the presence of the fasciotomy wounds the patient in fact took 3 to 4 weeks to fully weight bear. Thereafter his progress was uneventful and the fracture had united by 16 weeks (Fig. 25–5). He restarted his job 11 weeks after the injury, although it took over nine months before he could resume his soccer activities.

Discussion

Compartment syndrome is usually straightforward to diagnose and treat, although surgeons not infrequently do both badly. Traditionally, compartment syndrome is diagnosed by the presence of increased pain, particularly on passive dorsiflexion and plantarflexion of the toes, sensory abnormalities in the feet, muscle weakness, and absent peripheral pulses. However, these clinical signs often take many hours to become apparent and if the surgeon waits for the peripheral pulses to disappear, it will almost certainly be too late to save all of the leg musculature. Compartment pressure monitoring has been shown to detect compartment syndrome before the clinical symptoms become manifest.

The effects of compartment syndrome can be devastating. If it is missed or if the clinical signs are merely treated by increasing amounts of analgesia, amputation is the usual result. If the surgeon delays diagnosis by relying on the clinical signs, mus-

PITFALL

- The surgeon should remember that compartment pressures will vary relative to the distance between the fracture site and the tip of the catheter. It is important to measure the compartment pressure close to the fracture site and the catheter should be appropriately located. Compartment syndrome almost always affects the anterior and deep posterior compartments and pressure measurement of the anterior compartment is sufficient to diagnose the presence of a compartment syndrome.

cle weakness, soft tissue contractures, soft tissue infection, and permanent sensory abnormalities may well occur. In addition, compartment syndrome has a deleterious effect on bone union and delay in diagnosis has been shown to be associated with a high incidence of tibial nonunion in adults. In a recent publication McQueen et al. (1996) showed a statistically significant reduction in the sequelae that follow compartment syndrome through the use of compartment pressure monitoring.

There are two methods of directly measuring compartment pressure. A surgeon may use a "stick" method whereby a single pressure measurement is taken or, as already described, a continuous reading can be obtained using a slit catheter and recording equipment found in any anesthetic department. Ideally a continuous trace should be obtained because a surgeon should be aware of the pressure trend. A single pressure measurement may be high, but might represent one point on a pressure curve that is dropping after surgery. If a "stick" system is used, multiple pressures must be recorded, which is uncomfortable for the patient. McQueen (1996) has provided a description of the use of continuous pressure measurement.

Some surgeons are concerned that intramedullary nailing in general and reaming in particular raises intracompartmental pressure to a level that will induce compartment syndrome in some patients. There is no evidence that this is the case, but there is no doubt that the passage of any instrument down the intramedullary canal of a long bone will raise the intramedullary pressure and thereby the intracompartmental pressure. However, the pressure rise is transient and the intramedullary pressure will fall after the instrument has been withdrawn. At the end of an intramedullary nailing procedure it is not uncommon to find the intracompartmental pressure to be raised, with pressures of 40 or 50 mm Hg fairly common. In about 95% of cases the pressure will soon drop so that the difference between the diastolic pressure and the intracompartmental pressure is greater than 30 mm Hg. In these cases, the patient is safe and will not develop a compartment syndrome. In about 3 to 4% of cases the pressure will remain high and the compartment syndrome will require treatment. In a very small minority of patients the pressure will neither rise or fall but remain flat, usually recording a pressure reading of between 30 and 40 mm Hg. In these cases it is not uncommon to encounter myonecrosis when the leg is eventually explored. It is probable that the myonecrosis has followed a vascular injury at the time of the accident.

Neither reaming nor nailing causes the compartment syndrome that some surgeons associate with operative management of tibial fractures. Rather it is the fracture reduction with its associated muscle stretching that increases the compartment pressure. In Edinburgh, Scotland, where much of the clinical analysis of compartment syndrome and its pathogenesis has been carried out, surgeons have found a similar incidence of compartment syndrome with external fixation and intramedullary nailing in closed tibial diaphyseal fractures. The reason is that both methods of management require a closed reduction. The fact that the intracompartmental pressure rises after fracture reduction implies strongly that a delay in reducing the fracture is to be avoided. If the surgeon waits for two weeks until the soft tissues are contracted, then reduction of the fracture will be difficult and will be associated with a high intracompartmental pressure.

Some surgeons have used a single reading as their clinical basis for performing a fasciotomy. This is superficially attractive because it is quick and definitive. However, as already noted, it is the relationship between the diastolic blood pressure and the compartment pressure that is important and in hypertensive patients a compartment pressure of even 60 mm Hg may not be detrimental to the muscles. The relationship between the diastolic and intracompartmental pressures was first pointed out by Whitesides et al. in 1975. Since then, the optimal differential pressure has been a matter of debate, but a recent clinical study by McQueen and Court-Brown (1996) has confirmed that a pressure difference of 30 mm Hg between the diastolic and the intracompartmental pressures is appropriate.

Reamed intramedullary nailing using an interlocking nail is now widely used to treat closed tibial fractures regardless of the degree of soft tissue damage associated with the fracture. The technique is associated with high union rates and an infection rate of less than 2%. Analysis of the literature shows that the use of reamed tibial nailing in closed tibial diaphyseal fractures is associated with a union rate of 96.5%, with the remaining 3.5% uniting after exchange nailing. The relatively large nail size means that nail and screw breakage are uncommon and early weight bearing can be allowed. Thus it has been demonstrated that about 80% of patients who have closed tibial fractures treated with a reamed nail returned to work and their previous normal activities, apart from sport, before clinical union. About 93% of patients have normal hindfoot function (Court-Brown et al., 1990).

Alternative Methods of Treatment

The traditional method of managing closed tibial diaphyseal fractures was the application of a long-leg cast followed a few weeks later by the use of a functional cast or brace that theoretically allowed movement of the knee and hindfoot. A review of the literature suggests that the main problem associated with the cast management of tibial fractures is hindfoot stiffness with incidences of up to 45% being reported by a number of authors. The incidence of hindfoot stiffness does not appear to improve with the use of a functional brace. In addition, many surgeons report higher rates of malunion and nonunion, necessitating secondary surgery. Cast management of a patient who requires fasciotomies would be ill advised. Essentially, the requirement for fasciotomy converts the closed fracture into an open fracture and few surgeons would advocate nonoperative management for open fractures because of the high risk of infection and nonunion.

Unreamed Nailing

Unreamed nails have become popular for the management of open tibial diaphyseal fractures and many surgeons have adopted the technique on the grounds that smaller nails inserted without prior reaming are associated with less damage to the intramedullary vasculature. However, there are a number of drawbacks associated with the use of unreamed nails. These nails tend to be either 8 or 9 mm in diameter and consequently have smaller cross screws. There is therefore a higher incidence of both screw and nail breakage than encountered with reamed nails and to minimize the risk of this complication most surgeons ask their patients to remain nonweight bearing for 6 to 8 weeks after nailing. This is extremely inconvenient for the patient and in fact does not significantly reduce the incidence of screw and nail breakage.

The other main problems associated with the use of unreamed nails relate to the fact that reaming is undoubtedly osteogenic. Thus the incidence of nonunion and the requirement for secondary surgery to secure bone union are higher with unreamed nails than reamed nails. This was shown in a recent prospective randomized trial of Tscherne C1 closed tibial fractures (Court-Brown et al., 1996). The reamed fractures all united without any malunion or any requirement for secondary surgery, whereas the unreamed fractures took statistically longer to unite, required more secondary surgery, and had a higher incidence of malunion and metal breakage.

External Skeletal Fixation

External fixation for closed tibial fractures was popular in the 1980s. However, as with all diaphyseal fractures treated by external skeletal fixation, there was a high incidence of malunion and nonunion. This was lessened by the use of dynamic axial external fixators that allowed movement at the fracture site, but most reports of the use of external fixation in the management of closed tibial fractures report longer times to union than with intramedullary nailing, and higher incidences of nonunion and malunion. In addition, if the surgeon chooses to use a multiplanar or circular wire fixator to treat a closed tibial fracture, muscle penetration is inevitable and joint stiffness will result. If external fixation is used, a unilateral frame permitting axial movement should be employed.

Plating

Most surgeons have abandoned plating as a standard method for managing closed tibial fractures because considerable soft tissue dissection is required when compared with intramedullary nailing and external skeletal fixation. However, it could be argued that plating is reasonable in a closed tibial fracture that has had to be opened because of compartment syndrome. If a tibia is to be plated following a two incision fasciotomy, the medial incision will be used. It is ill advised to make a third anterior incision because a resulting skin bridge would be too narrow to ensure skin viability. Even though the skin is already open following a fasciotomy, plating will still require soft tissue stripping and it is advisable to use intramedullary nailing if it is available.

Type of Management	Advantages	Disadvantages	Comments
Cast traction	No advantage in the presence on compartment syndrome	Unstable fixation; infection; nonunion; joint stiffness	Nonoperative management should not be used for closed tibial fractures complicated by compartment syndrome
Reamed nailing	High union rate; low complication rate; good patient function	Knee pain	Method of choice for closed tibial fractures with or without compartment syndrome
Unreamed nailing	Low complication rate; good patient function	Lower union rate than reamed nailing; malunion; metal breakage; knee pain	Results are not as good as with reamed nailing but better than external fixation
External fixation	Speed of surgery	Nonunion; malunion; pin tract sepsis	Results are not as good as those obtained with intramedullary nailing; may be useful in multiply injured patients
Plating	None	Soft tissue stripping; joint stiffness	Inappropriate technique nowadays

Complications

The main complication of treating a closed tibial diaphyseal fracture associated with a compartment syndrome comes from failure to treat the compartment syndrome expeditiously. If a surgeon waits until the patient has motor weakness or absent pulses, then sequelae from the compartment syndrome are virtually inevitable. Common complications are muscle tightness secondary to myofibrosis, which often leads to pes cavus and claw toes. If the compartment syndrome is missed, much of the leg musculature will be replaced by fibrous tissue with consequent muscle weakness and hindfoot and forefoot deformities. The treatment of any residual sequelae of compartment syndrome depends on their severity. A missed compartment syndrome may well require amputation, but less severe problems such as claw toes may be amenable to reconstructive surgery.

One of the interesting complications of compartment syndrome is nonunion of the tibial fracture. Court-Brown and McQueen (1987) undertook a retrospective study to investigate the relationship between nonunion and compartment syndrome and demonstrated that if a surgeon relied on the clinical signs as a determinant of the requirement for fasciotomy in patients over 18 years of age, there was an increased incidence of nonunion compared with an equivalent population who had not had a compartment syndrome. Later work by McQueen et al. (1996) indicated that the use of compartment pressure monitoring reduced both the incidence of nonunion and the overall time to union. It is quite possible that a number of apparently inexplicable nonunions are caused by compartment pressures that are raised but do not reach a level whereby the clinical signs of compartment syndrome are evident.

As with any operatively managed closed tibial fracture, the surgeon may encounter problems with infection and nonunion. Infection of a nailed tibial fracture is treated the same way as osteomyelitis in any other area—with high dose antibiotics, drainage of infected foci, and exchange nailing. Nonunion is usually successfully treated by exchange nailing, although septic nonunion may require flap cover and bone grafting if treatment is delayed. The key to the successful treatment of tibial diaphyseal infection is early diagnosis and aggressive therapy.

A particular complication of tibial nailing is knee pain. This is usually felt over the proximal end of the nail and is exacerbated by physical activity, particularly by squatting or kneeling. It is rarely severe and usually relieved by nail removal, although occasionally nail removal itself may be difficult.

Suggested Readings

Court-Brown CM, Christie J, McQueen MM: Closed intramedullary tibial nailing. Its use in closed and type I open fractures. J Bone Joint Surg (Br) 1990; 72B:605–611.

Court-Brown CM, McQueen MM: Compartment syndrome delays tibial union. Acta Orthop Scand 1987; 58:249–252.

Court-Brown CM, Will E, Christie J, McQueen MM: Reamed or unreamed nailing for closed tibial fractures. J Bone Joint Surg (Br) 1996; 78B:580–583.

McQueen MM: How to monitor compartment pressures. Techniques in Orthopaedics 1996; 11:99–101.

McQueen MM, Christie J, Court-Brown CM: Compartment pressures after intramedullary nailing of the tibia. J Bone Joint Surg (Br) 1990; 72B:395–397.

McQueen MM, Christie J, Court-Brown CM: Acute compartment syndrome in tibial diaphyseal fractures. J Bone Joint Surg (Br) 1996; 78B:95–98.

McQueen MM, Court-Brown CM: Compartment monitoring in tibial fractures. The pressure threshold for decompression. J Bone Joint Surg (Br) 1996; 78B:99–104.

Tornetta P, Templeman D: Compartment syndrome associated with tibial fracture. J Bone Joint Surg (Am) 1996; 78A:1438–1444.

Whitesides TE, Haney TC, Morimoto K, Harada H: Tissue pressure measurements as a determinant for the need for fasciotomy. Clin Orthop 1975; 113:43–51.

Case 26

History and Physical Examination

A 32-year-old male was admitted to the emergency department having been involved in a traffic accident. He had been the rear seat passenger on a motorcycle that collided with a car. He had not lost consciousness and physical examination failed to show any evidence of chest, abdominal, pelvic, or spinal injuries.

Examination of the right leg showed a severe open tibial fracture. There was a 12 cm open wound overlying the anteromedial subcutaneous border of the upper tibia associated with obvious bony deformity. The soft tissues around the wound showed local epidermal damage, discoloration, and local swelling. Examination of the leg showed that he had distal pulses, good capillary return in the foot, and no evidence of abnormal neurological function.

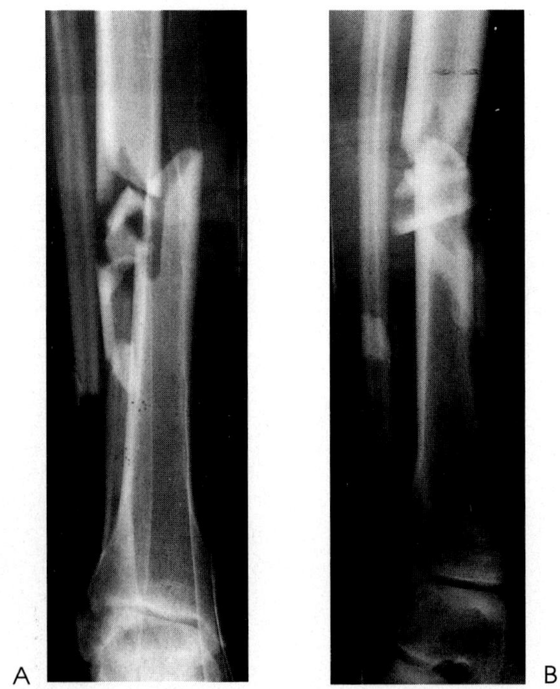

Figure 26–1. Anteroposterior (A) and lateral (B) radiographs taken in the emergency room before treatment. There is a fragmented wedge fracture of the tibial diaphysis. The lateral radiograph shows rotation of the proximal loose fragment.

Radiologic Findings

Anteroposterior and lateral radiographs confirmed that there was a severe fracture of the middle third of the tibial diaphysis (Fig. 26–1). The anteroposterior radiograph (Fig. 26–1A) showed two separate bone fragments and indicated that this was a fragmented wedge fracture. The fibular fracture was almost at the same level as the tibial fracture.

PEARL

- Gustilo defined his criteria for classifying open fractures in his 1976 and 1984 articles. The criteria are well known, but the most significant one concerns the extent of the soft tissue damage around the fracture site. Periosteal stripping is the main difference between IIIa and IIIb fractures and is responsible for markedly different prognoses for the two fracture types. In the tibia periosteal stripping is usually associated with bone fragmentation and it is not unusual to find one or more completely devitalized bone fragments in Gustilo IIIb open tibial fractures. These must be removed.

PITFALLS

- The use of saline lavage has become standard practice during debridement. There is little clinical evidence of its usefulness, but it seems logical to use lavage to clean the wound. However, the surgeon must never substitute lavage for a proper formal surgical debridement. Lavage can be used to clean the wound before debridement is undertaken, but it will be most effective if used after the damaged tissues have been exposed.

- The most frequent iatrogenic error during debridement is failure to remove all the devitalized bone. Each bone fragment should be carefully examined to assess its viability. If there is any doubt, the surgeon should remove the fragment.

The lateral radiograph (Fig. 26–1B) demonstrated that the more proximal of the two loose bone fragments had rotated by about 90 degrees and presumably had become at least partially detached from its soft tissue connections, thereby compromising its vascularity.

Diagnosis

Gustilo III open tibial diaphyseal fracture. AO classification: 42–B3.3. The rotation of the bone fragment shown on the lateral radiograph (Fig. 26–1B) suggested significant soft tissue stripping and that the fracture was probably Gustilo IIIb in severity. However, the final distinction between a Gustilo IIIa and IIIb fracture would be made at the time of surgery, based largely on the degree of soft tissue stripping and the presence of soft tissue and bone contamination.

Surgical Management

The two most important parts of the surgical management of any open fracture is the initial debridement. This should not be delayed and accordingly the patient was taken straight to the operating room where, after he had been anesthetized, the leg was thoroughly cleaned and the wound lavaged with saline. The patient was then

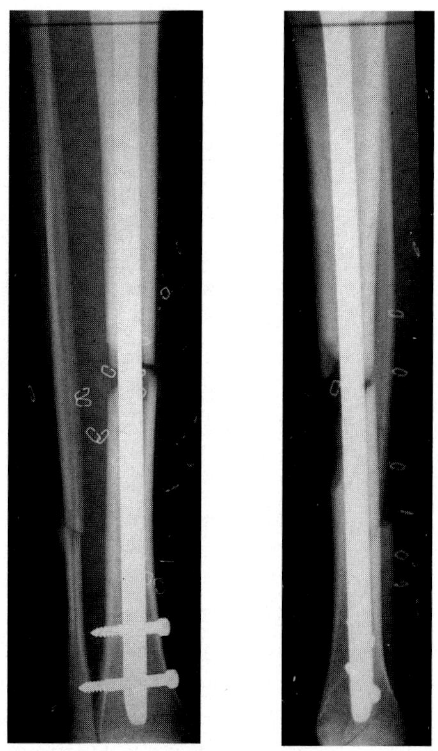
A B

Figure 26–2. Anteroposterior (A) and lateral (B) radiographs of the tibia after debridement, reamed nailing, and the application of a distally based fasciocutaneous flap. The skin staples indicate the area of the flap. Both loose bone fragments have been removed and there is an anterior bone defect measuring 4 cm in length.

placed on a nailing table using calcaneal traction and the leg was prepped and draped for a formal debridement and intramedullary nailing.

Initially the skin edges were excised. Inspection and digital palpation indicated no evidence of degloving and examination of the subcutaneous fat showed it to be normal. Thus no further skin was resected and the wound was subsequently extended to permit visualization of all the damaged soft tissues, bone fragments, and bone ends. Examination showed very little contamination, but there was significant periosteal stripping from both bone fragments that were consequently removed. At the end of the debridement it was thought that there was no residual contamination or devitalized tissue in the wound and the fracture was stabilized using a statically locked 11 mm reamed intramedullary nail.

After intramedullary nailing, a simple moist dressing using tulle was placed on the open wound and bandages applied. Two days after the initial surgical procedure the patient was returned to the operating room for a further wound inspection. No further contamination or devitalized tissue was seen and a distally based fasciocutaneous flap was used to cover the skin defect. Dressings were subsequently applied. Radiographs (Fig. 26–2) taken after the application of the fasciocutaneous flap not only show the extent of the flap but illustrate the size of the bone defect present after debridement and nailing. The bony gap measures about 4 cm anteriorly and extends over more than 70% of the diaphyseal circumference.

Postoperative Management

The flap was inspected 5 days after surgery and was noted to be satisfactory. Passive and active movement of the knee and hindfoot was allowed after 2 weeks, with the delay allowing the flap to heal. The patient was mobilized nonweight bearing using a protective foam pad over the flap with weight bearing gradually introduced after 6 weeks. Follow-up radiographs at 12 weeks showed some evidence of new bone formation (Fig. 26–3), but it was considered that the bone defect could not unite without corticocancellous bone grafting and this was undertaken 12 weeks after the injury. Graft incorporation was rapid and the fracture was clinically and radiologically united 32 weeks after the injury (Fig. 26–4). One year after the injury the patient had regained full ankle movement but still had some restriction of inversion and eversion that hindered some activities. The patient did not complain of knee pain at any time and the nail was not removed.

Discussion

There are a number of important considerations in the management of Gustilo type IIIb open tibial fractures. There is debate about which implant to use and surgeons currently favor unreamed intramedullary nails, reamed intramedullary nails, or external skeletal fixation. There is also discussion about the best method of flap cover for those fractures that require it; the main debate is between local flaps, usually a distally based fasciocutaneous flap, and free flaps that require microvascular anastomosis. The role of bone grafting, exchange nailing, and bone transport must be considered for the treatment of the inevitable nonunions that will follow some of these high energy injuries.

In recent years surgeons have increasingly used intramedullary nails to stabilize Gustilo IIIb fractures. Previously, plates or external skeletal fixation tended to be

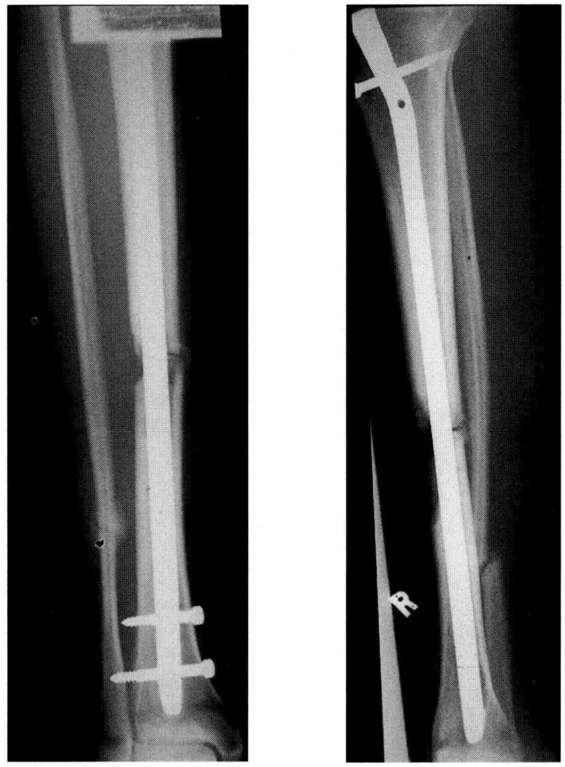

Figure 26–3. Anteroposterior (A) and lateral (B) radiographs taken 12 weeks after nailing show that new bone is present, but the bone defect is too extensive to unite without bone grafting.

used and there are still many surgeons who prefer external fixation, although the use of plates for the management of these difficult fractures has declined. The literature concerning the use of plates in open tibial diaphyseal fractures predates the evolution of modern plastic surgery techniques and it is unfair to compare the results of fracture fixation using bone plates in the 1970s with modern results using external skeletal fixation or intramedullary nails. Presumably better results would now be obtained with plating, but the fact remains that plating not only requires excessive soft tissue stripping but is technically difficult in the presence of bone the comminution that often occurs in Gustilo IIIb fractures.

External skeletal fixation was popularized in the 1980s and there is no doubt that it is a relatively safe method of managing complex tibial fractures. However, an analysis of the literature indicates that it is associated with higher rates of nonunion and malunion than intramedullary nailing and there is always the inevitable problem of pin tract sepsis. In addition, if small wire fixators are used, considerable problems occur with muscle penetration and consequent joint stiffness. Thus many surgeons will now use either an unreamed or reamed intramedullary nail to stabilize severe open tibial fractures.

Despite inevitable interest in the method of fixation it cannot be overemphasized that the most important operation is the initial debridement. This is described in detail in the section dealing with the open femoral fracture. It is vital that all contaminated and devitalized tissue is removed, including all bone fragments that either have no soft tissue attachment or are connected by devitalized soft tissue. There

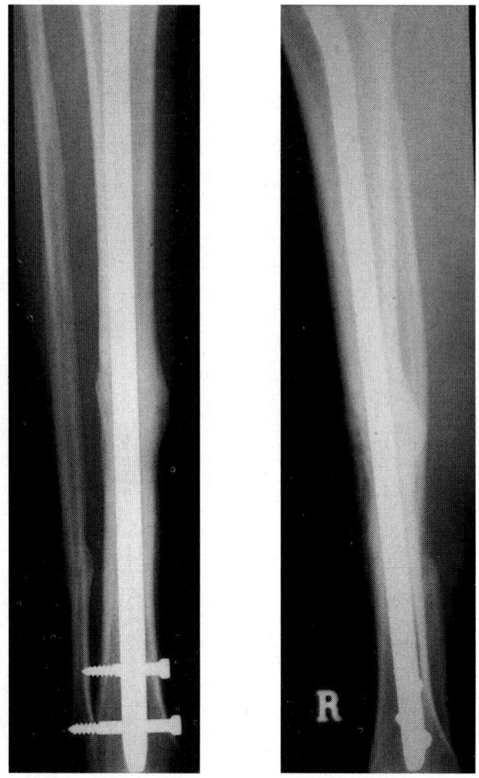

A B

Figure 26–4. Anteroposterior (A) and lateral (B) radiographs showing final union.

are a number of other important points that the surgeon should bear in mind when undertaking a debridement. Skin is remarkably resistant to direct injury but is very susceptible to damage from shearing injuries, which often cause significant degloving injuries. These injuries are particularly common in the older patient (Fig. 26–5) where the degloving may be circumferential. It is important that the surgeon carefully examines the skin in all open fractures for degloving. Degloved skin should be removed until dermal bleeding is encountered, even if this requires the excision of a considerable quantity of skin. However, the degloved skin should not be discarded because it may be an important source of split skin graft.

The surgeon should also examine the condition of the subcutaneous fat. It is not uncommon to find that the subcutaneous fat looks unhealthy even if the overlying skin appears viable. It is important to remember that some of the cutaneous blood supply will come through the subcutaneous fat layer; as it progressively becomes more avascular after injury, the skin vascularity also deteriorates. It is difficult to determine the resection margin for subcutaneous fat and it is always advisable to consult a plastic surgeon if there is doubt.

The surgeon should carefully examine the muscles in each affected compartment to assess the amount of damage caused by the injury. To facilitate this the wound must be extended longitudinally to expose all injured areas. It can be difficult to decide about muscle viability particularly if the patient is hypotensive or peripherally shut down. For this reason it is important to reassess the viability of the muscles at a follow-up procedure 36 to 48 hours after the initial debridement. Occasionally the

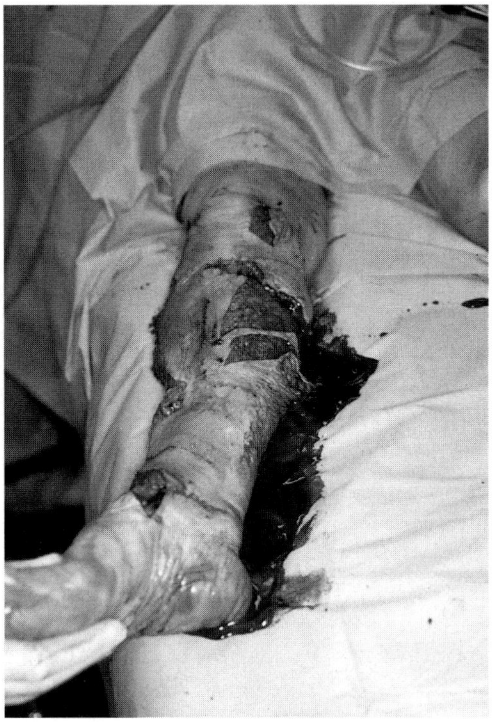

Figure 26–5. Major skin degloving in a 78-year-old female who sustained a tibial fracture in a motor vehicle accident. She was a pedestrian knocked down by an automobile. The degloved skin cannot be sutured, but split skin grafts can be harvested. Degloving injuries are becoming more common as the population ages.

surgeon will encounter muscles that have been exposed to a prolonged crushing force. This usually occurs in traffic accidents where the automobile body shell or engine has compressed the legs of the driver or front seat passenger for a prolonged period (Fig. 26–6). Under these circumstances the muscles will undergo a slow progressive myonecrosis that is often impossible to treat, even by serial debridements, and frequently amputation becomes inevitable.

After debridement the surgeon will select his or her method of bone stabilization. The current literature suggests that intramedullary nailing is preferable to external skeletal fixation. There is debate about the relative merits of reamed and unreamed nailing, but it is probable that the only difference between the two nail types is that unreamed nails are smaller and associated with a higher incidence of screw breakage. This view was confirmed by a prospective randomized trial carried out in Vancouver, Canada (Keating et al., 1997). Currently, most surgeons use small diameter nails but often undertaken limited reaming to ensure the easy passage of the nail down the tibia.

There is always a tendency for surgeons to want to close the open wound primarily. This must be avoided at all costs. There is no harm in leaving the wound open, but closure of the open wound may not only hide residual contamination or myonecrosis but can only be achieved by applying excessive tension to the skin edges. It is always good policy to reexamine the open fracture 36 to 48 hours after the initial operation. This allows for removal of any residual contamination or devitalized soft tissue. If residual contamination or devitalized tissue is encountered, another follow-up procedure should be undertaken after a further 36 to 48 hours.

Every attempt should be made to provide definitive soft tissue cover at the time of the initial follow-up procedure if possible. The literature is clear that the earlier definitive soft tissue cover is undertaken the better, although most authorities discour-

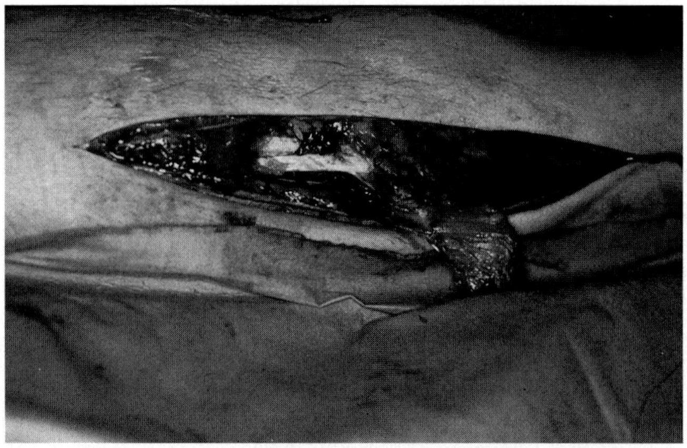

Figure 26–6. Myonecrosis in a 52-year-old truck driver. He was involved in an accident and his leg was crushed for over 1 hour. Successive debridements showed progressive muscle death and the leg was amputated 4 days after the accident.

age primary flap cover because of the risk of covering a contaminated wound. There is widespread agreement that the open wound should be covered by 5 days; logically, the best results are going to be obtained if soft tissue cover is undertaken by day two or three.

Plastic surgeons debate about the optimal method of providing definitive soft tissue cover, but a few basic principles apply. Split skin grafts should never be used to cover the anteromedial subcutaneous border of the tibia because failure is virtually inevitable and the risk of subsequent infection very high. Gastrocnemius muscle flaps can be used to cover proximal skin defects in the leg but they are difficult to raise again because they adhere to the underlying bone. This may prove troublesome for later bone grafting.

The choice of soft tissue cover for the more common defects in the middle and distal thirds of the leg lies between local flaps and free, microvascular flaps. In recent years surgeons have begun to favor local flaps, particularly the distally based fasciocutaneous flap, because they are successful and relatively easy to undertake. However, several factors will influence the surgeon's choice of flaps. These are the size and location of the defect, the need for a cosmetically satisfactory result, the presence of degloving, and the extent of associated bone loss. Larger skin defects can only be covered by free flaps regardless of their location. Most of these large defects occur in the distal tibia and hindfoot where free flaps are often favored by plastic surgeons. Free flaps also provide better cosmesis, but require specialist equipment and expertise and usually have to be undertaken in a plastic surgery operating room. Fasciocutaneous flaps are quicker and easier and can be performed in virtually any operating room. If there is significant degloving, surgeons may also elect to use a free flap because the local perforator vessels on which a fasciocutaneous flap is based may well be damaged and any local flap raised on damaged vessels is almost certain to fail. If there is bone loss, the surgeon may elect to use a microvascular osteocutaneous flap to close the bony defect.

Despite the apparent advantages of free flaps most soft tissue defects associated with open tibial diaphyseal fractures are readily amenable to closure with distally based fasciocutaneous flaps and surgeons now make considerable use of these and other local flaps. A recent survey in Edinburgh, Scotland, showed that all Gustilo IIIa fractures could be covered by local flaps or split skin grafting and only 15% of the Gustilo IIIb fractures required free flaps.

After flap cover has been undertaken, a rehabilitation program can begin. Usually joint movement is restricted for 2 to 3 weeks to allow the flap to heal fully. Thereafter weight bearing is dictated by the type of fixation and the extent of any other injury.

The time to union of Gustilo type IIIb fractures depends on the type of fixation device used by the surgeon, the adequacy of the soft tissue cover, whether or not prophylactic bone grafting is undertaken, and the presence of any bone defects. In this case bone grafting was undertaken 3 months after the injury, but many surgeons will bone graft a defect at about 6 weeks to shorten the time to union. This is a sensible course of action, particularly if external skeletal fixation is used as definitive fracture management.

Court-Brown et al. (1995) examined the role of exchange nailing in the management of open fractures treated with a reamed intramedullary nail. They showed it to be a very useful technique in all open fractures except for Gustilo type IIIb fractures associated with a bone loss of more than 2 cm and 50% of the circumference. When the bone defects were larger, they used early prophylactic bone grafting. It is suggested that if external skeletal fixation is used as a definitive management for a Gustilo IIIb open tibial fracture associated with bone loss, prophylactic bone grafting be carried out 6 to 8 weeks after the initial surgery once the soft tissues have healed. If intramedullary nailing is used, prophylactic grafting should be undertaken if there is a significant bone defect with exchange nailing being employed at 15 to 18 weeks if there is no sign of union in fractures that do not have a significant bone defect.

There is often discussion about the role of primary external fixation and secondary intramedullary nailing. This method of management has been discussed with reference to femoral diaphyseal fractures in the multiply injured patient. Analysis of the literature concerning sequential external fixation and intramedullary nailing in the tibia shows a lack of uniformity of opinion. Surgeons are polarized in their views, with many believing that the infection rate is unacceptably high and others stating that the technique can be used if care is taken with the application of the primary fixator. The technique is not often necessary, but if selected as the definitive treatment method, care must be exercised in assessing the external fixator pin tracts before a nail is inserted. It is unwise to insert an intramedullary canal into a tibia that has draining pin tracks and experience suggests that the results will be good if the pin tracks are allowed to granulate before the nail is inserted.

Amputation is always a possibility in Gustilo type IIIb fractures. This is discussed in more detail in the section dealing with the management of the Gustilo IIIc tibial fracture, but a number of IIIb fractures will inevitably result in below knee amputation. The high incidence of progressive myonecrosis following crushing injuries to the leg has already been mentioned. Failure to amputate the limb under these circumstances may be detrimental or even fatal for the patient because myoglobinuria and renal failure may ensue. The other cause of amputation of Gustilo IIIb fractures is osteomyelitis. The incidence of osteomyelitis in IIIb fractures has now dropped to about 5% in expert centers, but sporadic infection is inevitable and amputation may occasionally be required. The timing of amputation is discussed in the section dealing with Gustilo type IIIc open tibial fractures.

Alternative Methods of Management

The operation of debridement is fairly standard. However, there is debate about the optimal type of dressing for the open wound. If a follow-up procedure is planned within 48 hours, a simple moist dressing is satisfactory. However, the use of pig skin has been advocated as a temporary dressing. Recently surgeons have adopted the bead pouch technique. This involves placing antibiotic impregnated beads into the wound and then sealing the wound with a sterile plastic dressing.

The popular alternative to intramedullary nailing is external skeletal fixation. Some aspects of the use of external fixation in open tibial fractures have already been discussed, but there is debate about the type of fixator that should be used. The early unilateral frames used in the 1970s and 1980s were inadequate because they did not provide sufficient rigidity. However, modern external fixators are much improved and, where possible, a modern unilateral device should always be used. A multiplanar or circular frame will greatly restrict access to the soft tissues and any muscle penetration by pins will inevitably cause joint stiffness. In recent years there has been increased interest in the Ilizarov circular frame. It must be emphasized that this type of frame is designed for reconstructive surgery and its use is not required in the primary management of Gustilo type III open fractures.

Temporary external fixation has already been discussed. Some surgeons believe that the sequential use of external fixation followed by later intramedullary nailing is a good technique in severe open fractures. However, a major benefit of temporary external fixation is that if an inexperienced surgeon has to treat a difficult Gustilo type IIIb open tibial diaphyseal fracture, a thorough debridement, temporary external fixation, and transfer to an appropriate center constitute a sensible way of undertaking primary treatment.

Type of Management	Advantages	Disadvantages	Comments
Traction/casting	None	Poor fracture stability; high complication rates	Nonoperative management should not be used for management of open tibial fractures
Reamed intramedullary nailing	Good mechanical stability; good soft tissue access; rapid patient mobility; good results	Knee pain	Intramedullary nailing (reamed or unreamed) is the treatment of choice for open tibial diaphyseal fractures
Unreamed intramedullary nailing	Good soft tissue access; rapid patient mobilization; good results	Knee pain; mechanically less stable than reamed nailing	Intramedullary nailing (reamed or unreamed) is the treatment of choice for open tibial diaphyseal fractures
External fixation	Ease of application; good temporary fixation; quick	Poor definitive management; pin tract sepsis; nonunion	Higher complication rates than intramedullary nailing, but provides good temporary fixation
Plating	None	Soft tissue stripping; technically difficult; particularly in comminuted fractures	Rarely used

Few surgeons now use plates for open tibial fractures. In recent years new types of bone plate and indirect fracture reduction techniques have been developed to minimize soft tissue stripping but this still remains the main problem associated with plating. In addition long plates are required if the surgeon is spanning areas of extensive comminution and the results of the use of these plates are often poor. There is no place for the use of nonoperative management in Gustilo type IIIb open tibial diaphyseal fractures unless the surgeon does not have access to internal or external fixation equipment.

In this case corticocancellous bone grafting was used to fill the bone defect, an appropriate technique in this case. However, if the bone loss had been circumferential, bone transport or initial bone shortening and subsequent lengthening could have been used.

Complications

The most common complications of the management of open tibial diaphyseal fractures are osteomyelitis and nonunion. As with all complications, these are best avoided by adequate primary treatment and the incidence of osteomyelitis has fallen dramatically in the last 12 to 15 years. This is due to improved soft tissue handling and in particular to a better understanding of the need for cooperation between plastic surgeons and orthopedic trauma surgeons in the management of these difficult problems. In expert centers the infection rate of Gustilo type IIIb open tibial diaphyseal fractures is about 5%, regardless of which method of bone stabilization is used. Thus from time to time bone infection will occur. This should be treated by early recognition and appropriate aggressive therapy with high dose antibiotics, drainage of septic foci, and resection of devitalized tissues. Poor quality skin should be replaced by a healthy flap and bone defects treated by grafting or bone transport.

Nonunion should be predicted either from the size of the bone defect after the initial surgical treatment or from failure of serial radiographs to show signs of union by not later than 20 weeks. This can be treated by exchange nailing in previously nailed tibiae that do not have significant bone loss or by bone grafting or bone transport if there is significant bone loss. Malunion is treated by osteotomy and fixation using bone grafts as required.

There may well be other complications for which the surgeon has to consider treatment. Damage to the nerves in the leg may cause significant muscle weakness that may require the use of an orthosis or even reconstructive surgery. An insensate foot is a particular problem and the surgeon and patient may consider amputation; if this is not acceptable to the patient, the use of appropriate shoewear should be considered.

Suggested Readings

The severely traumatised lower limb: reconstruction versus amputation. Clin Orthop 1989; 243:1–99.

The treatment of tibial fractures. Clin Orthop 1995; 315:1–198.

Court-Brown CM, Keating JF, Christie J, McQueen MM: Exchange intramedullary nailing. Its use in aseptic tibial nonunion. J Bone Joint Surg (Br) 1995; 77B:407–411.

Court-Brown CM, McQueen MM, Quaba AA: Management of Open Fractures. Martin Dunitz, London, 1996.

Gustilo RB, Anderson JT: Prevention of infection in the treatment of 1025 open fractures of long bones: retrospective and prospective analysis. J Bone Joint Surg (Am) 1976; 58A:453–458.

Gustilo RB, Mendoza RM, Williams DM: Problems in the management of type III (severe) open fractures. A new classification of type III open fractures. J Trauma 1984; 24:742–746.

Keating JF, O'Brien PJ, Blachut PA, Meek RN, Broekhuyse HM: Locked intramedullary nailing with and without reaming for open fractures of the tibial shaft. A prospective randomised study. J Bone Joint Surg (Am) 1997; 79A:334–341.

Case 27

History and Physical Examination

A 27-year-old male was admitted to the emergency department after being involved in a motor vehicle accident. He had just gotten out of a taxi and was standing behind it when he was struck from the rear by another car traveling at approximately 30 miles per hour. He sustained a severe injury to his left leg and was taken to the emergency department where he arrived about 1 hour after the accident. He had no injury above his knees, but examination of the left leg showed massive soft tissue and bone damage with a massive posterior skin defect (Fig. 27–1). The viability of the musculature was difficult to determine from inspection of the soft tissues. Examination of the foot showed a patchy loss of sensation and Doppler examination of the posterior tibial and dorsalis pedis pulses showed no blood flow. Assessment of the patient's vital signs showed a blood pressure of 90/60 and tachycardia of 95/hour. The patient was resuscitated with crystalloids and red cell concentrate and transferred straight to the operating room.

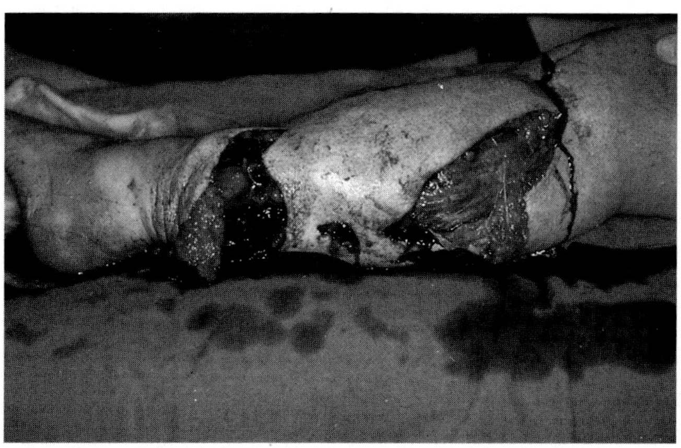

Figure 27–1. The appearance of the leg in the emergency department.

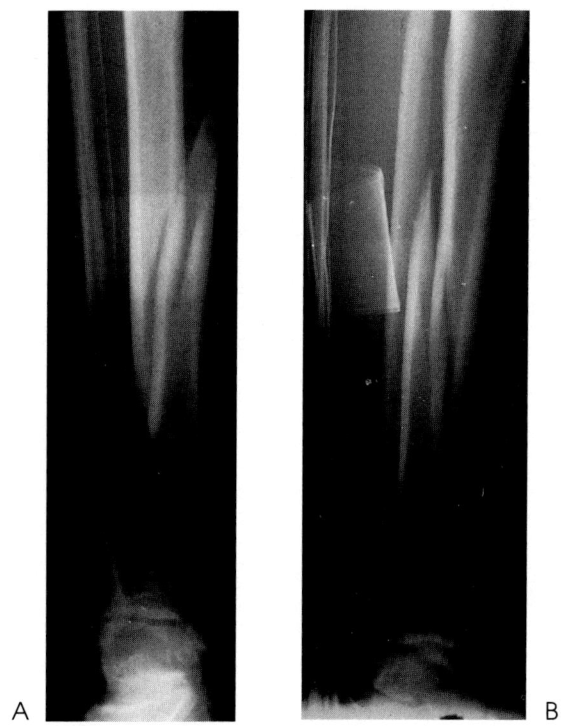

Figure 27–2. Anteroposterior (A) and lateral (B) radiographs of the tibia.

Radiologic Findings

Anteroposterior and lateral radiographs showed a segmental fracture of the tibia diaphysis (Fig. 27–2). The severity of the injury is highlighted by the fact that the segment has moved proximally by between 1 and 2 in, suggesting considerable soft tissue damage. There is also a fracture into the ankle joint.

PITFALL

- A tourniquet should not be used when assessing the soft tissue damage in these severe tibial fractures. The soft tissues have already been exposed to a prolonged period of ischemia and a tourniquet will certainly impede any residual blood flow in the leg. In addition, the surgeon will use tissue vascularity as a determinant for the extent of debridement and a requirement for amputation.

PEARL

- The surgeon should always strive to perform a below knee amputation if at all possible. It may well be easier and less time consuming to carry out an above knee amputation, but patients fare much better if they can use a below knee prosthesis. Modern below knee prostheses are easy to wear and the patient expends much less energy than when using an above knee prosthesis.

Diagnosis

Gustilo type IIIc open fracture of the tibial diaphysis. AO classification: 43–C2.1

Surgical Management

In the operating room the soft tissue wound of the left leg was cleaned using saline lavage. After prepping and draping the leg was reexamined. The muscles were devitalized and discolored, although there was little contamination. There was no evidence of contractility in any muscle group and bleeding was minimal. Both the anterior and posterior tibial arteries were damaged and the posterior tibial nerve was intact but stretched and extensively bruised. It was considered that even if blood flow to the foot could be reestablished using a vein graft, there would be little or no viable muscle in the leg and consequently function would be seriously impaired with very great risk of long term problems. Consequently, it was decided to amputate the limb. Fortunately, the extent of the soft tissue damage meant that a below knee amputation could be undertaken.

Postoperative Management

The stump healed well and a temporary prosthesis was fitted after 3 weeks. Subsequently, a definitive prosthetic limb was successfully fitted and the patient made an excellent recovery. He returned to his work as a self-employed businessperson 8 weeks after the injury. He stated that he was able to carry out all his professional activities, although he could not resume his previous interest in sports.

Discussion

As is often the case with orthopaedic classification systems, the term *Gustilo IIIc* can be interpreted in different ways. It would seem that the definition is straightforward in that *IIIc* applies to fractures that are associated with sufficient vascular damage to require vascular reconstruction if the limb is to be saved. However, in theory a patient might present with a Gustilo type III open tibial fracture and transection of the femoral artery. Therefore, for the purposes of discussion, it will be assumed that the term *IIIc* refers to vascular damage in the area of a tibial fracture. Most of these injuries are caused by traffic accidents or high energy bullets and the extent of the associated soft tissue damage is often very considerable.

The most important decision to be made in the management of Gustilo type IIIc open tibial fractures is whether the patient should have a primary amputation. There is always an understandable tendency for surgeons to wish to preserve the limb at all costs, but this is not always in the patient's best interests. In the case illustrated here the patient returned to work as well as several of his social activities at about 4 weeks, but had the leg been saved, it is likely that he would have encountered a number of complications resulting in infection, nonunion, and severe soft tissue problems. Inevitably, he would have had multiple reconstructive operations and the long term prognosis for the leg would have been poor. The literature suggests that only 10 to 15% of Gustilo type IIIc open tibial fractures are not eventually treated by amputation and a review of the IIIc open tibial fractures that were admitted to the orthopaedic trauma unit in Edinburgh, Scotland, over a 6 year period showed that all were eventually amputated. Some limbs survived for several years, but the considerable amount of reconstructive surgery and marked impairment of function, loss of earnings, and damage to the family unit usually encouraged the patient to seek amputation. Surgeons should be aware that they are often doing their patients a disservice when attempting to salvage these limbs.

The decision to perform primary amputation is difficult and ideally should be made by two experienced orthopaedic trauma surgeons if possible. Surgeons often consider the problems associated with the insensate foot that follows posterior tibial nerve damage when making such a decision, but in fact, the decision to amputate is more difficult if the foot is normal; and this is a frequent finding. There is no point in saving a leg that has little viable muscle tissue merely because the foot is sensate and potentially functional.

There are a number of factors that the surgeon should consider when deciding between amputation and salvage surgery. The age and occupation of the patient are not as important as one would initially believe. It is possible to make convincing arguments for and against amputation in any age group and there is no point in attempting limb salvage merely because the patient needs two good legs to undertake his or her job. No salvaged Gustilo type IIIc tibia will ever function perfectly and a good argument can be made for sacrificing limbs in young people who have demanding jobs because an early return to their employment is often beneficial. The main determinant of whether a primary amputation should be undertaken is damage to the musculature of the leg.

In Gustilo type IIIc fractures the musculature of the deep posterior compartment is usually extensively damaged. If this is combined with extensive anterior compartment muscle damage, much of the tibia will be denuded of muscle and not only will long term function be poor but the incidence of infection and nonunion will be high. Surgeons frequently underestimate the degree of muscle damage and attempt to salvage limbs that really should be amputated. Other considerations are the extent of associated nerve damage. It is highly unlikely that a limb in which there is significant damage to the posterior tibial nerve and severe muscle damage will ever function adequately. If there has been extensive additional damage to the hindfoot, amputation must be performed because the chances of successful salvage surgery are virtually nonexistent. The surgeon must also be aware of the nature and extent of other associated injuries. If the patient is seriously injured, amputation may well be a lifesaving operation.

In recent years a number of scoring systems have been devised to help surgeons decide on the requirement for amputation. An example is the Mangled Extremity Severity Score (MESS). This is a relatively simple rating scale for lower extremity trauma based on the extent of the skeletal or soft tissue injury, the severity of limb ischemia, the degree of hypervolemic shock, and the patient's age. The principle of all these scoring systems is that if the patient scores at or above a certain level (7 in the case of the MESS score), amputation may be required. As with all scoring systems, there are inherent problems in relying solely on an arithmetic figure to predict the need for an amputation. However, the use of a scoring system demands that the surgeon examine all aspects of the case and this attention to detail will certainly help in coming to a rational decision. It is suggested that systems such as the MESS score be used as an aid to decision making.

PEARL

- The patient should always be kept accurately informed about the state of his or her leg and the likely prognosis. Surgeons should resist the tendency to be consciously overoptimistic if it is not justified on clinical grounds. A number of the problems that follow amputation are caused by patients being given inaccurate information at an early stage.

The timing of amputation is particularly important. Amputation should always be performed early before the patient and the surgeon have invested too much time and effort in attempted reconstructive surgery. Ideally, the leg should be amputated primarily and under these circumstances the patient will usually blame the accident and the severity of the injury for the inevitability of the amputation. If a vascular repair is undertaken, the patient should be warned that the limb may not be considered salvageable at the time of the follow-up procedure and unless the surgeon is completely confident of success an amputation should then be undertaken. Amputation at this time will usually be accepted by the patient, but a later amputation may well be taken as a sign of surgical failure. There is little point in consulting the patient about whether they wish to retain the leg. Patients cannot be expected to have sufficient knowledge about the consequences of salvage or amputation and the decision must be always made by the surgeon, who should consult an experienced colleague.

If the surgeon opts for limb salvage, he or she must then decide whether the fracture should be stabilized before revascularization is undertaken. Clearly the prognosis will improve with early revascularization and it is unlikely that revascularization will succeed at all if it is delayed beyond about 6 hours. It is also obvious that stable fixation is required if the vascular repair is to be given any chance of being successful. Therefore it is suggested that the fracture be initially stabilized using a temporary unilateral external fixation device. This can be applied in a few minutes and vascular repair undertaken as a secondary procedure. If for some reason the fixation is likely to be prolonged, it is advisable to insert a temporary vascular stent into the artery to permit distal flow while the fracture is being fixed. However, the surgeon must remember that limb salvage is the priority and definitive fixation can be undertaken later.

Once the limb has been revascularized and the fracture fixed, the fracture should be treated as a IIIb fracture. There should be a follow-up procedure 36 to 48 hours after the initial procedure, at which time soft tissue cover and adjustment of the fracture fixation can be undertaken. As already stated, the follow-up procedure provides the surgeon with the last straightforward opportunity for amputation. Subsequent management will be as described in the section on Gustilo IIIb open tibial fractures.

Alternative Methods of Management

There are few rational alternatives to either primary amputation or temporary external fixation and revascularization followed by later definitive stabilization. Once the leg has been successfully revascularized, the surgeon can treat the fracture with whatever fixation device he or she wishes. As with Gustilo IIIb fractures, most surgeons would choose a reamed or unreamed intramedullary nail or external skeletal fixation as definitive treatment.

Complications

The most likely complication that surgeon and patient will encounter is that the decision to salvage the leg was wrong. By the time that this decision has been made the patient has usually undergone several operations and a considerable amount of time

Type of Management	Advantages	Disadvantages	Comments
Traction/casting	None	Poor stability; revascularization likely to fail; nonunion; malunion; infection	There is no place for nonoperative management in these serious fractures
Amputation	Definitive; early return to function	Phantom pain; stump symptoms	Frequently the only option in the Gustilo type IIIc fracture
External fixation	Useful temporary fixation	Pin tract sepsis; malunion; nonunion	Very useful for temporary management, but associated with complications if used definitively
Plating	None	Technically difficult; time consuming; difficult in comminuted fractures	A very small role in the management of Gustilo type IIIc fractures
Unreamed intramedullary nailing	Quick; early return to function	Time consuming if used primarily	Useful technique, but better undertaken secondarily after revascularization has been established
Reamed intramedullary nailing	Quick; early return to function	Time consuming if used primarily	Useful technique, but better undertaken secondarily after revascularization has been

and effort has been invested in salvaging the limb. Occasionally, the patient may ask for an amputation, but more commonly the surgeon will have to suggest that further surgery is unlikely to improve matters and the time has come for an amputation. Sometimes the patient may accept this advice, but not infrequently there is considerable hostility to the suggestion of an amputation and the implication is that the surgeon has failed to save the leg. The surgeon should always seek a second opinion from an experienced colleague at this time. It is also advisable to arrange for the patient to meet some amputees who can demonstrate the positive benefits of amputation. If the patient refuses an amputation, the surgeon has little option but to continue treatment, but it is likely that the professional relationship between the doctor and the patient will be permanently damaged.

If the limb is salvaged, there are likely to be a number of complications including osteomyelitis, nonunion and, malunion that will be treated in the same way as a Gustilo IIIb open tibial fracture. Not infrequently there are also psychological and social problems, including depression, marital difficulties, and employment difficulties. The orthopaedic surgeon is not usually able to deal with these problems, but should be aware of their existence and refer the patient appropriately.

It should always be remembered that amputation is not without its problems. Some of these can be minimized or avoided if the amputation is performed with care, but in a traumatic situation it may be impossible to fashion an ideal stump. Accordingly, stump problems including skin breakdown and ulceration as well as phantom pain and difficulties in fitting prosthesis may all occur and the patient should be referred to a specialized prosthetic service for supervision of these difficulties.

Suggested Readings

Gregory RT, Gould RJ, Peclet M: The mangled extremity syndrome: a severity grading system for multisystem injury of the extremity. J Trauma 1985; 25:1147–1150.

Gustilo RB: Current concepts in the management of open fractures. Instr Course Lect 1987; 36:359–366.

Helfet DL, Howey T, Sanders R: Limb salvage versus amputation. Clin Orthop 1990; 256:80–86.

Lange RH: Limb reconstruction versus amputation. Decision making in massive lower extremity trauma. Clin Orthop 1989; 243:92–99.

Makk SP, Voranen M, Seligson D: Amputation and late management of the severely injured limb. In Court-Brown CM, McQueen MM, Quaba AA (eds): Management of Open Fractures. Dunitz, London, 1996.

Pozo JL, Powell B, Andrews BG: The timing of amputation for lower limb trauma. J Bone Joint Surg (Br) 1990; 72B:288–292.

Case 28

History and Physical Examination

A 56-year-old woman experienced gradually increasing pain localized to her mid tibia. On physical examination, pain was limited to the mid tibial region; the ankle and knee were painless. The skin overlying the midshaft tibia showed changes compatible with radiation therapy (e.g., hair was absent, and its texture was smooth, almost rubbery). A well healed vertical midline scar extended from the patella distally to the tibial tubercle. Crepitation, angulation, and malrotation of the leg were not present.

The history was relevant in that the patient had been diagnosed with multiple myeloma and had recently finished a course of radiation therapy for an osteolytic lesion of the tibial diaphysis. The patient had also undergone a total knee arthroplasty 3 years earlier.

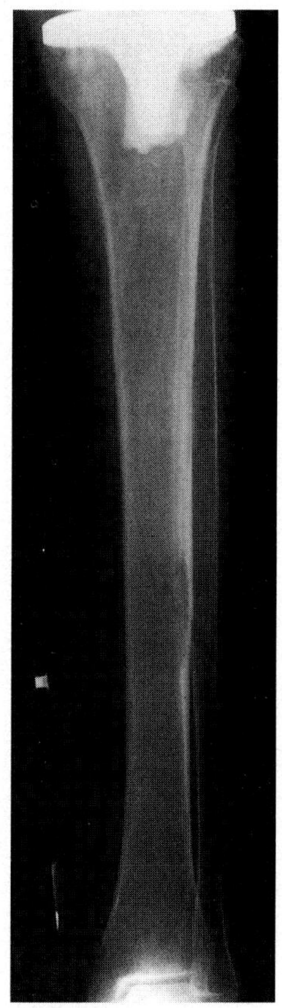

Figure 28–1. Radiograph of the tibia indicating a fracture of the middiaphysis. A cemented tibial component is visible proximally.

Radiologic Findings

Radiographs revealed an undisplaced transverse fracture through a lytic area in the tibial diaphysis. The fibula was not fractured. A cemented total knee arthroplasty in good position was present. The ankle and foot appeared to be normal, with no signs of tumor or arthritis (Fig. 28–1).

PEARL

- The key to successful retrograde nailing via the subtalar joint is the location of the entry portal. The location of the entry portal is determined fluoroscopically on anteroposterior and lateral projections. The portal must be aligned with the long axis of the tibia in both planes, so that when the nail, which is straight, is driven up the tibia, the calcaneus and talus will not be forced into varus, valgus, dorsiflexion, or plantar flexion.

Diagnosis

Undisplaced pathologic fracture of the tibial diaphysis with overlying radiated skin. An important additional factor was that the patient had undergone an ipsilateral total knee arthroplasty. AO classification: 42–A2.1.

Surgical Management

A short-leg removable cast was applied and the patient was instructed to be non-weight bearing. Follow-up was at monthly intervals. Six months after diagnosis of the fracture, there were no clinical or radiographic signs of healing. The fibula had fractured distal to the tibia fracture (Fig. 28–2). Pain with palpation was still present at the fracture site, and weight bearing was extremely painful.

The patient was taken to the operating room where an anesthetic was administered and the leg was prepped and draped. A retrograde reamed nail was inserted across the fracture via an entry portal in the calcaneus. A 2 cm incision was made on the plantar surface of the foot. A drill was used to perforate the cortex of the calcaneus.

A guidewire was inserted through the portal and driven across the subtalar joint, through the body of the talus, across the ankle joint, up the medullary canal of the

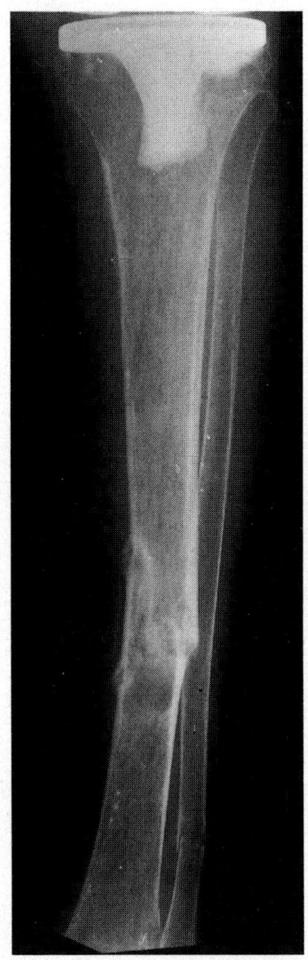

Figure 28–2. At 6 months the tibial fracture has angulated slightly. The fibula has fractured. Clinically, motion was present at the fracture site.

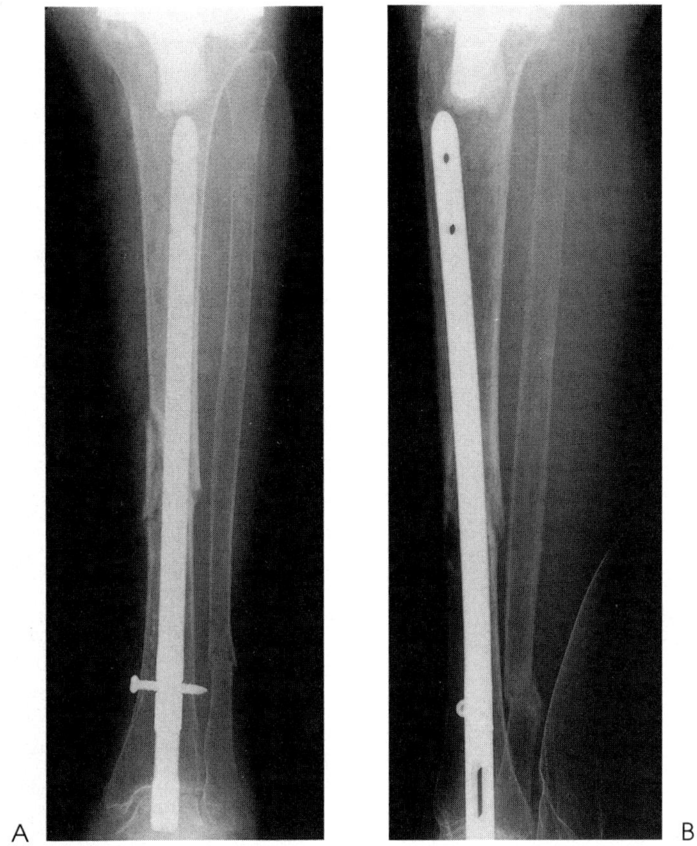

Figure 28–3. Anteroposterior (A) and lateral (B) radiographs obtained following stabilization with a retrograde nail.

tibia, and across the fracture. The calcaneus, talus, and tibia distal to the fracture were then sequentially reamed. The guide wire was removed. A femoral nail was driven across the fracture, positioned with the concave side of its bow facing anteriorly. The nail was locked dynamically with a single screw through the talus (Fig. 28–3).

Postoperative Management

Postoperatively the patient had normal sensation on the plantar aspect of her foot. Nonweight bearing was maintained for 6 weeks following nailing. Radiographs at 6 weeks indicated early healing. Clinically the patient had complete relief of her pain. Weight bearing was increased to full over the following month. At 6 months the fracture was healed (Fig. 28–4).

Discussion

This patient had a pathologic midshaft tibia fracture that did not respond to closed treatment. Management of the fracture was complicated by the course of radiation therapy and the presence of a total knee arthroplasty.

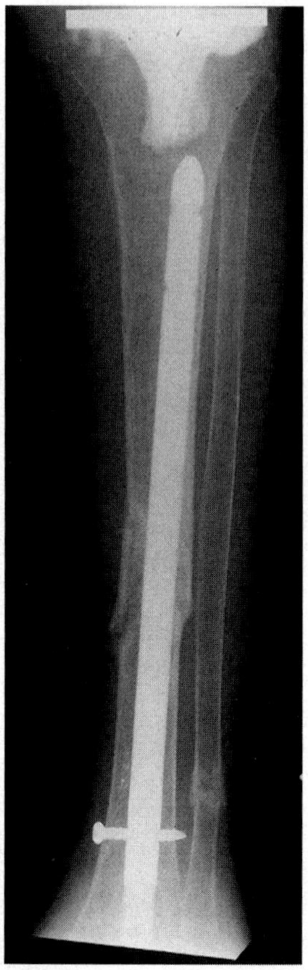

Figure 28–4. Six months following intramedullary nailing the tibia fracture is healing. The fibula fracture has healed.

Alternative Methods of Management

Alternatives to retrograde nailing as a method of management were external fixation, plating, cast immobilization and autologous bone marrow injection, and continued cast immobilization. Antegrade nailing was not an option because of the knee arthroplasty.

Retrograde nailing with a short statically locked nail has been described as a means of obtaining ankle or subtalar arthrodesis. We adapted the technique of retrograde nailing to this case. Because we were treating a middiaphyseal tibial fracture, a longer nail was required than for an ankle arthrodesis. We selected a femoral nail because, unlike tibial nails, femoral nails do not have a bend in the driving end that would potentially displace the subtalar or ankle joints during final impaction. The nail was locked distally to prevent it from backing out at the foot. It was not locked proximally to enable the fracture to impact. Because we only reamed the tibia up to and not across the fracture site good rotational stability was achieved without static locking. The advantages of retrograde nailing are that the radiated skin is not incised; the bone around the fracture is "reinjured" during reaming and healing is therefore stimulated; and the fracture is stabilized. The primary disadvantages of retrograde nailing are that the subtalar and ankle joint are arthrodesed and the plantar nerves of the foot are at risk of injury.

Management with external fixation has the advantage that the radiated skin is not incised and the fracture is stabilized. In addition, if a dynamic fixator is used, the fracture site can be compressed. External fixation has the disadvantage of limited patient acceptance and the risk of premature failure due to loosening of the pins in osteopoenic bone.

Plating exposes the patient to the risk of wound slough and subsequent infection. In addition, osteopenia limits stability of fixation. Because of the risk of a wound slough and the limited stability of fixation, plating is the least desirable management alternative.

Cast immobilization with autologous bone marrow injection has been described in the management of pathologic fractures that have gone on to delayed union. The advantages of the procedure are that the trauma to the overlying radiated skin is minimized and the bone marrow supplies osteoprogenitor cells that may increase the chance of consolidation of the fracture. The disadvantages are that prolonged casting is required and because this is a procedure with which there is minimal clinical experience, it is difficult to estimate the chance of success.

The only advantage of management with continued cast immobilization is that the patient is spared an operative procedure. The major disadvantage of cast immobilization is the low probability of consolidation of the fracture.

Type of Management	Advantages	Disadvantages	Comments
Retrograde nailing	Radiated skin is not incised; delayed union is reinjured	Subtalar and ankle joints are arthrodesed	Probably the best option
External fixation	Radiated skin is not incised; compression can be applied across the fracture	Limited patient acceptance; pin bone interface is likely to fail secondary to osteopenia	Patient acceptance limits this method of management
Plating	Anatomic reduction is achieved; early motion of surrounding joints is possible	Radiated skin is incised, exposing the patient to the risk of slough and infection; fixation is limited by osteopenia	Probably the least desirable alternative because it exposes the patient to the most risk with the least chance of success
Continued cast immobilization	Spares the patient a surgical procedure	Low probability of success	Indicated for nonambulatory patients or those with limited life expectancy
Cast immobilization and autologous bone marrow injection	Minimizes trauma to radiated skin; minimal operative procedure	Requires prolonged cast immobilization; impossible to assess chance of success	Excellent option if patient is willing to be casted indefinitely and wants to avoid an operative procedure

Complications

The potential complications of retrograde nailing of a pathologic midshaft tibial fracture with overlying radiated skin are nonunion and subsequent cut out or failure of the nail, breakdown of the skin, and injury of the plantar nerves of the foot. This fracture is more likely to go on to nonunion than most midshaft tibial fractures because it is pathologic and the bone has been radiated. Failure of the fracture to heal will eventually be followed either with cutout or fracture of the nail. Management of nonunion is either nonoperative (i.e., nonweight bearing and pulsed electromagnetic fields) or operative (i.e., nail exchange and autologous bone grafting).

Breakdown of the radiated skin is less likely to occur with closed retrograde nailing than with other methods of management. If the skin sloughs, the management options are directed at either salvage or amputation. Salvage will require a free soft tissue transfer to achieve coverage. Local procedures such as rotation of the soleus are doomed to failure because of the previous radiation. The chance of successful salvage is low because of the age of the patient, the local radiation, and the pathologic nature of the fracture. If the leg is amputated, the level of the amputation must be proximal to radiated tissue or the incisions will not heal. In this case because the patient has a total knee arthroplasty, knee disarticulation is not a possibility and the lowest possible level of amputation may be above the knee.

Injury to the medial and lateral plantar nerves can occur during retrograde nailing. Theoretically, both nerves are anterior and medial to the insertion site of the nail in the calcaneus. Therefore the most likely cause of injury is stretch from retraction of the soft tissues during nail insertion. Management is observation. The patient is educated regarding the danger of skin breakdown.

Suggested Readings

Bonargo BC, Rubin P: Nonunion of pathologic fracture after radiation therapy. Radiology 1967; 88(5):889–898.

Moore TJ, Prince R, Pochatko D, Smith JW, Fleming S: Retrograde intramedullary nailing for ankle arthrodesis. Foot and Ankle Inter 1995; 16(7):433–436.

Pochatko DJ, Smith JW, Phillips RA, Prince BD, Herick MR: Anatomic structures at risk: combined subtalar and ankle arthrodesis with a retrograde intramedullary rod. Foot and Ankle Inter 1995; 16(9):542–547.

Redmon BJ, Biermann JS, Blasier RB: Interlocking intramedullary nailing of pathological fractures of the humerus. J Bone Joint Surg 1996; 78A:891–896.

Case 29

History and Physical Examination

A 24-year-old man was admitted to the emergency department having jumped from a ledge about 6 feet off the ground. He had caught his left leg in some metal railings as he fell and on admission it was obvious that he had a deformed swollen left leg. There was no other injury. Examination showed normal neurovascular function in his leg. He was in considerable pain, but passive dorsiflexion of his toes did not cause a significant increase in his discomfort.

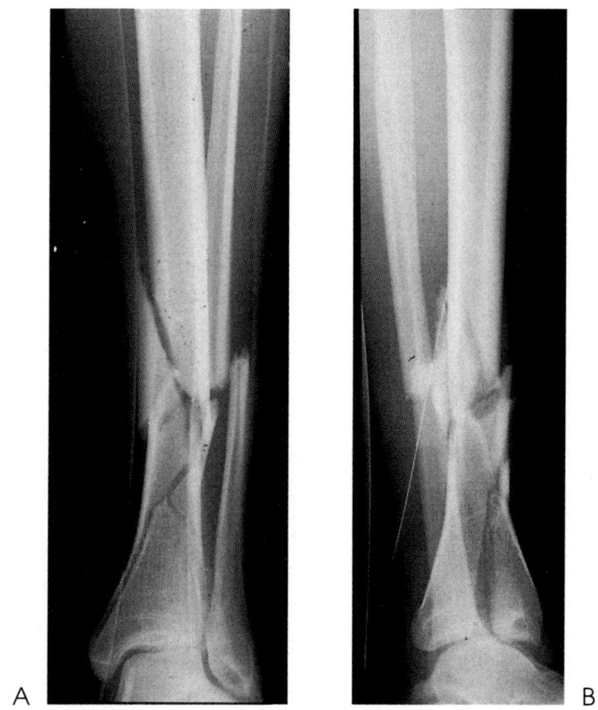

Figure 29–1. Anteroposterior (A) and lateral (B) radiographs of a complex fracture affecting the diaphysis and the tibial plafond.

Radiologic Findings

Anteroposterior and lateral radiographs showed a complex fracture of the lower half of the tibia associated with a transverse fibula fracture (Fig. 29–1). The lateral radiograph showed a simple articular fracture with considerable diaphyseal comminution.

Diagnosis

Fracture of the tibial plafond associated with considerable diaphyseal comminution. AO classification: 43–C2.3

Surgical Management

The leg was splinted in the emergency room to help relieve pain and minimize the extent of any further soft tissue or bone damage. The patient was taken to the operating room where a compartment pressure monitor was inserted with the patient under local anaesthetic. The tip of the slit catheter was placed in the anterior compartment midway between the diaphyseal and metaphyseal fractures. The initial pressure was 35 mm Hg but the diastolic blood pressure was 85 mm Hg and therefore blood flow in the muscles was not significantly impaired. The patient was given appropriate analgesia overnight, but the compartment pressure gradually rose and 8 hours after admission the compartment pressure was 60 mm Hg, with the diastolic blood pressure remaining at 85 mm Hg. Accordingly, the patient was taken to the operating room and the left leg was prepped and draped after removal of the compartment monitor.

Fluoroscopy was initially used to reduce the partial articular fracture of the tibial plafond. A good reduction was obtained by placing a percutaneous bone clamp across the fracture. Once the articular surface had been reduced it was held with two lagged interfragmentary screws. A semicircular external fixator bar was then placed around the distal fragment and held with three half pins that were inserted into the reconstructed metaphysis (Fig. 29–2). Two half pins were inserted into the diaphysis and joined in the metaphyseal construct by two side bars. A four compartment fasciotomy was then performed through medial and lateral incisions and dressings applied. Postoperative radiographs were satisfactory (Fig. 29–3).

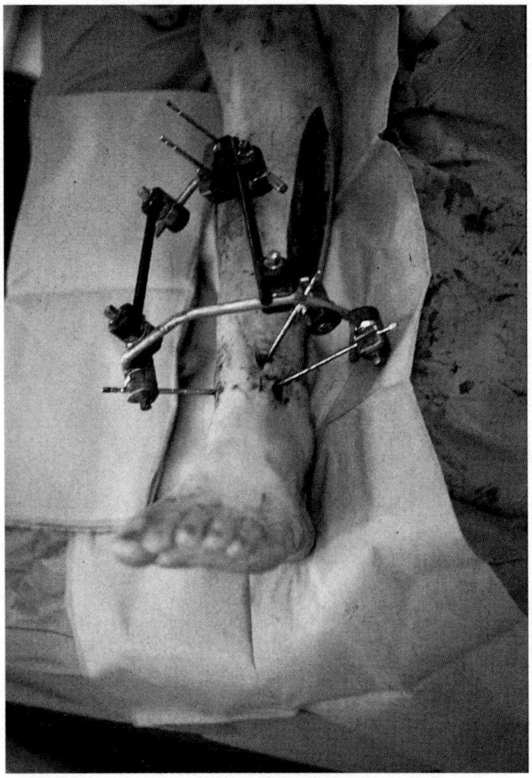

Figure 29–2. A semicircular external fixator was used to treat this fracture. Three distal pins provided good fixation and early joint movement was encouraged.

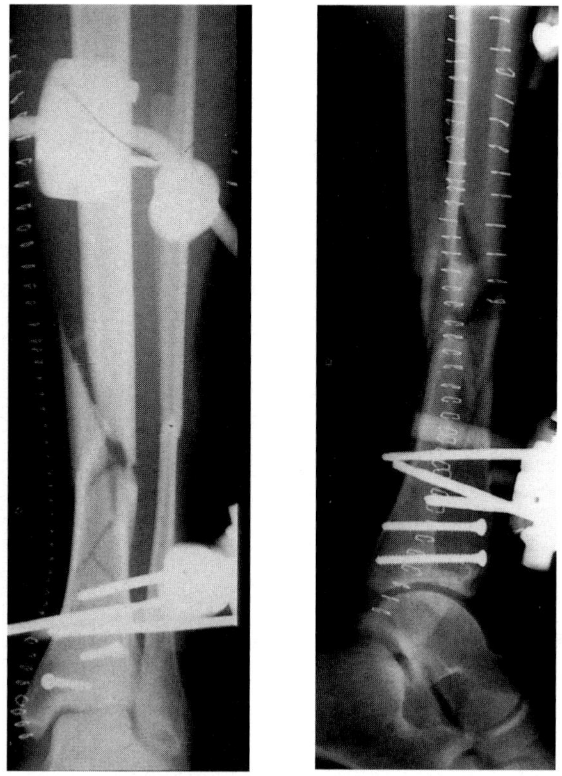

Figure 29–3. Anteroposterior (A) and lateral (B) postoperative radiographs show an excellent articular reduction and good alignment.

The patient was returned to the operating room 2 days later and the medial fasciotomy wound closed. The lateral fasciotomy was partially closed at that time, but it was thought that it could not be fully closed without tension; final closure was achieved 2 days later.

Postoperative Management

One week after the application of the fixation it was obvious that the patient could not maintain his foot in the plantar grade position and was developing an equinus contracture. Accordingly, the external fixator was extended down to his foot by placing two pins in the hallux metatarsal. The patient subsequently mobilized well with crutches.

Over the next 2 to 3 weeks the patient developed pin tract sepsis around the most medial of the three pins in the metaphyseal fragment. This was treated by local management including careful cleansing and a course of antibiotics. The pin did not need to be changed. The external fixator extension to the hallux metatarsal was removed after 3 weeks.

Seven weeks after the accident it was thought that the metaphyseal component of the fracture had united, but obviously the diaphyseal fracture had not. The patient was unhappy about wearing an external fixator for a prolonged period and it was therefore decided to treat the diaphyseal component of the fracture with a reamed intramedullary nail. The patient was readmitted and the three external fixator pins

PEARLS

- The development of an equinus contracture after internal or external fixation of a pilon fracture is not uncommon. Movement is painful for several days after surgery and the patient is usually more comfortable with the foot in equinus. If the foot is left in this position, it can be difficult to subsequently reestablish good ankle motion. If the equinus deformity persists for a prolonged period, a lengthening of the Achilles tendon may even be required. It is best controlled by applying a back slab or extending the external fixator to include the foot.
- Pin track sepsis is usually no more than a nuisance. It rarely gives rise to serious sepsis. One of the problems of external fixation is that pin care is very labor intensive and while the patient can undertake most of the care, pin sepsis requires nursing care. The incidence of pin track sepsis varies with the surgeon's definition of what it is, but in some series the incidence is over 40%. The greater the number of pins the greater the problem and thus small wire fixators frequently require considerable attention.

PITFALL

- When applying an external fixator to a diaphyseal fracture always make sure that the fracture is accurately reduced. It is usually very difficult to correct a deformity at a later date and the immediate postoperative fracture alignment often persists until union.

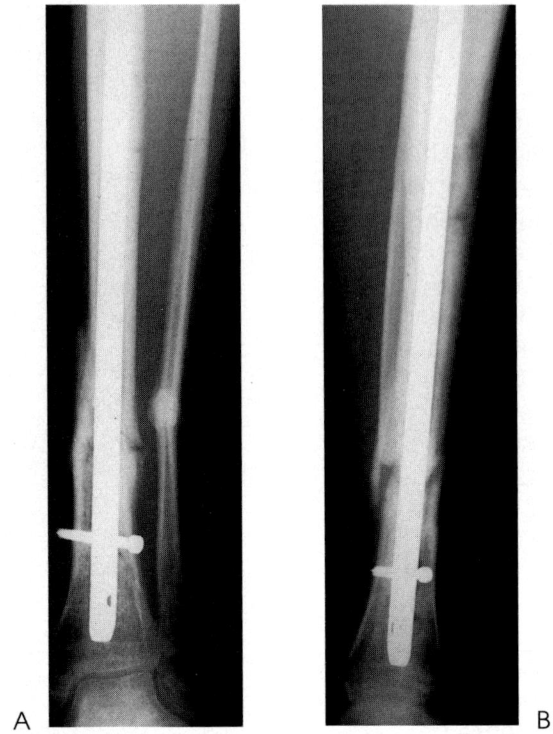

Figure 29–4. Union is proceeding. There is a degree of valgus but the patient had good function. Anteroposterior (A) and lateral (B) views.

and the two intrafragmentary screws were removed from the metaphyseal fragment. The pin tracts were curetted and the patient placed on antibiotics. The leg was supported in a back shell and the state of the pin tracts was monitored carefully. It took 8 days for the most medial pin tract to granulate, although the other two granulated quickly.

Once all the pin tracts had granulated it was considered safe enough to nail the tibia. A reamed nail of 12 mm diameter was inserted and statically locked. The patient was allowed to weight bear within a few days of nailing and a physiotherapy regime was organized. Twelve weeks after the nailing procedure was undertaken check radiographs showed that union was proceeding. The tibial fracture was in about 5 degrees of valgus, but the tibial plafond fracture was congruous and the patient had good hindfoot function (Fig. 29–4).

Discussion

There are two main methods of treating this type of fracture in which there is extensive diaphyseal comminution and fairly simple involvement of the lower tibial articular surface. The joint must be accurately reconstructed and rigidly fixed to allow early movement and minimize the risk of posttraumatic osteoarthritis. This can only be achieved with intrafragmentary screws. The real question is how to secure the reconstructed metaphyseal fragment to the diaphysis. Rüedi and Allgöwer (1979) highlighted the use of plates in the management of pilon fractures and achieved good results. However, the technique is difficult because it requires exten-

PITFALL

- Wound infection after plating of a pilon fracture is often attributed to the inherent problems of operating in the area. However, pilon fractures are high energy injuries associated with considerable soft tissue swelling and a high incidence of compartment syndrome. Once a plate is inserted it is usually very difficult to close the wound and attempts at closing it under tension cause the infection. If the wound cannot be closed without tension, it should be left open and closed at a later stage. Alternatively, a flap can be used.

sive soft tissue dissection. There is also a high incidence of wound infection after plating of pilon fractures. In this particular fracture plating would be very difficult because of the extent of the comminution. A very long plate associated with considerable soft tissue mobilization would be required.

In recent years the concept of minimally invasive surgery has become popular. The principle of this technique is that the fractures are either reduced closed or through small incisions that preserve the soft tissue attachments. Interfragmentary screws are used to fix the metaphyseal fragments and external fixation or intramedullary nailing is used for the reconstructed metaphysis to the diaphysis. The use of an intramedullary nail is attractive because the surgeon does not have to change fixation methods as in this case. If a nail is used, the surgeon must be careful to position the intrafragmentary screws such that the nail can be passed between them. If this cannot be done, it is probably wiser to use an external fixator. Some intramedullary nails have a distal anteroposterior screw hole and if so, this screw can be used to stabilize the metaphyseal fragments.

If an external fixator is used, the surgeon must elect whether to use it for definitive management of the diaphyseal fracture or temporary management until the metaphyseal fracture has united. Uncomplicated high energy tibial diaphyseal fractures may take up to 6 months to unite and patients often dislike wearing external fixators for this length of time. They often tolerate the fixator for about 3 months and then wish to have it removed. The other significant problem about using external fixation for definitive management is that the incidence of malunion tends to be higher.

The potential problem of changing from external fixation to intramedullary nailing is infection. Pin tract sepsis is common and the worry is that infection will seed in the intramedullary canal and cause widespread osteomyelitis after nailing. A review of the literature shows that surgical opinion is polarized about this technique, with some surgeons stating that it is safe and others claiming that the incidence of infection is high. Paradoxically, it seems that the higher rate of infection occurs in fractures where there is a prolonged delay between the removal of the external fixator and the insertion of the intramedullary nail. Whatever the merits of primary external fixation and secondary intramedullary nailing, many surgeons will be faced with having to use the technique from time to time and should be aware of how to minimize the incidence of infective complications.

Great care should be taken when inserting the external fixator pins at the time of the initial surgery. The pins should not be inserted through stab incisions but through incisions that minimize the risk of the skin or subcutaneous tissues being stretched by the pins. The pins should also not be inserted by power because this tends to burn the bone and damage the soft tissues.

Care should be taken about pin hygiene and the patient taught pin care techniques. However, expert supervision is also required. Of particular importance is the state of the pin tracts after pin removal. It is sensible to excise the pin tracts and curette the bone at the time of pin removal and then leave the tracts to granulate before inserting the intramedullary nail. If the pin tracts are uninfected, they will granulate very quickly.

Alternative Methods of Management

The obvious alternative treatment method is intramedullary nailing using either a reamed or unreamed nail. However, getting a nail past the intrafragmentary screws in the metaphysis is not always as easy as it appears and many surgeons who are inexperienced with intramedullary nailing may well opt for external fixation. The role of plating has been discussed. There is no role for nonoperative management in this difficult intraarticular fracture.

Type of Management	Advantages	Disadvantages	Comments
Traction/casting	None	Incongruous joint surface; joint stiffness; nonunion; malunion	Traction is required to try to reduce the articular surface and the results would be poor
Intramedullary nailing	Good joint movement; early mobilization; definitive management	Technically difficult	A good method in experienced hands
External fixation	Straightforward technique; allows joint motion	Pin tract sepsis; patient acceptability; malunion	Definitive external fixation is often difficult to maintain for the duration of union of a high velocity tibial diaphyseal fracture
External fixation and secondary intramedullary nailing	Technically straightforward; good joint motion	Risk of infection	A useful technique for surgeons inexperienced in intramedullary nailing
Plating	None	Soft tissue damage; joint stiffness; nonunion	Not suitable for this difficult intraarticular fracture

Complications

The most likely complications of this type of fracture are nonunion, malunion, and infection depending on the type of fixation employed by the surgeon. Nonunion of the metaphyseal component of the fracture is highly unlikely, but nonunion of the diaphysis may well occur. If nonunion occurs following external fixation, there may well be a malposition of the fracture and nailing may not be possible. The surgeon is then faced with either taking down the nonunion and nailing the fracture or merely using bone graft and maintaining the external fixator. If a nonunion has followed the use of an intramedullary nail, then exchange nailing should be undertaken.

In this case a malunion of the distal tibia did occur. Malunion is one of the most common complications of the use of a metaphyseal or diaphyseal external fixation. Ideally, a fracture malposition should be detected early and corrected, but this goal is not always achieved. In this case the malposition was noted at 12 weeks, by which time it was thought that it could not be corrected without open surgery. There is very little evidence that a malunion such as the one shown here causes significant functional disability. However, the literature concerning the late effects of hindfoot function following tibial diaphyseal malunion is all retrospective and consists mainly of analyses of patients who had tibial fractures many years earlier. Few patients complain of symptoms but most have, of course, forgotten about any alteration of gait or lifestyle engendered by the malunion. However, the available evidence does not support osteotomizing the tibia to correct the degree of tibial malalignment shown in this case.

Infection would be treated in the usual way with high dose antibiotics, drainage of any septic foci, and resection of bone and soft tissue as required. Bone grafting and soft tissue reconstruction may be needed.

The other depressingly common complication of pilon fractures is secondary posttraumatic osteoarthritis. In the AO type B fracture illustrated here the intraarticular component is easily treated and the incidence of posttraumatic osteoarthritis could be expected to be low, but in AO type C complete articular fractures accompanied by significant damage to the articular cartilage the incidence of osteoarthritis is high. If the patient is in intolerable pain, ankle arthrodesis is usually performed. The surgeon should be aware that this is a difficult operation and may not remove all the patient's discomfort because there may also be damage to the subtalar joint and the other joints of the hindfoot following the initial injury.

Suggested Readings

Barbieri R, Schenk R, Koval K, Aurori K, Autori B: Hybrid external fixation in the treatment of tibial plafond fractures. Clin Orthop 1996; 332:16–22.

Court-Brown CM, Pennig D (eds): Tibia. Butterworth Heinemann, Oxford, 1997.

Ovadia DN, Beals RK: Fractures of the tibial plafond. J Bone Joint Surg (Am) 1986; 68A:543–551.

Rüedi TP, Allgöwer M: The operative treatment of intraarticular fractures of the lower end of the tibia. Clin Orthop 1979; 138:105–110.

Teeny SM, Wiss DA: Open reduction and internal fixation of tibial plafond fractures. Clin Orthop 1993; 292:108–117.

Tornetta P, Weiner L, Bergman M, et al: Pilon fractures: treatment with combined internal and external fixation. J Orthop Trauma 1993; &:489–496.

Case 30

History and Physical Examination

A 66-year-old woman was admitted to the emergency department after a fall while hill climbing. She had felt extreme pain in her left ankle and was unable to weight bear. Examination showed the ankle to be deformed but with no evidence of distal neurovascular compromise. She had no other injury.

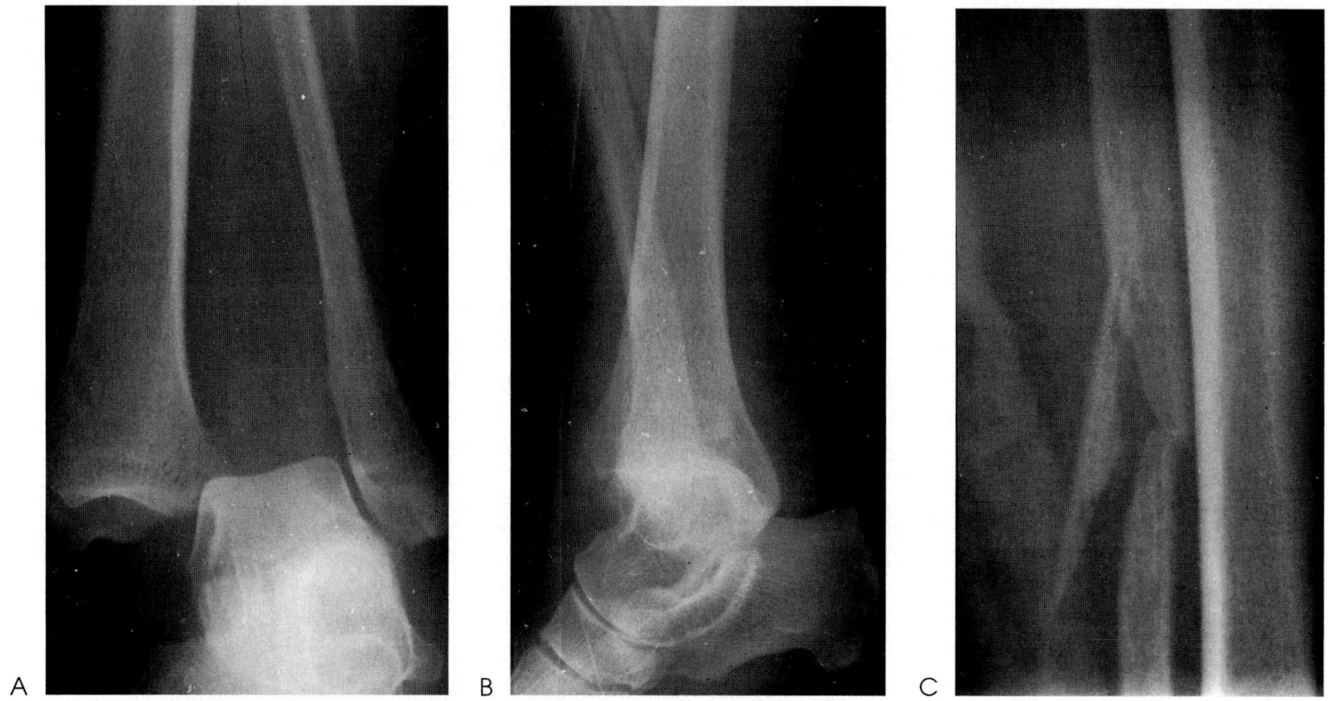

Figure 30–1. (A–C) Anteroposterior and lateral radiographs of an abduction ankle fracture dislocation.

Radiologic Findings

Anteroposterior and lateral radiographs (Fig. 30–1) showed a fracture dislocation of the left ankle. The anteroposterior view indicated a diastasis with disruption of the normal relationship between the distal tibia and fibula. The lateral view shows a suprasyndesmotic fracture of the fibula with a butterfly fragment.

Diagnosis

Suprasyndesmotic fracture dislocation of the ankle. AO classification: 44–C2.1 fracture.

Surgical Management

The ankle was manipulated in the emergency room to reduce the dislocation. A well padded light supportive cast was applied and the patient admitted to the orthopedic

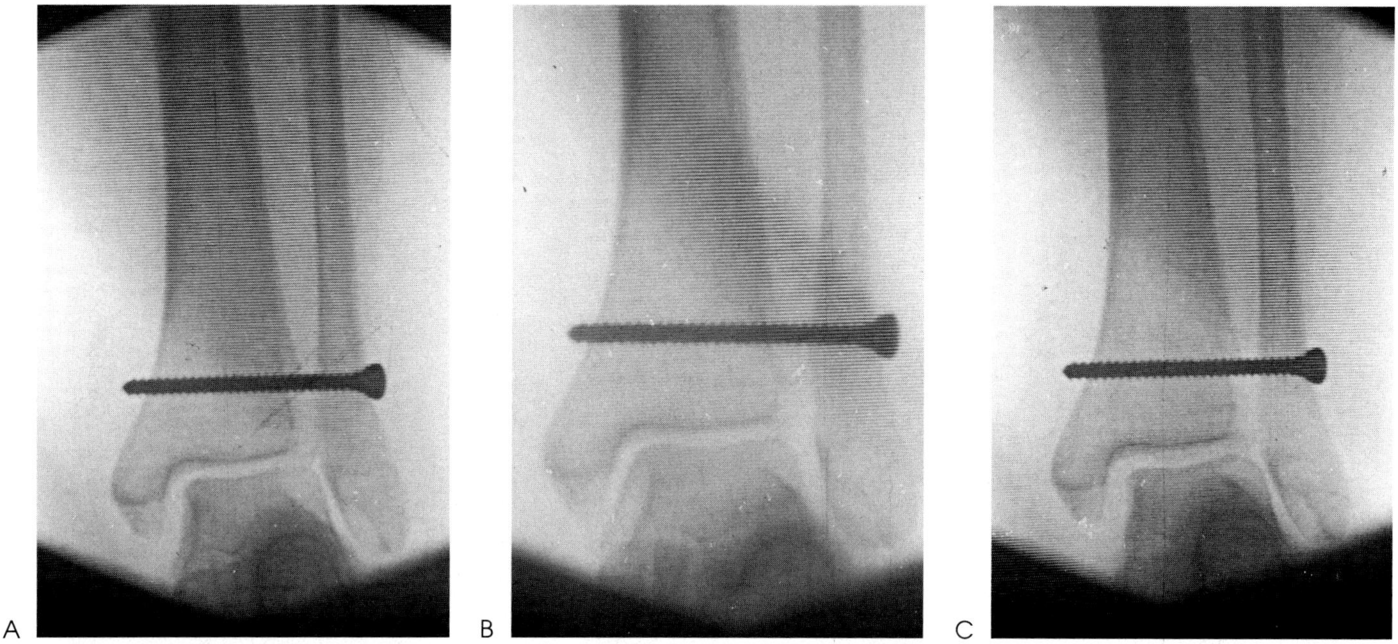

Figure 30–2. (A, B) After reduction and insertion of a diastasis screw some talar shift remains. The talar shift is reduced by inversion. (C) Plantarflexion of the foot opens the ankle medially and superiorly.

PITFALL

- The standard anteroposterior radiograph of the ankle does not demonstrate the true width of the syndesmosis. Figure 30-2 indicates that width. Surgeons must be careful not to interpret a syndesmosis view as showing a malreduced ankle. Closing a normal syndesmosis will merely restrict ankle function.

PEARL

- Persistent opening of the medial side of the ankle is often attributed to an infolded deltoid ligament. This can occur, but it is rare. The deltoid ligament is usually transected midsubstance and cannot infold. The radiologic appearance results from a persistent external rotation deformity.

trauma unit. On the following day the patient was taken to the operating room and the ankle was examined under fluoroscopy. It was clear that there was a diastasis with complete disruption of the syndesmosis and interosseous membrane. The distal fibula and tibia were reduced easily and one diastasis screw inserted. The ankle was then reexamined using fluoroscopy. This indicated that the syndesmosis was well reduced but with a degree of persistent talar shift (Fig. 30–2A). This was easily abolished by inversion of the ankle (Fig. 30–2B), which suggested considerable soft tissue damage around the ankle joint. Evidence of the extent of this damage was gained by plantarflexing the foot. This action caused the medial and superior joint lines to open (Fig. 30–2C), demonstrating that the medial and anterior ligamentous and capsular structures had been disrupted.

Postoperative Management

Because the ankle was congruous in inversion a below knee plaster was applied with the foot in sufficient inversion to reduce the talar shift. The patient was mobilized nonweight bearing and the plaster applied for 6 weeks. The patient was then allowed to weight bear and a physiotherapy program instituted. Nine months after the injury the patient had good function but had lost about 10 degrees of plantarflexion.

Discussion

In many ankle fractures the radiologic indication of soft tissue damage is talar shift, a lateral translation of the talus within the ankle mortice. Talar shift usually occurs

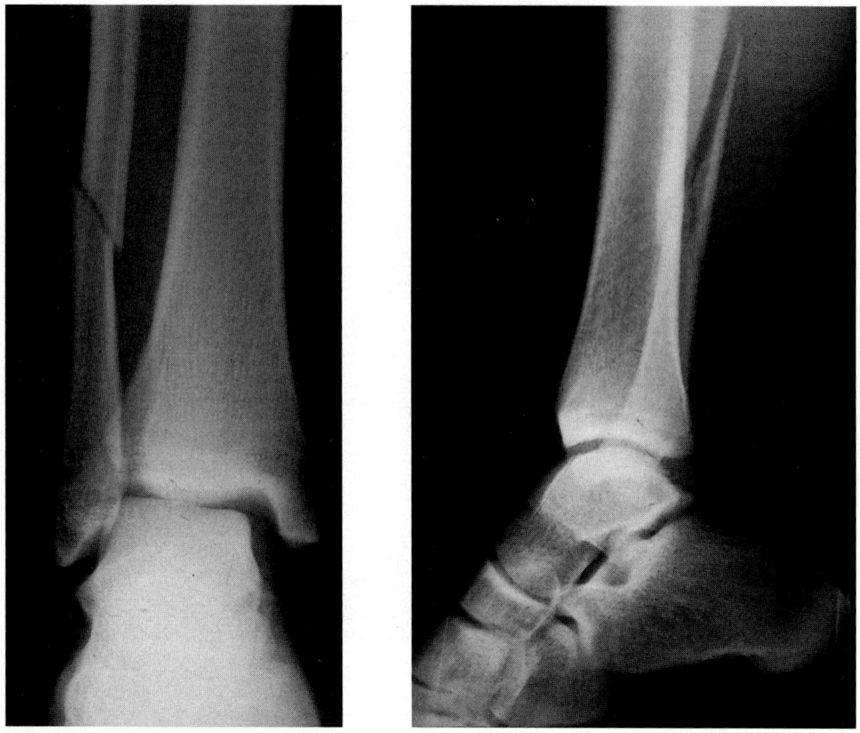

Figure 30–3. An external rotation suprasyndesmotic ankle fracture.

because of damage to the medial and anterior soft tissues around the ankle and is commonly seen in three types of fracture. The most severe talar shift occurs if an abduction force is applied to a pronated or everted foot. If this happens, the deltoid ligament and subsequently the anterior and posterior capsule will tear. If the deforming force continues, the syndesmosis and the interosseous membrane also tear and a suprasyndesmotic fracture of the fibula occurs. Because the deformation is caused by an abduction force the fibular fracture tends to be transverse or comminuted. An example is shown in Figure 30–1.

Talar shift is more commonly seen if an external rotation force is applied to a supinated or inverted foot. If this occurs, the deltoid ligament ruptures; the anterior capsule may also rupture. However, in this type of fracture the deforming force is rotational and the posterior syndesmosis acts as the fulcrum. Thus the posterior syndesmosis and the interosseous ligament remain intact and the suprasyndesmotic fibular fracture tends to be spiral or oblique (Fig. 30–3). The last type of ankle fracture commonly associated with talar shift is the transsyndesmotic spiral or oblique fibular fracture (Fig. 30–4). It is also caused by external rotation, but the anterior capsule is usually, but not invariably, intact.

The importance of external rotation in the pathogenesis of talar shift cannot be overemphasized. There is a belief among a number of orthopedic surgeons that talar shift always represents a lateral shift of the talus within the ankle mortise brought on by an abduction or valgus force. This view presumably persists because of the appearance of the anteroposterior radiographs. However, most suprasyndesmotic and transsyndesmotic fibular fractures associated with talar shift have a spiral configuration and it is clear that the talar shift has followed an external rotation force. As the

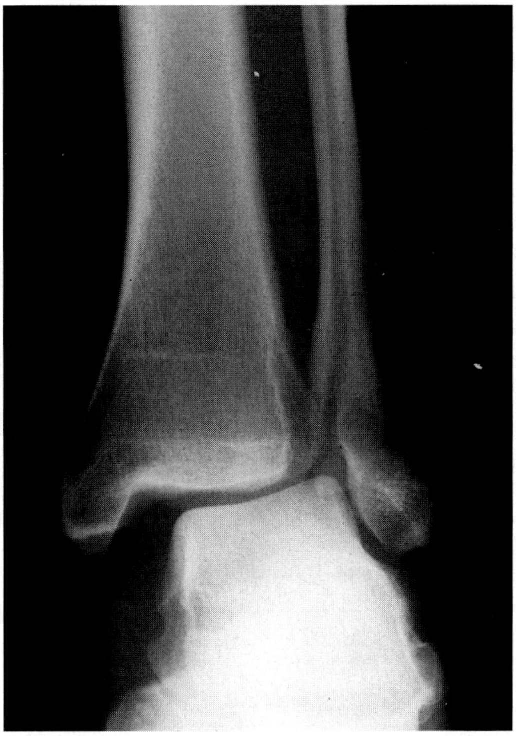

Figure 30–4. An anteroposterior radiograph of a transsyndesmotic ankle fracture with talar shift.

talus externally rotates in the ankle mortise it appears to move away from the medial malleolus on the anteroposterior radiographs. It is interesting to note that a transsyndesmotic fibular fracture with a minor degree of talar shift can be associated with attenuation of the deltoid ligament and it is therefore possible to see talar shift in the presence of an intact deltoid ligament and anterior capsule.

The soft tissue damage associated with talar shift in suprasyndesmotic fractures may be very extensive and surgical examination of the medial side of the ankle joint will show a completely transected deltoid ligament with a tear in the anterior capsule of the ankle joint that extends as far laterally as the anterior syndesmosis and may include the complete syndesmosis and the interosseous membrane. The posterior soft tissue defect is often more difficult to define, but usually the capsular tear passes behind the tibialis posterior into the back of the ankle joint. For the soft tis-

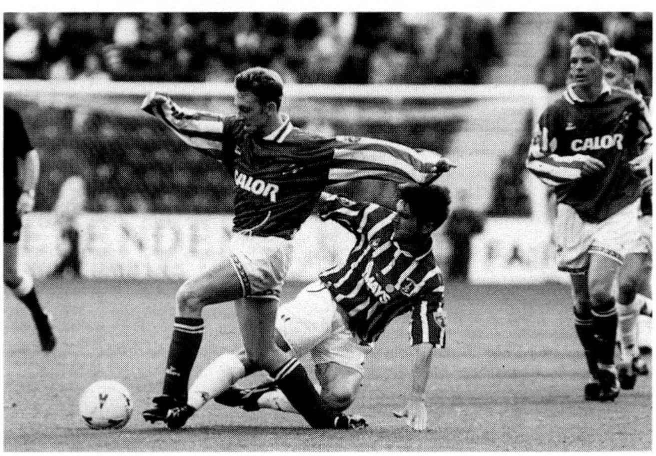

Figure 30–5. The injury that caused the fracture seen in Figure 30–3. Note that the foot is fully externally rotated.

sues to be so extensively damaged the ankle must have been virtually dislocated at the time of maximum deformity. In abduction injuries such as the case illustrated in Figure 30–1 the patient often presents with a dislocated ankle. However, in external rotation injuries the natural recoil of the tissues may have reduced the dislocation; the severity of the soft tissue injury may not be obvious from radiographs. This is well illustrated in Figure 30–5, which shows the position of the foot of a professional soccer player at the time of maximal deformity. This patient's radiographs are shown in Figure 30–3 and it is obvious that they do not indicate the true extent of the damage.

With this degree of soft tissue damage it is impossible to guarantee full correction of the ankle subluxation merely by plating the fibula or inserting a diastasis screw and the surgeon should always examine the congruity of the ankle mortise using fluoroscopy after fibular fixation. If, as shown in Figure 30–2, the ankle joint opens up with an external rotation force, the surgeon must choose between applying a cast with the foot in inversion and repairing the medial and anterior soft tissues. It may be impossible to repair a posterior capsular defect, but a good repair of the anterior capsule and deltoid ligament will greatly enhance the stability of the ankle joint. Postoperatively the fixation should be protected by the use of a cast for 6 weeks and the surgeon should take regular radiographs to examine the congruity of the ankle joint. There is no good data on which to base a choice between operative and nonoperative management of the medial and anterior soft tissues, but it seems reasonable to treat the soft tissue component of ankle fractures in the elderly nonoperatively and suture the soft tissues in younger patients, particularly if they play sports at a high level.

Alternative Methods of Management

The treatment of the abduction and external rotation types of suprasyndesmotic fracture is similar. In the case illustrated here the surgeon chose to use a diastasis screw to maintain the relationship between the distal fibula and tibia until the fracture had united and the soft tissues healed. A diastasis screw is particularly useful for high suprasyndesmotic, external rotation fibular fractures where the fibula is in alignment. In suprasyndesmotic abduction fractures the fibular fracture is more distal and the use of a fibular plate and supplementary diastasis screw is recommended. It has been suggested that in low suprasyndesmotic fractures a fibular plate without a supplementary diastasis screw provides adequate stability because the plate takes over the function of the damaged interosseous ligament. This is true in a number of fractures, but if the surgeon is unsure about the need for a diastasis screw, he or she should apply an abduction force to the internally fixed distal fibular under fluoroscopy to see if the syndesmosis opens. If it does, a diastasis screw should be inserted.

Transsyndesmotic ankle fractures do not require a diastasis screw and most only need de-rotation and plating of the distal fibular fracture. Very occasionally, even transsyndesmotic fractures are associated with significant damage to the deltoid ligament and anterior capsule and in these cases the surgeon will have to consider the need for operative repair of the soft tissues.

The two other methods of management that might be selected by surgeons for the treatment of these fractures are nonoperative management or the use of less rigid forms of internal fixation. Nonoperative management of ankle fractures with talar shift can be undertaken, but is very labor intensive and necessitates a number

PEARL

- There is debate about the number and location of the diastasis screws. Some surgeons recommend two diastasis screws, but clinically it does not seem to matter if one or two is used. The purpose of the diastasis screw is to maintain tibiofibular alignment while the soft tissues unite.

of anaesthetics and plaster changes to maintain the position of the talus in the ankle mortise. With care, however, reasonable results can be achieved.

The other technique of internal fixation using less rigid implants is helpful in older patients with osteoporotic bone. Surgeons may use a Rush pin or other similar device to immobilize the fibular fracture. A recent alternative is the locked intramedullary fibular nail, but as yet there is little evidence of how useful this device is. An intramedullary device can be passed into the fibular through a distal stab incision. However, surgeons should be aware that unlocked intramedullary devices will not confer any rotatory stability to the fibular fracture and thus a cast is necessary. The other disadvantage of using a fibular intramedullary nail is the resulting difficulty of inserting a diastasis screw if that is required.

Type of Management	Advantages	Disadvantages	Comments
Cast	Straightforward method; no anesthetic	Labor intensive; multiple anaesthetics; expensive; malunion	Less popular now; difficult technique to get right
Plate fixation	Straightforward surgery; good results	May require soft tissue surgery; not applicable for type C abduction fractures	The surgeon needs to use fluoroscopy to examine the stability of a fracture
Plate and diastasis screw	Good results in type C abduction fractures	Care must be taken with diastasis screw placement	This is the method of choice for abduction type C fractures
Intramedullary fibular nail	Useful in osteoporotic bone	No rotational stability	Can be useful in older patients

Complications

The most difficult complication of the management of ankle fractures with talar shift is a recurrence of the problem after removal of the diastasis screw. Conventionally, diastasis screws are removed after about 6 weeks, but it is self-evident that the soft tissues will not be healed by that time. Thus in ankle fractures with severe soft tissue damage the talar shift may recur. If it is not detected, ankle function can be seriously compromised. If late talar shift occurs, it will almost always have arisen because of an external rotation deformity. Treatment is thus directed at internally rotating the ankle. This cannot be achieved merely by performing a transsyndesmotic internal rotational osteotomy of the distal fibula; the anterior capsule and deltoid ligament also have to be tightened. The results are not always satisfactory. Failure to gain a good reduction of the ankle joint may well result in posttraumatic osteoarthritis. It has been demonstrated that even minor incongruity of the ankle is associated with abnormal loading and an increased risk of osteoarthritis. Unfortunately, symptomatic osteoarthritis may have to be treated by an ankle arthrodesis.

Other more common complications of this type of ankle fracture are persistent ankle pain and instability. The pain is often difficult to define and may arise from the inferior tibiofibular joint, anterior capsule, medial ligament, or from the fibular plate and screws. Usually the treatment is symptomatic, although physiotherapy can help the ankle instability and plate removal after bone union may help local discomfort.

Suggested Readings

Harper MC: The deltoid ligament: an evaluation of need for surgical repair. Clin Orthop 1988; 226:156–168.

Kelikian H, Kelikian AS: Disorders of the Ankle. WB Saunders, Philadelphia, 1985.

Lauge-Hansen N: Fractures of the ankle. Analytic history survey as basis of a new experimental roentgenologic and clinical investigations. Arch Surg 1948; 56:259–317.

Lauge-Hansen N: Fractures of the ankle II. Combined experimental-surgical and experimental-roentgenological investigations. Arch Surg 1950; 60:957–985.

Pankovitch AM: Maisonneuve fracture of the fibula. J Bone Joint Surg (Am) 1976; 58A:337–342.

Trafton PG, Bray TJ, Simpson LA: Fractures and soft tissue injuries of the ankle. In Browner BD, Jupiter JB, Levine AM, Trafton PG (eds): Skeletal Trauma. WB Saunders, Philadelphia, 1992.

Case 31

History and Physical Examination

A 32-year-old man fell feet first into a 50 gallon drum of hydrochloric acid. He was immediately pulled from the drum and his pants, shoes, and socks removed and his legs and feet washed with water. He arrived in the emergency department 20 minutes later. He complained of pain secondary to the acid burns, and obvious deformity of the distal right extremity at the ankle was present. First and second degree burns were present over both lower extremities up to the knees. The neurovascular examination of the lower extremities was within the limits of normal.

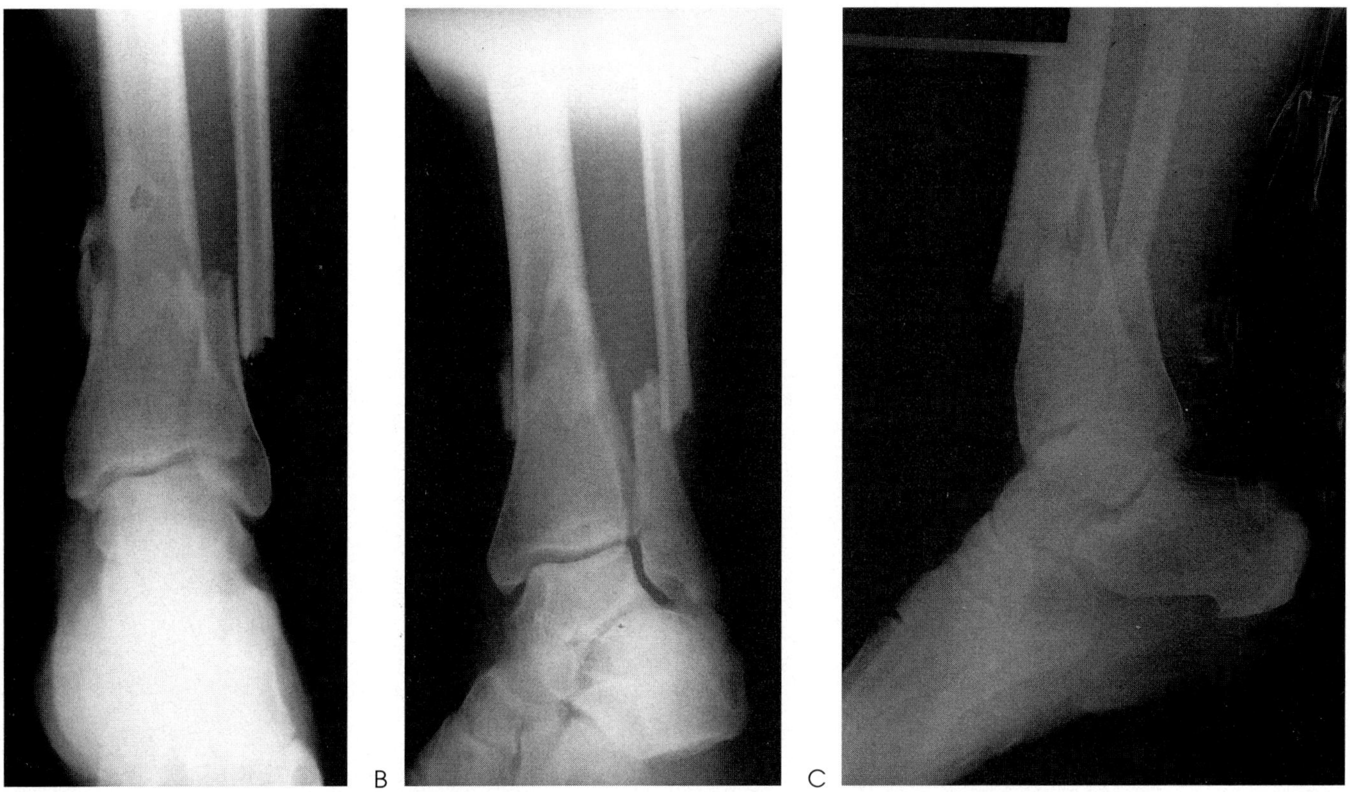

A B C

Figure 31–1. (A–C) Anteroposterior, oblique, and lateral radiographs of the distal tibia obtained at admission. The fracture is extraarticular.

Radiologic Findings

Radiographs of the right lower extremity revealed an extraarticular fracture of the distal tibia and fibula (Fig. 31–1).

Diagnosis

Closed extraarticular fracture of the distal tibia and fibula with overlying first and second degree acid burns. AO classification: 42–A2.3.

Surgical Management

Both lower extremities were gently irrigated with physiologic saline. The burns were covered with silvadene and a soft dressing. The fracture was reduced with manual traction while the patient was sedated, and a short leg splint was applied.

The patient was taken to the operating room 4 hours after injury. A general anesthetic was administered and the splint and dressings were removed from his right lower extremity. The skin was prepped by spraying it with povidone iodine solution. A small wire circular frame was applied to the leg. The ankle joint was precisely located using fluoroscopy and two small wires were inserted just proximal to the subchondral bone. Two small wires were inserted proximally, just distal to the tibial plateau. The fracture was reduced and a two ring frame was applied and tightened, holding the reduction. A drop pin was added to the proximal ring to increase the stability of the fixation (Fig. 31–2).

Postoperative Management

Postoperative burn care consisted of daily dressing changes with silvadene ointment. The burns epithelialized without skin grafting. Pin care was performed daily by irrigating the pin sites with physiologic saline and removing serum and blood with a cotton applicator. The fracture healed with hypertrophic callus and the frame was removed at 8 weeks. Cast immobilization was not necessary following frame removal (Fig. 31–3).

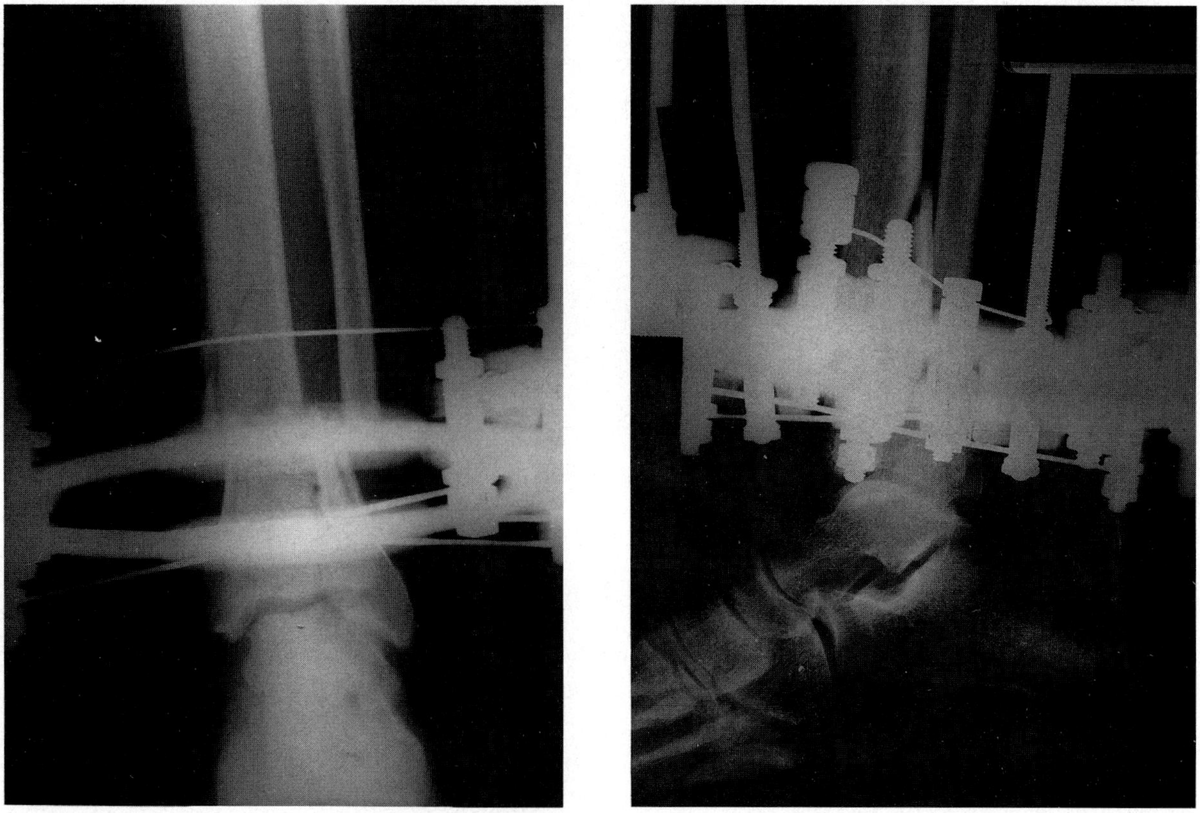

A B

Figure 31–2. Anteroposterior (A) and lateral (B) radiographs obtained after stabilization with a small wire circular frame. It is difficult to assess the fracture through the frame.

PEARL

- The most conclusive sign of fracture consolidation is the ability to bear weight without pain at the fracture site. Small wire circular frames allow some stresses across the fracture site. Therefore if the fracture is not healed, weight bearing is painful. Patients will frequently have pain at the pin sites. Pin site pain must be distinguished from pain at the fracture site.

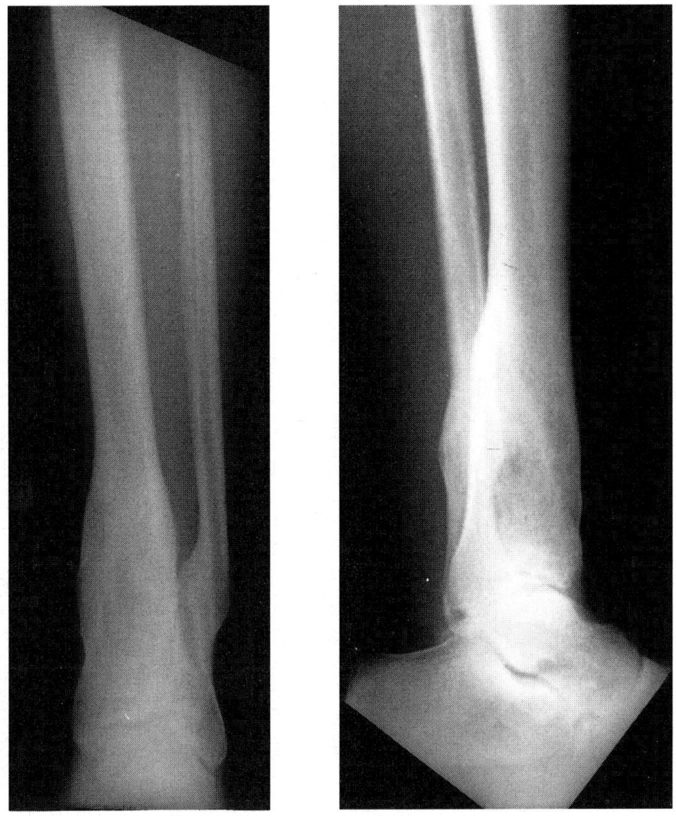

Figure 31–3. Two years postinjury the fracture is solidly healed. Anteroposterior (A) and lateral (B) views.

Discussion

A burned surface is rapidly colonized with bacteria and is impossible to sterilize. To minimize the risk of pin tract infection, the fracture was reduced and stabilized with an external fixator emergently. Following stabilization of the fracture routine burn care was performed on the skin and the pin sites were cleaned daily to minimize the risk of pin tract infection. The fracture healed with hypertrophic callus. This is unusual following a metaphyseal fracture, and may have resulted from the burn or the micromotion allowed by the small wire fixator. In most cases, it is difficult to determine the optimum time for frame removal. This is because the frame frequently obscures the fracture site radiographically and it is difficult to follow the progression of healing. In this case, because of the hypertrophic callus, the timing of frame removal was not difficult. The fracture was clearly healed at 8 weeks and the frame removed.

Alternative Methods of Management

Alternatives to external fixation in the management of this fracture were immediate or delayed open reduction and internal fixation with a plate; closed reduction and intramedullary nailing; closed reduction and stabilization with a large pin cantilever external fixator; and closed reduction and immobilization in a cast. The risk of infection following immediate open reduction and internal fixation outweighs the benefits of early motion without external support. The burned surface of the skin is rapidly colonized with bacteria. Delayed epithelialization of the wound gives these bacteria access to the fracture site and postoperative hematoma. Delaying fixation until the skin has healed minimizes the risk of infection. However, weeks or even months may be required for the skin to heal, and during this time measures must be taken to hold the fracture out to length otherwise reduction without shortening of the tibia and fibula may not be possible. Two methods of holding the fracture out to length following a closed reduction are external fixation and casting. Once these methods of management have been undertaken the surgeon should wait and see if they result in healing before subjecting the patient to a second operative procedure. Closed reduction and intramedullary nailing, in this case, were not indicated because the nail would have been inserted through damaged skin and the fracture was too distal. If the nail could have been inserted through uninjured skin and if the fracture had been more proximal, nailing would have been an ideal method of management. Closed reduction and stabilization with a large pin cantilever frame have the advantage of having the frame smaller than a small wire circular frame with consequent improved patient acceptance. In this case the fracture was so distal that fixation of the distal fragment would not have been possible without the pins being in the zone of injury and thus increasing the chance of inoculation of the fracture site with bacteria. Closed reduction and immobilization in a cast minimize the risk of infection of the fracture site, but the disadvantage is that the skin is not accessible for burn care.

Type of Management	Advantages	Disadvantages	Comments
Immediate ORIF	Anatomic reduction; fracture stability; access to skin for burn care	Risk of infection of fracture	The risk of infection outweighs the benefits
Delayed ORIF	Minimizes risk of infection; anatomic reduction possible; stable fixation	Fracture must be held out to length with cast or external fixator while skin heals	Requires additional operative procedure to hold fracture out to length
Closed intramedullary nailing	In this case no advantages	Nail is inserted through burn; fracture not stabilized adequately	May be ideal procedure if site of insertion is not injured, and if fracture is more amenable to nailing
Large pin cantilever frame	Frame is well tolerated by patient	Due to small size of distal fragment, may not be able to place pins out of zone of injury	Excellent method if fracture were more proximal
Casting	Closed procedure minimizes risk of infection	Restricts access to skin for burn care	Not a good method of management because skin cannot be cared for
Small wire circular frame	Allows pin placement out of zone of injury; fracture stability	Bulky frame poorly tolerated by patients	Despite limited patient acceptance may be best method of management.

Complications

Complications of fractures with overlying burns managed with a small wire external fixator are nonunion and pin tract infection. In cases in which nonunion becomes evident prior to frame removal, nonoperative measures such as pulsed electromagnetic fields are indicated. In cases in which the frame has been removed and a nonunion is present, delayed internal fixation is performed. The nonunion is immobilized in a removable splint. The splint is removed several times a day for skin care; when the pin tracts have healed, the surgeon performs internal fixation and autogenous bone grafting.

The radiographic sign of pin tract infection is osteolysis around the pin. The clinical signs are redness, pain, and increased drainage. This is a potentially very serious complication that can lead to septic arthritis if the pins communicate with the joint, infection of the fracture if the pins are in the zone of injury, or chronic osteomyelitis and ring sequestrum of the cortical bone surrounding the pin. The risk of pin tract infection is minimized by meticulous pin tract care. Once pin tract infection has occurred, a short course of conservative therapy, including broad spectrum antibiotics and daily whirlpool debridement, is attempted. If this does not result in suppression of infection, the pin or pins are removed, and new pins inserted.

Suggested Readings

Maiocchi AB, Aronson J (eds): A.S.A.M.I Group Operative Principles of Ilizarov. Williams and Wilkins, Baltimore, 1991.

Case 32

History and Physical Examination

A 31-year-old female was admitted to the emergency department following a traffic accident. She had been a front seat passenger in a car involved in a collision and her foot had been forced into dorsiflexion by the impact of the crash. She had a painful left hindfoot and was unable to weight bear. The only other injury was an undisplaced fracture of the terminal phalanx of her left ring finger.

Radiologic Findings

Anteroposterior and lateral radiographs show a comminuted fracture of the talar neck (Fig. 32–1). There is evidence of comminution between the body and head of the talus and the body has rotated within the ankle mortise. The talonavicular joint is congruous. The anteroposterior view suggests the presence of a triangular fragment in the neck of the talus, with the base of the triangle lying medially.

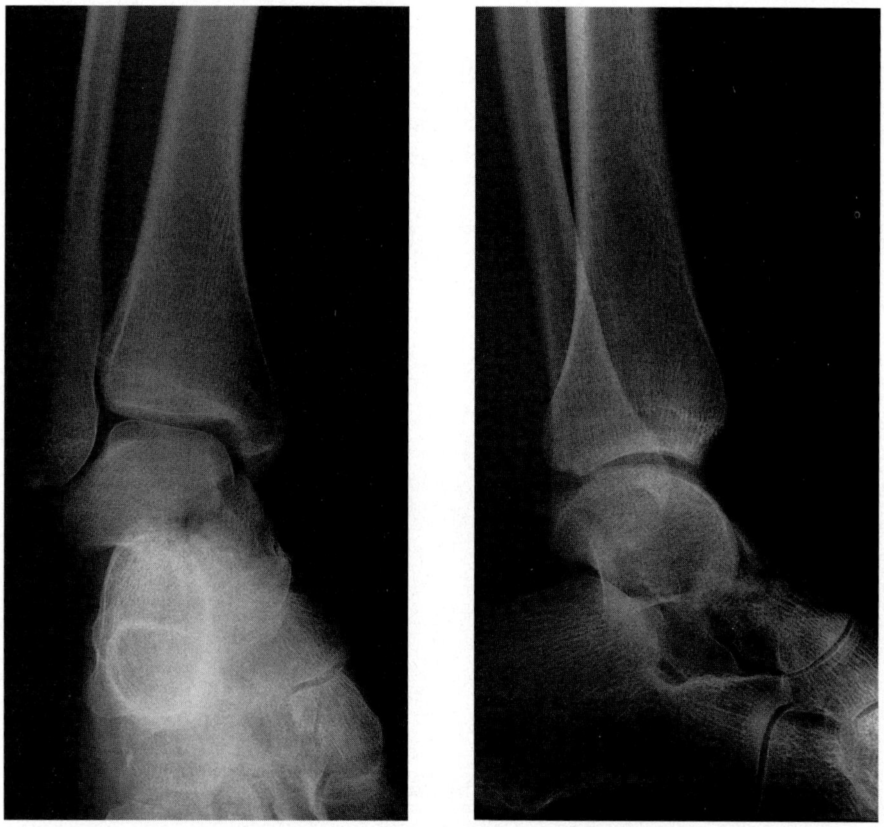

A B

Figure 32–1. Anteroposterior (A) and lateral (B) radiographs of a Hawkins type II fracture of the talar neck. There is comminution and subtalar involvement.

Diagnosis

Comminuted fracture of the talar neck with involvement of the subtalar joint. A Hawkins type II fracture. OTA classification: 72–A1.2.

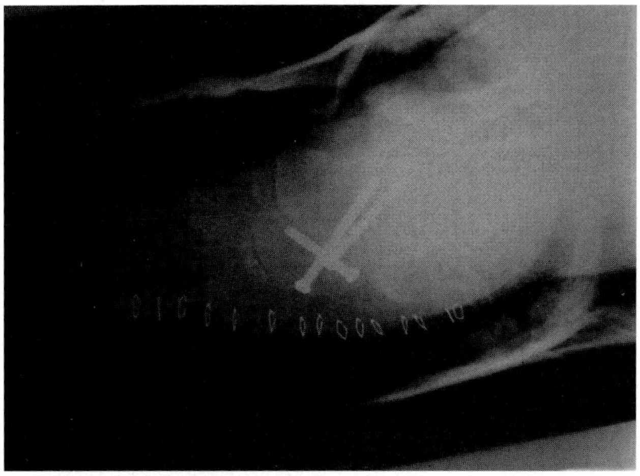

A

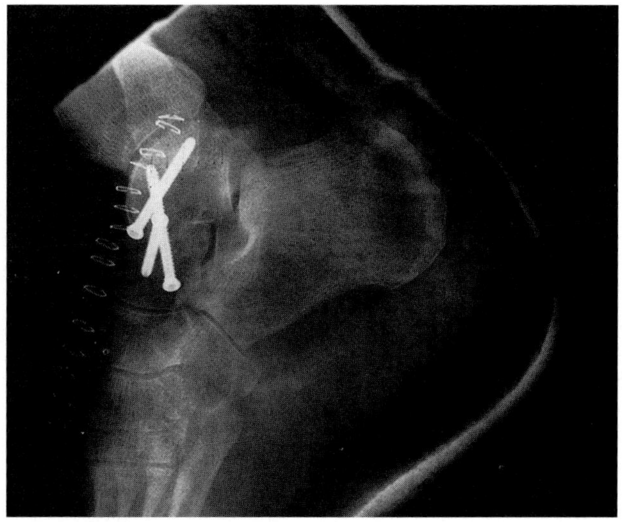

B

Figure 32–2. Postoperative anteroposterior (A) and lateral (B) radiographs showing that a good reduction has been achieved.

PEARLS

- The Hawkins classification of talar neck fractures has the merit of being relatively easy to apply. There are three categories depending on the involvement of the subtalar and ankle joints. Type I fractures are undisplaced and involve neither joint. Type II fractures are displaced and involve the subtalar joint; type III fractures are associated with dislocation of the body of the talus and consequent disruption of both joints.
- The two common approaches to the talus are anteromedial and anterolateral. Both can be extended by osteotomizing the adjacent malleolus. The anteromedial approach protects the blood supply but does not allow visualization of the subtalar joint. In comminuted fractures it may be necessary to use both approaches.

Surgical Management

The patient was taken to the operating room where the leg was prepped and draped. An anteromedial incision was made from the level of the medial malleolus to the midfoot area. The fracture was approached through the space between the tendons of tibialis anterior and tibialis posterior. Inspection of the fracture showed that there was a triangular fragment in the talar neck. Three small fragment bone screws were used to internally fix the talus and rigid fixation was achieved (Fig. 32–2).

Postoperative Management

The patient was left in a plaster back shell for 2 weeks to allow the soft tissue swelling to settle. A physiotherapy program was then instituted, but because of discomfort the patient used the back shell as a resting splint for a further 6 weeks. Weight bearing was allowed at 10 weeks and radiographs taken 1 year after the fracture showed good union with excellent reconstruction of the subtalar joint and no evidence of avascular necrosis (Fig. 32–3). At that time the patient had normal ankle function and 5 degrees of inversion and eversion. Walking over rough ground was still uncomfortable, but the patient could perform all her other activities without discomfort.

Discussion

The talus is an unusual bone in that about 60% of its surface is articular. There are no tendons or muscles attached to the talus and the blood supply is consequently poor. The vascular supply to the talus comes from the three main vessels of the leg through a periosteal vascular network that covers all of the cartilage free surfaces of the bone. In addition, there are two discrete vessels that enter the bone through the tarsal sinus and the tarsal canal. This tenuous blood supply means that avascular necrosis is the most frequent complication of fractures of the talus. The overall incidence of avascular necrosis is reported to be about 50%, but it obviously will vary

PITFALL

- It is surprisingly difficult to diagnose an undisplaced fracture. Many fractures that are said to be undisplaced are in fact minimally displaced. The difference is important because truly undisplaced fractures usually have little associated soft tissue damage. Any displacement suggests more damage and a worse prognosis.

A 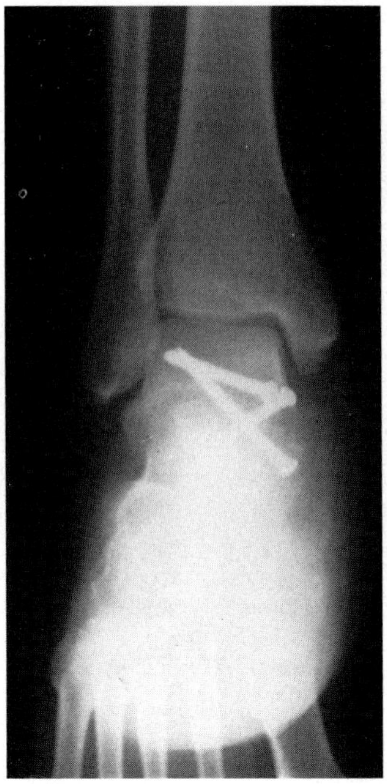

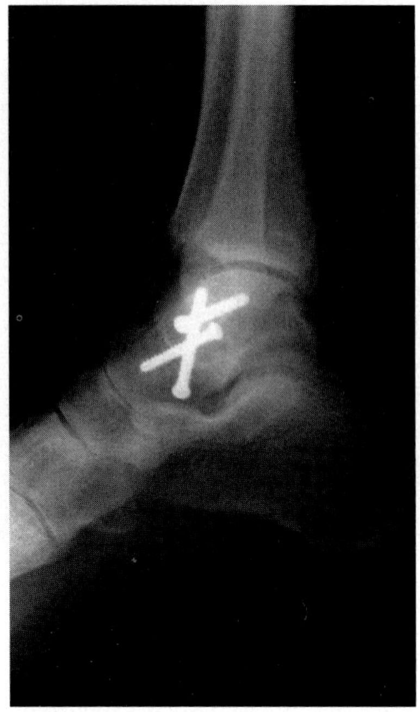 B

Figure 32–3. At one year there is good union and no evidence of avascular necrosis. (A) Anteroposterior and (B) lateral views.

with the severity of the fracture and any associated disruption of the blood supply. An undisplaced (Hawkins type I) talar neck fracture will not significantly interfere with talar vascularity and the incidence of avascular necrosis of these fractures varies between 0 and 15%. In Hawkins type II fractures, where there is subtalar involvement, the incidence of avascular necrosis lies between 16 and 60%, and in Hawkins type III fractures, where the talar fragments are completely displaced such that both ankle and subtalar joints are involved, the incidence of avascular necrosis lies between 33 and 100%.

The optimal treatment for all talar neck fractures is internal fixation. There is evidence that immediate compression fixation of talar neck fractures will reduce the incidence of avascular necrosis even in fractures that are described as undisplaced. Where there is any displacement at all the fracture should be treated as displaced intraarticular fracture and rigid internal fixation using intrafragmentary screws should be used.

In undisplaced or minimally displaced fractures it is reasonable to attempt closed reduction and percutaneous screw fixation. Minimal displacement may be corrected by plantar flexing and inverting the foot and then compressing the fracture while returning the foot to the neutral position. Two Kirschner wires inserted posteriorly under fluoroscopic control should be used for internal fixation (Fig. 32–4). Once the reduced position has been confirmed by fluoroscopy these can be substituted by cancellous screws. If canulated cancellous screws are available, they should be used.

Displaced fractures require open reduction and internal fixation. The most common approach is the anteromedial one used in this case. If lateral visualization is required to reduce and fix loose bone fragment or gain access to the lateral side of the talar dome, a supplementary lateral approach will be required.

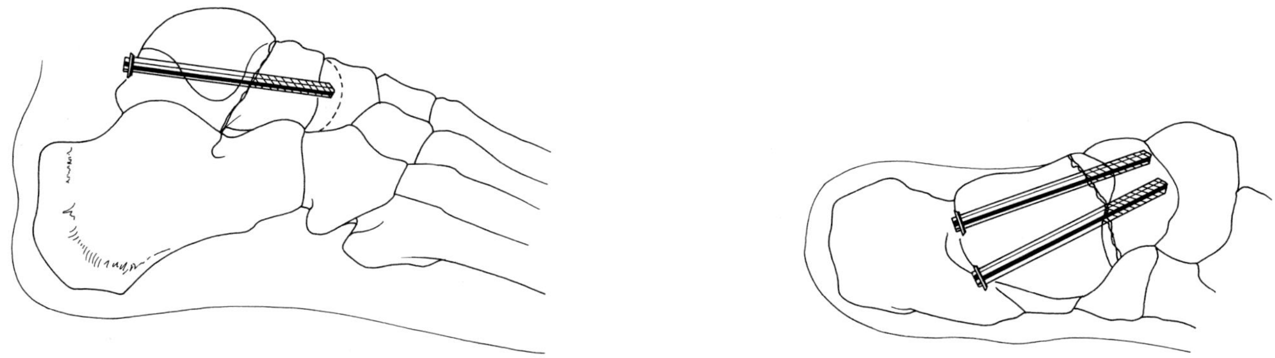

Figure 32–4. Lateral (A) and axial (B) views of the correct positions of the two screws used to fix a talar neck fracture. Where possible, these should be placed from posterior to anterior to prevent articular damage.

Open reduction of a simple neck fracture is usually straightforward. Once reduction has been achieved, K wires can be used to maintain the reduction and again two cancellous screws can be inserted. The problem with placing screws from anterior to posterior is that it is difficult to avoid placing the screws into an articular surface. The screws can be countersunk, but ideally articular damage should be avoided and the surgeon should consider placing the screws from posterior to anterior under fluoroscopic control in the manner already described and illustrated in Figure 32–4. In this case the comminution meant that three screws were required to gain stability. Where this occurs, it is likely that the surgeon will need to insert one or more screws through an articular surface and care must be taken to countersink these below the level of the articular surface.

In cases in which the talar body fragment has been extruded from the ankle mortise it must be reduced and fixed. The risk of avascular necrosis and secondary osteoarthritis in the ankle and subtalar joints is fairly high, and the incidence and treatment of avascular necrosis of the talus are discussed in the next section dealing with talar body fractures.

Alternative Methods of Management

The role of nonoperative management has been discussed. If used, it should be restricted to the treatment of undisplaced talar neck fractures. However, nonoperative

Type of Management	Advantages	Disadvantages	Comments
Cast management	Occasionally useful in undisplaced fractures	Joint stiffness; pain; nonunion; avascular necrosis	Rarely indicated as internal fixation is a more appropriate technique
Internal fixation	Early joint movement; lower incidence of avascular necrosis	Technically difficult	This is the method of choice for talar neck fractures

management requires the prolonged use of a cast. The other method of internal fixation that can be employed is the use of Kirschner wires to immobilize the bone fragments instead of bone screws. These will usually maintain the fracture position, but the patient needs to use a cast for a prolonged period and a higher incidence of avascular necrosis is likely. There is no place for external skeletal fixation.

Complications

Common complications of talar neck fracture are avascular necrosis and secondary osteoarthritis. The incidence of avascular necrosis has already been noted. Secondary osteoarthritis is said to occur in about 35% of talar neck fractures; the incidence depends on the severity of the fracture. The treatment of these conditions is discussed in the next case. Other complications include Sudeck's atrophy, which is said to be three times more common after nonoperative treatment, as well as mild pain and stiffness, which is usually treated by nonsteroidal antiinflammatory drugs and physiotherapy.

Suggested Readings

Canale ST, Kelly FB: Fractures of the neck of the talus. J Bone Joint Surg (Am) 1978; 60A:143–156.

Grob D, Simpson LA, Weber BG, Bray T: Operative treatment of displaced talus fractures. Clin Orthop 1985; 199:88–96.

Haliburton RA, Sullivan CR, Kelly PJ, Peterson LFA: The extra-osseous and intra-osseous blood supply of the talus. J Bone Joint Surg (Am) 1958; 40A:1115–1120.

Hansen ST: Foot injuries. In Browner BD, Jupiter JB, Levine AM, Trafton PG (eds): Skeletal Trauma. Philadelphia, WB Saunders, 1992.

Sangeorzan BJ, Mayo KA, Hansen ST: Intraarticular fractures of the foot. Clin Orthop 1993; 292:135–141.

Szyszkowitz R, Reschauer R, Seggl W: Eighty-five talus fractures treated by ORIF with five to eight years of follow up study of 69 patients. Clin Orthop 1985; 1993:97–107.

Case 33

History and Physical Examination

A 28-year-old man who had been involved in a motor vehicle accident was admitted to the emergency department. He had been the driver of an articulated truck that collided with an automobile; he had not been wearing any form of restraint at the time of the accident.

On arrival at the emergency department it was noted that he had a Glasgow coma scale of 15 and there was no evidence of cervical, thoracolumbar, intraabdominal, or pelvic injuries. He had a tachycardia of 100/minute with a blood pressure of 150/90 mm Hg. Examination showed an open fracture of the right humeral diaphysis, a closed fracture of the right forearm, and a severe open fracture of the right hindfoot. Examination of the hindfoot showed that the foot had been displaced so that it lay medial to the lower end of the tibia. There appeared to be good capillary return in his toes with only a slight generalized reduction of sensation noted on the dorsum and sole of his foot. There was a 15 cm contaminated wound over the lateral aspect of the ankle joint.

A

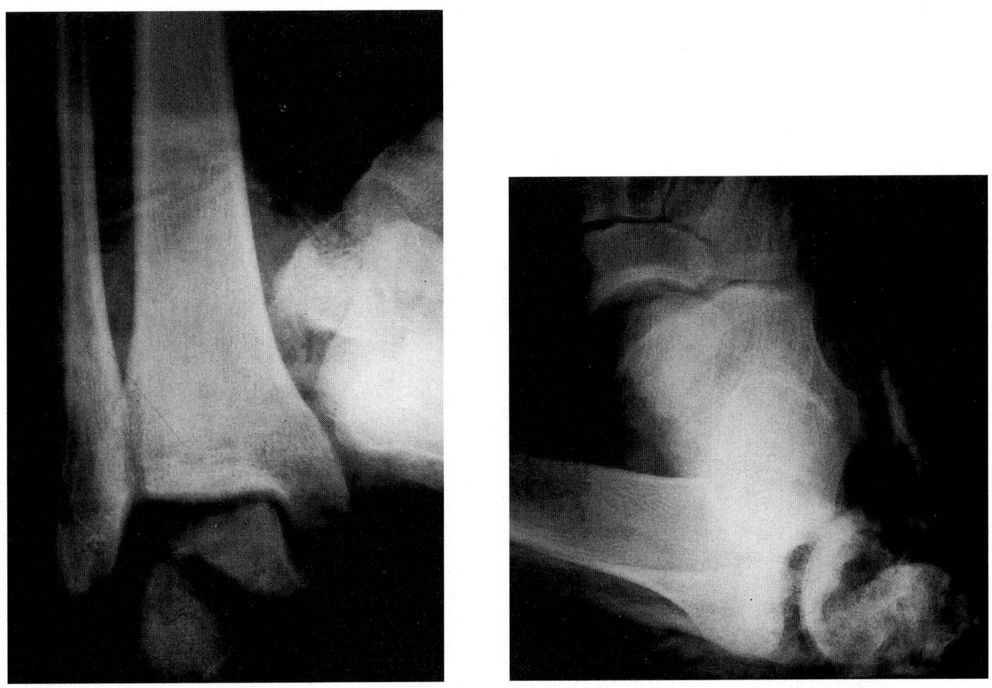

B

Figure 33–1. Anteroposterior (A) and lateral (B) radiographs showing the damage to the talus.

Radiologic Findings

An anteroposterior radiograph (Fig. 33–1A) showed that the body of the talus had been fractured into two major fragments. The lateral radiograph (Fig. 33–1B) suggested greater comminution of the body fragment but also showed a talar neck fracture. It also indicated that the foot had been dislocated medially, with evidence of damage to the talonavicular joint.

Diagnosis

A comminuted fracture of the talar body and neck with dislocation of the foot. OTA classification: 72–C2.2.

Surgical Management

The patient was taken to the operating room where the fracture was reduced and the dorsalis pedis pulse noted to be present. The right leg was then prepped and draped and the wound explored. The neurovascular supply to the foot was seen to be intact. The lateral wound was debrided and lavaged with normal saline. The fragments that constituted the head of the talus were reduced and fixed with two canulated intrafragmentary screws. An anteromedial approach was then made to expose the neck and the talus and the talonavicular joint. The talar neck fracture was stabilized with two further intrafragmentary cancellous screws. There was minor damage to the talonavicular joint. The medial wound was closed and the lateral wound left open. The forearm fracture and the open humeral diaphyseal fracture were plated. Postoperative radiographs of the hindfoot were satisfactory (Fig. 33–2).

The patient was returned to the operating room 36 hours later and the lateral wound was examined by both orthopedic and plastic surgeons. The soft tissue defect on the lateral side of the ankle measured 7 by 5 cm, but it was noted that the lateral malleolus was covered with periosteum and a layer of viable soft tissue. A split skin graft was therefore used to cover the defect.

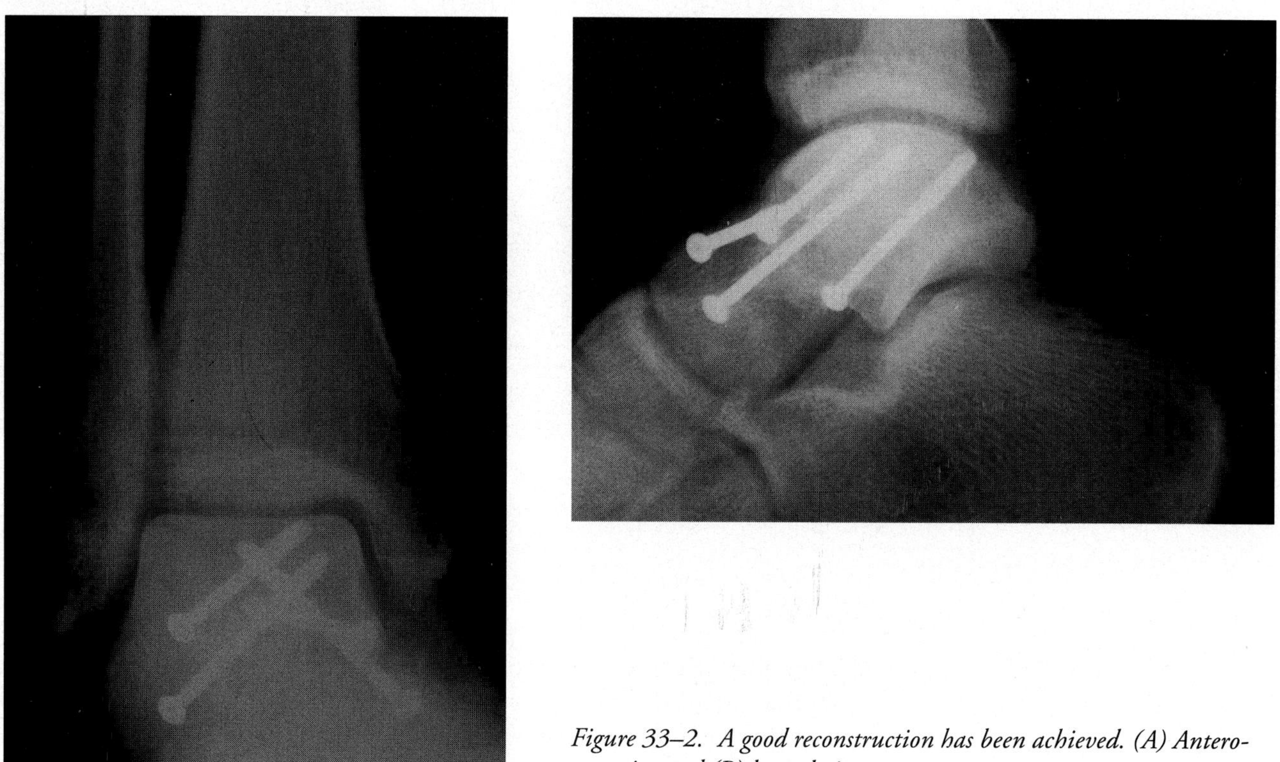

A

B

Figure 33–2. A good reconstruction has been achieved. (A) Anteroposterior and (B) lateral views.

PEARL

- Over 50% of open fractures of the hindfoot require plastic surgery to close the soft tissue defect. The combination of severe soft tissue injury and comminuted displaced fractures inevitably leads to a poor prognosis.

PITFALL

- Great care must be taken when the surgeon is exposing the fracture fragments. The talus is already devascularized and inappropriate surgery will further damage the blood supply.

Postoperative Management

Postoperatively the patient mobilized nonweight bearing on the right leg. An AFO was applied to rest the soft tissues and maintain the foot in a plantargrade position. All the wounds healed well, but radiographs taken two months later (Fig. 33–3) showed early signs of avascular necrosis of the head of the talus. Four months after the injury it became obvious that the foot was assuming an equinovarus position. At that time it was possible for the patient to actively dorsiflex his foot into the neutral position and he retained 30 degrees of plantar flexion. However, over the next 2 months the foot became progressively stiffer and it was clear that he was developing a fixed equinovarus deformity. The AFO failed to control the position of the hindfoot and radiographs showed evidence of posttraumatic osteoarthritis of both the ankle and subtalar joints (Fig. 33–4).

The patient was followed up for an additional 6 months but his hindfoot pain increased and successive radiographs continued to show avascular necrosis of the talus. The equinovarus deformity was fixed and he complained of pain that appeared to be related to the ankle and the subtalar and talonavicular joints. Accordingly, a pantalar arthrodesis was performed using corticocancellous autograft. Even though the arthrodesis was successful radiologically, the patient continued to complain of significant hindfoot pain to the extent that he never returned to his employment or his preoperative social activities.

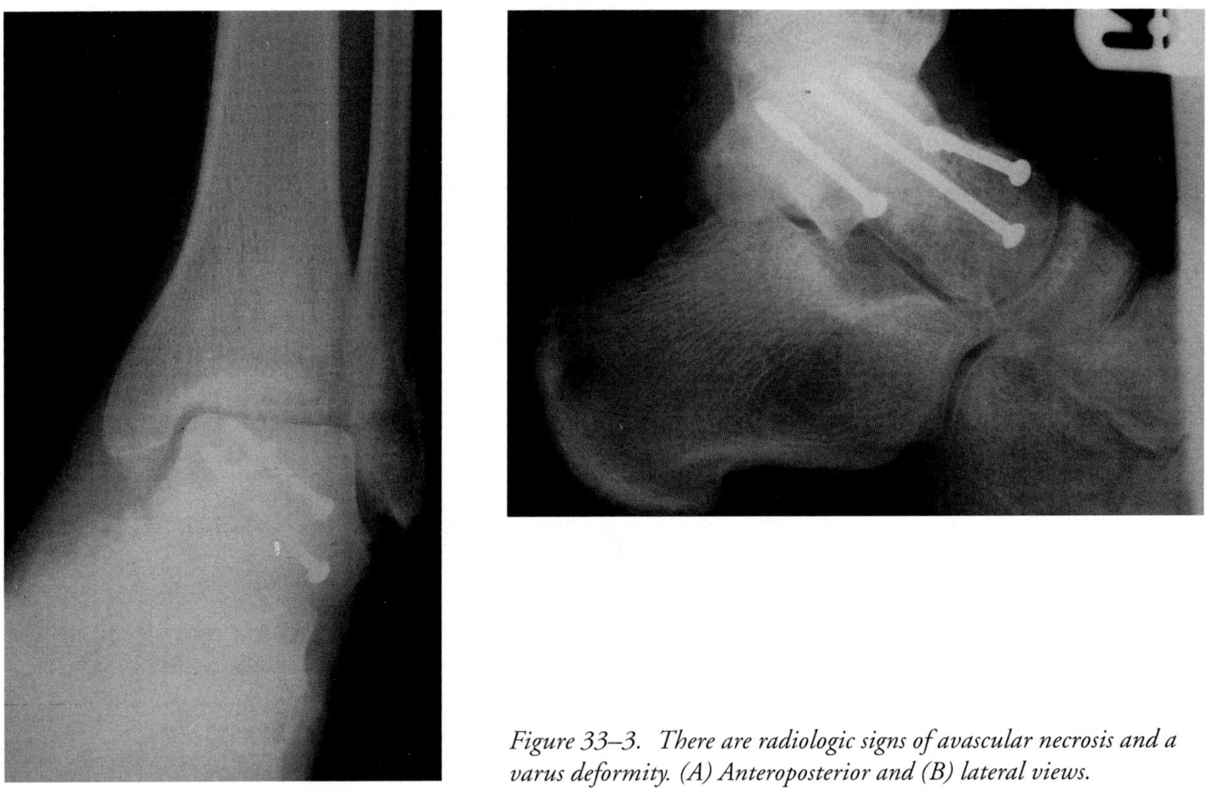

A

B

Figure 33–3. There are radiologic signs of avascular necrosis and a varus deformity. (A) Anteroposterior and (B) lateral views.

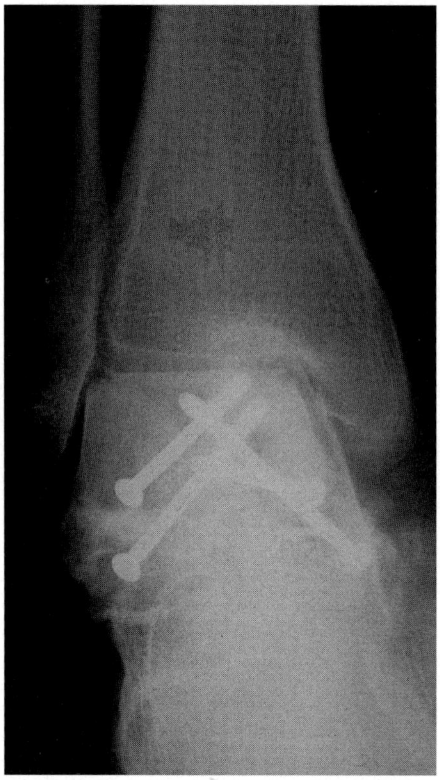

A

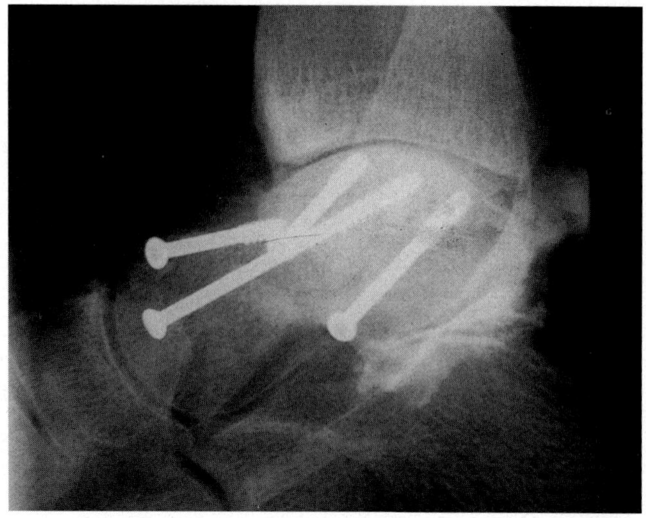

B

Figure 33–4. The equinovarus deformity has become fixed and there are signs of posttraumatic osteoarthritis. (A) Anteroposterior and (B) lateral views.

Discussion

Fractures of the body of the talus are highly uncommon. They always follow high energy injuries and are therefore associated with considerable soft tissue damage. There are very few series detailing the results of their management; consequently, no uniformity of opinion exists about how to treat the almost inevitable avascular necrosis or posttraumatic osteoarthritis. As with other rare fractures, much of the literature precedes the era of internal fixation and therefore is not particularly relevant.

Sneppen et al. (1977) reviewed 51 patients with talar body fractures. In cases in which significant talar compression occurred they found that 50% of patients had ankle osteoarthritis; if the talus exhibited a shearing pattern of injury, as in this case, the incidence of posttraumatic osteoarthritis in both the ankle and subtalar joints was 41%, with a further 24% of patients having osteoarthritis in either the ankle or subtalar joints. These two types of talar body fracture also showed the highest incidence of avascular necrosis. Their conclusion was that rigid fixation should be used for displaced talar body fractures and few surgeons would disagree.

The problem with the management of these difficult fractures is not the primary treatment but the management of the almost inevitable complications. Because the incidence of avascular necrosis and posttraumatic arthritis of the ankle and subtalar joints is high surgeons are faced with having to undertake fusion of the ankle as well as the subtalar and occasionally the talonavicular joints.

It is often difficult to identify the source of hindfoot pain. In addition to the damage to the talus and the adjacent joints there may well have been damage to other parts of the hindfoot and midfoot. Thus the pain may be multifocal in origin. Even if no other foot damage is present, the surgeon may find it difficult to distinguish between ankle and subtalar pain. Usually both joints will be stiff and it is un-

PEARL

- The combination of a severe hindfoot fracture with significant fractures of the midfoot or forefoot can be very difficult to treat. Amputation should be considered in these patients.

likely that active or passive movement of either joint will be pain free. Radiographs and more sophisticated imaging techniques are notoriously unreliable in determining the source of pain and the surgeon may have to use local anesthetic blocking techniques to aid diagnosis. These techniques may be successful, but unfortunately there is a high incidence of false positive results.

It is advisable to fuse the joint that is considered most symptomatic unless, as in this case, the surgeon is convinced that more than one joint is giving rise to symptoms. A successful ankle or subtalar fusion may reduce the level of discomfort to a tolerable level and remove the need for fusion of the other joints.

Alternative Methods of Management

An alternative to secondary arthrodesis is primary arthrodesis of either the ankle or subtalar joint. The rationale behind this treatment method is to encourage vascularization of the talus. There is, however, little evidence concerning the usefulness of either primary ankle or subtalar arthrodesis.

A further technique of ankle fusion was described by Blair (1943). He excised the talar body and then used a sliding graft from the distal anterior surface of the tibia. The graft was embedded in the neck of the talus. Reasonable results have been reported using this and similar techniques, but few surgeons today employ this method. The other classical method of treating complex talar fractures that has fallen into disfavour is talectomy. Removal of the talus leads to a flattened disorganized hindfoot and late pain.

Type of Management	Advantages	Disadvantages	Comments
Casting	None	Avascular necrosis; osteoarthritis; pain	High complication rate; no indication currently
Internal fixation	Better talar reconstruction	Avascular necrosis; osteoarthritis; pain	Better results; nonoperative management, but still high complication rates
Primary arthrodesis	Unknown	Technically difficult	Very few results available
Talectomy	None	Hindfoot deformity; pain	Probably no indication currently

Complications

The major complications of talar body fractures are avascular necrosis and posttraumatic osteoarthritis. These have already been described.

Suggested Readings

Blair HC: Comminuted fractures and fracture dislocations of the body of the astralagus. Operative treatment. Am J Surg 1943; 59:37–43.

Heckman JD: Fractures and dislocations of the foot. In Rockwood CA, Green DP, Bucholz RW, Heckman JD (eds): Rockwood and Green's Fractures in Adults. 4th ed. Lippincott-Raven, Philadelphia, 1996.

McKeever FM: Treatment and complications of fractures and dislocations of the talus. Clin Orthop 1963; 30:45–52.

Pennal GF: Fractures of the talus. Clin Orthop 1963; 30:53–63.

Ritsema GH: Total talar dislocation. J Trauma 1988; 28:692–694.

Scranton PE: An overview of ankle arthrodesis. Clin Orthop 1991; 268:96–101.

Sneppen O, Bach Christensen S, Krogsøe O, Lorentzen J: Fracture of the body of the talus. Acta Orthop Scand 1977; 48:317–324.

Case 34

History and Physical Examination

A 28-year-old male fell one story from a roof, landing on his feet. Although he was wearing work boots, it was clear that a significant deformity of the foot and ankle was present. He was immediately taken to an outside hospital where the boot was cut off, exposing a laceration on the lateral side of the foot through which a fragment of bone was extruded. Radiographs were obtained and the patient was splinted and transferred. He arrived in the emergency department approximately 6 hours after injury. There were no injuries other than that to the foot and ankle. Examination indicated an extruded fragment of the head of the talus on the lateral side of the foot with inversion of the forefoot. The toes had normal sensation and good capillary refill (Fig. 34–1).

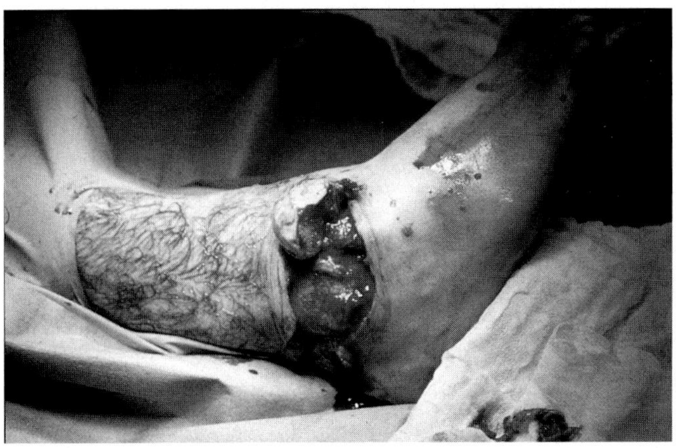

Figure 34–1. Clinical appearance of the foot at admission. The head of the talus is lying on the skin.

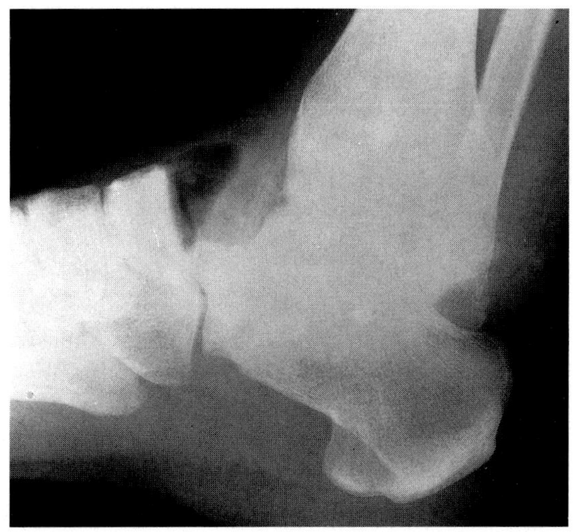

Figure 34–2. Lateral radiograph of the foot. There is a dislocation of the talocalcaneal articulation and subluxation of the tibiotalar joint.

Radiologic Findings

Radiographs were difficult to interpret but indicated a dislocation of the talocalcaneal and talonavicular articulations with subluxation of the tibiotalar articulation (Fig. 34–2). There was also a displaced fracture of the neck of the talus. No other injuries were evident radiographically. The bones of the forefoot and ankle mortise appeared within the limits of normal.

Diagnosis

Open pantalar dislocation of the talus with a fracture of the neck of the talus.

PEARL

- The key point in the diagnosis is that the injury is 6 hours old. The prognosis rapidly worsens with further delay in debridement and reduction due to increased swelling, increasingly compromised vascular supply, and increasing risk of infection. Expeditious surgical debridement and reduction are necessary.

Surgical Management

The leg was scrubbed and draped. The open wound was extended proximally and distally. The head of the talus was grossly contaminated with particles of debris impacted into its surface. It was avascular, with only a thin strand of synovial tissue remaining attached to it. The head was removed. The remainder of the wound was debrided of damaged soft tissue. Several free osteochondral fragments were identified and removed, and the wound was irrigated with 6 liters of saline. The body of the talus was reduced into the ankle mortise and subtalar joint by distracting the ankle and applying traction through the heel and forefoot and manipulating the body fragment. The reduction of the talus body in the ankle mortis was stable; however, the talocalcaneal articulation was easily subluxed. A large dead space was present proximal to the navicular, where the head of the talus would have been. Two smooth Steinmann pins were driven from the calcaneus into the talus, stabilizing the talocalcaneal articulation. The ankle did not require stabilization. The dead space between the navicular and body of the talus was packed with polymethylmethacrylate antibiotic beads (Fig. 34–3). The original wound was closed loosely over a gauze wick. The extensions of the wound were closed with skin sutures only, and the foot and leg were splinted.

The patient was brought back to the operating room on the first postoperative day for a second look. The wound appeared clean. The antibiotic beads were removed and the wound was irrigated. New antibiotic beads were placed in the dead space and the wound was closed.

Postoperative Management

The patient was nonweight bearing on the injured extremity. Ankle range of motion exercises were initiated at 7 days. Systemic antibiotics were continued for a total of 10 days. At 3 weeks the patient was taken back to the operating room and the antibiotic beads were removed. The medial border of the foot appeared shortened and the forefoot appeared inverted because of collapse of the dead space occupied by the

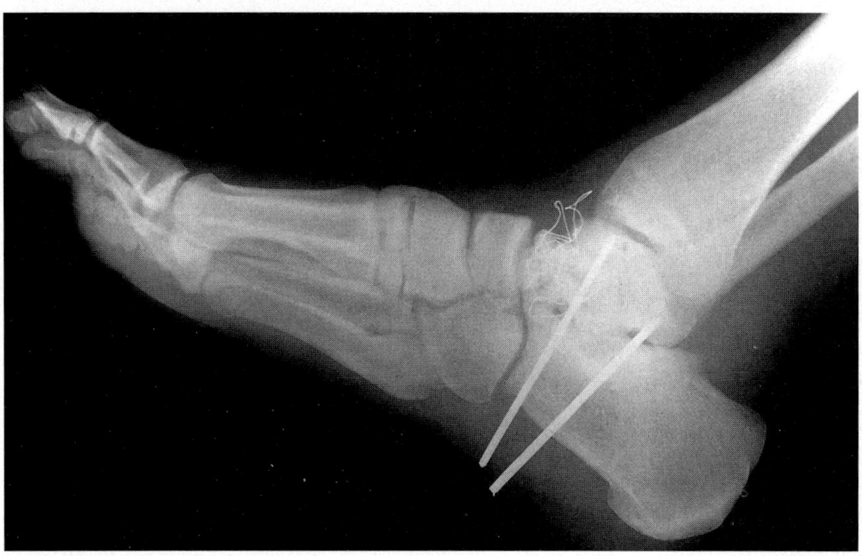

Figure 34–3. Lateral radiograph following reduction of the talus, removal of the head of the talus, and packing of the dead space with antibiotic beads.

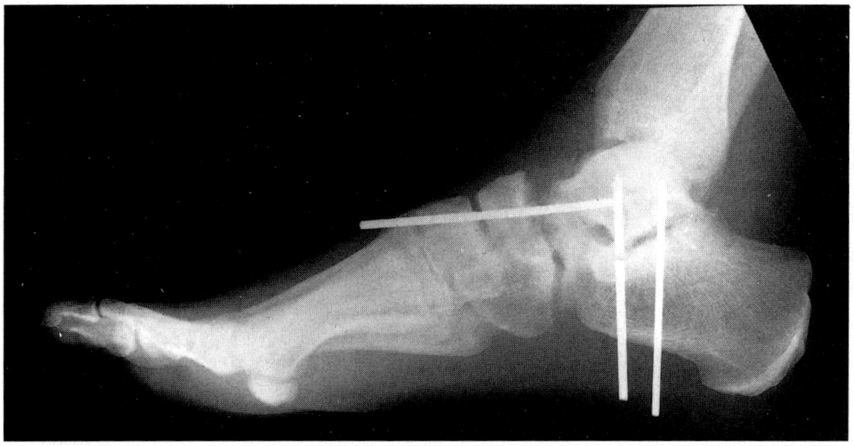

Figure 34–4. Lateral radiograph following autogenous bone grafting and stabilization of the medial column of the foot with a pin.

beads. A threaded Steinmann pin was driven from the navicular into the body of the talus while the medial side of the foot was distracted, thus restoring medial length of the foot. The cartilage was curetted from the posterior aspect of the navicular. Autogenous cancellous bone graft was harvested from the ipsilateral femoral condyles, mixed with Tobramycin, and used to fill the defect (Fig. 34–4).

The talonavicular pin and talocalcaneal pins were removed 12 weeks after bone grafting. Despite consolidation of the bone graft, there were no signs of revascularization of the talus at 6 months after injury. Partial weight bearing in a patellar tendon bearing ankle foot orthosis with a stiff soled shoe and a molded arch support was initiated and gradually advanced to full weight bearing. At 1 year the body of the talus still appears avascular (Fig. 34–5).

Discussion

The three keys to the acute management of this injury are debridement, reduction and stabilization of the fracture dislocation, and dead space management. The head of the talus was avascular and grossly contaminated. It was *debrided.* The body of the talus that was presumed to be avascular was not debrided. Thus one of the rules of open fracture management was broken—for example, all necrotic tissue was not removed. Salvage of the body of the talus maximizes the potential for near complete recovery, at the risk of increasing the risk of infection. If posttraumatic osteomyelitis had occurred, a talectomy would have been necessary.

Reduction was confirmed by direct visualization of the talus through the open wound and radiographically. *Stability* of reduction was augmented with pin fixation. A threaded Steinmann pin was selected to maintain the length of the medial column because the threads prevent sliding of the bone on the pin.

Removal of the head of the talus left a large *dead space.* This dead space was filled with antibiotic beads. The beads act as a spacer, minimizing the amount of hematoma that accumulates, and as a drug delivery system, delivering high local concentration of antibiotics into the wound.

The keys to subacute management are early bone grafting of the defect, maintenance of motion of surrounding joints, and prolonged nonweight bearing. *Autogenous bone graft* was harvested from the ipsilateral femoral condyles. We have found that harvesting bone graft from the femoral condyles is less painful than harvesting

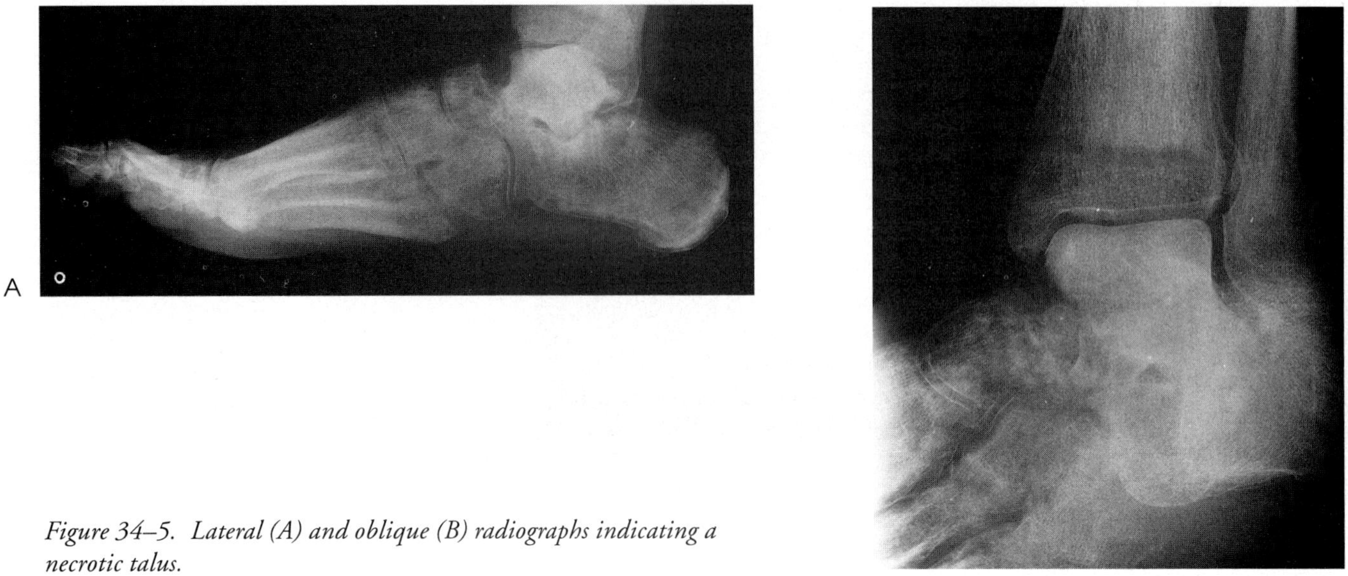

Figure 34–5. Lateral (A) and oblique (B) radiographs indicating a necrotic talus.

it from the iliac crest. Use of the femoral condyles as a donor site requires that the patient be nonweight bearing on that extremity for 6 weeks postsurgery. Therefore in cases such as this, in which the patient will be nonweight bearing, we use the femoral condyle as our source of autogenous graft.

Physical therapy is initiated when incisional pain becomes tolerable. Therapy is directed to *maintenance of motion* and prevention of contractures of the toes and ankle.

Prolonged nonweight bearing is necessary to minimize the possibility of collapse of the talar body. Fractures of the neck of the talus are classified according to a system described by Hawkins and expanded by Canale. In this system, the fracture is classified by the amount of displacement of the fracture and the status of the subtalar and ankle joints. A Hawkins I fracture denotes a minimally displaced fracture of the talar neck. A Hawkins II denotes a displaced fracture of the talar neck and a subluxed or dislocated subtalar joint. A Hawkins III denotes a displaced fracture of the talar neck with the body of the talus dislocated from the subtalar joint and ankle. Canale added a fourth type of fracture in which the neck is fractured, the body is dislocated from the ankle and subtalar joint, and the head is dislocated from the navicular. Avascular necrosis of the body of the talus and nonunion of the neck of the talus are more likely with the more displaced fracture types. The incidence of avascular necrosis increases from 0 to 5% with a Hawkins I injury to near 100% with a Hawkins-Canale IV. This patient had sustained a type IV fracture dislocation and is certain to develop avascular necrosis. To prevent collapse while vascular ingrowth is occurring nonweight bearing is maintained.

Alternative Methods of Management

Alternative methods of management are Boyd's amputation or talectomy; reduction and fixation of the head and body; and reduction of the body, excision of the head, and delayed bone grafting of the head defect. Boyd's amputation or talectomy has the advantages of possibly being one definitive procedure and minimizing the possibility of multiple surgeries. Boyd's amputation and talectomy have the disadvantage of resulting in permanent significant loss of function and shortening of the extremity. Reduction of the head and stabilization of the head fragment to the body of the talus are combined with stabilization of the talocalcaneal and talonavicular articulations. Theoretically, this method minimizes loss of function; however, practically, the risk of infection is so great that it precludes this method of management for open fracture dislocations.

Excision of the head and delayed bone grafting is a reasonable compromise between these two methods. It minimizes the risk of infection because the exposed avascular head fragment is excised and the resulting defect is filled temporarily with antibiotic beads. However, this method does not eliminate the possibility of infection because the avascular head fragment is left in the wound. Loss of function is minimized and the length of the extremity is preserved because the body of the talus is retained and the head and neck are replaced with bone graft.

Type of Management	Advantages	Disadvantages	Comments
Boyd's amputation or talectomy	Definitive, 1 stage, procedure; relatively short recovery	Results in significant loss of function	May be optimum management when patient cannot undergo prolonged convalescence
Reduction and fixation of the head and body	If successful, will result in least loss of function	Increased risk of infection	Risk of infection is so high that procedure may not be warranted
Reduction of body only and grafting of defect	Minimal loss of function; minimizes risk of infection	Prolonged recovery; may develop shortening of medial column of foot	Does not eliminate risk of infection (necrotic body fragment is left in situ)

Complications

Complications are nonunion, infection, arthritis, and shortening of the medial column of the foot. Nonunion of the graft to the body of the talus or failure of fusion of the talonavicular joint is managed with repeat bone grafting.

Infection usually involves the avascular body of the talus. Management is either an amputation (Boyd's or below knee) or attempted salvage of the foot. Salvage is most reliably accomplished with staged procedures. These procedures are debridement of the body of the talus and all avascular tissue, management of dead space with antibiotic beads, stabilization and maintenance of length with an external fixator or threaded pins, culture specific systemic antibiotics, and frequently, a free soft tissue transfer.

Arthritis is often a sequelae of avascular necrosis of the talar body. Both the talocalcaneal articulation and the tibiotalar articulation may be involved. The incidence of arthritis is minimized by delaying weight bearing until there is clear evidence of revascularization of the talar body. The problem is that it may take years for revascularization to occur. Management is arthrodesis of the involved articulations.

Shortening of the medial column of the foot occurs because the bone graft replacing the head and neck of the talus shortens. Management is operative and consists of intraoperative reestablishment of length with a distracter, repeat bone grafting, and maintenance of length with threaded pins or an external fixator.

Suggested Readings

Canale ST, Kelly FB: Fractures of the neck of the talus. J Bone Joint Surg 1978; 60-A:143–156.

Comfort TH, Behrens F, Gaither DW, Denis F, Sigmond M: Long term results of displaced talar neck fractures. CORR 1985; 199:81–87.

DeLee JC, Curtis R: Subtalar dislocation of the foot. J Bone Joint Surg 1982; 64-A:433–437.

Edmonds I, Elliott D, Nade S: Open subtalar dislocation. Aust NZ J Surg 1991; 61:681–686.

Hawkins LG: Fractures of the neck of the talus. J Bone Joint Surg 1970; 52-A:991–1002.

Henderson RC: Posttraumatic necrosis of the talus: the Hawkins sign versus magnetic resonance imaging. J Orthop Trauma 1991; 5(1):96–99.

Heppenstall RB, Farahavar H, Balderston R, Lotke P: Evaluation and management of subtalar dislocations. J Trauma 1980; 20(6):494–497.

Monson ST, Ryan JR: Subtalar dislocation. J Bone Joint Surg 1981; 63-A:1156–1158.

Mulfinger GL, Trueta J: The blood supply of the talus. J Bone Joint Surg 1970; 52-B:160–167.

Case 35

History and Physical Examination

A 64-year-old man was the driver of an automobile involved in a traffic accident. The floor of the car was driven upwards, imparting an axial compression force to his inverted left hindfoot. Following the accident he was unable to weight bear and on admission to the emergency department it was clear that he had a significant injury to his left hindfoot. Examination showed no evidence of neurovascular abnormality in the left forefoot. He was able to flex and extend his toes, although all movements of the foot were painful.

A

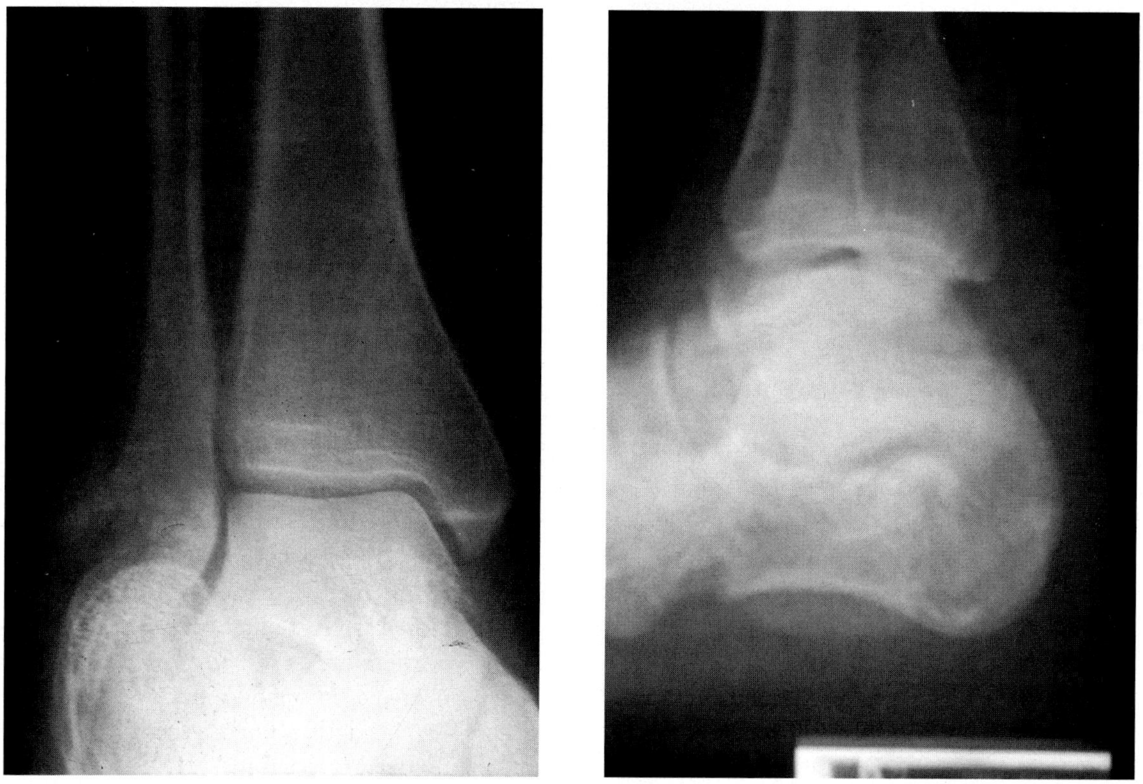

B

Figure 35–1. Anteroposterior (A) and lateral (B) radiographs of a calcaneal fracture dislocation.

Radiologic Findings

Anteroposterior and lateral radiographs indicated an unusual appearance of the hindfoot (Fig. 35–1). The lateral radiograph showed that Bohler's angle appeared to be maintained but was sited near the top of the talus. The upper half of the calcaneus was more radioopaque than usual, suggesting either impaction, which was unlikely in view of the intact Bohler's angle, or that the calcaneus and talus were overlapping. On the anteroposterior view bone is just overlapping the distal fibula. There is also minor damage to the talus and the lateral malleolus.

PITFALL

- Operative management of calcaneal fractures is often stated to be associated with a high incidence of wound complications for two main reasons. First, surgeons often wait until the swelling around the hindfoot has settled before operating on the calcaneus. During this period the soft tissues contract and it is therefore difficult to close the skin incision after the calcaneal height has been restored. Second, surgeons often open the various tissue planes when exposing the lateral wall of the calcaneus. This should be avoided because it devascularizes the tissues. The skin incision should be continued down to the bone and the upper and lower flaps raised with subperiosteal dissection. Care should be taken to avoid damage to the sural nerve and the peroneal tendons.

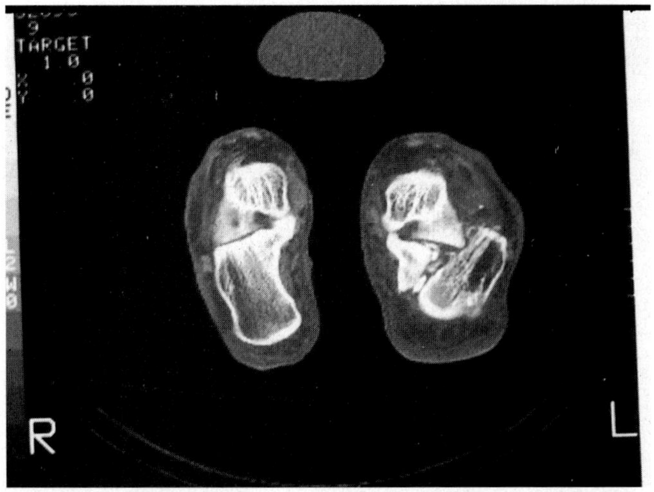

Figure 35–2. A CAT scan indicating the fracture dislocation (left). The normal side (right) is included for comparison.

A computerized axial tomography (CAT) scan was obtained (Fig. 35–2). This clearly shows that the talus and the anteromedial portion of the calcaneus have dropped down to lie lateral to the residual posterolateral calcaneal fragment.

Diagnosis

Fracture dislocation of the calcaneus. OTA classification: 73–C1.2.

Surgical Management

The patient was taken to the operating room and the left leg prepped and draped. A curved lateral incision was made starting 2 in. above the lateral malleolus. It passed under the lateral malleolus and along the body of the calcaneus as far as the calcaneocuboid joint. The soft tissues were dissected subperiosteally from the upper two thirds of the calcaneus and it was confirmed that the lateral ligamentous complex had been completely disrupted. Unfortunately, reduction of the fracture proved difficult. A small medial incision was therefore made and a few small intraarticular bone fragments removed. This permitted a successful reduction and the fracture was then stabilized with lagged screws placed through a two hole plate. The lateral malleolar fracture was also internally fixed (Fig. 35–3).

Postoperative Management

The patient wore a supportive cast for 3 weeks and thereafter full mobilization of the hindfoot was encouraged. Weight bearing was delayed for 3 months until the fracture had united. One year after surgery the patient had no pain but felt slightly unbalanced when walking over rough ground. At that time he had 5 degrees of dorsiflexion, 30 degrees of plantar flexion, 5 degrees of inversion, and 10 degrees of eversion.

Discussion

The location and orientation of calcaneal fractures are often difficult to appreciate because of the unusual shape of the bone. This case illustrates the primary fracture

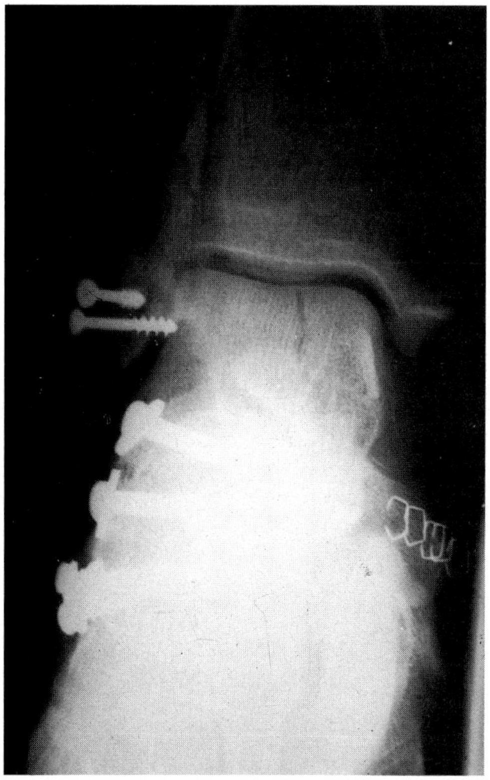

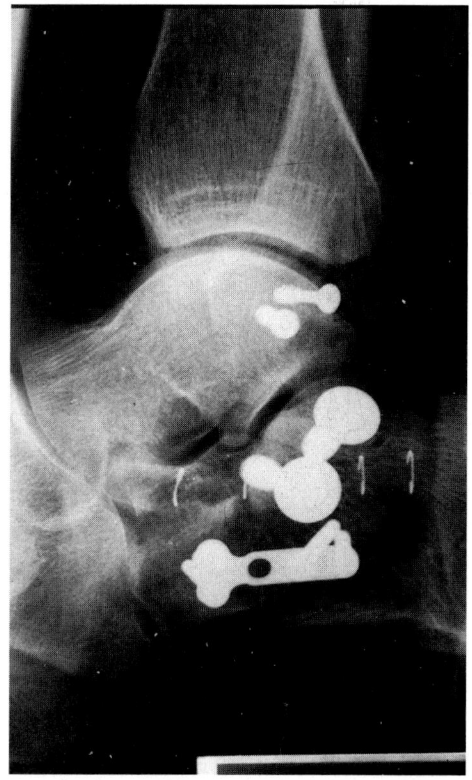

Figure 35–3. *Anteroposterior (A) and lateral (B) radiographs showing the postoperative result. A good reconstruction has been obtained.*

that was first described by Essex-Lopresti (1952) and Warwick and Bremner (1953). This fracture line is a constant feature of all intraarticular calcaneal fractures, although its exact position may vary. The primary fracture runs forward and laterally from a point on the medial side of the calcaneus at a variable distance behind the sustentaculum tali, dividing the calcaneus into anteromedial and posterolateral fragments (Fig. 35–4). Intraarticular calcaneal fractures where only the primary fracture occurs are rare because the considerable axial load applied to the calcaneus usually causes more damage to the bone. If there is an associated disruption of the lateral ligamentous complex, then the injury pattern shown in this case may occur (Fig. 35–4).

Usually, however, the lateral ligamentous complex remains intact and the posterolateral calcaneal fragment is prevented from moving laterally. Under these circumstances the continuing axial force causes further disruption to the posterolateral fragment. It is depressed and rotated downward into the metaphyseal bone of the body of the calcaneus. If the primary fracture enters the sulcus, the complete posterior articular facet will be driven downward. This type of fracture was referred to as a joint depression fracture by Essex-Lopresti. When the depressed articular cartilage is continuous with the upper part of the body of the calcaneus, which is split longitudinally, an Essex-Lopresti tongue type fracture ensues. Usually the lateral wall of the calcaneus is comminuted and there is a fracture line running vertically through the lateral wall to involve the inferior surface of the calcaneus.

It is important that surgeons appreciate the types of calcaneal fractures they may encounter. Many surgeons adopt a policy of nonoperative management of

PEARL

- Surgeons frequently underestimate the difficulty in operating on calcaneal fractures. Like the acetabulum, the calcaneus has a complex three-dimensional structure and the learning curve in calcaneal surgery is significant. It is advisable to send complex calcaneal fractures to a specialist trauma or foot surgeon if the initial surgeon lacks the necessary expertise.

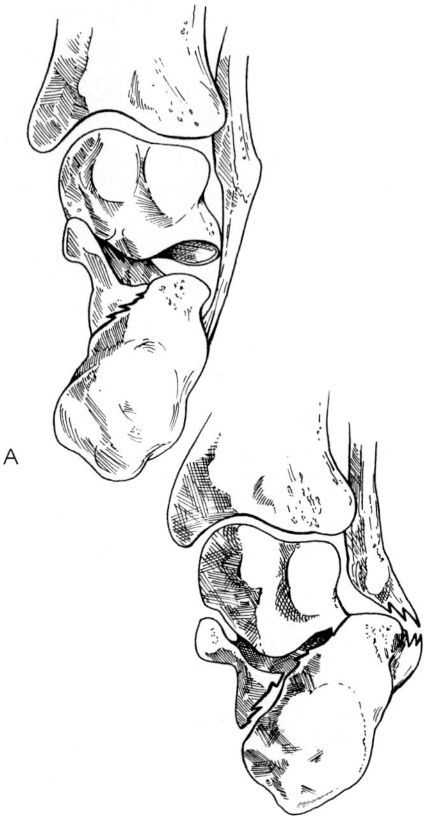

Figure 35–4. The aetiology of a calcaneal fracture dislocation. The primary fracture is caused in the usual manner (A). The lateral ligament tears and the posterolateral fragment moves laterally to lie beside the talus (B).

calcaneal fractures regardless of their type because they find the surgery very difficult. Failure to operate on a straightforward fracture as illustrated in this case would be inappropriate. If the fracture is treated nonoperatively, it would certainly unite but the heel would be widened and there would be a marked loss of heel height. The subtalar joint would be incongruous and secondary osteoarthritis inevitable. There might also be peroneal tendon impingement accompanied by pain and residual disability. More difficult calcaneal fractures are illustrated elsewhere in this book. Although surgeons debate the benefits of internal fixation of these more complex fractures, straightforward fractures such as the one illustrated here require internal fixation.

Alternative Methods of Management

The two main methods surgeons will employ to treat this type of fracture are internal fixation and nonoperative management. The problems of nonoperative management have already been outlined and it is strongly advised that this type of two fragment fracture be internally fixed. The rigid fixation used in this case allows early joint movement; less rigid fixation provided by methods such as Kirschner wire fixation can be used if a postoperative cast is applied for about 6 weeks. There would be no advantage in using external fixation for this fracture.

Type of Management	Advantages	Disadvantages	Comments
Cast management	None	Deformed hindfoot; joint stiffness; pain; osteoarthritis	Should not be used for this type of two fragment calcaneal fracture
Internal fixation	Accurate reduction; early movement; improved results	Difficult if done late	The method of choice. Rigid fixation is better. Should be performed early

Complications

The complications of the operative management of calcaneal fractures are skin healing and posttraumatic osteoarthritis. The problems of skin healing are usually resolved by early surgery and correct attention to surgical technique when raising the skin flaps. If a superficial wound infection occurs, it should be treated aggressively with rest and elevation of the foot and high dose antibiotics. If the infection persists, early soft tissue resection and subsequent flap cover are indicated.

Posttraumatic osteoarthritis occurs because of a failure to adequately reduce the articular surface and from damage to the articular cartilage at the time of the injury. If the discomfort that accompanies the arthritic change is too severe to be adequately treated by analgesics and nonsteroidal antiinflammatory drugs, a subtalar arthrodesis is indicated. This operation is easier to perform if the calcaneus has been reconstructed after the fracture.

Suggested Readings

Biga N, Thomine JM: La fracture-luxation du calcaneum. A propos de 4 observations. Rev Chir Orth 1977; 63:191–197.

Court-Brown CM, Boot DA, Kellam JF: Fracture dislocation of the calcaneus. Clin Orthop 1986; 213:201–206.

Essex-Lopresti P: The mechanism, reduction technique and results in fractures of the os calcis. Br J Surg 1952; 39:395–419.

Palmer I: The mechanism and treatment of fractures of the calcaneus: open reduction with the use of cancellous grafts. J Bone Joint Surg (Am) 1948; 30A:2–8.

Pozo JL, Kirwan E O'G, Jackson AM: The long term results of conservative management of severely displaced fractures of the calcaneus. J Bone Joint Surg (Br) 1984; 66B:386–390.

Warwick CK, Bremner AE: Fractures of the calcaneum. J Bone Joint Surg (Br) 1953; 35B:33–49.

Case 36

History and Physical Examination

A 45-year-old farmer was brought to the emergency room after falling 12 feet and landing on his heels. He was unable to weight bear on his left foot, which was swollen. Examination showed no other injury and in particular there was no evidence of any spinal injury. He had normal neurovascular function in his left forefoot, although toe flexion and extension was restricted because of pain.

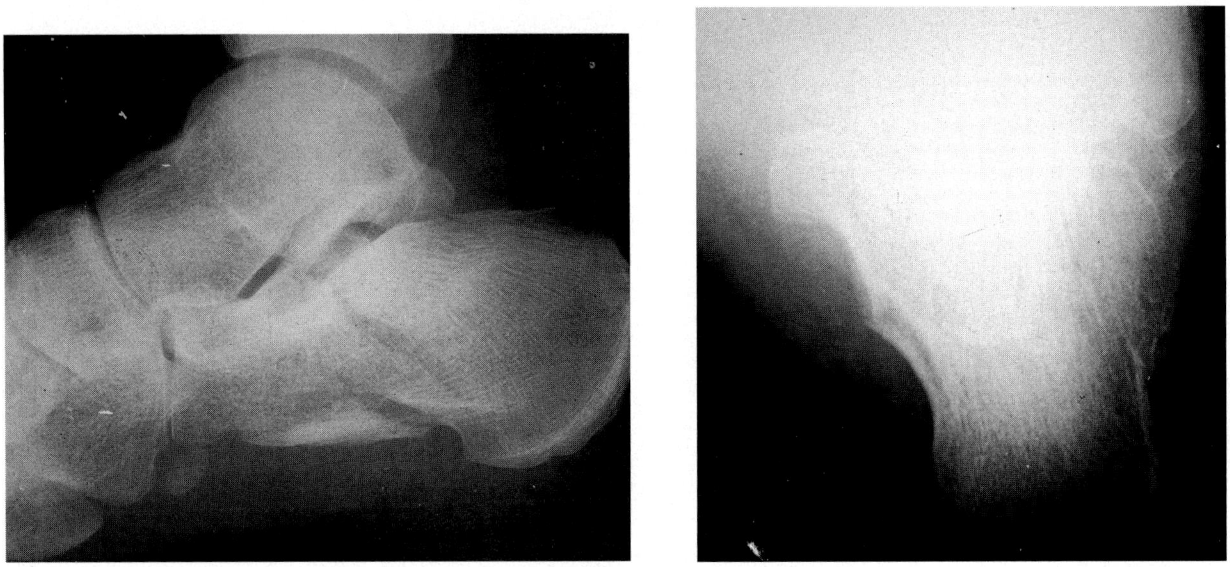

A B

Figure 36–1. Lateral (A) and axial (B) views of the calcaneus showing a comminuted intraarticular fracture.

Radiologic Findings

Anteroposterior, lateral (Fig. 36–1A) and axial (Fig. 36–1B) views were taken of the left heel. The anteroposterior view was not helpful. The lateral radiograph indicates a loss of Bohler's angle. There is a double shadow in the area of the posterior articular facet indicating that the facet is in at least two fragments. The bone just under the facet is less radiolucent than usual, suggesting that the facet has been depressed downward by the force of the impact. The lateral wall and the base of the calcaneus are also fractured and the lateral wall fracture runs forward to the area of the calcaneocuboid joint. The axial view shows the primary fracture under the lateral wall is slightly expanded.

A computerized axial tomography (CAT) scan (Fig. 36–2) confirmed the fracture and showed that the posterior articular facet was in fact in three fragments, although the medial two fragments were probably functioning as one. There was a step between the two main fragments. The CAT scan failed to delineate the amount of depression of the articular facet, but it must be remembered that each section of the CAT scan only supplies information about a limited area of the fracture.

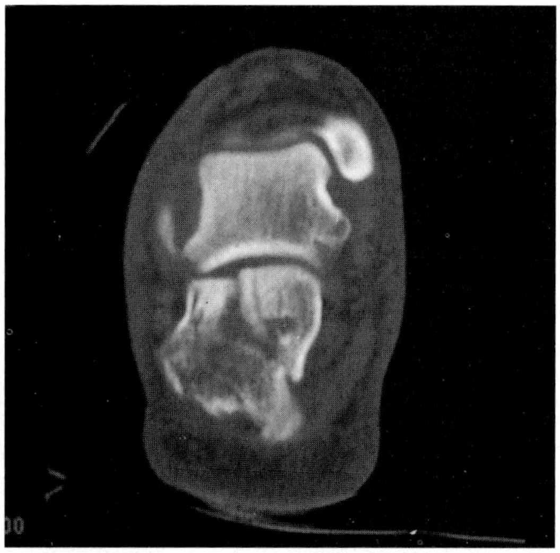

Figure 36–2. A CAT scan showed the intraarticular fracture as well as the varus heel alignment and the widening of the calcaneus.

Diagnosis

Intraarticular fracture of the calcaneus. The posterior articular facet is in two main fragments and is depressed. OTA classification: 73–C1.1.

Surgical Management

On the day after admission the patient was taken to the operating room. The leg was prepped and draped. A long curved lateral incision, commencing above and behind the lateral malleolus and extending down to the body of the calcaneus and then forward to the calcaneocuboid joint, was used to expose the calcaneus. The resection was continued down to the calcaneus and soft tissue flaps were elevated using subperiosteal sharp dissection. None of the intermediate soft tissue planes were dissected. The dissection was continued proximally until the subtalar joint was exposed. The lower flap was then elevated to expose the inferior part of the calcaneus

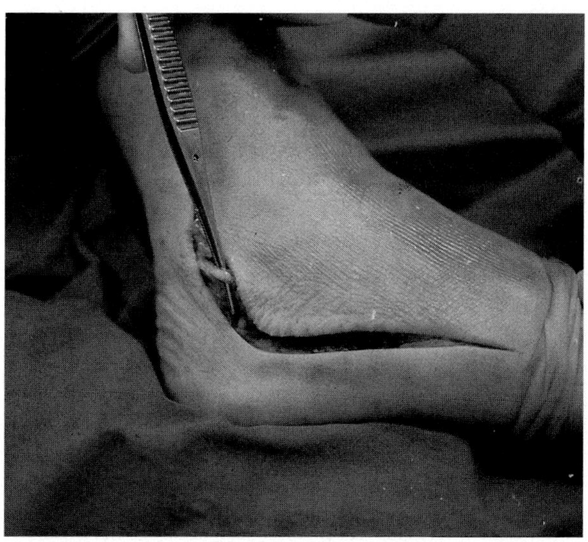

Figure 36–3. The sural nerve is easily damaged as it runs across the incision. It should be turned upward with the superior soft tissue flap.

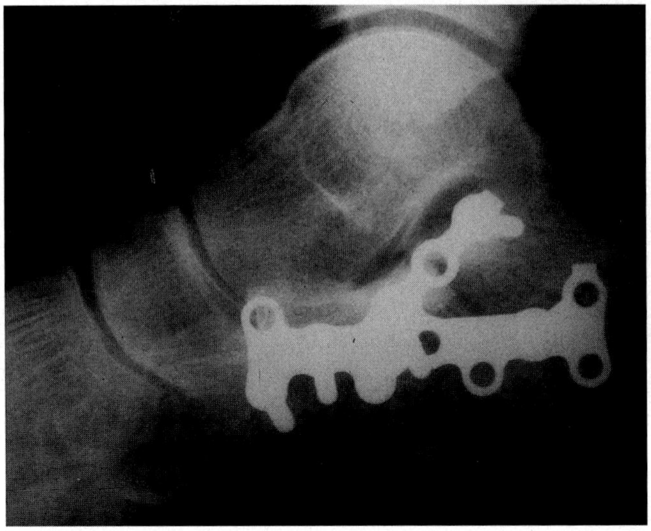

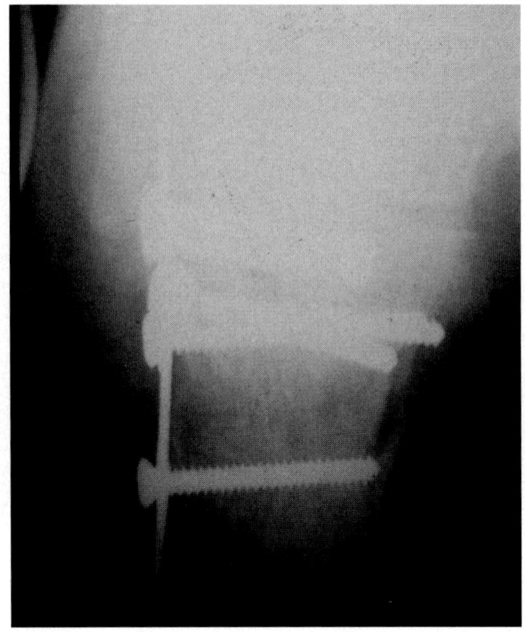

Figure 36–4. Postoperative radiographs showing good articular reconstruction. Lateral (A) and axial (B) views.

PITFALL

- It is remarkably easy to damage both the sural nerve and the peroneal tendons. The sural nerve should be mobilized upward within the upper skin flap. However, great care must be taken in making the initial skin incision in case the nerve is damaged. A sural neuroma can be very troublesome for the patient.

PEARL

- Counterclockwise derotation is the key to reducing the posterior facet. This is relatively easy if the facet is in one or two fragments. If it is in more than two fragments, the facet should be reconstructed sequentially starting with the most medial fragment and rebuilding the facet using temporary Kirschner wires prior to applying a plate.

and the dissection was taken as far forward as the calcaneocuboid joint. Care was taken to identify and preserve the sural nerve and avoid damaging the peroneal tendons (Fig. 36–3).

Inspection confirmed that the posterior facet was in two main fragments. These were reduced and held with a temporary Kirschner wire and then de-rotated to their reduced position. The lateral wall was then reconstructed and a calcaneal plate applied and screwed home. The side arm of the plate allowed a screw to be placed in the posterior facet fragment. Postoperative radiographs were satisfactory (Fig. 36–4).

Postoperative Management

A back shell was applied to the leg and maintained for about a week to allow the soft tissue swelling to diminish. Passive and active physiotherapy was then encouraged and the patient remained nonweight bearing for 3 months. Gradual weight bearing was then commenced and he was weight bearing after a further month. One year after the fracture he reported minimal pain and that he was functioning well, although he was still wary of climbing ladders. Examination showed normal ankle movement with 5 degrees of subtalar inversion and 10 degrees of eversion. His heel alignment was good and he walked well without a limp. The radiograph (Fig. 36–5) showed good alignment and that Bohler's angle had been maintained.

Discussion

Many surgeons are wary of internally fixing the calcaneus. It is technically demanding and until relatively recently there were no adequate classification systems to as-

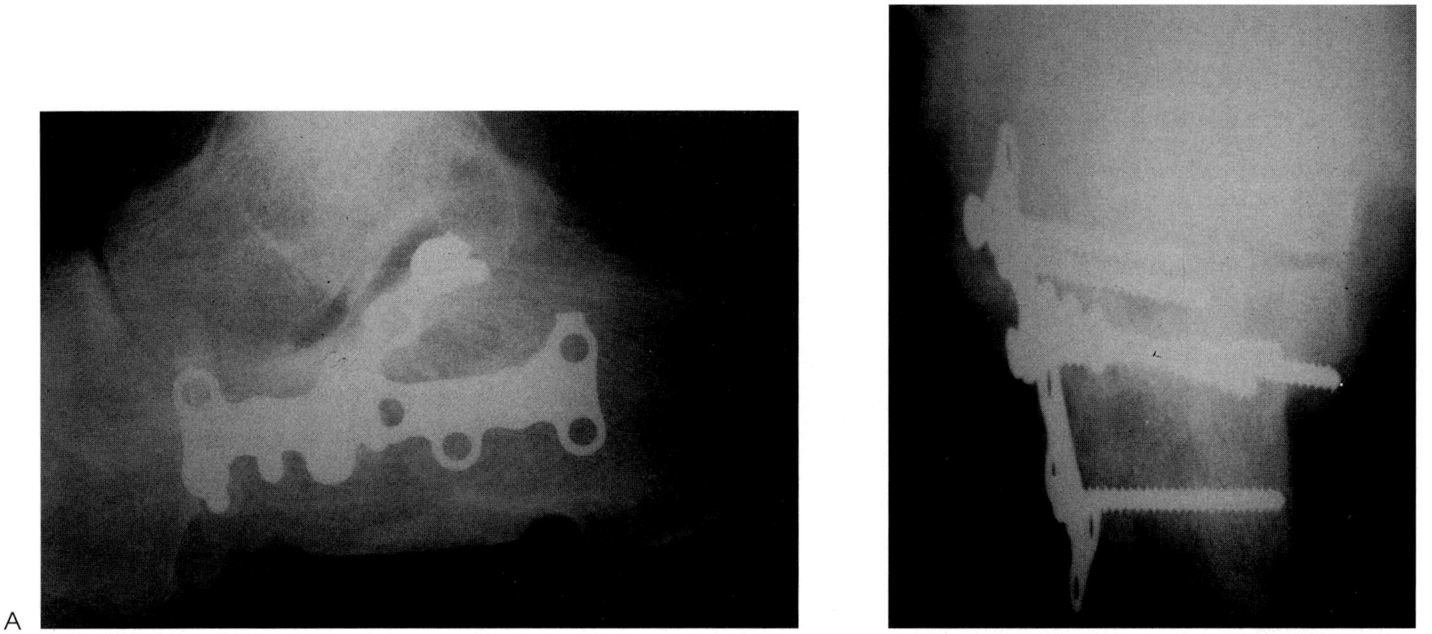

Figure 36–5. At 1 year Bohler's angle has been maintained and the subtalar joint looks satisfactory. Lateral (A) and axial (B) views.

sist the surgeon in deciding which fractures to operate on. In addition, the recent introduction of plates specifically designed for the calcaneus has helped improve the results of operative treatment. There is, however, still great debate about whether these fractures should be fixed. Much of the information on which the debate is based is unfortunately historic and comes from the time when these fractures were fixed by Kirschner wires and then placed in plaster for a prolonged period. The results of this type of management were usually poor. However, with modern reconstructive techniques utilizing plates and screws good fixation can be achieved and early motion facilitated.

The problem most surgeons encounter with calcaneal fracture fixation is not actually reducing the fracture but maintaining the posterior facet in the reduced position. There is always a tendency for it to re-displace by rotating back to lie within the body of the calcaneus. In this case the re-displacement of the posterior facet has been prevented by the use of a specially designed calcaneal plate. However, many surgeons have used bone grafting and a laterally applied straight reconstruction plate. Unfortunately, bone graft does not usually maintain the position of the facet and the correct heel height is rarely maintained with this technique. To avoid this surgeons have placed the lateral plate diagonally or have used two plates, one of which is a six or seven hole third tubular plate placed along the axis of the calcaneus that is supplemented by a small plate running at 90 degrees to the first plate, which is used to maintain the position of the posterior facet. However, the use of a specially designed calcaneal plate is an improvement on these earlier techniques.

Surgeons should always be aware of why a CAT scan might be useful in the type of complex fracture. Ordering a CAT scan has almost become a reflex action and frequently surgeons derive little more information from the scan than they could have by correctly reading the radiographs. Sanders (1992) devised a careful calcaneal fracture classification based on the appearance of the CAT scan but it is unlikely that the decision to operate will be based solely on the number of posterior facet fragments shown on the scan. Sanders correctly indicated that the results obtained by operating on calcanei shown to be multifragmentary on the CAT scan would not be as good, but this does not mean surgery should be avoided. It is also unlikely that the CAT scan will be used to define the surgical approach because few surgeons now routinely use the medial approach.

The CAT scan is, however, helpful in assessing calcaneal damage preoperatively. It is particularly useful in assessing the degree of varus of the heel and the presence of any comminution between the main fragments of the posterior facet. The CAT scan is also useful in highlighting the extent of the fracture outwith the posterior facet. Thus calcaneocuboid damage will be visualized along with injuries to the other bones of the hindfoot.

It is important to have an adequate exposure of the complete calcaneus. At surgery the surgeon will usually be faced with a very standard appearance. After the soft tissue flaps have been elevated the surgeon sees the bulging lateral wall but cannot see the posterior articular facet. The lateral wall is usually fractured and the surgeon can therefore hinge open the lateral wall to expose the posterior articular facet that frequently lies within the body of the calcaneus. If the posterior articular facet is in one piece, it can be elevated fairly easily and held temporarily with a Kirschner wire. If the articular facet is fractured, the fragments can usually be reduced and held with temporary wires until definitive fixation can be undertaken. Once the facet has been placed in the correct position the lateral wall is reconstituted and a calcaneal plate applied. Surgeons should be careful to place the screws through the plate into the medial wall of the calcaneus to compress the medial and lateral walls together.

A review of the recent literature suggests that well reconstructed calcaneal fractures can have a good prognosis. Surgeons who advocate nonoperative management should stop to consider the effects of this treatment. The posterior facet will remain depressed in the metaphyseal bone of the body of the calcaneus and the calcaneus will therefore remain widened and the heel height will be reduced. Function is irretrievably lost quite quickly.

Hindfoot function is vital and if the heel height is reduced and the width of the calcaneus increased, it is impossible to regain anything resembling adequate function. Pain is virtually inevitable and many patients will eventually have a subtalar fusion. Unfortunately, however, this does not restore heel height and the sad fact is that many people never return to their jobs after a severe calcaneal fracture. Even if good articular reduction is not obtained at surgery, realignment of the heel and maintenance of heel height will allow a later subtalar fusion to be more successful. Early fracture fixation of operable calcaneal fractures is strongly advocated.

Alternative Methods of Management

The problems associated with nonoperative management have already been described. However, some surgeons advocate external skeletal fixation for the management of severe intraarticular calcaneal fractures. This concept is not new and superficially the idea of distracting the hindfoot to regain heel height is attractive. However, it betrays a lack of appreciation of the mechanics of the fracture. Distraction external fixation relies on the principle of ligamentotaxis. Unfortunately, the soft tissue connections to the posterior facet fragments are poor and the fragments are embedded in the metaphyseal bone of the body of the calcaneus. Axial traction will not succeed in reducing the posterior facet and maintaining its alignment.

Recently the Ilizarov external fixation has been used in conjunction with open reduction and K wire fixation of the intraarticular fragments. Unfortunately, this technique does not allow early joint movement and seems to confer no real advantage over internal fixation techniques.

Type of Management	Advantages	Disadvantages	Comments
Casting/traction	None	Malunion; joint stiffness; secondary osteoarthritis; loss of heel height; increase of heel width	Cast management of intraarticular calcaneal fractures provides no advantage over modern fixation methods
Internal fixation (plates)	Early motion; maintenance of heel height; maintenance of heel width; improved results	Technically difficult; some risk of infection and wound breakdown	This is the method of choice for intraarticular calcaneal fractures but should be done by experienced surgeons
Internal fixation (K wires)	May help preserve heel height	Maintained broad heel; requires a cast; joint stiffness	Has many of the problems of nonoperative management
External fixator (without internal fixation)	None	Does not correct heel deformities; secondary osteoarthritis; joint stiffness	No advantage over nonoperative management
External fixation and internal fixation	Preserves heel height; may reduce heel width	Immobilization; joint stiffness; pin tract sepsis	Confers no advantage over appropriate internal fixation

Complications

The usual complications of intraarticular calcaneal fractures are pain, subtalar stiffness, and secondary posttraumatic osteoarthritis. If nonoperative management is used, the patient will often complain of heel deformity, an inability to wear normal shoes, abnormal gait, and peroneal tendon impingement. The incidence of pain, subtalar stiffness, and secondary osteoarthritis in operatively managed fractures varies with the surgeon's ability to reduce the posterior facet fragments and maintain the reduced position of the reconstructed fragment. Obviously, this will depend on the severity of the injury and the experience of the surgeon. However, it is likely that there will be damage to the articular cartilage and thus even perfectly reconstructed calcanei may present with hindfoot pain after a time. If the symptoms are intolerable and cannot be treated by nonoperative means, then subtalar arthrodesis is usually undertaken. The surgeon should try to ascertain that the symptoms are from the subtalar joint before undertaking a subtalar arthrodesis. Because calcaneal fractures follow axial loading there may be damage to the ankle joint and the other joints in the hindfoot as well as to the subtalar joint. After a few years this occult intraarticular damage may give rise to pain that will persist after a successful subtalar arthrodesis has been performed. Local anesthetic blocking of the various joints can be undertaken to try to identify which hindfoot joint is most painful.

It is impossible to gain heel height after a nonoperatively managed depressed intraarticular fracture has united. The soft tissues contract quickly and the patient is left with a depressed os calcus. The widening of the bone can be treated by a lateral wall osteotomy undertaken through a posterior incision. This has the twin benefit of reducing bony encroachment on the peroneal tendons and narrowing the calcaneus. However, once the calcaneus is deformed, it is impossible to restore its normal shape and the patient usually has troublesome symptoms.

PEARL

- Unfortunately it is not always easy to determine with certainty which hindfoot joint is the source of the pain. Indeed, more than one joint may be incriminated. Local anesthetic intraarticular injections to block the pain may help, but not infrequently the surgeon may have to guess as to the source of the discomfort and act appropriately. Understandably, the results of treatment are poor and equally understandably most surgeons resist fusing joints other than the subtalar joint unless it is absolutely necessary.

Suggested Readings

Benirschke SK, Sangeorzan BJ: Extensive intraarticular fractures of the foot: surgical management of calcaneal fractures. Clin Orthop 1993; 292:128–134.

Essex-Lopresti P: The mechanism, reduction technique and results in fractures of the os calcis. Br J Surg 1952; 39:395–419.

Hildebrand KA, Buckley RE, Mohtadi NGH, Faris P: Functional outcome measures after displaced intra-articular calcaneal fractures. J Bone Joint Surg (Br) 1996; 78B:119–123.

Sanders R: Intraarticular fractures of the calcaneus: present state of the art. J Orthop Trauma 1992; 6:252–265.

Stephenson JR: Treatment of displaced intraarticular fractures of the calcaneus using medial and lateral approaches, internal fixation and early motion. J Bone Joint Surg (Am) 1987; 69:115–130.

Zwipp H, Tscherne H, Wülker N, Grote R: Der intraartikuläre fersenbeinbruch. Klassification, bewertung und operationstakit. Unfallchirurg 1989; 92:117–129.

Case 37

History and Physical Examination

A 32-year-old male was the unrestrained driver in an automobile accident and his air bag deployed on impact. He was extracted from the automobile and arrived in the emergency department approximately 30 minutes after the accident. He was alert and conscious, complaining of bilateral foot pain. His shoes and socks were cut off. Obvious deformity of the right foot was present. There was a stellate laceration on the plantar aspect of the right foot. The laceration involved almost the entire plantar surface of the hind foot, and fragments of bone were visible in the wound and lying on the skin. The plantar skin of the foot distal to the open wound was insensate; however, brisk capillary refill of the nail beds was present.

Obvious deformity of the left foot was not present. However, it was diffusely and tensely swollen and painful to palpation. Lacerations or defects in the skin were not present. The neurovascular examination was within the limits of normal on the left. The patient also complained of right knee pain. The skin over the right knee was intact, but a tense hemarthrosis was present. Ligamentous stability and active range of motion were not determined because of pain.

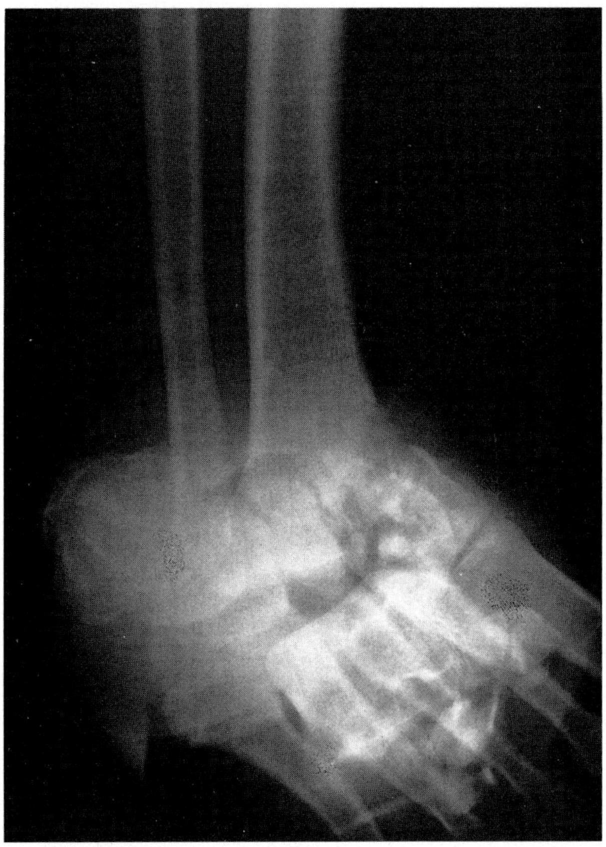

Figure 37–1. Radiograph of the right foot indicating a fracture dislocation of the calcaneus talus and distal tibia. The talus is seen superimposed on the metatarsals.

PEARL

- Insensate plantar skin indicates disruption of the posterior tibial nerve or of its terminal branches, the medial and lateral plantar nerves. Because of the extent of the injury it is not possible to localize where the disruption occurred. Insensate palmar skin mitigates for amputation, but is not an absolute indication for it.

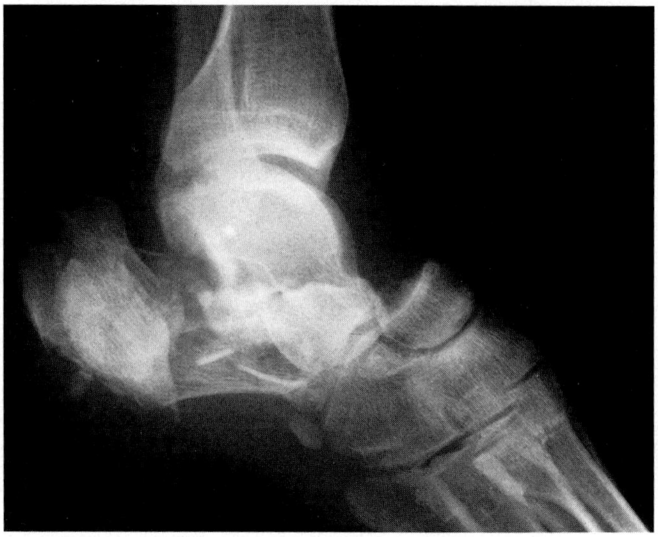

Figure 37–2. Lateral radiograph of the left foot indicating a fracture of the calcaneus and dislocation of the talocalcaneal and talonavicular articulations.

Radiologic Findings

Lateral radiographs of both feet indicated severely displaced comminuted fractures of the calcanei. The fracture of the right side was not able to be classified; however, it appeared as if the likely mechanism of injury was the talus being driven through the plantar aspect of the foot. In addition to the calcaneus fracture, there was a comminuted fracture of the distal tibia with impaction of the articular surface and dislocation of the talus from the ankle mortise with a displaced fracture of the talar neck (Fig. 37–1). The fracture of the left calcaneus appeared to be a tongue type fracture with an associated subtalar dislocation (Fig. 37–2). Radiographs of the right knee indicated a comminuted, displaced fracture of the distal pole of the patella.

Diagnosis

Right open calcaneus fracture with associated tibial plafond fracture, fracture dislocation of the talus, and injury to the posterior tibial or medial and lateral plantar nerves; closed left calcaneus fracture with an associated subtalar dislocation; and fracture of the distal pole of the patella with possible ligamentous injury of the knee.

Surgical Management

The open wound of the right foot was cultured, irrigated, and covered with a sterile dressing. A second generation cephalosporin was administered intravenously. When the patient had been cleared for surgery he was taken emergently to the operating room.

In the operating room, a general anesthetic was administered and both lower extremities were scrubbed. The open wound on the right side was debrided of all nonviable tissue. Loose fragments of bone, including portions of the talus tibia, and calcaneus were removed. Crushed and avascular soft tissue was excised and specimens sent for culture. The plantar nerves were not seen. The wound was irrigated. An external fixator with two pins in the tibia, one pin in the tuberosity of the calcaneus,

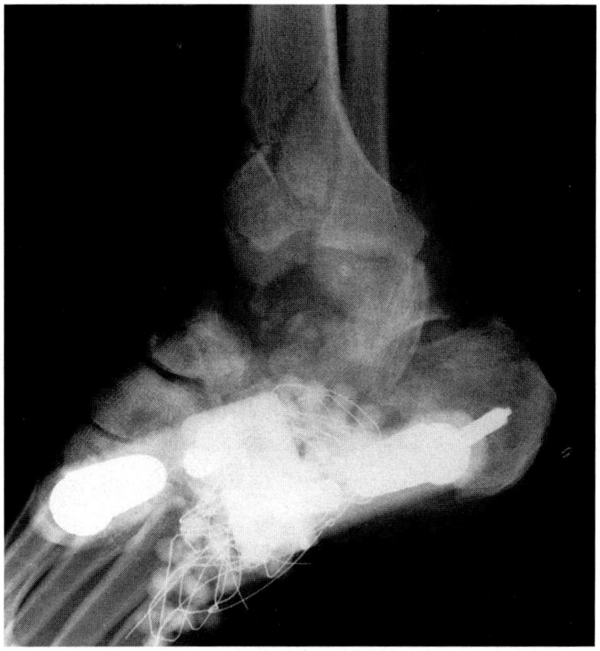

Figure 37–3. Lateral radiograph of right foot after stabilization with an external fixator and insertion of antibiotic beads.

and one pin in the forefoot was utilized to stabilize the foot. The defect was packed with antibiotic beads and covered with an impermeable plastic drape (Fig. 37–3).

The left foot was placed in a compression dressing and splinted. The knee was examined and the collateral and cruciate ligaments were intact. The patella fracture was exposed through a vertical midline incision, reduced, and stabilized with pins and screws.

The options for the right foot were discussed with the patient and his family. They were opposed to any type of amputation and wanted to salvage the forefoot. The patient was taken back to the operating room at 2 days and at 4 days for a second and third look. In these procedures, the wound was debrided and the beads were exchanged. After the third look, the skin was closed loosely over the beads. At 2 weeks the defect on the right side was grafted with autogenous cancellous bone harvested from the iliac crest. The graft was mixed with 1.2 grams of Tobramycin (Fig. 37–4). The left calcaneus was exposed via an extensile lateral incision. The subtalar joint was reduced and stabilized with a transarticular pin, and the remainder of the calcaneus was reconstructed as accurately as possible and stabilized with screws and pins (Fig. 37–5).

Postoperative Management

The intraoperative cultures obtained the night of injury were positive for pseudomonas and therefore Gentamicin was added to the antibiotic regimen and continued for 6 weeks. The right foot continued to drain and cultures were positive for pseudomonas. Four months postinjury the right foot was debrided once more. A large amount of what appeared to be necrotic cancellous bone from the first grafting was removed. The defect was packed with antibiotic beads, and antibiotics were administered systemically. Three weeks later the foot was again grafted with autogenous cancellous bone mixed with Tobramycin. The drainage ceased. The fixator was removed 6 months after injury. Nonweight bearing was maintained a total of 8

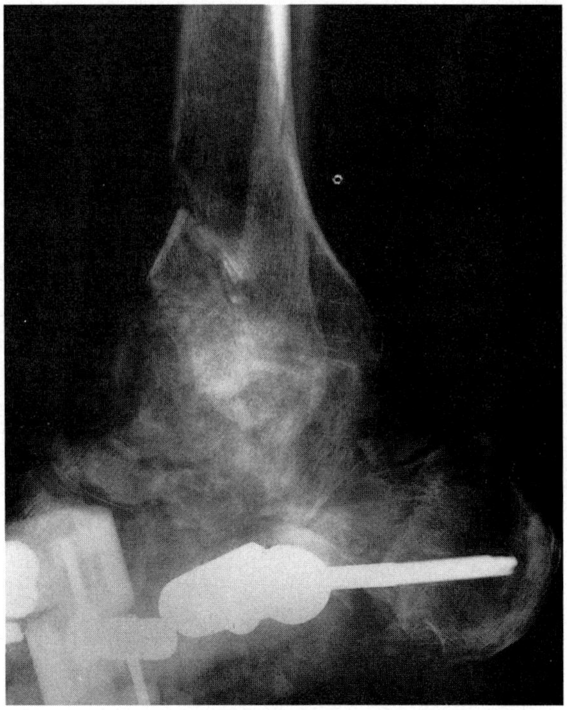

Figure 37–4. Lateral radiograph of right foot after bead removal and grafting with autogenous bone.

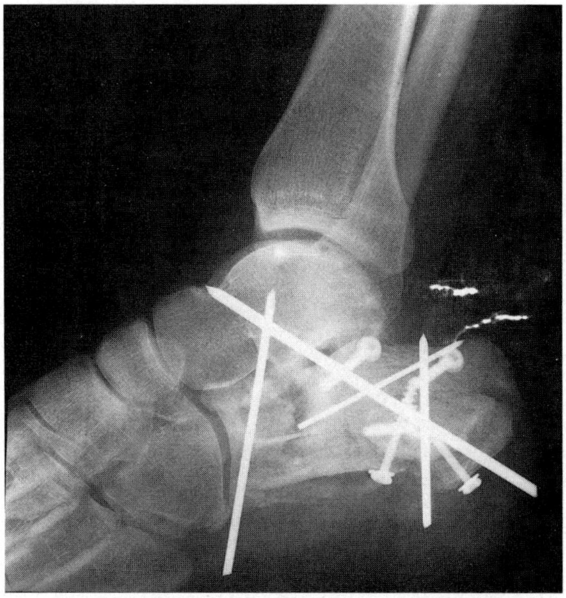

Figure 37–5. Lateral of the left foot following attempted reduction and internal fixation. The talocalcaneal articulation has been accurately reduced.

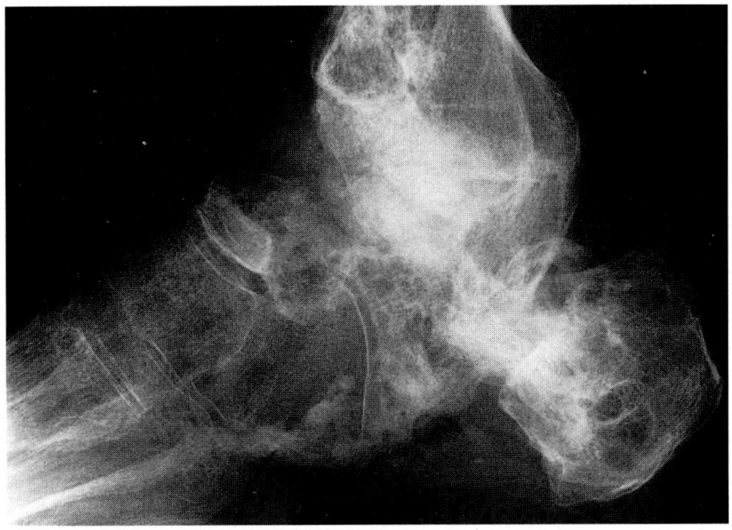

Figure 37–6. Lateral radiograph of the right foot at 1 year. At this point the patient has been bearing weight in a molded shoe.

months and then slowly advanced in a custom molded shoe. The sole of the foot distal to the injury remains insensate, but has not broken down (Fig. 37–6).

On the left side, nonweight bearing was maintained for 12 weeks, and then advanced as tolerated. Despite the extended period of nonweight bearing, reduction was lost (Fig. 37–7). The patient is able to bear weight without pain in a custom molded shoe. The patella healed without complications.

Discussion

Below knee amputation was considered because of the severity of the bony injury and associated injury of the posterior tibial nerve or its branches. An insensate foot

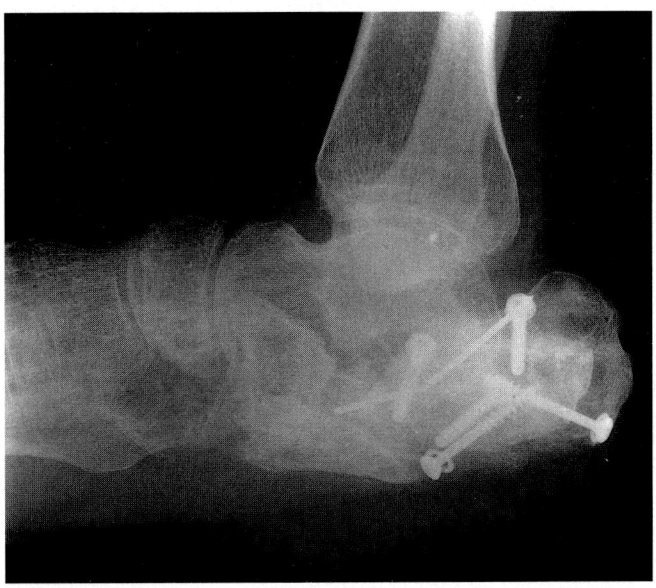

Figure 37–7. Lateral radiograph of left foot. Reduction has been lost, and the calcaneus has collapsed.

is not an absolute indication for amputation, but the patient is susceptible to the development of neurotrophic arthritis and skin breakdown.

Alternative Methods of Management

The patient refused to undergo amputation. If the patient had not insisted on salvage, alternative methods of management would have been below knee amputation or Pirigoff amputation. In this case below knee amputation has the advantages of being a quick permanent solution to the problem. It is technically the simplest solution, but has the disadvantages of significant loss of function and all the problems of stump and prosthesis management.

The Pirigoff amputation consists of amputating the foot anterior to the tuberosity of the calcaneus. The tuberosity is rotated 90 degrees opposing its cut surface to the distal tibia. This procedure results in a stump on which the patient can bear weight. The stump is not as durable as one resulting from a Boyd amputation because the heel pad is anterior and not on the distal end of the stump. However, in this case, because the anterior portion of the heel pad was destroyed in the accident, a Boyd amputation would not have been possible. The distal tibia fracture would add to the difficulty of performing a Pirigoff amputation and obtaining a solid calcaneal tibial fusion.

Once the decision was made to attempt salvage of the foot, the major concern was the optimum method of stabilizing the bones of the foot. Alternatives to stabilization with an external fixator are accurate open reduction and fixation with screws and plates, internal splinting with Kirschner wires, and an external plaster splint. External fixation has the advantage of stabilizing the major fragments without leaving a foreign body in the wound; thus the risk of infection is lower with this method than with others. An external fixator also allows access to the wound.

Open reduction and internal fixation with screws and plates would seem to be the ideal alternative; however, it was not possible because of the extensive bony comminution and soft tissue injury. Open reduction would have exposed the patient to additional surgical trauma and increased the risk of postoperative complications of infection and nonunion.

Type of Management	Advantages	Disadvantages	Comments
Salvage of the foot	Preserves the forefoot	Subjects the patient to multiple procedures; foot may be painful and not functional	Performed in this case because of patient's refusal to undergo amputation
Below knee amputation	Technically the least demanding option	Significant loss of function	Probably the most commonly used method
Pirigoff amputation	Results in a weight bearing stump	Technically demanding; the fracture of the distal tibia makes this even more difficult	The added difficulty of the distal tibia fracture mitigates against this option

Type of Management	Advantages	Disadvantages	Comments
External fixation	Does not leave a foreign body in the wound; allows access to the wound	Limited patient tolerance	Probably the best method to achieve stability
Accurate internal fixation with screw and plates	Would give the best result if it were technically possible	Not possible due to bone loss and comminution; increases the risk of postoperative complications	Technical difficulty prevents this from being an option
Internal splinting with threaded Kirschner wires	Would provide stability with minimal surgical trauma	Technically difficult to stabilize foot and ankle because of extensive fractures; an external plaster splint would be required to augment stability	A possible alternative to external fixation
External plaster splint	Minimal operative trauma	Would not maintain reduction; does not allow access to wound	External fixation or internal splinting with Kirshner wires are better alternatives

Theoretically, threaded Kirschner wires could have been used to hold the major fragments in place. However, in light of the distal tibial fracture and debridement of the talus, it would have been extremely difficult to achieve a stable construct and a plaster splint would be required.

An external plaster splint has the advantage of being minimally invasive. It has the disadvantage of not allowing access to the wound. In addition, an external splint would not immobilize the fragments and deformity is likely to be more pronounced with this method of management.

Complications

The complications of this injury are infection, nonunion, and a painful dysfunctional foot. Infection occurred in this case and is managed with repeat debridement, management of dead space (usually with beads and delayed autogenous bone graft), and systemic antibiotics directed at the pathogenic organisms.

Nonunion may be difficult to diagnose. The presenting symptom is usually pain. The pain from nonunion is distinct from that caused by arthritis in that increased activity increases the severity of the pain. Pain caused by arthritis is usually worse after periods of immobility and gradually lessens with activity. Radiographic studies that may confirm the diagnosis are CAT scans and stress studies under fluoroscopy. Injections of surrounding joints or the area in question with long acting anesthetic agents may be helpful in differentiating posttraumatic arthritis from nonunion. Conservative management of a nonunion involves application of pulsed electromagnetic fields and immobilization. Operative management consists of grafting with autogenous bone and internal fixation or immobilization with a cast or external fixator.

PEARL

- A patient with pain secondary to arthritis will typically relate that the pain is most severe in the morning before he "gets going." A patient with pain secondary to a nonunion will feel good in the morning, but as the day wears on the pain becomes more and more severe.

The most difficult, and perhaps most common, problem following the type of injury this patient sustained is a painful dysfunctional foot. In cases in which the pain is due to compression of a nerve, exostosis, malunion, or posttraumatic arthritis, the management is obvious (i.e., decompression of the nerve, excision of the exostosis, osteotomy of the malunion, or arthrodesis of the arthritic joint). Unfortunately, in the majority of cases there is a major component of the pain and dysfunction for which a cause cannot be determined. This component is often diagnosed as reflex sympathetic dystrophy. Pain management services, physical therapy for gait training along with flexibility exercises, nonsteroidal antiinflammatories, and custom molded shoes may afford some relief.

Suggested Readings

Ebrahim NA, Savolaine ER, Paley K, Jackson WT: Comminuted fracture of the calcaneus associated with subluxation of the talus. Foot and Ankle 1993; 14(7):380–384.

Gregory P, DiPasquale T, Herscovici D, Sanders R: Ipsilateral fractures of the talus and calcaneus. Foot and Ankle Inter 1996; 17(11):701–705.

Sclamberg EL, Davenport K: Operative treatment of displaced intraarticular fractures of the calcaneus. J Trauma 1988; 28(4):510–516.

Case 38

History and Physical Examination

A 43-year-old woman was the unrestrained driver in an automobile accident. She arrived in the emergency department approximately 20 minutes after injury, complaining of left ankle and foot pain. On physical examination obvious deformity was present and it appeared that the forefoot was medially displaced. The neurovascular examination of the foot was within the limits of normal. The injury was closed, although the skin on the lateral aspect of the foot was tented over a bony prominence, probably the calcaneus. Injuries to other organ systems were ruled out, and the medical history was not relevant.

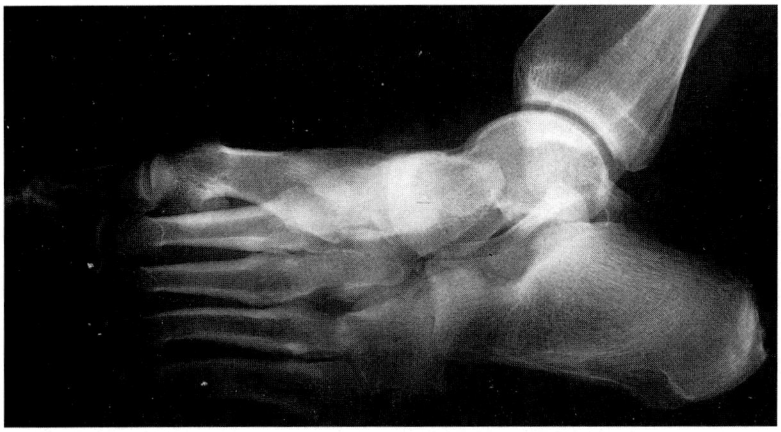

A

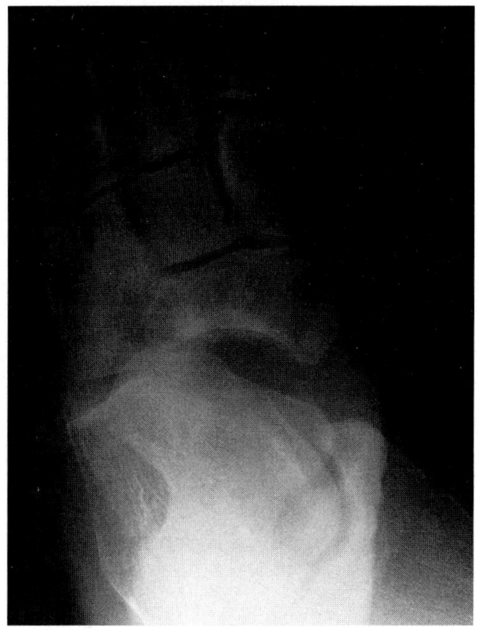

B

Figure 38–1. Oblique (A) and anteroposterior (B) radiographs indicating a dislocation of midtarsal, or Chopart's, joint. The navicular and cuboid are displaced medially and dorsally in relation to the talus and calcaneus. In addition, the calcaneal talar joint is subluxed.

Radiologic Findings

Radiographs of the foot indicated dorsomedial dislocation of the midtarsal, or Chopart's, joint. In addition, the talocalcaneal articulation appeared subluxed. No other fractures were evident (Fig. 38–1).

Diagnosis

Closed dislocation of the midtarsal joint and subluxation of the talocalcaneal articulation.

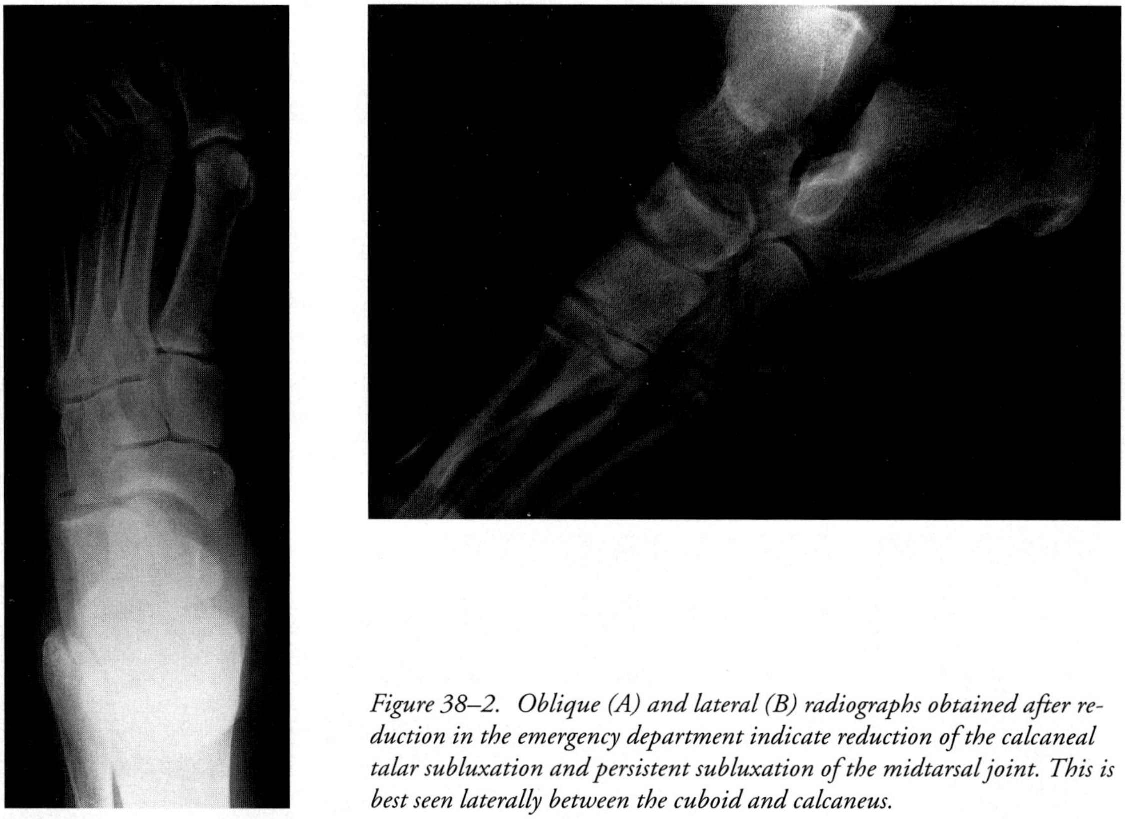

A B

Figure 38–2. Oblique (A) and lateral (B) radiographs obtained after reduction in the emergency department indicate reduction of the calcaneal talar subluxation and persistent subluxation of the midtarsal joint. This is best seen laterally between the cuboid and calcaneus.

PEARL

- Although this was a closed injury, the skin that was tented laterally over the calcaneus was at risk for necrosing. To minimize the chances of necrosis, reduction must be performed as soon as possible. If it had not been possible to correct the deformity in the emergency department, immediate open reduction in the operating room would have been indicated.

Surgical Management

A closed reduction was performed in the emergency room with intravenous sedation. The reduction was performed by applying traction to the forefoot in line with the deformity and then abducting the forefoot. This corrected the gross deformity. Radiographs indicated a reduced talocalcaneal articulation joint with persistent subluxation of the midtarsal joint (Fig. 38–2). The extremity was immobilized in a well padded, short leg, posterior splint.

The day after injury, the patient was taken to the operating room. An anesthetic was administered, and the foot and leg were scrubbed and draped. The midtarsal joint was reduced with the aid of fluoroscopy. Reduction of talocalcaneal articulation was confirmed with fluoroscopy. Large Kirschner wires were inserted across the talonavicular and calcanealcuboid articulations (Fig. 38–3). The extremity was splinted.

Postoperative Management

The first postoperative day, a short leg cast was applied and the patient was discharged nonweight bearing. At 6 weeks the pins were removed and the patient was allowed to weight bear as tolerated in a stiff soled shoe with an arch support (Fig. 38–4).

Discussion

Midtarsal joint injuries are rare, and discussion in the literature is limited. Kenwright and Tylor (1970) reported 58 injuries involving the talus and peritalar joints.

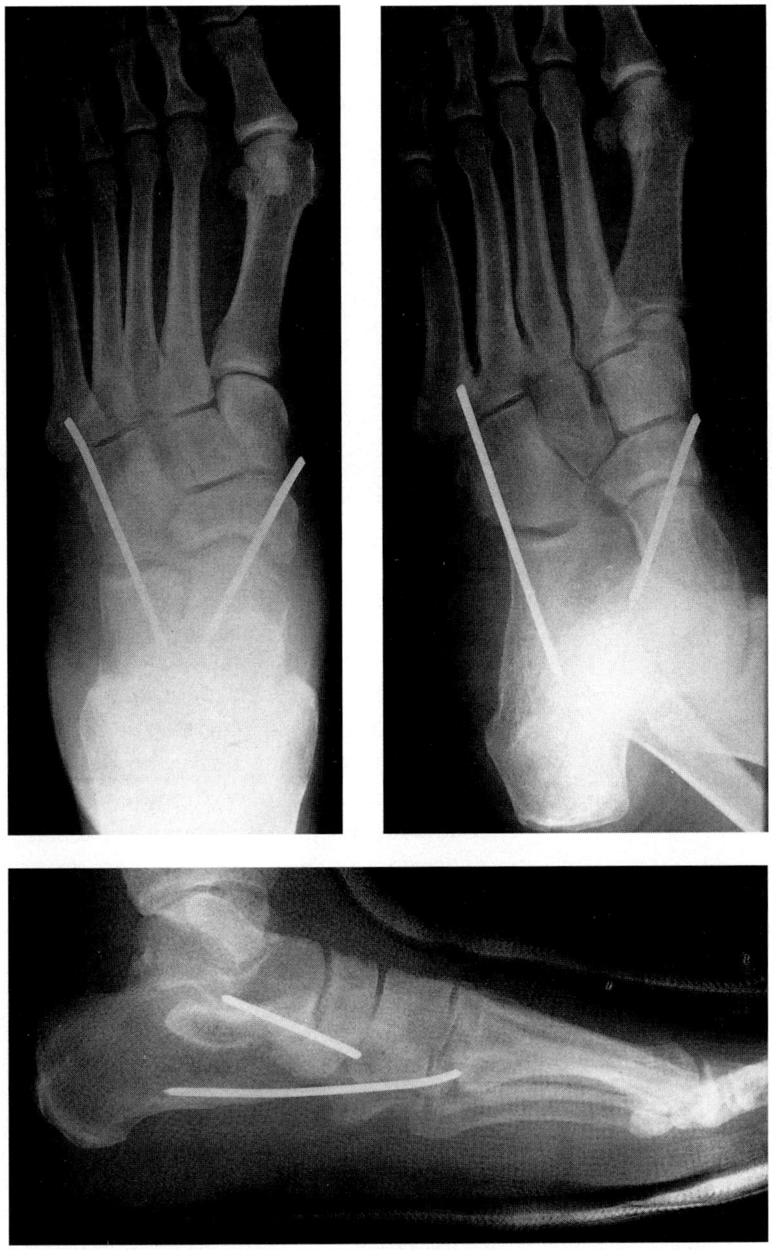

A B C

Figure 38–3. (A–C) Radiographs obtained after reduction of the midtarsal joint and stabilization with Kirschner wires. The midtarsal joint is aligned anatomically.

Of these, only 10 involved the midtarsal joint. Minimally displaced midtarsal dislocations did well with nonoperative treatment. In their review of 71 cases of midtarsal injury, Main and Jowett (1975) identified five patterns of injury based on the direction of the deforming force: medial, lateral, longitudinal, plantar, and crush. Included in the medial and lateral patterns was a "swivel" type injury. This patient sustained a swivel injury of the midtarsal joint. In this type of injury, the forefoot rotates around an axis roughly parallel with the second metatarsal. The talocalcaneal articulation was subluxed. The talonavicular and calcanealcuboid articulations, comprising the midtarsal joint, were dislocated.

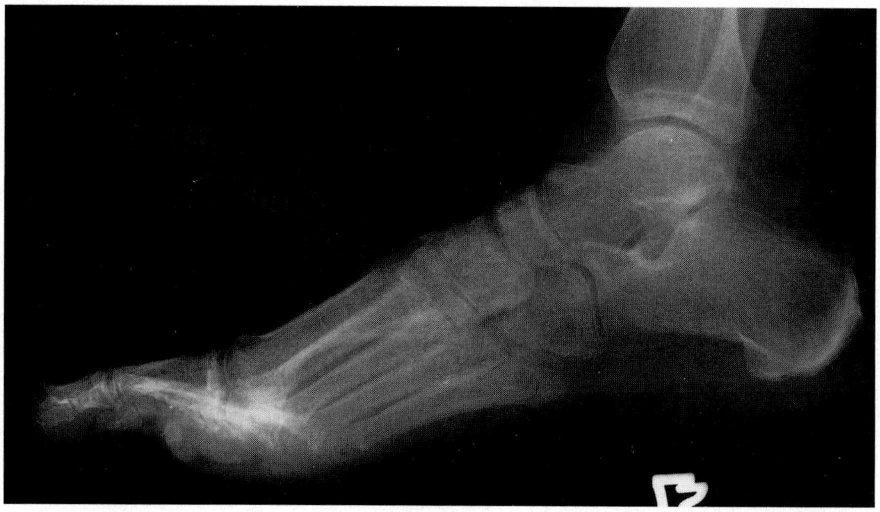

Figure 38–4. Radiograph obtained 6 months after injury indicates maintenance of alignment.

Alternative Methods of Management

Alternatives to closed reduction and percutaneous pinning are closed reduction and immobilization, and open reduction. Closed reduction and immobilization has the advantage of sparing the patient an operation; however, there is a definite risk of redislocation. Internal fixation decreases this risk. Open reduction has the advantage of ensuring accurate alignment of the articular surfaces; however, it has the disadvantage of exposing the patient to the risk of infection. The patient is more liable to develop a wound slough when the overlying skin has been damaged or, as in this case, when tented over the bone.

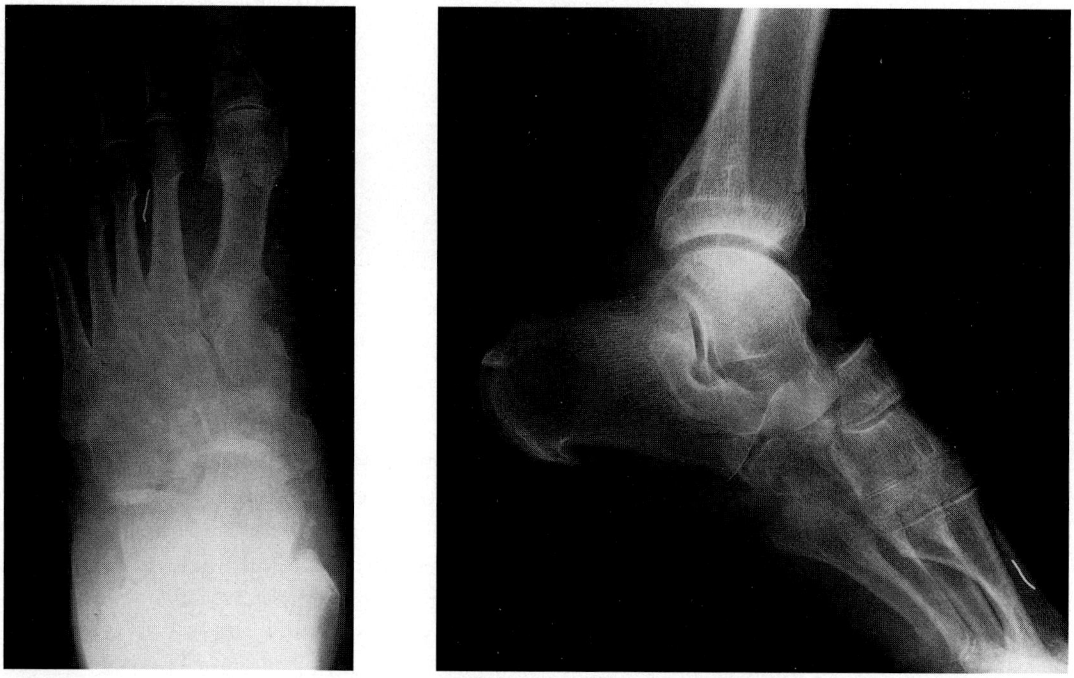

A B

Figure 38–5. Oblique (A) and lateral (B) radiographs of a midtarsal dislocation with a fracture of the navicular.

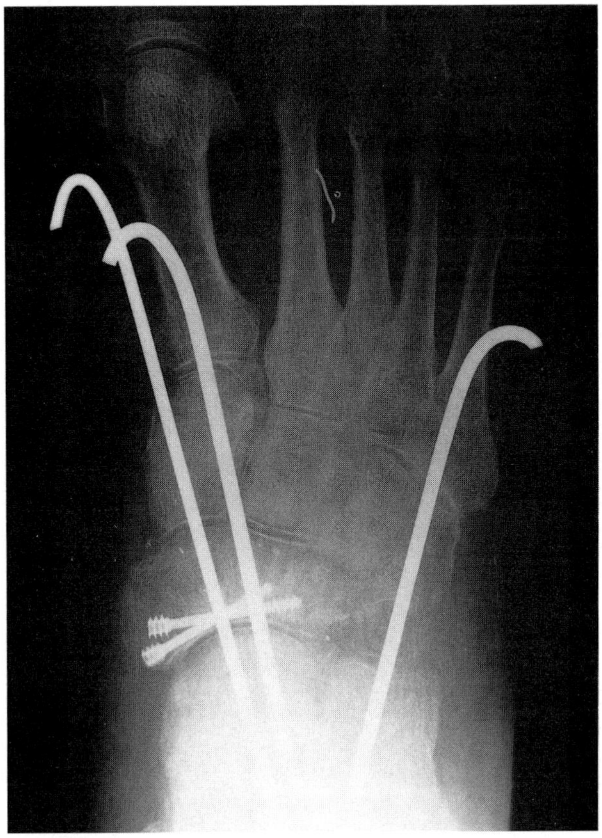

Figure 38–6. Radiograph following reduction and fixation of the navicular and reduction and stabilization of the midtarsal joint with Kirschner wires.

When there is an associated intraarticular fracture of the navicular, talus, cuboid, or talus, open reduction is required to accurately reduce the fracture or remove small fragments from between articular surfaces (Figs. 38–5 and 38–6). Prolonged immobilization and nonweight bearing are necessary whenever there is a pin spanning a joint. Attempted early motion or weight bearing may be complicated by pin breakage.

Type of Management	Advantages	Disadvantages	Comments
Closed reduction and percutaneous pinning	Minimizes the risk of infection; prevents redislocation	Requires an operative procedure	Often the optimum method of management for displaced injuries
Closed reduction and cast immobilization	Spares the patient an operative procedure	Risk of redislocation	Optimum method for minimally displaced injuries
Open reduction and internal fixation	Ensures anatomic reduction	Increases risk of infection	Optimum method when there is associated intraarticular fracture

Complications

Complications include loss of reduction and arthritis. If diagnosed prior to healing, loss of reduction is managed with open reduction and stabilization of the articulations with large pins. If the dislocation has healed in a subluxed position, conservative management consists of modifications of footwear. If conservative management fails, realignment and arthrodesis of the involved articulations are indicated. Post-traumatic arthritis can occur due to the extent of the original injury or because the original injury was not diagnosed accurately and treated appropriately. Arthritis is managed conservatively with shoe inserts, nonsteroidal antiinflammatory medication, and local injections of steroids. If these measures fail, limited fusions of the symptomatic articulations are performed.

Suggested Readings

Howie CR et al: Occult midtarsal subluxation. CORR 1986; 209:206–209.

Kenwright J, Taylor RG: Major injuries of the talus. J Bone Joint Surg 1970; 52B: 36–48.

Main BJ, Jowett RL: Injuries of the midtarsal joint. J Bone Joint Surg 1975; 57B:89–97.

Tountas AA: Occult fracture subluxation of the midtarsal joint. CORR 1989; 243:195–199.

Case 39

History and Physical Examination

A 48-year-old male injured his foot when his shoe was caught in a grain auger. He arrived in the emergency department 90 minutes after injury. The forefoot and midfoot were crushed and degloved with exposed bone and tendon. The wound was extensively contaminated with debris from the auger. The plantar skin was intact from the instep proximally, including the heel pad. The toes were insensate and capillary refill was not present (Fig. 39–1).

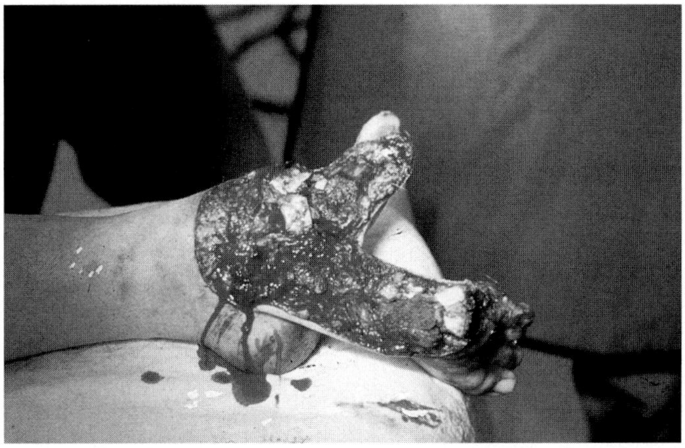

Figure 39–1. Appearance of the foot at admission to the emergency department. There is obvious contamination and devitalized tissue.

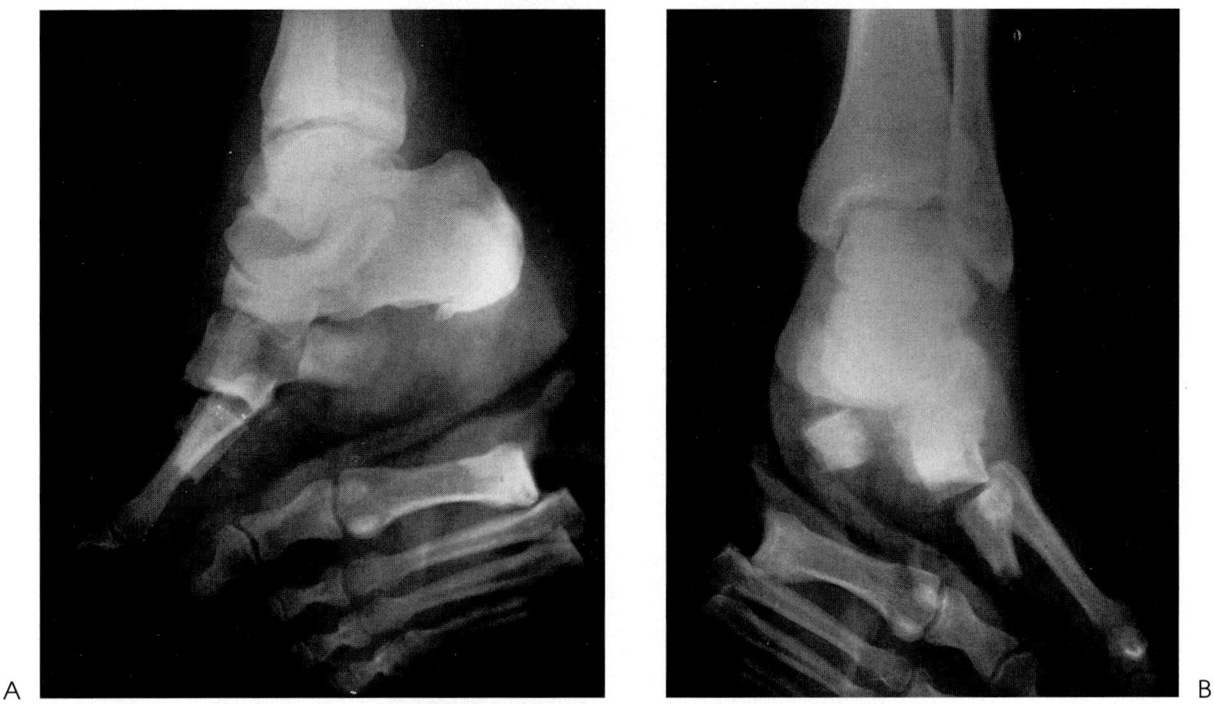

Figure 39–2. (A,B) Radiographs indicate destruction of the forefoot and midfoot.

Radiologic Findings

Radiographs indicated that the bony injury was limited to the forefoot and midfoot. The distal tibia, distal fibula, talus, and calcaneus appeared intact (Fig. 39–2).

Diagnosis

Fracture dislocation of the forefoot. Because of the extensive contamination and destruction of tissue this injury was classified as a grade 3 fracture dislocation of the midfoot. Because of the neurovascular compromise to the forefoot the injury was further classified as a grade 3-C injury.

Surgical Management

Large fragments of plant material, cloth, and shoe leather were removed from the wound. The wound was swabbed to obtain material for aerobic, anaerobic, and fungal cultures. When material for culture had been obtained, the wound was gently irrigated with physiologic saline and covered with a bulky compressive sterile dressing. Tetanus toxoid, a second generation cephalosporin, metronidazol, and an aminoglycoside were administered.

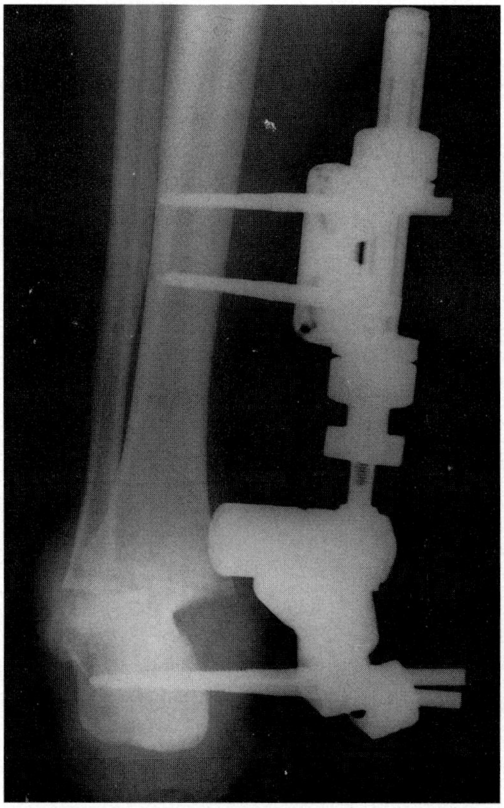

Figure 39–3. An anteroposterior radiograph obtained after a Boyd's amputation and stabilization of the calcaneus to the tibia with a dynamic external fixator.

PITFALL

- There is a temptation to preserve as much of the foot as possible. This can result in the attempted salvage of a portion of the foot that not only is not functional, but is detrimental in that it complicates fitting a prosthesis to the stump, is painful, and is prone to break down. In most cases of traumatic amputation in young patients, amputation at one level (i.e., transmetatarsal, Lisfrancs joint; or Boyd's or Syme's) will yield a more functional extremity than an amputation that crosses several levels in an effort to salvage parts the forefoot or midfoot.

The patient was taken to the operating room where a Boyd's amputation of the foot was performed. Specimens of tissue were obtained for culture. The forefoot and midfoot were amputated, the talus, articular surface of the distal tibia, and the distal fibula were excised through the wound. The cortical bone of the superior surface of the calcaneal tuberosity was removed with an osteotome. The calcaneus was displaced anteriorly beneath the distal tibia, and the superior surface of the calcaneus was compressed against the inferior surface of the tibia with a large pin dynamic external fixator. The fixator was applied with two pins in the calcaneus and two pins in the tibia (Fig. 39–3). The skin and subcutaneous tissue were loosely approximated. On the first postinjury day, the wound was opened, redebrided, and reapproximated.

Postoperative Management

The postoperative course was complicated by swelling that impinged on the fixator. The swelling was managed with constant elevation and gradually resolved over the first 3 weeks. Cultures of material from the wound were positive for gram negative organisms and gram positive rods. Antibiotics were continued for 2 weeks. Compression was applied across the fusion site at a rate of .25 mm per day starting on the seventh postinjury day and continuing for 2 weeks. A split thickness skin graft was used to cover an open area on the anterior aspect of the stump at 4 weeks. The external fixator was removed at 10 weeks. Four months after injury, weight bearing as tolerated was started, and a below knee prosthesis with an end bearing socket was fit

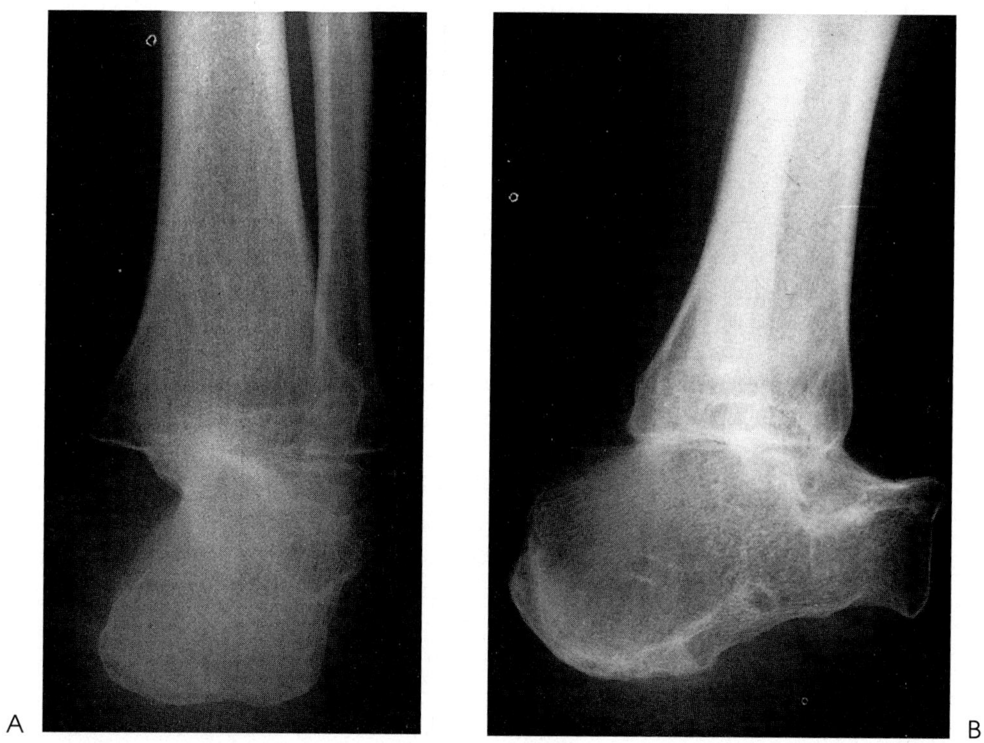

Figure 39–4. (A,B) Radiographs obtained 1 year after injury indicating consolidation of the calcaneus to the tibia.

to the stump. At 6 months the patient was full weight bearing, and at 9 months he returned to farming (Fig. 39–4).

Discussion

This patient sustained a grade IIIC injury of his foot. The most important and first step in management is debridement of devitalized tissue and foreign material as soon as possible. Because this injury occurred in a farming accident and was grossly contaminated, the patient is at risk for developing an extremely aggressive infection (e.g., clostridium perfringens or clostridium tetani) or an infection caused by unusual pathogens (e.g., sporotrichosis or nocardia). Therefore material for culture is obtained in the emergency department and broad spectrum antibiotics are administered. In the operating room more tissue is sent for culture of aerobic, anaerobic, fungal, and mycotic organisms. This is done with the knowledge that antibiotics have been initiated and therefore the cultures may be negative; however, the material obtained for culture in the operating room is from the depths of the wound and may identify pathogens in addition to those identified from the cultures obtained in the emergency department. In the first week postinjury, antibiotic therapy is modified based on the cultures obtained in the emergency department and operating room.

Alternative Methods of Management

Once the wound has been debrided, reconstruction can proceed. The goal of reconstruction is to return as much function as possible to the extremity, minimize chronic pain, and minimize the possibility of infection. Often, when there is an extensive wound that cannot be completely excised, the wound is initially debrided. Several days later when it is clear that the wound is not infected, the reconstructive procedure is performed. In this case, the wound was completely excised, therefore the reconstructive procedure could be performed at the same surgery. The levels of amputation that were considered were transmetatarsal, Lisfranc's, Chopart's, Syme's, Boyd's, and below knee. Transmetatarsal amputation and amputation through the tarsal-metatarsal joint (Lisfranc's joint) result in a functional extremity with little or no morbidity other than loss of push off. Deformity seldom occurs, and the heel pad is preserved. Because the heel pad is preserved, there is minimal pain with weight bearing and the length of the extremity is also preserved. The extent of the injury precluded either of these amputations.

Amputation through the tarsals or the talonavicular and calcaneal cuboid joints (Chopart's joint) is often unsatisfactory. Push off is completely lost. The heel pad is preserved, but a severe equinovalgus deformity develops rapidly due to the unopposed action of the ankle plantar flexors. As the deformity progresses, the heel pad moves posteriorly and proximally, and the anterior aspect of the tarsals or navicular and cuboid become the weight bearing surface. Because of the poor prognosis, amputation at this level is seldom performed.

In 1843 Syme described the amputation that bears his name. Syme's amputation is a technically simple procedure. The ankle is disarticulated and the distal tibia and distal fibula excised. The heel pad is preserved, taking care to protect its blood supply, and is used to cover the end of the stump. Pain with weight bearing is minimized because the heel pad is retained. The most frequently encountered causes of an unsatisfactory Syme's amputation are posterior migration of the heel pad and excessive shortening of the extremity.

In 1939 Boyd described a modification of Syme's amputation in which the forefoot, midfoot, and talus were disarticulated. The heel pad and calcaneus were preserved and the calcaneus was fused to the tibia. Boyd made no recommendations regarding the method of fixation of the calcaneus to the tibia; however, most authors have reported using a large Steinmann pin passed from the heel through the calcaneus into the tibia. The advantages of a successful Boyd's amputation over a Syme's amputation are relative preservation of length and a heel pad that is firmly anchored to the end of the stump. The major disadvantage of Boyd's amputation has been difficulty in achieving tibiocalcaneal fusion. Use of a large pin dynamic external fixator, as in this case, may result in more reliable and rapid tibiocalcaneal-calcaneal fusion than the traditional method of Steinmann pin fixation. Reliable tibiocalcaneal-calcaneal fusion coupled with prevention of heel pad migration and preservation of limb length makes Boyd's amputation the procedure of choice when midfoot amputation is contemplated.

Type of Management	Advantages	Disadvantages	Comments
Amputation distal to Lisfranc's joint	Preserves heel pad and some push off, but often is not proximal to the zone of injury	No disadvantages if the level of amputation is proximal to the zone of injury	Not applicable in this case because of level of injury
Amputation at the midtarsal or Chopart's joint	Preserves heel pad and results in end bearing stump	Severe equinovalgus deformity rapidly develops	Equinovalgus deformity is an overriding disadvantage which makes this method unsuitable
Syme's amputation	Preserves heel pad and is end bearing	Greater loss of length than with Boyd's technique and posterior heel pad migration can occur	Boyd's amputation is a better alternative because of preservation of length and stability of heel pad
Boyd's amputation	Preserves heel pad and length; results in end bearing stump	Loss of function	Selected as the best alternative in this case
Below knee amputation	Is well above the zone of injury, and is a simple procedure	Loss of function	Loss of function due to the stump not being weight-bearing is an overriding disadvantage

Below knee amputation would have been necessary if the heel pad had been destroyed. It has the advantage of definitively removing all damaged tissue; however, it also causes serious permanent disability.

Complications

The complications and morbidity of partial foot amputations are loss of push off, deformity, pain, shortening of the extremity, and infection.

All partial foot amputations proximal to the metatarsal-phalangeal joints result in some loss of push off. In general, the more proximal the level of amputation, the greater the loss of push off.

Pain with weight bearing is most frequently due to loss of the normal cushioning provided by the heel pad. This is either because the heel pad is absent (e.g., it has migrated posteriorly), or because it is no longer functioning due to rupture of the fibrous septa. Posterior migration of the heel pad is best prevented by fusing part or all of the calcaneus to the distal tibia. To relieve pain from the loss of the heel pad, the patient is fit with a patellar tendon bearing prosthesis.

Shortening of the extremity is not a factor in amputations distal to the hind foot. Functional shortening is an inevitable part of amputations involving the hindfoot or proximal to the hindfoot. Resection of the talus results in 2 to 3 cm of shortening; resection of the calcaneus results in an additional 2 to 4 cm of shortening.

Infection usually occurs when, in an effort to preserve more of the foot, too distal an amputation is performed. In cases in which the foot is functioning well and the infected area is localized, local debridement and systemic antibiotic therapy may be successful. In most cases, however, the definitive management of infection is revision of the amputation to a more proximal level.

Suggested Readings

Alldredge RH, Thompson TC: The technique of Syme amputation. J Bone Joint Surg 1959; 41-A:1267.

Boyd HB: Amputation of the foot with calcaneotibial arthrodesis. J Bone Joint Surg 1939; 21:997.

Kornah B: Modified Boyd amputation. J Bone Joint Surg 1996; 78-B:149–50.

Lindquist C, Riska EB: Chopart, Pirogoff and Syme amputations. Acta Orthop Scand 1966; 37:110–116.

Mills KL: Guide to Orthopedics, p. 285. Vol I. Churchill Livingston, Edinburgh, 1981.

Nakhgevany KB, Rhode JE: Ankle level amputation. Surgery 1984; 95:549.

Pederson HE, Day AJ: The transmetatarsal amputation in peripheral vascular disease. J Bone Joint Surg 1954; 36-A:1190.

Sarmiento A: A modified surgical-prosthetic approach to the Syme's amputation: a follow-up report. Clin Orthop 1972; 85:11.

Syme J: Amputation at the ankle joint. The London and Edinburgh Monthly J Med Sci 1843; 26:93.

Thompson RG: Amputation in the lower extremity. J Bone Joint Surg 1963; 45-A:1723.

Index

Acetabulum, posterior lip of, fracture, 196–202
Acid burns, overlying extraarticular fracture, 381–385
Allograft struts, with supracondylar femoral fracture, 297
Amputation
calcaneus fracture, with tibial plafond fracture, 415–422
Chopart's joint, forefoot fracture dislocation, 429–434
forefoot fracture dislocation, 355–360
Lisfranc's joint, distal to, forefoot fracture dislocation, 429–434
tibial diaphysis, Gustilo type IIIc open fracture, 355–360
Ankle, suprasyndesmotic fracture dislocation, 374–380
Arthritis
calcaneal fracture, 407
humerus, Gustilo type III fracture, 96
Pagetic femur, 232
radius
comminuted intraarticular fracture, 162–163
head fracture, 109
talar neck fracture, 390
tibial plateau fracture, bicondylar, 311
Austin Moore prosthesis, subcapital fracture, displaced, 178
Autologous bone marrow injection, pathologic fracture, with overlying radiated skin, 365
Avascular necrosis, talar neck fracture, 390

Bicondylar tibial plateau fracture, 305–312
Bleeding, with supracondylar fracture, in hemophiliac, 272–277
Bone grafting, osteomyelitic bone, subtrochanteric fracture, 213
Boyd's amputation
forefoot fracture dislocation, 355–360
pantalar talus dislocation, 401
Bridging frame, with intraarticular tibial fracture, 313
Burn, acid, overlying extraarticular fracture, 381–385

Calcaneus fracture
dislocation, 403–407
intraarticular, 408–414
counterclockwise derotation, 410
operational difficulty with, 406
with tibial plafond fracture, 415–422
Cantilever frame, large pin, extraarticular fracture, with overlying acid burns, 384
Circular frame, wire
extraarticular fracture with overlying acid burns, 384
intraarticular tibial fracture, 313

Clavicle fracture
comminuted, 21–26
complications, 25–26
external fixation, 25
intramedullary pinning, 25
nonoperative management, 25
nonunion, 25
plating, 25
fixation, 19
interligamentous, 27–31
arthritis, acromioclavicular joint, 29
complications, 29–31
with corocoid process avulsion, 27–31
interosseous wires, 29
intramedullary pin, 29
Kenny Howard sling, 29
management, 29
nonunion, 29
operative management, with plating, 29
physis, displacement of clavicle end, 13
Closed head injury, 8
Colles' fracture, 148
bone substitutes, 154
intrafocal pinning, 154
intramedullary flexible pinning, 154
management, 154
percutaneous dorsal pinning, 154
periarticular fixation, 154
plating, 154
re-manipulation, 154
transarticular external fixation, 154
Colostomy, Malgaingne dislocation and, 168
Contracture, equinus, after fixation of pilon fracture, 369
Corocoid process avulsion, 27–31

Deltoid ligament, infolded, suprasyndesmotic fracture dislocation, 375
Discrepancy in leg length, following Salter-Harris II femoral fracture, 291

Elbow dislocation
with closed fracture, 118
complications, 124–125
external fixation, 124
intramedullary nailing, 124
management, 124
nonoperative management, 124
open reduction and internal fixation, 124
with epicondylar fracture, 88
complications, 91
epicondyle fixation, cast management, 91
management, 91
myositis ossificans, 91
neurovascular dysfunction, 91
recurrent dislocation, 91
soft tissue repair, 91
with radial head fracture, 98
collateral ligament repair, 103
complications, 104

Elbow dislocation, with radial head fracture, (*continued*)
  dynamic external fixation, 103
  management, 103
  open reduction, internal fixation, 103
  silastic prosthesis, 103
Ender nails, with femur fracture, peritrochanteric, reverse, 186
Epicondylar fracture, elbow dislocation with, 88
  complications, 91
  epicondyle fixation, cast management, 91
  management, 91
  myositis ossificans, 91
  recurrent dislocation, 91
  soft tissue repair, 91
Equinus contracture, after fixation of pilon fracture, 369

Fasciotomy, fracture stabilization, order of performance, with tibia, fibula fracture, 336
Femoral bilateral fracture, 238–245
  complications, 244
  external fixation, 243
  hypovolaemia, 238
  management, 243
  osteomyelitis, 244
  plating, 243
  pulmonary dysfunction, 244
  reamed intramedullary nailing, 243
  traction casting, 243
  unreamed intramedullary nailing, 243
Femoral diaphysis
  neck, ipsilateral fracture, 216–221
    antegrade nailing, 221, 228
    avascular necrosis, 220
    bone grafting, 224
    cancellous screws, 221
    external fixation, 228
    femoral nails, 218
    infection, 229
    management, 221, 228
    pelvic donor site morbidity, 227
    plates, 228
      fixation of, 221
    radiographs, 216
    reconstruction nailing, 221
    retrograde nailing, 221, 228
    screw fixation, 221
    spinning loose diaphyseal segment, 218
    traction, 221
      cast, 228
  transverse fracture, 8
Femoral intercondylar fracture, with displacement of articular surfaces, 267–271
Femoral midshaft fracture, 55
Femoral open fracture
  grade III, 196–202
    first generation locked nail, 205
    fracture table, advantages of, 204
    infection, 206
    management, 205
    plate, 205
    reconstruction nail, 205
    screws, 205
    side plate
      95 degree, 205
      135 degree, 205
    visceral injuries with, 204
  in hemophiliac, 278–286
Femoral peritrochanteric fracture, reverse, 182–188
  antegrade reconstruction nail
    long, 186
    short, 186
  collapse through fracture site, 187
  compression hip screw, 186
  guidewire, 184
  management, 186
  retrograde nail, 186
Femoral physeal fracture, Salter-Harris II, 287–292
Femoral subcapital displaced fracture, 174–181
  Austin Moore prosthesis, 178
  bipolar procedures, 180
  complications, 180
  hemiarthroplasty, 180
  hemiarthroplasty prostheses, 175
  hip pain, 181
  management, 180
  mobilization, 176
  multiple screw fixation, 180
  nonoperative management, 180
  total hip replacement, 180
Femoral subtrochanteric fracture, 203–207
  osteomyelitic bone, 208–215
    amputation, 213
    bone grafting, 213
    culture material, obtaining, 209
    debridement, 209
    external fixation, 213
    free soft tissue transfer, 213
    infection, 213–214
    intercalary lengthening, 213
    management, 213
    necrotic bone, 209
    traction, 213
  Pagetic, 230–237
    casting, 237
    complications, 237
    external fixation, 237
    hemorrhage, 237
    intramedullary nailing, 237
    management, 237
    osteoarthritis, 232
    plating, 237
    traction, 237
Femoral supracondylar fracture
  displaced, 258–266
  low energy, above well-aligned prosthesis, 293–299
  with undisplaced intraarticular extension, 246–252
Fibula
  closed fracture, 335–343
  extraarticular fracture, with overlying acid burns, 381–385
Foot, forefoot, fracture dislocation, 429–434
Forearm
  open fracture, with radius fracture, 136

complications, 141
external fixation, 140
infection, 141
intramedullary nailing, 140
management, 140
nail in radius, 140
plates, 140
on ulna, 140
screws, 140
rotation block, radial head fracture, 106
arthritis, 109
complications, 109
fragment excision, 108
management, 108
open reduction and internal fixation, 108
with prosthetic replacement, 108
radial head excision, 108
Fracture table, advantages of, 204

Gamma nail, femur fracture, peritrochanteric, reverse, 186
Glenoid
inferior half, fracture from gunshot, 3
closed management, 6
debridement
with open reduction, internal fixation, 6
reconstruction, with bone block, 6
stabilization, 6
neck
displaced fracture, 16–20
fixation of, 19
Grafting of bone, in hemophiliac, 285
Growth arrest, partial, trauma and, 290
Gunshot injury
glenoid fracture, inferior half, 3
humerus, Grade III B fracture, 59–65
Gustilo type III fracture
humerus, 92
complications, 96
internal fixation, 96
management, 96
nonoperative management, 96
posttraumatic osteoarthritis, 96
transarticular external fixation, 96
tibial, diaphyseal, 344–354
Gustilo type IIIc fracture, tibial diaphysis, 355–360

Hawkins classification, talar neck fractures, 387
Head injury, closed, 8
Hemiarthroplasty
humerus
four part fracture, 53
translated two part fracture, 45
humerus fracture, 38
intertrochanteric fracture, three-part, 194
subcapital fracture, 175
Hemipelvis dislocation, hypovolemia secondary to, 167–173
anterior fixator, 171
colostomy, 168
complications, 172
hemorrhage, 172
hypovolemia with, 169
management, 171
percutaneous screws, 171
sepsis, 172
Steffe plates, 171
symphysis
anterior external fixator, 171
plate to stabilize, 171
Hemophiliac, comminuted supracondylar fracture in, 272–277
Hemorrhage, with Malgaingne dislocation, 169
Hip replacement, total, subcapital fracture, displaced, 180
Humeral fracture
diaphyseal, 238–245
complications, 244
external fixation, 243
hypovolaemia, 238
management, 243
osteomyelitis, 244
plating, 243
pulmonary dysfunction, 244
with radial nerve palsy, 55
reamed intramedullary nailing, 243
traction casting, 243
unreamed intramedullary nailing, 243
four part, 47
complications, 52
hemiarthroplasty, 53
internal fixation, 53
management, 53
nonoperative management, 53
Grade III B, from gunshot, 59–65
Gustilo type III, 92
complications, 96
internal fixation, 96
management, 96
nonoperative management, 96
posttraumatic osteoarthritis, 96
soft tissue repair, 96
transarticular external fixation, 96
hemiarthroplasty, 38
intercondylar, 66
complications, 72–73
management, 72
with metaphyseal bone loss, 79
arthroplasty, 85
complications, 86
external fixation, nonbridging, 85
infection, 86
internal fixation, 85
intramedullary nailing, 85
joint stiffness, 86
management, 85
nonoperative managemnt, 85
open reduction, 85
subscapularis transfer, 38
surgical neck, lesser tuberosity, 32–39
translated two-part, 41
complications, 45–46
external fixation, 45
hemiarthroplasty, 45
management, 45
nonoperative management, 45
rigid fixation, 45
tuberosity transfer, subscapularis transfer, 38

Humeroulnar articulation, radioulnar, subluxation, 111
  complications, 116
  instability, chronic, 116
Hypovolaemia, femoral fracture, bilateral, 238

Infolded deltoid ligament, suprasyndesmotic fracture dislocation, 375
Intercalary lengthening, subtrochanteric fracture, osteomyelitic bone, 213
Intercondylar fracture
  femur, with displacement of articular surfaces, 267–271
  humerus, closed, 66
Interligamentous fracture, clavicle, 27–31
Intertrochanteric fracture, three-part, 189–195
  alternative implants, 194
  anatomic reduction, 194
  hemiarthroplasty, 194
  infection, 195
  management, 194
  osteotomy, medial displacement, 194
  polymethylmethacrylate, 193
    augmentation with, 194

Kenny Howard sling, clavicle, interligamentous fracture, 29
Kirschner wire
  complications with, 14
  displaced transverse fracture, ulna, 146
  radius fracture, 162
Knee joint, open injury of, 196–202
Knee prosthesis, low energy fracture of tibia distal to, 329–334

Length discrepancy, leg, following Salter-Harris II femoral fracture, 291
Lengthening of bone, in hemophiliac, 285
Lesser tuberosity, humerus, fracture, 32–39
Lung contusion, with fractured ribs, 16–20

Malgaingne dislocation, 167–173
  anterior fixator, 171
  colostomy, 168
  complications, 172
  hemorrhage, hypovolemia with, 169
  management, 171
  percutaneous screws, 171
  Steffe plates, 171
  symphysis
    anterior external fixator, 171
    plate to stabilize, 171
Marrow injection, autologous, pathologic fracture, with overlying radiated skin, 365
Metaphyseal bone loss, with humeral fracture, 79
  arthroplasty, 85
  complications, 86
  external fixation, nonbridging, 85
  infection, 86
  intramedullary nailing, 85
  management, 85
  nonoperative managemnt, 85
  open reduction, 85
Midtarsal joint, dislocation, 423–428

Monteggia fracture dislocation, arm, 127
  complications, 134
  heterotopic ossification, 134
  internal fixation of ulna, 133
  management, 133
  nonoperative management, 133
  posterior interosseous neuropraxia, 134
  radial head, closed reduction of, 133
  ulna, internal fixation, 133
Myositis ossificans, with epicondylar fracture, elbow dislocation, 91

Necrosis, avascular, with talar neck fracture, 390

Osteoarthritis
  bicondylar tibial plateau fracture, 311
  calcaneal fracture, 407
  humerus, Gustilo type III fracture, 96
  Pagetic femur, 232
  radius
    comminuted intraarticular fracture, 162–163
    head fracture, 109
  talar neck fracture, 390
  tibia, bicondylar plateau fracture, 311
Osteomyelitis
  femoral fracture, bilateral, 244
  Gustilo III tibial diaphyseal fracture, 353
  subtrochanteric fracture
    amputation, 213
    bone grafting, 213
    external fixation, 213
    free soft tissue transfer, 213
    infection, 213–214
    intercalary lengthening, 213
    traction, 213
Osteopenia, with transcondylar fracture, 74–78
  arthroplasty, 77
  closed management, 77
  complications, 78
  management, 77
  open reduction and internal fixation, 77

Paget's disease, femur, subtrochanteric fracture, 230–237
  complications, 237
  external fixation, 237
  hemorrhage, 237
  intramedullary nailing, 237
  management, 237
  osteoarthritis, 232
  plating, 237
  traction, 237
Partial growth arrest, trauma and, 290
Patella
  grade III open fracture, 300–304
  tendon laceration, 196–202
Peritrochanteric fracture, reverse, femur, 182–188
  antegrade reconstruction nail
    long, 186
    short, 186
  collapse through fracture site, 187
  compression hip screw, 186

guidewire, 184
management, 186
retrograde nail, 186
Pirigoff amputation, calcaneus fracture with tibial plafond fracture, 420
Plafond fracture, tibial, with diaphyseal comminution, 367–373
PMMA. *See* Polymethylmethacrylate
Polymethylmethacrylate
intertrochanteric fracture, three-part, 193, 194
supracondylar femoral fracture, augmentation with, 297
Pubic rami, fracture, 196–202

Radial fracture
Colles' fracture, extraarticular, distal, 148
bone substitutes, 154
complications, 155–156
intrafocal pinning, 154
intramedullary flexible pinning, 154
malunion, 155
management, 154
percutaneous dorsal pinning, 154
periarticular fixation, 154
plating, 154
re-manipulation, 154
transarticular external fixation, 154
comminuted, intraarticular, 158
complications, 162–163
external fixator, 162
Kirschner wire, 162
management, 162
nonoperative management, 162
plating, 162
posttraumatic osteoarthritis, 162–163
elbow closed fracture dislocation, 118
complications, 124–125
external fixation, 124
intramedullary nailing, 124
management, 124
nonoperative management, 124
open reduction and internal fixation, 124
forearm, open fracture, 136
complications, 141
external fixation, 140
infection, 141
intramedullary nailing, 140
management, 140
plate on ulna, 140
plates, 140
transverse, displaced, 143
cast, traction, 146
complications, 146–147
joint contractures, secondary, 146
Kirschner wires, 146
management, 146
muscle damage, irreversible, 146
neurological sequelae, 146
plating, 146
rush pins, 146
traction, 146
Radial head dislocation, 118
Radial head fracture
with block to forearm rotation, 106
arthritis, 109
complications, 109
fragment excision, 108
management, 108
open reduction and internal fixation, 108
with prosthetic replacement, 108
radial head excision, 108
synovitis, following silastic prosthesis insertion, 109
displaced intraarticular, 98
elbow dislocation with, 98
collateral ligament repair, 103
complications, 104
dynamic external fixation, 103
management, 103
open reduction, internal fixation, 103
silastic prosthesis, 103
Radial nerve palsy, with humeral diaphysis, 55
Radiated skin, overlying tibial diaphysis fracture, 361–366
Radioulnar dissociation, with humeroulnar articulation subluxation, 111
complications, 116
instability, chronic, 116
Reamed nailing
Gustilo III tibial fracture, 352, 355–360
in tibia, fibula fracture, 341
Retrograde nail, supracondylar femoral fracture, 297
Rib, fractured, with lung contusion, 16–20
Rush pins, displaced transverse fracture, ulna, 146

Salter-Harris II femoral physeal fracture, 287–292
Scapula, displaced extraarticular fracture, 8
Schatzker type VI tibial fracture, with elevated pressures, 313–320
Shortening of bone, in hemophiliac, 285
Shoulder, nonunion, loss of motion, 11
Silastic prosthesis, radial head fracture, elbow dislocation with, 103
Skin, radiated, overlying pathologic fracture, 365
Spiral blade, femur fracture, reverse peritrochanteric, 186
Steffe plates, Malgaingne dislocation, 171
Sternoclavicular joint, anterior dislocation of, 13
Surgical neck, humerus, fracture, 32–39
Syme's amputation, forefoot fracture dislocation, 355–360

Talar neck fracture
comminuted, with foot dislocation, 391–396
Hawkins classification, 387
with pantalar dislocation, 397–402
with subtalar joint involvement, 386–390
Talectomy, 395, 401
Tibial fracture
closed, 335–343
diaphyseal
Gustilo III, 344–354, 355–360
with overlying radiated skin, 361–366
distal to knee prosthesis, 329–334
extraarticular

Tibial fracture, extraarticular, (*continued*)
with comminution of tibial diaphysis, 321–328
with overlying acid burns, 381–385
intraarticular, with elevated pressures, 313–320
Tibial plafond fracture, with diaphyseal comminution, 367–373
Tibial plateau fracture, bicondylar, 305–312
osteoarthritis after, 311
Total hip replacement, subcapital fracture, displaced, 180
Transcondylar fracture with intraarticular extension, 74–78
arthroplasty, 77
closed management, 77
complications, 78
management, 77
open reduction and internal fixation, 77
Tuberosity transfer, humerus fracture, 38

Ulnar fracture
communication, with elbow closed fracture dislocation, 118
complications, 124–125
external fixation, 124
intramedullary nailing, 124
management, 124
nonoperative management, 124
open reduction and internal fixation, 124
displaced, transverse, 143
cast, traction, 146
complications, 146–147
joint contractures, secondary, 146
Kirschner wires, 146
management, 146
muscle damage, irreversible, 146
neurological sequelae, 146
plating, 146
rush pins, 146
traction, 146
Unreamed nailing
femur fracture, reverse peritrochanteric, 186
fibula, tibia fracture, 341
Gustilo III tibial fracture, 352, 355–360
Urethra disruption, with hemipelvis dislocation, 167–173

Visceral injuries, with high-energy injury, 204

Wire circular frame, with intraarticular tibial fracture, 313